Fundamental Aspects of ANATOMY

Dr. P. Sreedevi M.D
Principal
Sree Mookambika Institute of Medical Sciences, Kulasekharam,
Kanyakumari Dist, Tamil Nadu.
Formerly
Professor and Head, Department of Anatomy,
Kasturba Medical College, Manipal, Karnataka State.
Professor, Medical College, Trivandrum, Kerala State.

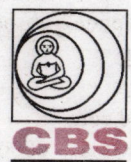

CBS

CBS PUBLISHERS & DISTRIBUTORS PVT. LTD.

NEW DELHI • BANGALORE • PUNE • COCHIN • CHENNAI (INDIA)

ISBN : 978-81-239-1603-3

First Edition : 2008
Reprint : 2010, 2012, 2014

Published by Satish Kumar Jain and produced by V.K. Jain for
CBS Publishers & Distributors Pvt. Ltd.,
CBS Plaza, 4819/XI Prahlad Street, 24 Ansari Road, Daryaganj,
New Delhi - 110002, India.   • Website: www.cbspd.com
e-mail: delhi@cbspd.com, cbspubs@airtelmail.in
Ph.: 23289259, 23266861, 23266867   • Fax: 011-23243014

Branches:

• **Bengaluru:** Seema House, 2975, 17th Cross, K.R. Road,
  Bansankari 2nd Stage, Bengaluru - 560070
  • Ph.: +91-80-26771678/79 • Fax: +91-80-26771680
  • E-mail: cbsbng@gmail.com, bangalore@cbspd.com
• **Pune:** Bhuruk Prestige, Sr. No. 52/12/2+1+3/2,
  Narhe, Haveli (Near Katraj-Dehu Road By-pass), Pune - 411041
  • Ph.: +91-20-64704058/59, 32342277   • E-mail: pune@cbspd.com
• **Kochi:** 36/14, Kalluvilakam, Lissie Hospital Road,
  Kochi - 682018, Kerala • Ph.: +91-484-4059061-65
  • Fax: +91-484-4059065 • E-mail: cochin@cbspd.com
• **Chennai:** 20, West Park Road, Shenoy Nagar, Chennai - 600030
  Ph.: +91-44-26260666, 26208620   • Fax: +91-44-42032115
  • E-mail: chennai@cbspd.com

Printed at :
R.B. Printers, Delhi

Dedicated to
Goddess Devi Mookambika
My Family
My Professional Colleagues
My Students.

Foreword

A composition is effective only when it is the result of a heartfelt need. As the author has expressed in her preface, the problem of finding a single source textbook of Anatomy for the paramedical courses has been long felt by generations of Anatomy teachers. Basic knowledge of the structure of the body is essential for all who take up any of the health science courses.

Dr. Sreedevi, a brilliant and popular Anatomy teacher for over three decades, one who got recognition as the best teacher award by Manipal Academy of Higher Education has taken it upon herself the task of filling this deficiency of a simple text book of Anatomy suitable for all paramedical courses. Her empathy with the teachers and students alike for effective understanding of the subject has made her eminently suitable for this difficult task.

The facts are presented in a simple language easy to follow by any +2 student. Illustrations are imperative for any text book of Anatomy. Many text books incorporate photographs or the work of professional artists for illustrations. Here the author has herself prepared the diagrams which are simple yet accurate and easy to follow and remember/reproduce. She has used them in the course of her teaching and carry just the necessary details for a particular lesson, e.g., The laryngeal muscles are so nicely depicted that one can visualise their actions easily.

On the whole Dr. Sreedevi has succeeded in her aim to make Anatomy "digestible" for the students. I hope the cost will also be "swallowable".

Although meant for paramedical courses, the book is comprehensive enough in its coverage for the use of MBBS students also. The questions given at the end of each chapter are apt and cover all important aspects of the portion. Thus it would be very useful for revision prior to examination.

I have known Dr. Sreedevi ever since she joined the Anatomy department of the Trivandrum Medical College as a tutor in 1972. She has impressed me as an all rounder with varied interests who would successfully complete any task she undertook surmounting all difficulties. It was a pleasure to be her guide for MD Anatomy in her research work on the development of the human retina.

I am very happy to introduce and recommend this book as a basic text book of Anatomy.

Dr Sreedevi is now principal of Sree Mookambika Institute of Medical Sciences, Kulashekharam of Kanyakumari District. I wish her all success and hope she will venture into new pastures for the enhancement of medical services to the public.

Dr. N Sarada Devi
MBBS, MSc, MRCP, DGO
Formerly
Professor and Director of Anatomy
Trivandrum Medical College
Retired Principal
Kerala Medical College

Preface

Human Anatomy is a subject of study for all the students of all the Medical and Paramedical and allied health science courses, in the 1st year itself. Knowledge of basics of Anatomy is essential throughout their professional career. Majority of the students find the subject difficult. Being an Anatomy teacher for more than 35 years, it has been my endeavour to make the subject more digestable and interesting as possible to the students.

It is a known fact that Anatomy teachers experience the helplessness in prescribing a single Anatomy textbook for the students of the courses like B.Sc Nursing, BPT, BOT, BRTT, BASLT, BMLT, BNMT, BME, BBT etc. I realised this need to its core while I was working as the H.O.D of Anatomy in K.M.C, Manipal, and decided to make a simple Anatomy textbook that can be of use to such students. Now as the book is formed, I sincerly hope that with this book, the students of Ayurvedic, Homeopathic, Dental and Medical will find Anatomy an easy and interesting subject.

Dr. P Sreedevi

Acknowledgement

While I was working in KMC, Manipal, the idea of writing a simple Anatomy Textbook struck to my mind. I shared my feeling with my friends, Dr. K.Sasidharan, Professor and HOD of Urology, KMC, Manipal, and his wife Mrs. Sathi Sasidharan. They urged me earnestly to do it at the earliest. But for their constant encouragement and persuasion I might not have made this book at all. In this regard both of them deserve my special thanks. My sincere thanks are due to my colleagues Ms. Sheena, Ms. Jessy, Dr. Lenin and Ms. Indulekha for giving me regular encouragement.

In computer processing of my work and layout and positioning of the figures, Mr. Jayasankar and Mrs. Sobha Jayasankar, Mr. Nipin Niravath and Mrs. Sunnisa Niravath and Mrs. Suchitra Reghuram played the major role. I extend my sincere thanks to them. My special thanks are due to Mr. Chand Singh for designing the cover pages. The DTP work, scanning and redraw the diagrams and page layout were arranged in the office of Limited Colors, Delhi by Ms. Nishi Verma and Mr. Chand Singh Naagar. I am greatful to team of Limited Colors who took sincere effort for the design and layout of the book.

Without the motivational and inspirational support extended by Mr. Gopakumar, my husband, Dr. Reghuram Gopakumar, my son and Mrs. Suchitra Reghuram, my daughter-in-law, I could not have completed this work.

I also wish to express my sincere heart felt thanks to Dr. Velayudhan Nair (Chairman) and Dr. Mrs. Rema V. Nair (Director) of Sri Mookambika Institute of Medical Sciences - Padanilam Welfare Trust, Padanilam, Kulasekharam, Kanyakumari District, Tamil Nadu, whose constant encouragement and appreciation have been instrumental in the making of this book.

I feel it an honour to have Prof. N. Sarada Devi, MBBS, M.Sc, MRCP, DGO, the former Director and Professor of Anatomy, Medical College, Trivandrum and retired as Principal from Kerala Medical College Service, to write a foreword for my book. She was my teacher, my guide and always I had been following her advice in my academic career. I extend my heart felt thanks to her.

I am thankful to Dr. Rajagopal Shenoi, Professor of Surgery, K.M.C, Manipal for introducing me to M/s. CBS Publishers and Distributors. I am grateful to Mr. Satish Kumar Jain, and Mr. B.R. Sharma of CBS Publishers and Distributors, New Delhi for publishing the book.

Dr. P Sreedevi

Contents

1 Cell and Tissues of the Body

INTRODUCTION

Anatomy forms the basis of practice of medicine. It includes the gross structure of various parts that make up the human body and also the microscopic structure.

Descriptive terms in Anatomy

Anatomical position:

Body in erect posture with feet together, hands by the side, palms of hands and face directed forwards.

Anatomical planes:

1. **Sagital plane-Median plane:** A vertical plane that divides the body into right and left halves.
2. **Coronal plane:** A vertical plane that passes at right angles to the sagital plane.
3. **Horizontal or transverse plane:** Passes horizontally separating the body into upper and lower parts.

Other terms:

1. **Anterior or ventral and posterior or dorsal:** Parts and structures in front of the body and on the back of the body.
2. **Medial and lateral:** Some part or structure nearer the midline and farther from the midline.
3. **Superior (Cranial, Rostral) and inferior (caudal):** Some part or structure nearer to head region and some part, nearer to lower part of body or away from head region.

GENERAL ANATOMY

CELL AND TISSUES OF THE BODY

Structure of Cell

Cell is the unit structure of human body. The structure, size and other features of human cells get modified according to their position and function. But all cells have some basic features in common. Generally a cell has cytoplasm, surrounded by cell membrane (plasma membrane). Has a nucleus, cell organelles and inclusions. (Fig. 1.1)

Plasma Membrane

Electron Microscopic appearance shows, it is a trilaminar membrane. It has a semipermeable layer of lipid with inner and outer protein layers. Free surface of certain cells at some location show tiny regular vertical projections of cell membrane called microvilli. This causes a brush border or striated appearance to the cells. Microvilli help to increase the surface area of the cell exposed, hence seen in regions where absorption is required as in intestine.

Some cells have motile fine cilia on their surfaces. They function to remove secretions or foreign particles from their surface. A single thread like motile process is called flagellum- in spermatozoa. When the cells form tissues *e.g.,* epithelium, they will be closely arranged and are joined by different types of cell junctions- tight

1

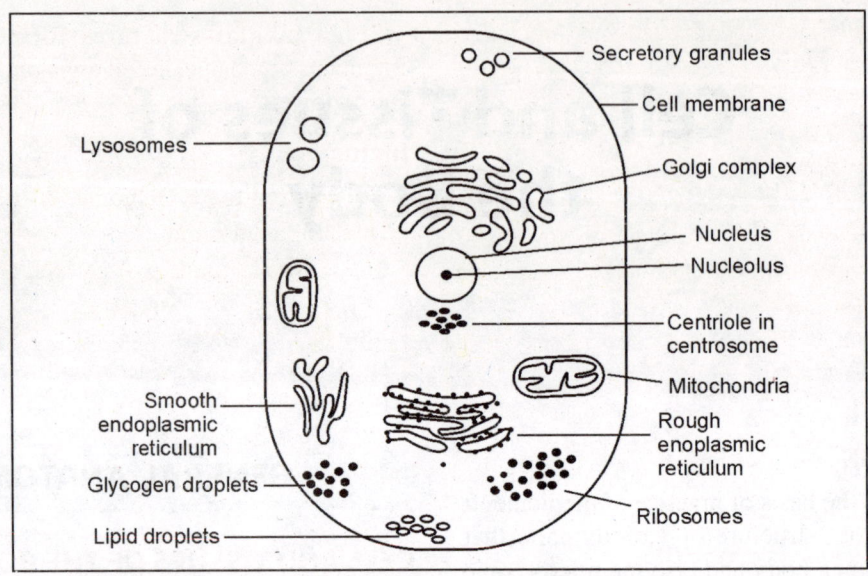

Fig. 1.1: Structure of cell

junctions (desmosomes), gap junctions or leaky tight junctions, according to the functional necessity.

Cytoplasm

It is a semifluid substance, most part formed of water, remaining part by protein, lipids, carbohydrates, organic and inorganic salts.

Nucleus

Present in all cells except RBCs and platelets of blood. Usually single, some are multinucleated. Position is generally central. Shape corresponds to shape of cell- rounded, oval, elongated or lobulated.

Nucleus is enveloped by a nuclear membrane which also is trilaminar and has tiny pores. It contains nucleoplasm and predominantly seen structure is chromatin material. Chromatin contains DNA and proteins. In resting cells, they are highly coiled and appear as small masses or granules. During cell division, they change into chromosomes- 46 in each somatic cell.

In female cell which contains 2 X chromosomes, 1 X chromosome is condensed into a small concavoconvex mass of chromatin and is seen on the inner surface of nuclear membrane. It is called Barr Body.

Nucleuolus is a highly refractile rounded body at the centre of nucleus. Contains RNA. It disappears at prophase of mitosis and reappears at telophase.

Apart from nucleus, cells contain Organelles- which are essential elements of biologically active cell and also some inert nonliving elements- Inclusions.

Organelles

1. Centrosome: Seen near the nucleus as a small clear area of cytoplasm. Contains usually two dark particles, centrioles- They become active at cell division.

2. Mitochondria: they are rod like or filamentous. Bounded by a double membrane. From the inner layer, incomplete foldings project in- cristae. They are centres of oxidation activity in the cell. Contains a number of enzyme systems. It is the site where chemical energy is derived by breakdown of organic compound i.e., source of energy in a cell.

3. Golgi apparatus: they appear as broad, flat membranous cisterns, piled one over the other, with vesicles. Proteins synthesized in the RER are received, aggregated,

chemically modified, packed and targeted to the cell surface in vesicles for secretion or storage.

4. Endoplasmic reticulum: branching and anastamosing flat tubules or vesicles. Ribosomes are sites of protein sythesis from amino acids. They occur free or in groups-(Polyribosomes) or seen attached to surface of endoplasmic reticulum. So endoplasmic reticulum is of 2 types:

(a) Smooth- with no ribosomes.

(b) Rough- with ribosomes attached-concerned with protein synthesis.

Smooth endoplasmic reticulum has varying functions in different cells. In muscle cell, release and recapture of calcium ions. In liver, concerned with lipid and cholesterol metabolism.

5. Lysosomes: Membrane bound particles containing hydrolytic enzymes. Active in breakdown and digestion of injured cells; and intracellular digestion of foreign materials i.e.They are responsible for intracellular digestion.

6. Microtubules.

Fine tubular structures formed of protein. Maintains cell shape, in cell division, helps in spindle formation.

Inclusions

1. Stored food: Glycogen or lipid droplets
2. Pigment granules: *e.g.,* melanin in skin
3. Stored products of cell metabolic activity.

CELL DIVISION

Cell division is an essential feature of development and growth. The 2 types of cell division are Mitosis and Meiosis. In Mitosis, the 2 daughter cells get the same number of chromosomes (46) as the parent cell. In meiosis, The daughter cells have only half the number (23) of chromosomes. So this occurs only for the formation of germ cells, Gametes.

Mitosis (Fig. 1.2)

Resting cell at interphase has its chromosomes as chromatin material.

(a) Prophase: before mitosis, chromosomes become linear structures, replicate their DNA. They get coiled and shortened. Each chromosome has now 2 chromatids, connected at centromere. The centrioles

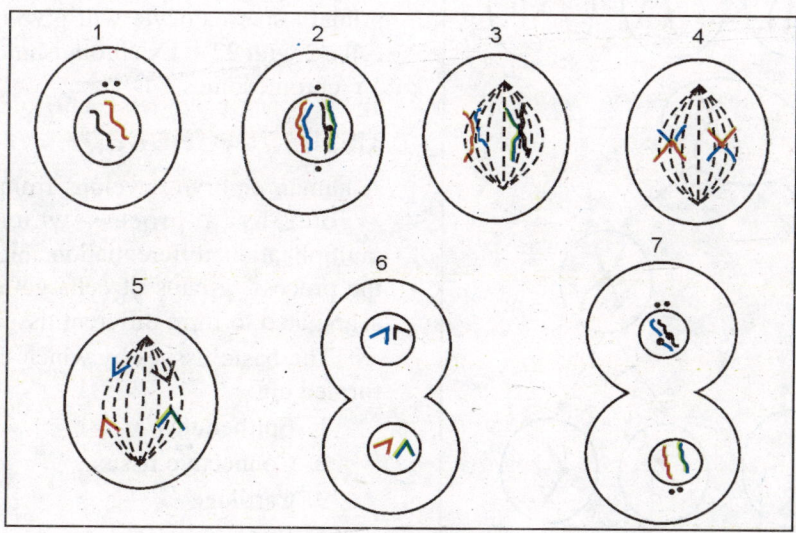

Fig. 1.2: Mitosis

move to the 2 poles of the cell and spindles are formed. Nucleolus disappears. Nuclear membrane breaks down.

(b) Metaphase: the double structured chromosomes get arranged at the equator and get attached to the spindles at centromeres.

(c) Anaphase: at the beginning of anaphase, the centromere divides. During anaphase, the chromatids migrate along the spindles to the poles.

(d) Telophase: the chromosomes uncoil and lengthen. Nuclear membrane and nucleoli reappear and cytoplasm also divides equally into 2 halves. Then each daughter cell gets half of the doubled chromosomes-thus same chromosomal pattern of the mother cell.

Meiosis (Reduction division) (Fig 1.3)

Has two stages: 1st meiosis and 2nd meiosis. Meiosis is undergone by the primary oocyte and primary spermatozyte, the primitive germ cells. The primitive germ cells replicate the DNA and chromosomes become double structured.

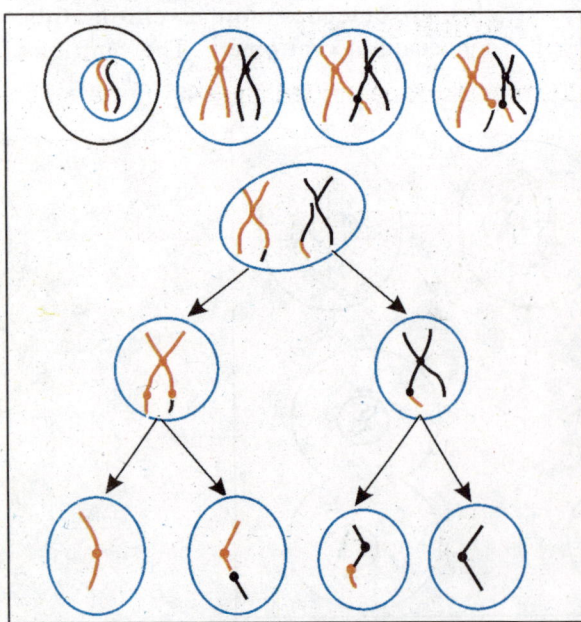

Fig. 1.3: Meiosis

Prophase is prolonged and has different stages: Leptotene, Zygotene, Pachytene, Diplotene and Diakinesis. As in early prophase, the chromosomes become thickened. By zygotene stage, there is pairing of homologous chromosomes and pair is point to point except for X and Y chromosomes. During pachytene stage, there is crossing over of the segments of chromatids of each pair. This is called chiasma formation. By this, segments are exchanged between the two chromatids ie, blocks of genes are exchanged between homologous chromosomes. During metaphase, each member of the pair gets attached to the spindle. During anaphase, each member of the homologous pair moves towards the poles of the cell. During telophase, the 2 daughter cells are formed with 23 double structured chromosomes.

2nd meiotic division

There is no DNA replication. Further it is like the mitosis itself. The 23 double structured chromosomes divide at the centromere and when the second division is over, 2 daughter cells of 23 single chromosomes with ½ the amount of DNA are formed.

Due to meiosis, primary oocyte gives rise to 4 daughter cells, each with 22 + 1X chromosomes. A primary spermatocyte will give rise to 4 daughter cells, 2 with 22 + 1X chromosomes and 2 with 22 + 1Y chromosomes.

TISSUES OF THE BODY

A human embryo develops from a fertilized egg-zygote, by a process which includes cell multiplication, differentiation, migration etc. During the process, groups of cells get differentiated and segregated to form different tissues of the body.

The basic tissues by which the human body is formed are:

1. Epithelium
2. Connective tissue
3. Cartilage
4. Bone

5. Muscle tissue
6. Vascular tissue
7. Nervous tissue
8. Glandular tissue

1. EPITHELIUM

Epithelium forms the coverings or linings of the external or internal surfaces of the body- as outer surface of skin, internal lining of the blood vessels, the digestive, respiratory and urogenital systems, the closed serous cavities of body (as pleural, pericardial and peritoneal cavities).

Epithelium consists of a layer or layers of cells arranged regularly over a basement membrane with no intercellular space. Adjacent cells are connected by different types of cell junctions.

The epithelial cells with the basement membrane and underlying minimum amount of connective tissue form a membrane. When there is a thin film of mucous moistening the surface of the membrane, it is called mucous membrane. *e.g.,* in digestive, respiratory, urogenital systems.

When there is a film of watery fluid moistening the surface of membrane, it is called serous membrane. *e.g.,* in peritoneum, pleura etc.

Classification of epithelium

Based on the number of layers of cells that form the epithelium, 2 types.

(a) Simple
(b) Compound or stratified

Based on the shape of cells, they are subdivided into

(a) Simple
  (i) simple squamous
  (ii) simple cuboidal
  (iii) simple columnar
(b) Compound or stratified
  (i) stratified squamous- non keratinised
  (ii) stratified squamous- keratinised
  (iii) stratified cuboidal
  (iv) stratified columnar
  (v) transitional

(c) Pseudo stratified epithelium
  This comes between simple and stratified types.
(d) Glandular epithelium:
  Invaginations from the epithelium.

(a) Simple Epithelia (Fig. 1.4 a - c)

1. Simple squamous (Fig. 1.4a): Cells are flat. Nucleus at the broadest part of the cell.
   e.g., In alveoli of lungs, in the inner lining of blood vessels, loop of Henle in kidney.
2. Simple cuboidal (Fig. 1.4b): Height and width of cells are equal. Nucleus rounded, at the centre.
   e.g., Lining of thyroid follicles, Ducts of glands
3. Simple columnar (Fig. 1.4 C_1–C_3): Cylindrical cells, nucleus oval, nearer the base of cells. *e.g.,* stomach, gall bladder.

At certain sites, free surface of the columnar cells show tiny projections of cell membrane called microvilli. They give a striated or brush border appearance to the epithelium. Found in epithelium which has absorptive functions. *e.g.,* Small intestine, certain renal tubules. Certain other sites, free surfaces of the cells show longer projections -cilia which are motile. They help in sweeping foreign bodies from the surface or help in transferring secretion. *e.g.,* respiratory tract, fallopian tube.

(b) Stratified epithelia (Fig. 1.4 d–f)

1. Stratified squamous: Nonkeratinised. Basal cells are columnar. Above that, 3–8 layers of polygonal cells. Surface cells are squamous. Seen lining wet surfaces *e.g.,* Cornea, oesophagus, mouth.(Fig.1.4d)
2. Stratified squamous: Keratinised - similar to the above type. But over the surface there is a layer of scale like non nucleated dead cells, which form keratin or cornification. *e.g.,* epidermis of skin. (Fig.1.4e)
3. Stratified cuboidal: Over the basement membrane two or more layers of cuboidal

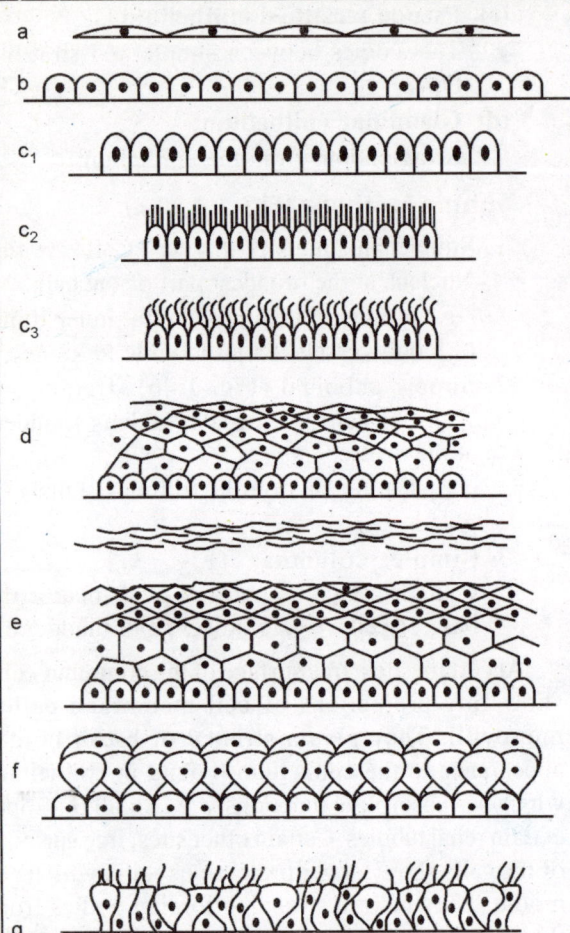

Fig. 1.4: (a to c): Simple epithelia (d to f): Stratified epithelia (g): Pseudo stratified columnar epithelium

cuboidal, above that, pear shaped cells and surface cells are faceted cells. (Fig.1.4 f)

(c) Pseudostratified epithelium. (Fig.1.4g)

This comes between stratified and simple types.

e.g., Trachea. Cells are of different heights and shapes. Similates a stratified epithelium, but all cells reach the basement membrane.

(d) Glandular epithelium

They are invaginations from the epithelium and often described as glandular tissue.

2. CONNECTIVE TISSUE

It is widely distributed in different forms in the body. Seen beneath the skin as fascia, forms packing material among organs or muscles or vessels and nerves, forms coverings for organs as capsules, forms tendons, ligaments, aponeurosis etc.

Generalised form of connective tissue is connective tissue proper and specialized forms of connective tissue are cartilage and bone.

Basic structure of connective tissue

It has cells and matrix. Matrix comprises a gel like ground substance in which fibers are embedded. Ground substance is formed of soluble complexes of glycosaminoglycans, linked to protein molecules. i.e., It is proteoglycans. Fibres are insoluble protein filaments – three types are there, Collagen, Elastic (elastin) and Reticulin fibres. (Fig. 1.5)

cells. *e.g.,* large ducts of glands, membrana granulosa of ovarian follicle.

4. Stratified columnar: More than two layers of columnar cells. *e.g.,* In parts of pharynx and penile urethra.

5. Transitional or urothelium. *e.g.,* ureter and urinary bladder. Cells are 2–3 layered in distended bladder. Number of layers becomes 4–8 in contracted bladder. Cells are able to rearrange themselves according to the conditions of the organ, because deep cells do not have tight cell junctions. Basal cells are

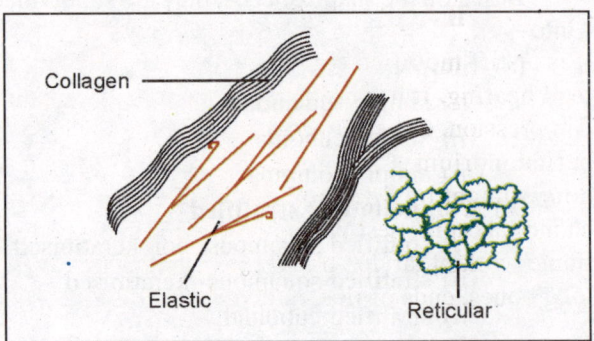

Fig. 1.5: Connective Tissue Fibres

FIBRES

Collagen: White in fresh state, generally seen in bundles. Not extensible.

Elastic: Yellow in fresh state, generally run singly, they are extensible, individual fibers show branching. Cut ends curl up due to elasticity.

Reticulin: Similar to collagen, but thin fibrils which branch and anastamose.

CELLS

- **Fibroblasts**
- **Macrophages**
- **Mast cells**
- **Plasma cells**
- **Fat cells**

Fibroblasts are large cells with cytoplasmic processes. They produce the fibers in the tissue.

Macrophages have irregular processes. Involved in engulfing foreign or unwanted materials from tissues.

Mast cells contain large granules, they produce heparin and histamine.

Plasma cells are involved in immunity.

Fat cells store extra fat in the tissues.

Ground substance has the nature of binding water. Most of extra cellular fluid in the body is in the form of bound water in the matrix of connective tissue.

Proportion of cells, fibres and ground substance differ in different organs or different locations.

3. CARTILAGE

It is a stiff modified connective tissue, capable of load bearing. It has high resistance to tension and compression. Generally covered by a fibrous layer, perichondrium. Cartilage is avascular, it gets its nourishment by diffusion of nutrients from perichondrial capillaries. Widely distributed in the bodyframe work of larynx, trachea, external ear, ends of long bones, ends of ribs, intervertebral disc etc.

General structure

As in any connective tissue, cartilage has cells- Chondrocytes, in a matrix. Matrix varies in its nature and composition, in different types of cartilages. It is composed of collagen or elastic fibres in a stiff ground substance.

Ground substance is a meshwork of proteoglycan molecules, holding water and dissolved salts. Here proteoglycans have chondroitin sulphates and keratin sulphates.

Types

Hyaline, Elastic and White fibrocartilage.

Hyaline cartilage (Fig. 1.6)

Has a glassy homogenous appearance. Found in - trachea, costal cartilage, ends of long bones, epiphysis..Covered by perichondrium. Matrix is clear and transparent like glass. Electron microscopic appearance shows, it has fine collagen fibres which are not visible by ordinary microscope- the refractive index of matrix and fibers is same.

In the matrix, chondrocytes are arranged in spaces called lacunae. Typically in Hyaline cartilage they form groups of 2 or more- cell nests- inside lacunae. Underneath perichondrium flat immature cells – Chondroblasts are seen, singly in smaller lacunae. Chondroblasts are involved in growth of cartilage and get converted into chondrocytes.

Elastic cartilage (Fig. 1.7)

Seen in eustacian tube, epiglottis, external ear. Here cells are singly arranged in the lacunae. Matrix is traversed by elastic fibers which ramify around the lacunae.

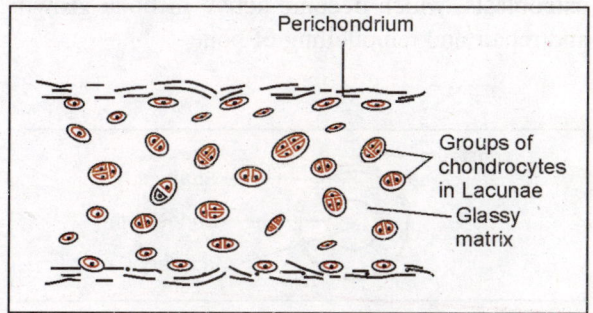

Fig. 1.6: Hyaline Cartilage

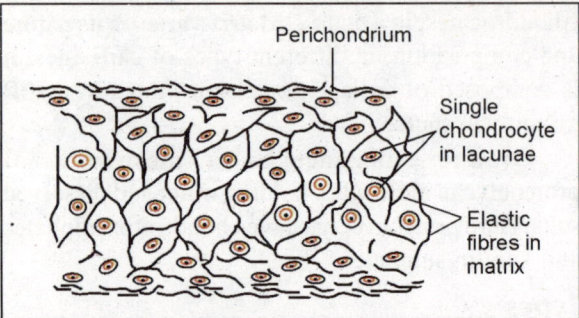

Fig. 1.7: Elastic Cartilage

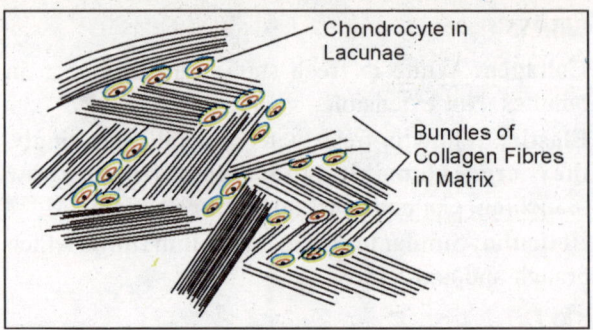

Fig. 1.8: Fibrocartilage

Fibrocartilage (Fig 1.8)

Found in intervertebral disc, intra articular discs. Matrix is traversed by dense fascicles of white collagenous fibres. Hence also called White fibrocartilage. Chondrocytes are arranged in the interfascicular matrix in rows, inside lacunae.

4. BONE

Like cartilage it is a specialized connective tissue, but made hard due to deposition of calcium salts in the matrix. Unlike cartilage, it is vascular.

Periosteum

The fibrous layer which covers the bone, except at its articular ends. It has an outer fibrous highly vascular layer and inner cellular layer which is less vascular. To the outer layer, the tendons and ligaments get attached. From the sites of attachments, strong thin fibers pass into the compact bone as fibers of Sharpey.

Cells of the inner layer are osteoclasts and osteoblasts, which become active in bone growth and repair and remodelling of bone.

Gross structure of bone

In gross appearance, 2 types of bones can be distinguished-

(a) Spongy or cancellous

(b) Dense or compact

In a long bone at the ends spongy bone is seen- as trabeculae of bone with spaces among them which contain bone marrow. Shaft of the bone is formed of dense or compact bone with no intervening spaces, but through the middle of the shaft, the medullary cavity runs which contains bone marrow.

As the outer surface of bone is covered by periosteum, inner surface – medullary cavity is lined by endosteum (Fig. 1.9).

Parts of a long bone (Fig 1.10)

In a young bone the long middle part is shaft or diaphysis and the 2 ends are epiphysis. Part of

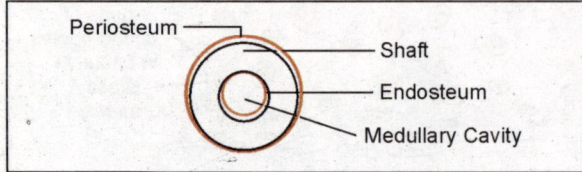

Fig. 1.9: C. S. of Long Bone

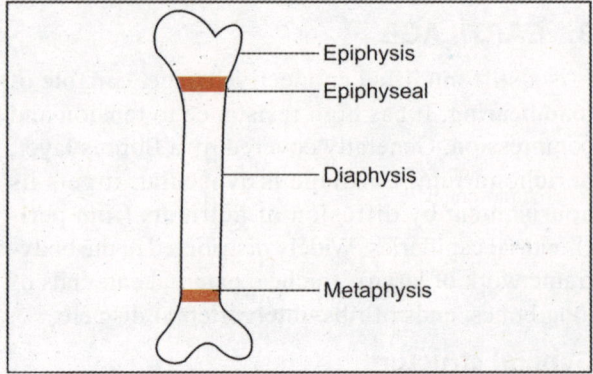

Fig. 1.10: Parts of Long Bone

diaphysis near the epiphysis is metaphysis. Between the metaphysis and epiphysis, a piece of hyaline cartilage is present in a growing bone- Epiphyseal plate.

Microscopic structure (Fig. 1.11 a,b)

Vertical channels called Haversian canals traverse through the calcified matrix of compact bone. They are interconnected by horizontal or oblique channels. Haversian canals are connected to endosteal and periosteal surfaces by channels called Volkman's canals.

Haversian canals and their connecting channels contain blood vessels and nerves of bones. Characteristic feature of compact bone is that the calcified matrix is arranged in layers- lamellae and lamellae contain lacunae in which bone cells-osteocytes are lodged.

Haversian canals are surrounded by a number of lamellae, concentric lamellae with osteocytes in lacunae. This forms the structural unit of the tissue – Haversian system or osteon. Among the Haversian systems, the lamellae present are interstitial lamellae. Near the outer and inner surfaces of the bone, outer and inner circumferential lamellae are seen.

Structure of bone is the same in cancellous bone also, but Haversian systems are not very typical.

OSSIFICATION

Ossification means bone formation or bone development. There are two ways in which bone is formed.

1. Intramembranous ossification.
2. Intracartilagenous or endochondral ossification.

Generally flat and irregular bones develop by intramembranous method and long bones develop by endochondral ossification.

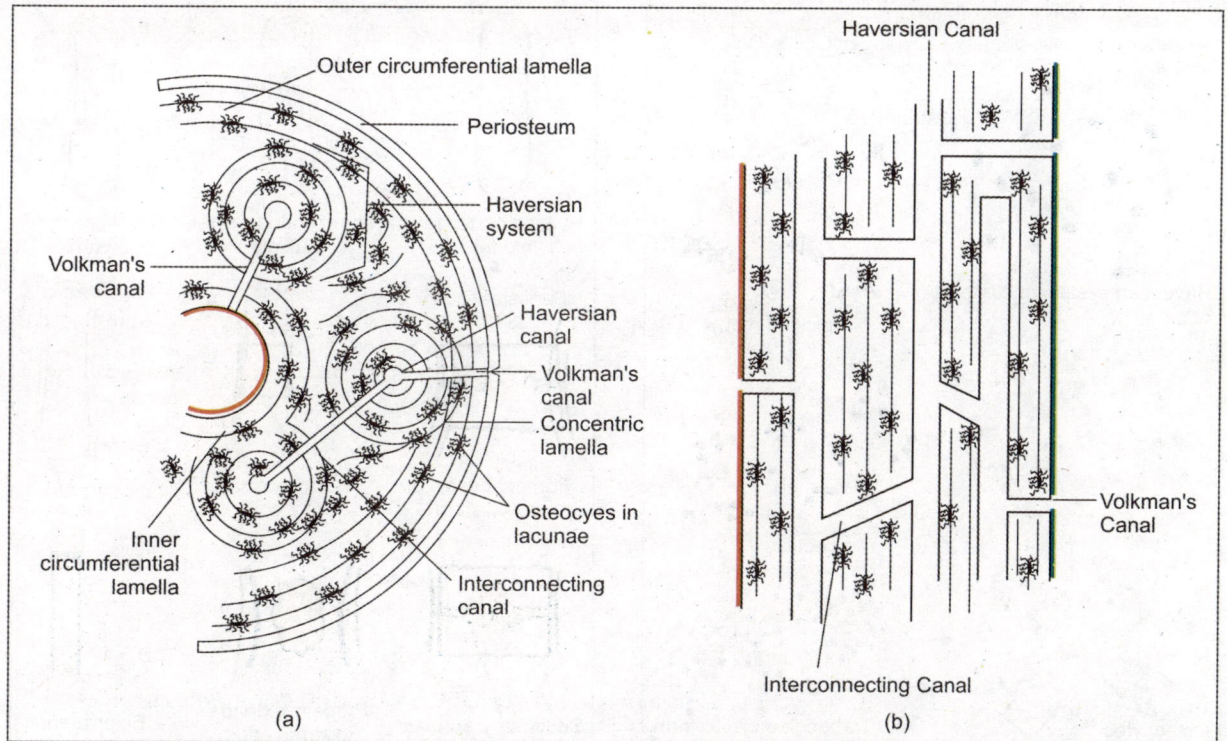

Fig. 1.11: (a) Microscopic Structure of C.S. of Bone (b) Microscopic Structure of L.S. of Bone

Intramembranous ossification (Fig. 1.12)

In the embryo, bone develops in a membrane of embryonal connective tissue, Mesenchyme. At the site where a bone is to be formed, the mesenchymal cells multiply and the area becomes highly vascular. This is the primary centre of ossification. The cells become ostogenic- osteoblasts. They secrete matrix around them which gets calcified. Thus many spicules of bone are formed. Cells which get trapped inside the calcified matrix change to mature bone cells, osteocytes. Osteoblasts are still seen on surface of spicules.

Spicules join to form a network of bony tissue- A trabeculum. Spaces among them contain blood vessels. Osteoblasts on the surfaces of the spicules continue to secrete bone matrix in anular fashion and the trabecular bone is converted into compact bone.

Endochondral ossification (Fig. 1.13)

A hyaline cartilagenous model of the bone is 1st laid down in the mesenchyme which is replaced by bone. The cartilaginous model is covered by perichondrium. Chondrocytes at the centre of the model multiply and enlarge. The matrix among them gets calcified.

Cells die and Clear spaces called primary areolae are formed.

Deep to the perichondrium, a layer of bone tissue is formed around the centre of the model- Subperiosteal bony collar. There the periochondrium changes to periosteum.

Tiny sprouts from the periosteum containing osteoblasts, osteoclasts and blood vessels, called periosteal buds grow into primary areolae. This region is the primary centre of ossification.

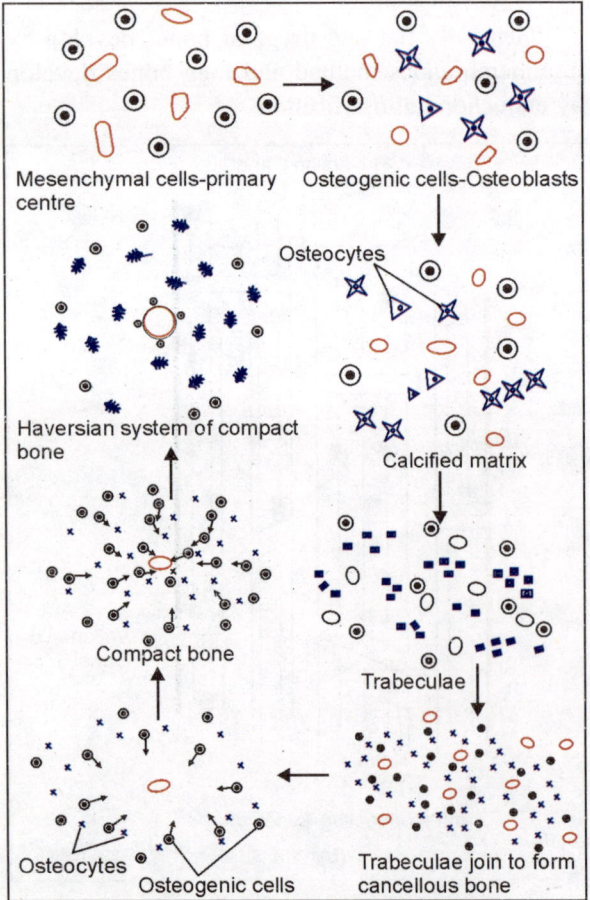

Fig. 1.12: Intramembranous Ossification

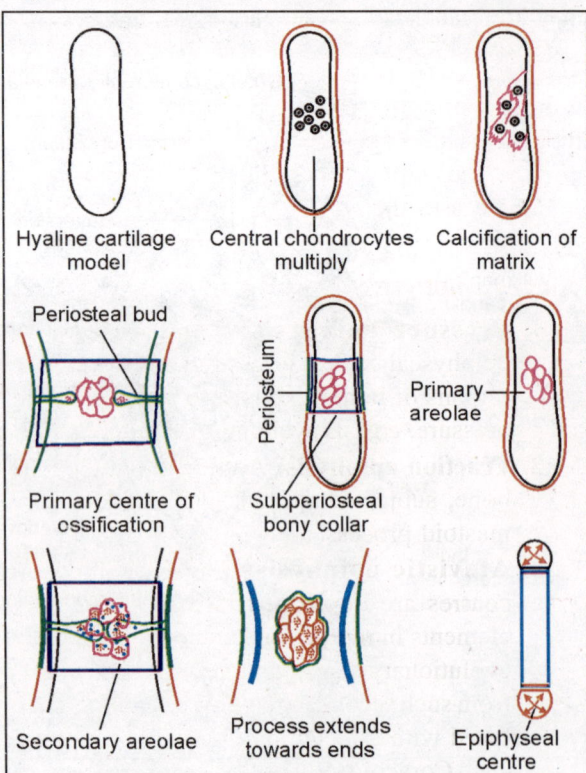

Fig. 1.13: Endochondral Ossification

Osteoclasts destroy the calcified walls of primary areolae and larger spaces- secondary areolae are formed. On to them, osteoblasts deposit new bone. This continues and larger space, medullary cavity is formed, which contains bone marrow. The process extends towards ends of bone. Part of shaft of the bone, formed from primary centre of ossification is diaphysis. At the 2 ends, epyphisial centres (secondary centres) appear and there also, bone formation starts. Between bone formed by primary centre and secondary centre, there is a plate of original hyaline cartilage, epiphyseal plate. It continues to grow until 18-22 years of age. Then growth of the bone is stopped and epiphyseal plates disappear. Thickness of bone increases by growth of subperiosteal bone.

Blood supply of bone

Periosteal arteries, nutrient arteries, epiphyseal arteries and metaphyseal arteries supply the bone. They are branches from neighbouring arteries.

Epiphysis

In long bones, between the metaphysis and epiphyseal ends of bones, there is a plate of hyaline cartilage, the epiphyseal cartilage. As the growth of the bone ceases the epiphyseal plate is replaced by bone.

Types of epiphysis .

1. **Pressure epiphysis:** Some secondary epiphyseal centres of ossification develop in regions of bones exposed to much articular pressure. *e.g.,* Lower end of femur.
2. **Traction epiphysis:** Appear in parts of the bone, subjected to muscular traction. *e.g.,* mastoid process.
3. **Atavistic epiphysis:** These epiphyseal centres are developed into separate bony elements in reptiles and amphibians of early evolutionary stages. In mammals bony parts from such secondary epiphyseal centres have fused with a neighbouring bone as its part. *e.g.,* Coracoid process of scapula, Parts of sphenoid, Occipital bone, Temporal bone.

JOINTS

Joints are regions where bones are joined or connected to each other. Joints are classified in 3 different ways.

A. Based on the range of movements possible at a joint

1. Synarthrosis: A joint where no movement is possible.
2. Amphiarthrosis: Limited amount of movements are possible.
3. Diarthrosis: A freely mobile joint.

B. Based on the number of axes around which movements take place.

1. Uniaxial joint
2. Biaxial joint
3. Multiaxial joint

C. Based on the form and gross structure of the joint

1. Fibrous joint
2. Cartilagenous joint
3. Synovial joint

1. Fibrous joints

Here the facing ends of bones are joined together by a minimum amount of fibrous (connective) tissue. These are generally immobile joints.

Types:

(a) Sutures
(b) Gomphosis
(c) Syndesmosis

(a) **Sutures (Fig 1.14)**

They are present among skull bones. Different varieties of sutures are:

Plane: between horizontal plates of palatine bones.

Serrate: between parietal bones.

Denticulate: lambdoid suture.

Squamous: between temporal and parietal bones.

Schindylesis: (wedge shaped) - between vomer and sphenoid.

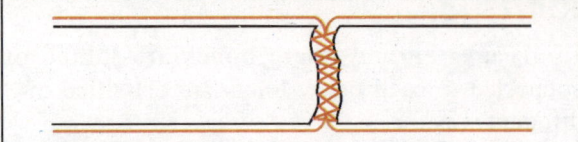

Fig. 1.14: Fibrous Joint - Suture

(b) Gomphosis (Peg and socket): Joint between tooth and its socket.

(c) Syndesmosis: Here the connecting fibrous tissue is more than at the sutures, so that a limited amount of mobility is permited. *e.g.,* Tibiofibular syndesmosis.

2. Cartilagenous joints (Fig 1.15.)

Bones are joined by a piece of cartilage: Two types.

(a) Primary cartilagenous joint (synchondrosis): Bones are connected by a piece of hyaline cartilage. They are not permanent, present during growing stage only. Bony union occurs when growth is over. No mobility is possible. *e.g.,* epiphyseal plate, neurocentral joint.

(b) Secondary cartilagenous joint (Symphysis)

Bony ends are covered by a piece of hyaline cartilage and they are joined by fibrocartilage. They are generally permanent. Certain degree of movement is possible. *e.g.,* Pubic symphysis, joints between vertebral bodies.

3. Synovial joint

Generally freely mobile joints. (Fig. 1.16.) Facing ends of Bones are covered by a piece of hyaline cartilage—Articular cartilage. Connected together by a sleeve of fibrous tissue-capsule. Inner surface of capsule is lined by a thin serous membrane-Synovial membrane which also lines the nonarticular parts of bones inside the joint cavity. It secretes a thin film of fluid- synovial fluid which lubricates and nourishes the joint cavity. At regions, there are localized thickenings of fibres of the capsule which form ligaments. They strengthen the capsule and limit the movements at the joint.

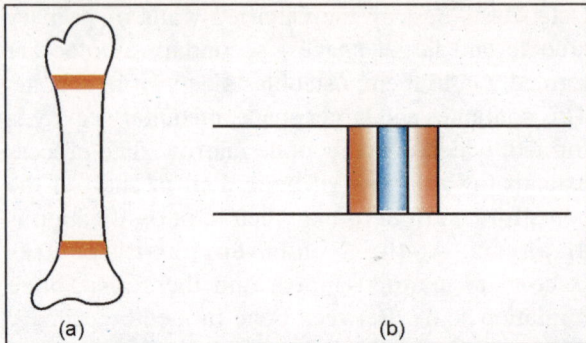

Fig. 1.15: (a) Primary Cartilagenous Joint (Synchondrosis) (b) Secondary Cartilagenous Joint (Symphysis)

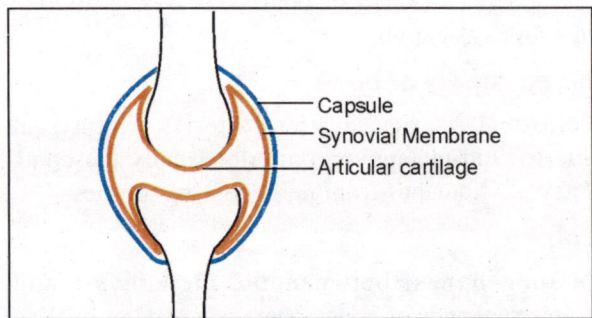

Fig. 1.16: Typical Synovial Joint

Types (Fig 1.17 a to f)

(a) Plane: The facing surfaces are plane. *e.g.,* intercarpal joints.

(b) Saddle: Facing surfaces are reciprocally concavoconvex. *e.g.,* First carpometacarpal joint, sternoclavicular joint.

(c) Hinge joint: Articular parts simulate hinge of the lid of a box. Movements are possible only around a single-transverse axis. *e.g.,* Elbow joint.

(d) Pivot joint: A cylindrical pivot of bone rotates in a ring formed by bone and fibrous tissue- as in the gate of compound wall. Here also movement is possible only around a single vertical axis—Rotation. *e.g.,* superior radioulnar joint, Median atlanto axial joint.

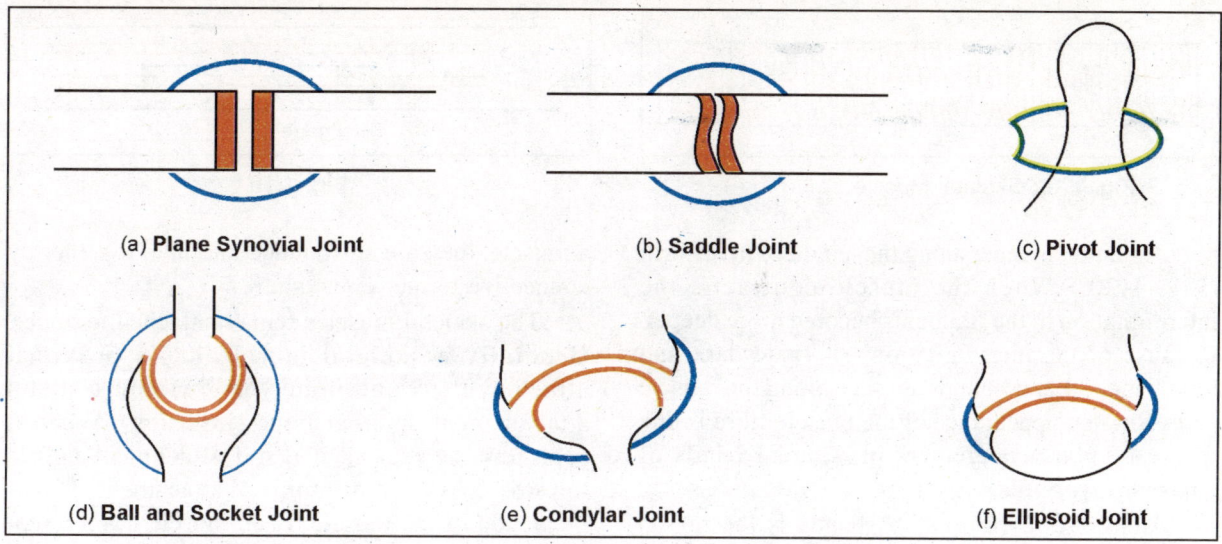

(a) **Plane Synovial Joint**   (b) **Saddle Joint**   (c) **Pivot Joint**

(d) **Ball and Socket Joint**   (e) **Condylar Joint**   (f) **Ellipsoid Joint**

Fig. 1.17

(e) **Ball and socket joint:** Wide range of movements are possible around a number of axes. A spherical end of bone is joined to a socket or cup shaped bone. *e.g.,* Shoulder joint, hip joint.

(f) **Condylar joint:** Instead of a spherical surface, an oblong convex condyle articulates with a concave socket. *e.g.,* Temporomandibular joint, knee joint.

(g) **Ellipsoid joint:** An oval convex ellipsoid articulates with a concave socket. *e.g.,* Wrist joint.

5. MUSCLE TISSUE

Basic structural unit of a muscle is the muscle cell-myocyte which is usually known as muscle fibre because many of the muscle cells are thin and long. Three types of muscle tissue are present in the body.

1. **Skeletal-Striated, voluntary.** Seen attached to bones of the body.
2. **Cardiac-Striated, involuntary.** Muscle tissue of the heart.
3. **Smooth-Nonstriated, involuntary.** Seen in the walls of organs of GIT, urinary tract, reproductive organs, in the walls of blood vessels, in the trachea, bronchi, in the dermis of thin skin.

Special characteristic nature of the muscle tissue is its ability to contract- contractility on stimulation. This is effected by the presence of fine protein filaments in the cells- myofilaments- **Actin** and **Myosin** filaments.

Structure

1. **Skeletal muscle:** When seen under light microscope, a muscle fibre appears as a long cylindrical structure which shows transverse dark and light lines: striations and the flat elongated nucleus is peripherally placed. The cell is multinucleated. Cell membrane is called Sarcolemma and cytoplasm is called sarcoplasm. (Fig.1.18.) Ultrastructure shows that sarcoplasm contains parallelly arranged thin myofibrils. (Fig. 1.19.)

Each myofibril has a dark line – Z line at regular intervals. The distance between two Z lines is the contractile unit – Sarcomere.

The sarcomere part of the myofibril consists of two types of myofilaments – Thin actin and thick myosin filaments. They are arranged in

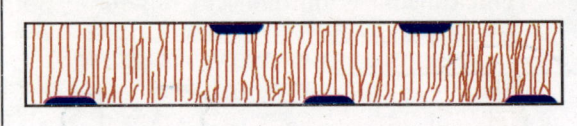

Fig. 1.18: Skeletal Muscle Cell (Fibre)

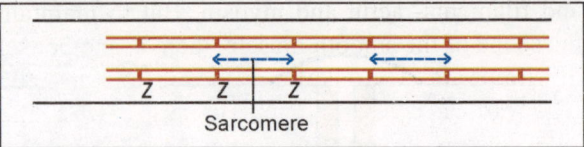

Fig. 1.19

interdigitating manner along the length of myofibril. (Fig. 1.20.) When the muscle contracts, the interdigitation of the filaments become more deeper. Because of the interdigitation, alternate dark and light bands- **A** and **I** bands are seen along the muscle cells. Striated appearance of the muscle fibre is due to the regular arrangement of A and I bands of adjacent myofibrils.

Along the myofibrils, "A band" is the region occupied by thick myosin filaments, the ends of which are overlapped by the actin filaments.

"H band" is the central paler major part of A band where actin filaments do not overlap.

"M line"- At the central points, the myosin filaments are linked together by a material. This is the M line.

"I band"- Consists of adjacent parts of two neighbouring sarcomeres, where thin actin filaments are not overlapped by myosin filaments. It is bisected by Z line.

"Z line"-line along which thin actin filaments of adjacent sarcomeres overlap and are anchored.

Individual muscle fibres are covered by delicate connective tissue- endomysium. Fasciculi of muscle fibres are surrounded by connective tissue, perimysium. Fasciculi when grouped together form a muscle, they are surrounded and held together by connective tissue- epimysium.

The skeletal muscles remain attached to bones. Generally a skeletal muscle has a proximal attachment to one bone (origin) and a distal attachment to another bone (insertion). When it contracts the region of distal attachment moves towards the region of proximal attachment. This is the action of the muscle. Each muscle has a motor nerve supplying it.

2. Cardiac muscle: (Fig. 1.21) Forms myocardium.

Striated. Cells have one or two centrally placed nuclei. They branch and get connected with the adjacent cells. Cell junctions are called intercalated discs. Striations are not as prominent as seen in skeletal muscle, because of the abundance of mitochondria among the myofibrils.

3. Smooth muscle (Fig. 1.22.). Unstriated. Present in skin, walls of blood vessels, intestinal tract, uterus, bladder etc. Spindle shaped. Oval nucleus is at the centre. Cytoplasm has myofibrils

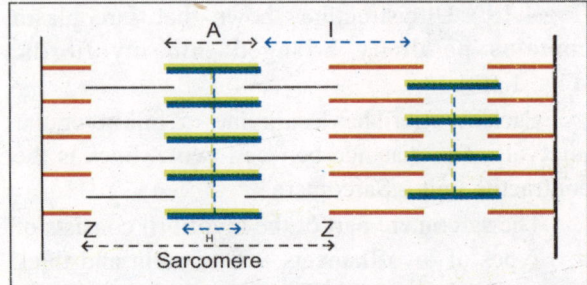

Fig. 1.20

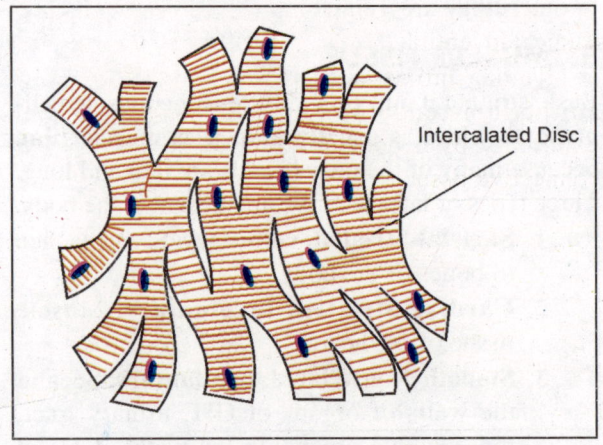

Fig. 1.21: Cardiac Muscle

and filaments- actin and myosin. But to maintain the shape of the smooth muscle, there is another set of filaments- Cytoskeleton. Actin and myosin filaments are arranged at an angle with the cytoskeleton and so they do not have the regular alternate light and dark bands. Hence smooth muscle.

6. VASCULAR TISSUE

Blood vascular tissue

The blood vascular system consists of the heart and blood vessels. Leaving the heart, the blood is distributed through a series of large tubular structures- the arteries. The largest artery leaving the heart with pure blood is the aorta, having a diameter of about 2.5 cm. The arteries ramify in various parts of body, they subdivide to form smaller vessels, arterioles. They also undergo further repeated division and smallest tubules, capillaries or sinusoids are formed, depending on the functional requirement. These narrowest thin walled vessels are in intimate contact with the tissues. From the tissues, venous blood is collected through venous capillaries, conveyed to larger venules, then to veins. Veins converge to form large veins which return the venous blood to heart.

Structure (Fig. 1.23)

The basic structure of the wall of a blood vessel shows that it has three zones or layers- from inner to outer, they are Tunica intima, Tunica media and Tunica adventitia.

Tunica intima consists of simple squamous epithelium- endothelium which is supported externally by a delicate layer of subendothelial connective tissue.

Tunica media is fibromuscular- with smooth muscle cells and connective tissue. (elastic, collagen or reticular)

Tunica adventitia is the outermost layer, formed of connective tissue.

Structure of large arteries (Elastic arteries)

e.g., Aorta, subclavian artery, common iliac arteries. Fig 1.24.

Tunica intima: Endothelium and subendothelial connective tissue which contain elastic and collagen fibers. Outside this, there is a fenestrated elastic layer- internal elastic lamina. It is not sharply demarcated because the media also contains elastic tissue.

Tunica media: Consists of number of layers of fenestrated elastic lamellae. Between the elastic layers, there is minimum amount of connective tissue and a few smooth muscle cells. The number of elastic lamellae increase with age.

Tunica adventitia is formed of elastic, collagen and reticular fibres.

As the walls of the large arteries are thick, its outer region is nourished by branches from same artery or neighbouring arteries. They are called vasa vasorum.

Medium sized arteries (Muscular arteries)

e.g., Radial artery, facial artery. (Fig. 1.25)

Tunica intima has the same structure as that of large artery.

Tunica media is a muscular layer formed of number of layers of smooth muscle cells, arranged circularly around the lumen. The muscle fibers are separated by minimum amount of connective tissue.

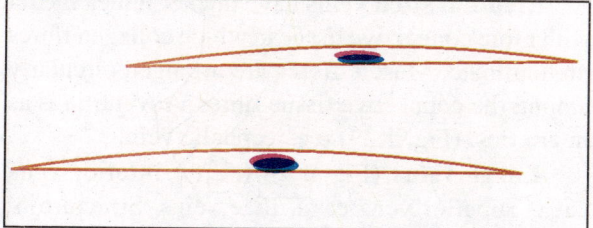

Fig. 1.22: Smooth Muscle (Nonstriated)

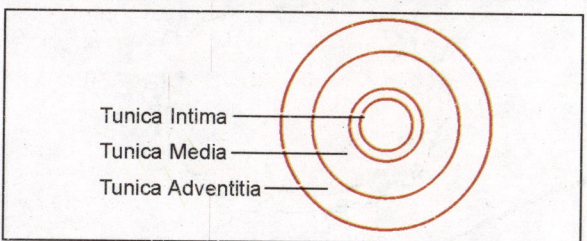

Tunica Intima
Tunica Media
Tunica Adventitia

Fig. 1.23

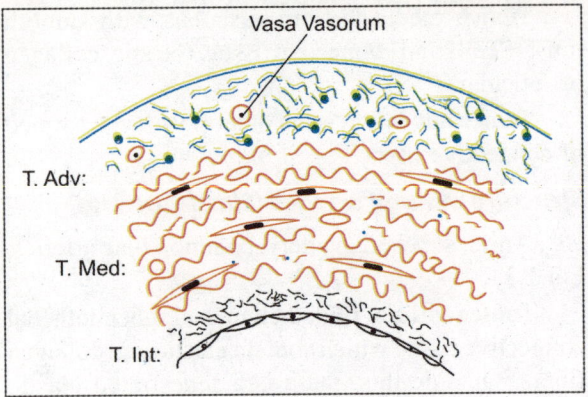

Fig. 1.24: Large Artery

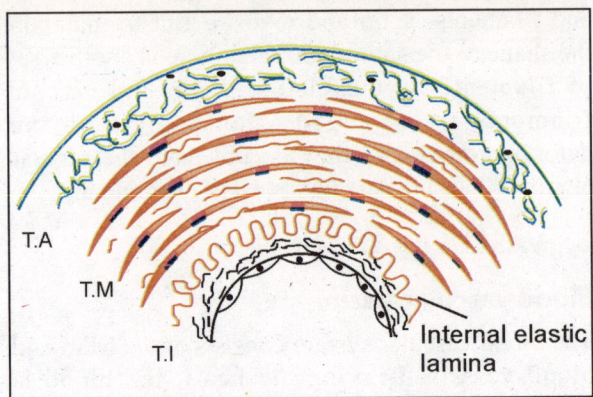

Fig. 1.25: Medium Sized Artery

Between the intima and media, there is a prominent internal elastic lamina. It is bright and refractile and thrown into wavy folds.

Tunica adventitia is formed of connective tissue. Between the media and adventitia, the elastic tissue in adventitia condenses to form an external elastic lamina.

Arterioles

Smallest muscular arteries are arterioles. Their wall thickness is less and contains only very few layers of muscle fibers.

Capillaries (Fig 1.26)

Very thin walled. Has an endothelium surrounded by delicate fibres and cells, a basal lamina. In certain capillaries, there will be tiny pores between the narrow parts of endothelial cells and there are no tight junctions between the endothelial cells. They are called fenestrated capillaries. This structural peculiarity is the basis of capillary permeability.

Sinusoids

In organs like liver, spleen and endocrine glands, the smallest vessels differ from true capillaries. They have wider irregular lumen and thinner walls. There is no subendothelial connective tissue separating the vessels from the tissue. Hence there is more contact between the tissue and the blood.

Structure of veins

Structure of the walls of veins also is similar to arteries, with three tunics. But the main difference between arteries and veins in the structure is, the thinner tunica media- elastic and muscle content is less. Lumen is not circular as in arteries.

Venous capillaries

Continuous with arterial capillaries and they continue as venules. Large venules show the three tunics, with very few muscle fibers in the media.

Medium sized veins have thicker tunica media with more connective tissue in which collagen fibres predominate. Muscle fibres are arranged circularly among the connective tissue fibres. Adventitia is as in arteries. (Fig. 1.27) *e.g.,* cephalic vein.

Large veins (Fig. 1.28.): *e.g.,* Inferior vena cava, Superior vena cava, Iliac veins. Structure of intima and media are similar to that in medium sized

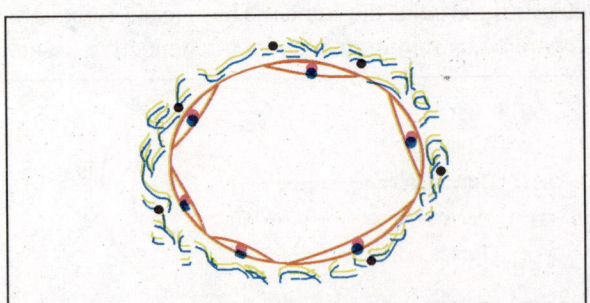

Fig. 1.26: Capillary

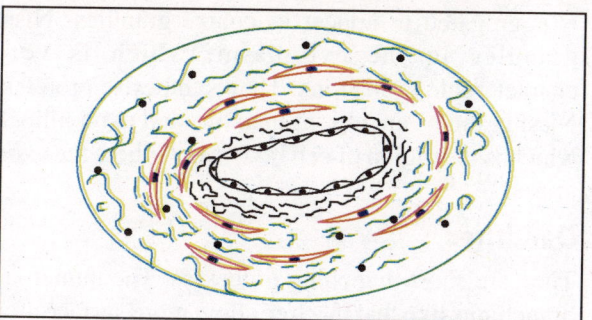

Fig. 1.27: Medium Sized Vein

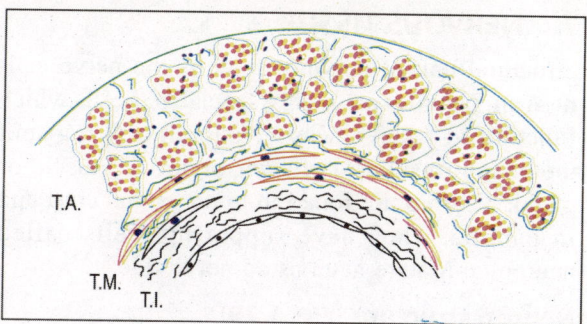

Fig. 1.28: Large Vein

veins. The thickest tunic is tunica adventitia which contains many bundles of smooth muscle fibres longitudinally arranged around the lumen, among fibrous tissue. Most veins have valves inside, which prevent reflux of blood. Semilunar in shape, they are formed of reduplication of intima. Veins of lower limb contain numerous valves. Valves are absent in very small veins, and in some large veins.

LYMPHATIC TISSUE

Lymphatic tissue or lymphoid tissue is not one of the fundamental tissue types of the body, but is a special type of reticular tissue, infiltered by lymphocytes. Consists of a system of vessels permiating most of the tissues of the body and lymphatic organs as lymph nodes, thymus, tonsil, spleen and lymph follicles in the mucous membrane, especially of alimentary tract.

Most of the tissue fluid returns to blood circulation through the venous ends of capillaries and they take up only soluble crystalloids. About 10–20% of tissue fluid is transported through lymphatic vessels which absorb particulate matter and colloid materials from tissue spaces. Lymph is a clear fluid except that from alimentary tract, which appears milky due to the presence of absorbed fat.

Lymph vessels begin as a plexus of fine capillaries which have blind ends, in tissue spaces. Structure of capillaries is similar to blood capillaries, but are more permeable to substances of greater molecular size- colloid materials, cell debris, micro organisms. Lymph vessels are absent in CNS, bone marrow, and avascular structures as epidermis, hair, nail, cornea and cartilage.

Lymph capillaries join to form larger vessels and they have numerous valves, hence have beaded appearance. Their walls have all the three tunics, but much thinner than those of blood vessels.

The lymph vessels pass through groups of lymph nodes. Lymph is filtered in a series of lymph nodes in its course. The large lymph vessels- Thoracic duct and right lymphatic duct pour the lymph finally into the large veins at the root of neck.

Function

In addition to transporting and clearing the lymph, lymphatic system is involved in phagocytosis, immune responses and contributing to the cell population of blood and lymph.

Lymphocytes

They differentiate from bone marrow and thymus. (B lymphocytes and T lymphocytes). B lymphocytes produce antibodies and T lymphocytes remove particulate matter, viruses, bacteria etc.

From their sites of origin, the lymphocytes pass in circulation to reach the peripheral lymphoid organs. They multiply there and migrate to other tissues as needed.

Applied aspects

In the limbs, superficial lymphatic vessels get blocked by the invasion of vessels by filarial parasites. There is swelling and signs of inflammation of the affected part.

7. NERVOUS TISSUE

Structural unit of nervous tissue is the nerve cell-**neuron**. Neurons are highly specialized cells which function to receive sensory stimuli and transmit motor information to effector organs – muscle or gland. Neurons are found in brain, spinal cord and in ganglia. They have supporting cells called neuroglia. Mature neurons do not divide.

Neuron structure (Fig. 1.29)

Cell body of the neuron called perikaryon has processes from its surface – neurites. Shorter and branching processes are dendrites which receive information or stimuli. A single long process that conducts impulses away from the neuron is axon. Axons of neurons together form nerve fibers. Nucleus of the neuron is pale with a prominent nucleolus. All the cell organelles and inclusions are present with numerous microtubules, microfilaments and neurofilaments. Rough endoplasmic reticulum

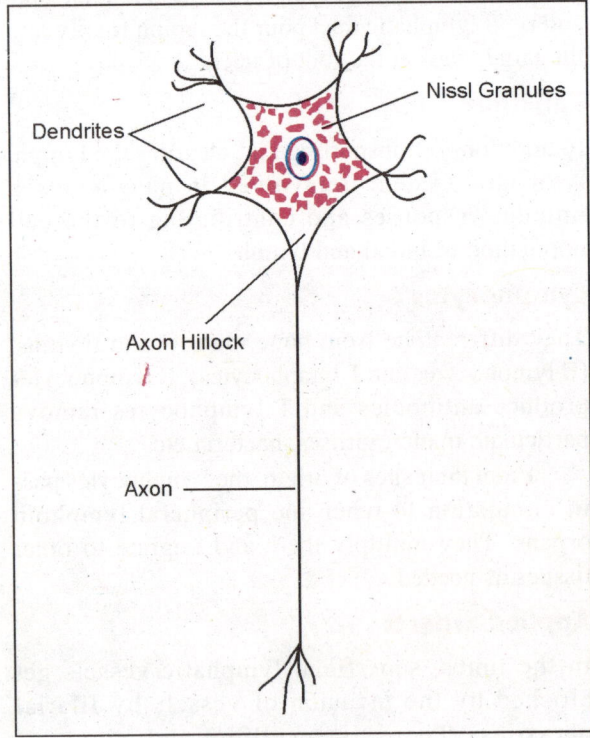

Fig. 1.29: Neuron

is aggregated to appear as coarse granules- Nissl granules in the cytoplasm, which is very characteristic to neurons. They synthesise proteins. Nissl granules are absent in axons and axon hillock which is the region of cell body from where the axon arises.

Dendrites

They are short branching processes. The numerous branchings like that in a tree allow more surface area to receive stimuli.

Axon

A single long process arising from the cell body at the axon hillock. It branches only at its terminal part and there branches will be numerous. Collaterals may be seen. Length of axons vary from 0.1 mm to 2–3 metres. Axons send impulses away from the cell body. Synapses are special cell contacts between nerve cells or between nerve cells and effector organs.

Types of neurons (Fig. 1.30)

1. *Multipolar neurons.* They have number of dendrites and a single short or long axon. *e.g.,* Anterior horn cells of spinal cord, Pyramidal cells of cerebral cortex, Purkinje cells of cerebellum.
2. *Bipolar neurons.* Cell body is slightly elongated, from both ends of which a single process arises. *e.g.,* Bipolar cells of retina.
3. *Unipolar neurons.* From the cell body, a single process arises and divides into a central process and a peripheral process. *e.g.,* Sensory ganglion cells (dorsal root ganglion cells).
4. *Anaxonic neurons.* They have only dendrites. *e.g.,* Amacrine cells of retina.

Neuroglia

They are nonexcitable cells unlike neurons. But provide structural and metabolic support to neurons. They are more numerous than neurons. Four types are described.

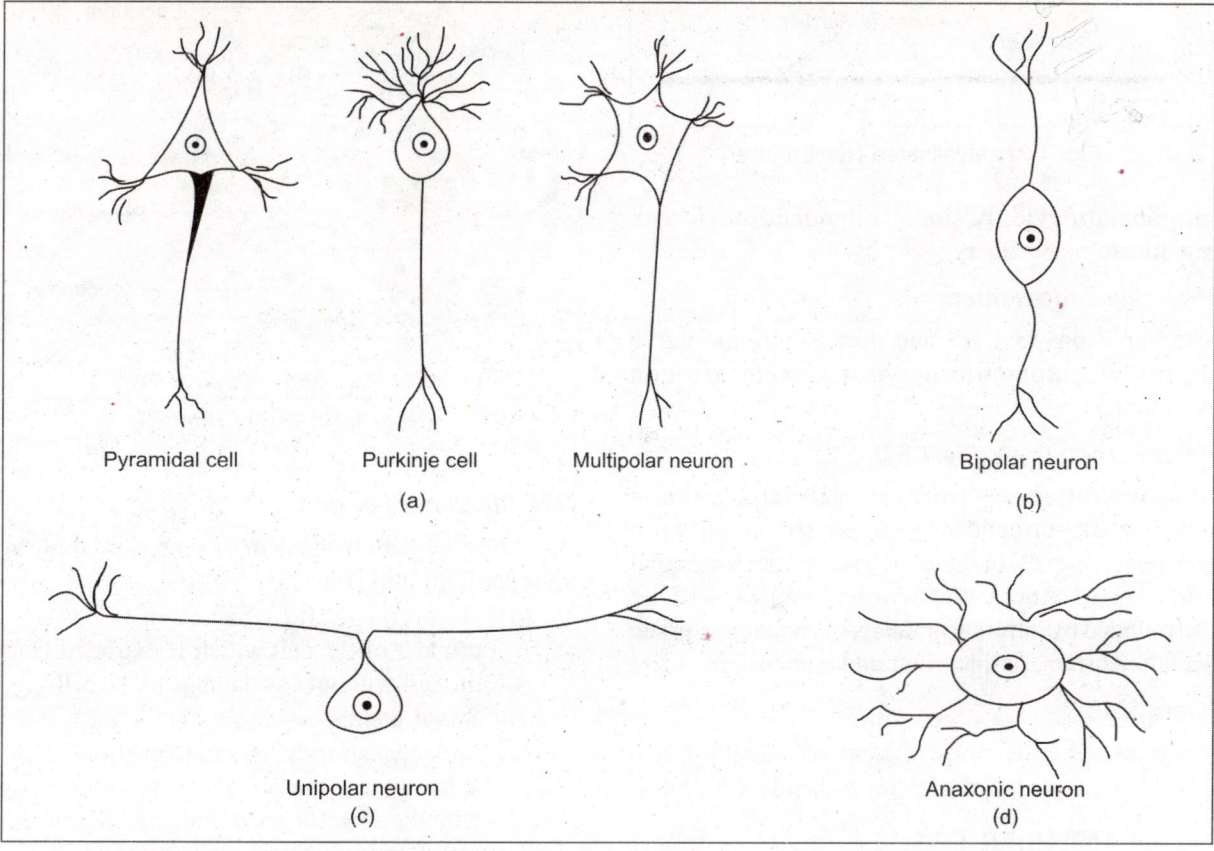

Fig. 1.30: (a) Multipolar Neurons (b) Bipolar Neuron (c) Unipolar Neuron (d) Anaxonic Neuron

1. *Astrocytes.* Small cells with numerous branching processes in all directions. They form supporting frame work for cells and fibres.
2. *Oligodendrocytes.* Smaller cells with fewer delicate processes. They form the myelin sheath for nerve fibres of CNS.
3. *Schwann cells.* They form myelin sheath for peripheral nerves.
4. *Microglia.* Smallest of the group. They are inactive in normal healthy condition. In degenerative or inflammatory conditions, they become active, migrate to the site of lesion and become phagocytic.
5. *Ependymal cells.* They line the cavities of brain and central canal of spinal cord.

Nerve fibre

Nerve fibres are formed by axons. Bundles of axons in CNS form nerve tracts. In peripheral nervous system (PNS), they form nerves.

Myelinated nerve fibre (Fig 1.31)

Nerve fibres are ensheathed by myelin sheath. Myelin sheath is formed by Schwann cells in PNS. Schwann sheath is a discontinuous sheath seen as adjacent segments, separated by nodes of Ranveir.

Myelin formation

In peripheral nerve, the schwann cells surround (encircle) the axon so that its cell membrane forms several layers around the axon. Most of the cytoplasm is squeezed to the outer layer and also the nucleus. In CNS, myelin formation is formed by

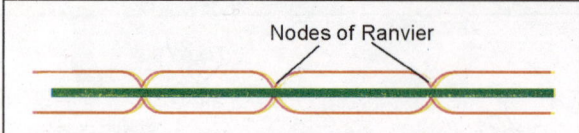

Fig. 1.31: Myelinated Nerve Fibre

oligodendrocyte. A single oligodendrocyte can myelinate many fibers.

Non myelinated fibers

Shorter axons of CNS and post ganglionic nerve fibers of autonomic nervous system are non myelinated.

Peripheral nerves (Fig.1.32)

Bundles of nerve fibres- myelinated or non myelinated, surrounded by connective tissue form peripheral nerves. In them each nerve fibre and small bundles of fibers and whole bundles will be surrounded by different amounts of connective tissue - endoneurium, perineurium and epineurium.

Ganglia

Ganglia are collections of neurons outside CNS. Nuclei are collections of neurons inside the CNS.

8. GLANDULAR TISSUE

Certain cells of the body manufacture specific substances and pour them out as secretions which are to be used elsewhere in the body. Such cells constitute glands. Glands are modified tissues derived from epithelia.

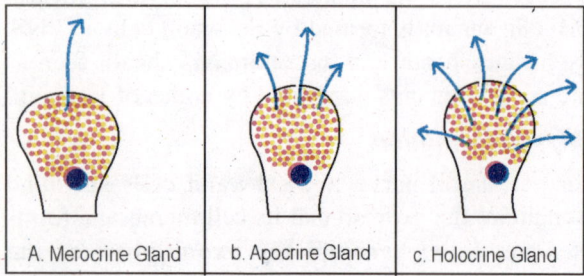

A. Merocrine Gland   b. Apocrine Gland   c. Holocrine Gland

Fig. 1.33

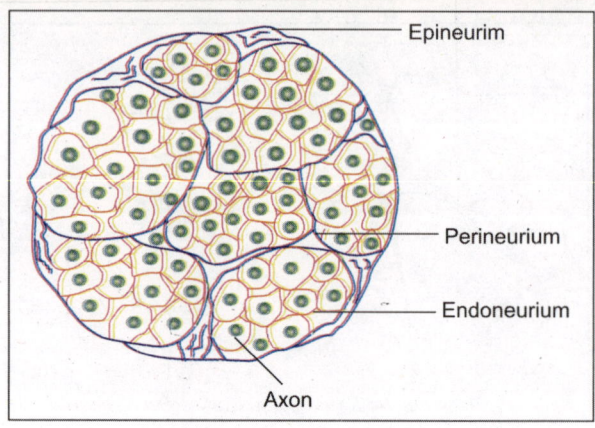

Fig. 1.32: C.S of Nerve

Classification of glands

I. Based on the mechanism of secretion, they are classified into (Fig. 1.33)

   (a) *Merocrine glands.* Secretion is merely a product of the cell which is extruded from the cell,without any damage to the cell. *e.g.,* Sweat glands

   (b) *Apocrine glands.* A small portion of the apical part of the cell also is released along with the secretory material. *e.g.,* Mammary gland, modified sweat glands of axilla and circum anal region.

   (c) *Holocrine glands.* Cells get filled with secretory products, then they disintegrate and whole content is extruded as secretion. *e.g.,* Sebaceous glands.

II. Based on the nature of secretion, glands are classified into:

   (a) *Mucous glands.* Produce thick viscous secretion. *e.g.,* Goblet cells, Glands of palate, pharynx sublingual glands.

   (b) *Serous glands.* Produce thin watery secretion. *e.g.,* Parotid, Pancreas.

   (c) *Mixed glands.* Produce both types of secretion. *e.g.,* submandibular salivary gland.

III. Based on the mode of transfer of secretion, glands are classified into: (Fig 1.34)

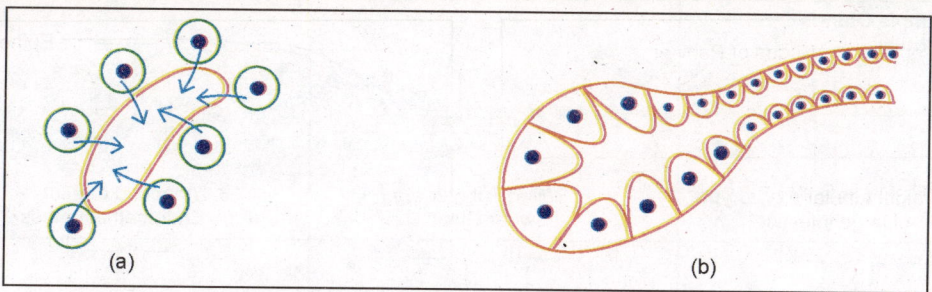

Fig. 1.34: (a) Endocrine Gland (b) Exocrine Gland

(a) Endocrine glands (ductless glands): They pour the secretion directly into blood stream. *e.g.,* Thyroid, Pituitary.

(b) Exocrine glands- Generally they do have ducts, to convey the secretion to the epithelial surface. So exocrine glands have a secretory part and conducting part or ducts.

Secretory part is lined by some modified columnar cells- as cylindrical or pyramidal cells. Ducts lined by cuboidal or columnar or stratified type.

Exocrine glands which have ducts are subdivided according to their duct system into- (Fig1.35)

I. **Simple glands:** The secretory part opens into an unbranched duct.

II. **Compound glands:** Have a branched duct system.

Based on the shape and form of the secretory part they are further classified as follows:

Simple

(a) Tubular- Secretory part is tubular

  1. Simple straight tubular. *e.g.,* Crypts of Leiberkuhn.

  2. Coiled tubular. *e.g.,* Sweat gland

  3. Branched tubular. *e.g.,* Endometerial glands.

(b) Alveolar or acinar- Secretory part is dilated as a sac

  1. Simple acinar. Not seen in humans but only in amphibians

  2. Branched alveolar *e.g.,* Sebaceous glands.

(c) Tubuloalveolar

Secretory part has tubular and alveolar form. *e.g.,* Brunner's glands, Oesophageal glands.

Compound Glands

(a) Compound tubular- *e.g.,* Kidney, Testes

(b) Compound tubuloalveolar. *e.g.,* Parotid, Pancreas

(c) Compound alveolar- *e.g.,* Mammary gland

SKIN

Skin is not purely a sensory organ, because it has other important functions also. It covers the body, involved in regulation of body temperature, has limited excretory and absorptive functions. As it contains many sensory nerve endings, it is an organ of general sensation.

Skin consists of a deeper larger part of vascular connective tissue – dermis covered by an outer avascular epithelium, epidermis. Epidermis is thicker in thick skin as in palm, sole etc and thin in thin skin, elsewhere in the body.

Structure

Thick skin (Fig. 1.36)

Epidermis is made of stratified squamous epithelium that has different layers.

Basal layer (stratum basale or germinative layer). Formed of columnar cells. Here cells undergo

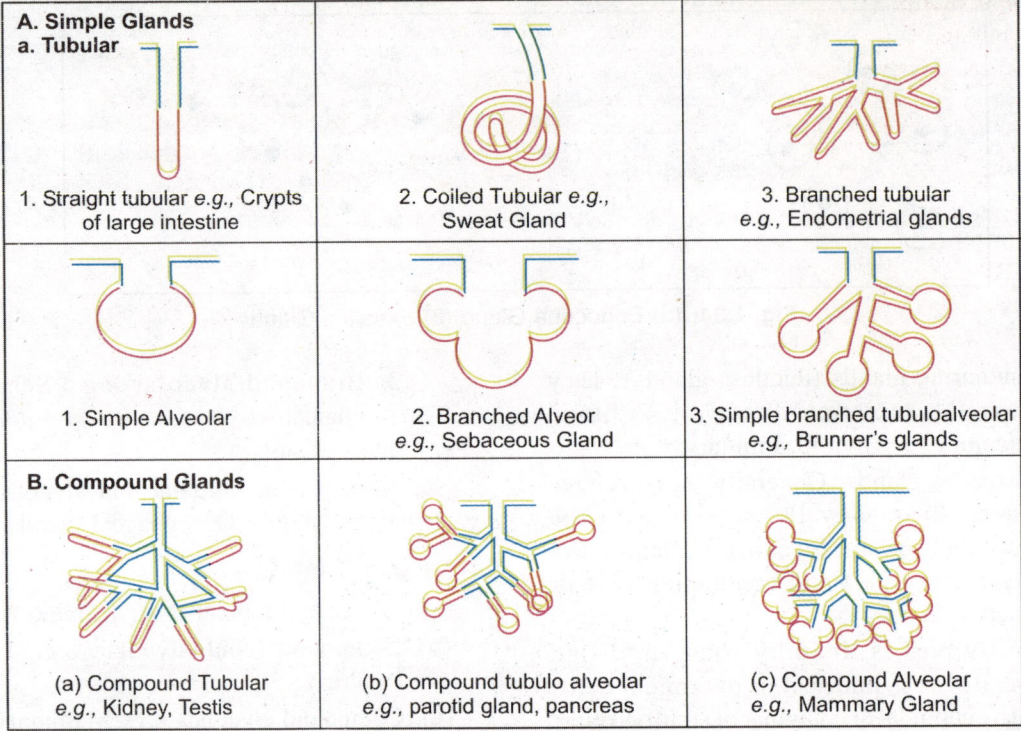

A. Simple Glands
a. Tubular

1. Straight tubular *e.g.,* Crypts of large intestine

2. Coiled Tubular *e.g.,* Sweat Gland

3. Branched tubular *e.g.,* Endometrial glands

1. Simple Alveolar

2. Branched Alveor *e.g.,* Sebaceous Gland

3. Simple branched tubuloalveolar *e.g.,* Brunner's glands

B. Compound Glands

(a) Compound Tubular *e.g.,* Kidney, Testis

(b) Compound tubulo alveolar *e.g.,* parotid gland, pancreas

(c) Compound Alveolar *e.g.,* Mammary Gland

Fig. 1.35: Classification of Exocrine Glands

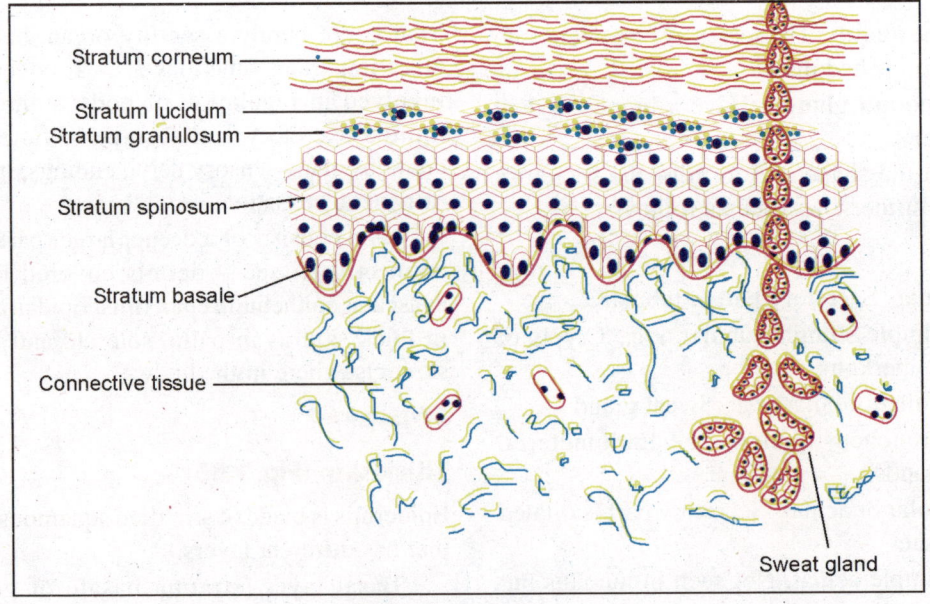

Stratum corneum

Stratum lucidum
Stratum granulosum

Stratum spinosum

Stratum basale

Connective tissue

Sweat gland

Fig. 1.36: Thick Skin

mitotic division and contain melanin and other pigment granules that give colour to the skin.

Next is stratum spinosum or prickle cell layer made of several layers of polyhedral cells. There are desmosomes or tight junctions among the cells of this layer, which give a thorny or spinous appearance to the layer.

Outer to this, there is the stratum granulosum formed of 2 or 3 layers of fusiform cells with plenty of keratohyaline granules.

Next is the clear stratum lucidum that contains traces of dying cells.

Outermost is the stratum corneum which contains several layers of horny dead epithilial cells with no traces of cytoplasm and nuclei, but keratin.

Dermis: Formed by felted connective tissue, contains blood vessels, nerves, lymphatics and sweat glands. Its deeper part is called reticular layer, where strong interlacing bands of collagen fibre predominate and a few elastic fibres. Here the glands are situated.

Superficial part of dermis is called papillary layer containing collagen and elastic fibres. Papillary layer shows projections called papillae into the epidermis. They contain capillaries and terminal nerve capsules for sensation- Tactile (Meissner's) corpscles, Crause's end bulbs, Ruffini end organs etc.

Hair, nail, sweat glands and sebaceous glands are appendages of skin.

Thin skin (Fig 1.37)

Epidermis is thin and the keratin also is less. From the surface of epidermis, invaginations go into the dermis- Hair follicles, in an oblique direction. Hair follicles lodge the roots of hairs, which end at the bottom of the follicle as hair bulb.

Thin bundles of involuntary (smooth) muscle fibres are connected to the hair follicle, on its slanding side. The muscle is called arrectores pilorum (arrector pile) and originates from the superficial layer of dermis. Contraction of arrector pili muscle causes appearance of 'goose skin' on exposure to cold and in emotional reactions. The muscle is supplied by sympathetic nerves.

Sebaceous glands are holocrine glands and are situated between the arrector pili and hair follicle. Their ducts open into the hair follicle. Contraction of arrector pili muscle helps to squeeze the secretion of the glands through ducts into hair follicle. Action of the sebaceous glands is controlled by hormones and not nerves.

Sweat glands are simple coiled tubular glands, situated deep in the dermis. Their ducts traverse the dermis and epidermis and open into the surface of skin. They are merocrine by nature of secretion and supplied by sympathetic nerve fibres.

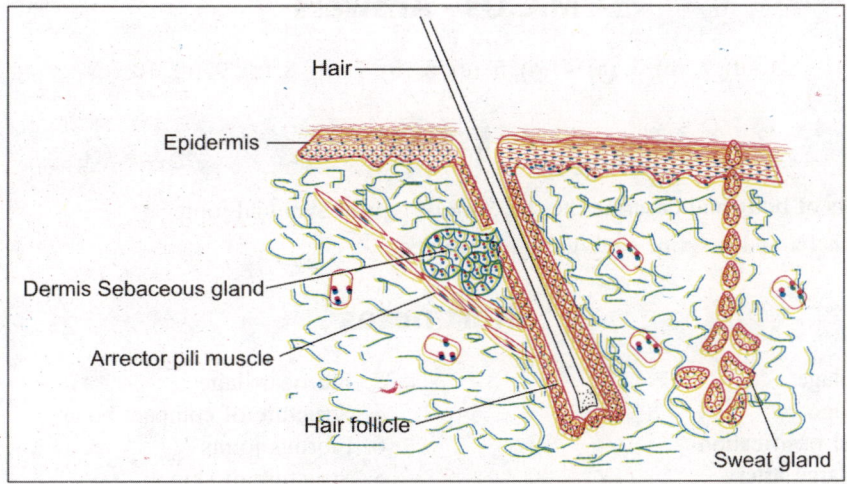

Fig. 1.37: Thin Skin

Single Best Response M.C.Qs

1. Source of energy in a cell is
   (a) Ribosomes
   (b) Lysosomes
   (c) Golgi apparatus
   (d) Mitochondria

2. Site of protein synthesis in a cell is
   (a) Lyosomes
   (b) Ribosomes
   (c) Mitochondria
   (d) Golgi apparatus

3. Striated border of absorptive epithelial cells is due to
   (a) Microvilli
   (b) Cilia
   (c) Flagella
   (d) Glycocalyx

4. Simple squamous epithelium is seen in
   (a) Alveoli of lungs
   (b) Inner lining of stomach
   (c) Inner lining of urinary bladder
   (d) Inner lining of Trachea

5. Sebaceous glands belong to the type of
   (a) Endocrine gland
   (b) Merocrine gland
   (c) Holocrine gland
   (d) Apocrine gland

6. Hyaline cartilage is present in
   (a) Inter vertebral disc
   (b) Epiphyseal plate
   (c) Epiglottis
   (d) Auricle

7. Dermis of thick skin has
   (a) Arector pili muscle
   (b) Hair follicle
   (c) Sweat gland
   (d) Sebaceous gland

8. Nissl granules are found in
   (a) Neurons
   (b) Muscle cells
   (c) Cartilage cells
   (d) Bone cells

9. Wrist joint is an example of
   (a) Ball and socket joint
   (b) Pivot joint
   (c) Saddle joint
   (d) Ellipsoid joint

10. Following are erect about cardiac muscle except
    (a) It shows branching
    (b) It is striated
    (c) Nuclei are peripherally placed
    (d) Intercalated discs are present.

M.C.Qs - Answers

1. (d), 2. (b), 3. (a), 4. (a), 5. (c), 6. (b), 7. (d), 8. (a), 9. (d), 10. (c)

Essays

I. Classify joints of body and describe the structure of typical synovial joint.
II. Classify Epithelia and describe each giving examples.

Short notes

1. Hyaline cartilage
2. Fibrocartilage
3. Elastic cartilage
4. Structure of compact bone
5. Endochondral ossification
6. Fibrous joints
7. Structure of large artery
8. Structure of skin
9. Meiosis
10. Structure of cell.

2 Skeletal System

The Skeleton forms the framework of the body. It is divided into

1. Axial skeleton – formed of bones of head, neck and trunk.
2. Appendicular skeleton – formed of bones of upper and lower limbs.

Study of bones of the body is Osteology.

AXIAL SKELETON

Axial skeleton has kull, vertebral column, sternum and ribs.

SKULL

The bony framework of the head is formed of 26 bones. Skull has the cranium which has a large cavity that contains brain and the lower jaw bone, the mandible.

Cranium has a number of flat irregular bones, joined by fibrous joints, sutures. Apart from the cranial cavity, the skull has orbital cavities, nasal cavities and oral cavity.

Bones of skull (Fig. 2.1, 2.2)

1. One frontal bone – anteriorly – contains frontal air sinus.
2. 2 parietal bones - behind frontal bone and both joined by sagital suture. Coronal suture is between frontal and 2 parietal bones.
3. One occipital bone, behind parietals, the suture between occipital and parietals being lambdoid suture. Articulates below with Atlas vertebra.
4. Two temporal bones on the sides, below parietals. Articulate with head of mandible at Temporo- Mandibular Joint (TMJ).
5. 2 maxillae, on the face – contains maxillary air sinuses.
6. 2 zygomatic bones, on the prominence of cheek.
7. 2 small nasal bones.
8. 2 small lacrimal bones.
9. 2 inferior nasal conchae in the nasal cavities.
10. One sphenoid bone, at the base of the skull, contains sphenoidal air sinus.
11. 2 ethmoid bones above and behind maxilla, contain ethmoidal air sinuses.
12. One vomer on the base.
13. 2 palatine bones.
14. Three ossicles – incus, malleus, stapes – in middle ear.
15. One mandible, the lower jaw bone. Its head articulates with mandibular fossa of temporal bone.
16. One hyoid bone- a U shaped bone, does not form part of skull, but placed in front of upper part of neck.

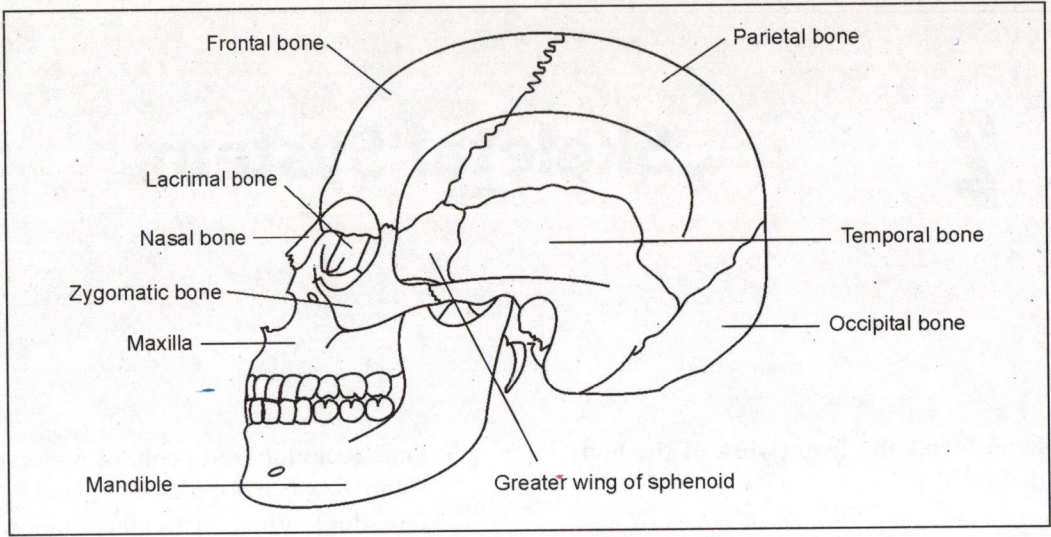

Fig. 2.1: Skull - Lateral View

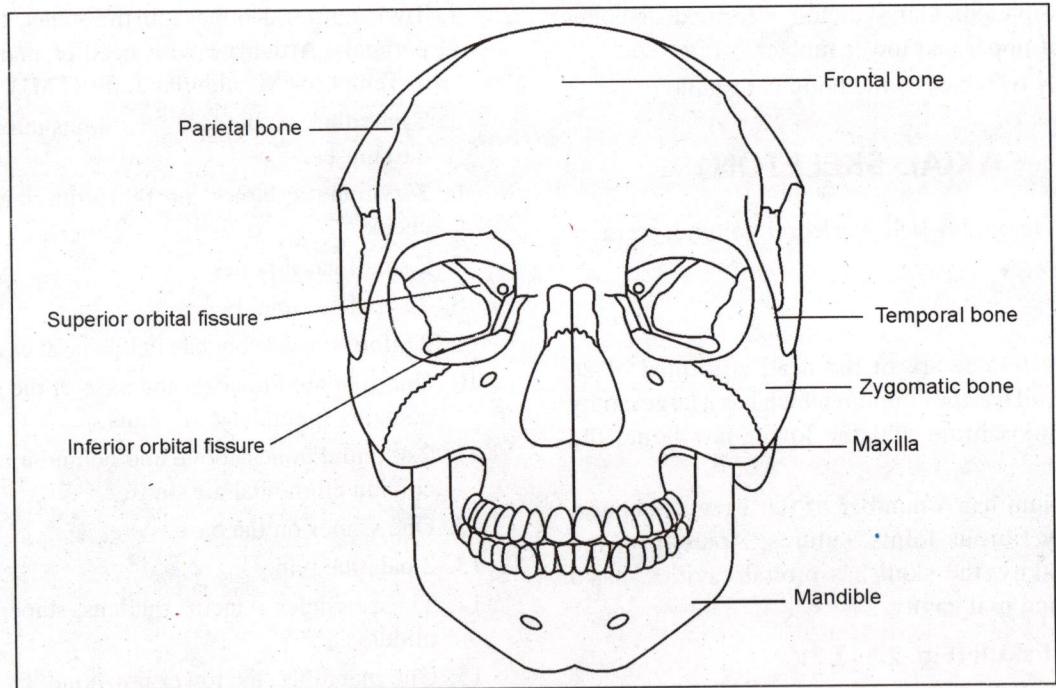

Fig. 2.2: Skull - Anterior View

Mandible (Fig. 2.3., 2.4)

The strong bone of face, forms the lower jaw. It has a 'U' shaped flat body with upper and lower borders and inner and outer surfaces. Its upper border bears alveolar sockets for teeth.

Posteriorly body projects up into the flat ramus. Angle of mandible is the junction between lower border of body and posterior border of ramus. Upper

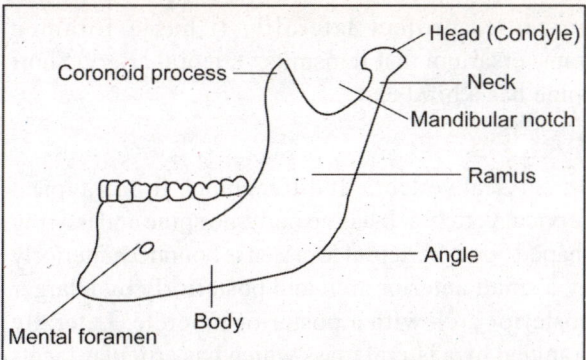

Fig. 2.3: Mandible - Lateral Surface

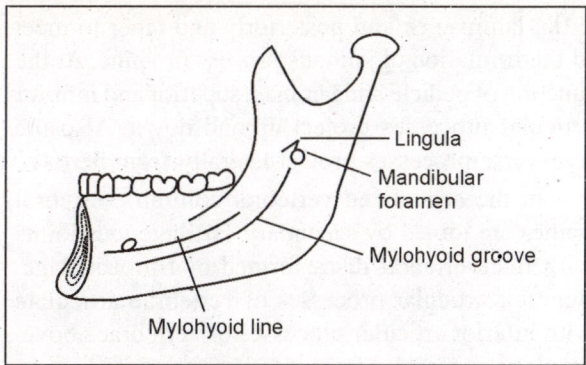

Fig. 2.4: Mandible - Medial Surface

end of ramus shows an anterior triangular process, coronoid process and a posterior process, the head or condylar process which articulates with temporal bone at TMJ (Temporo Mandibular Joint). A constricted part below the head is neck, the anterior surface of which has an impression – pterygoid fovea. Between Coronoid and condylar processes, a deep notch is seen, the mandibular notch.

Near the upper part of medial surface of ramus of mandible, mandibular foramen is seen which is guarded by a small triangular spicule of bone, lingula. Starting from the mandibular foramen, downwards on the medial surface of the body, there is a groove, mylohyoid groove in which the mylohyoid nerve and vessels run. Above and in front of it, mylohyoid line gives attachment to mylohyoid muscle. On the anterior part of the outer surface of body, mental foramen transmits the mental nerve and vessels.

In new borns, the body of mandible is seen as right and left halves, joined at symphysis menti, which later fuse to form the single body.

VERTEBRAL COLUMN

Vertebral column, the central axis of the body is formed of 7 cervical vertebrae, 12 thoracic vertebrae, 5 lumbar vertebrae, sacrum formed by fusion of 5 vertebrae, and a small coccyx formed by fusion of 4 rudimentary vertebrae, forming a total of 26 bones.

Common features of vertebrae (Fig. 2.5 and 2.6)

Vertebra has a ventral short cylindrical or oval massive part – body and a dorsal neural arch, both together enclosing the vertebral foramen. A short and thick pedicle is seen at the region where neural arch fuses with body. From the region of the pedicle,

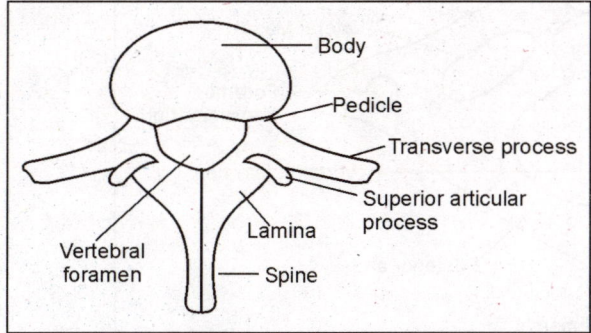

Fig. 2.5: Vertebra - Seen from above

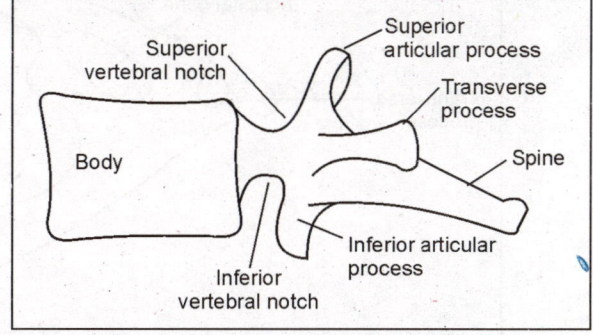

Fig. 2.6: Vertebra - Seen from side

2 flat laminae extend posteriorly and taper to meet in the formation of spinous process or spine. At the junction of pedicle and laminae, superior and inferior articular processes project up and down. Also the transverse processes project laterally from here.

In the articulated vertebral column, vertebral bodies are joined by secondary cartilagenous joints with intervertebral discs formed of fibrocartilage. Superior articular processes of vertebrae articulate with inferior articular processes of vertebrae above, by plane synovial joints.

Above and below the pedicles, there are superior and inferior vertebral notches, which when articulated, forms intervertebral foramen.

In the vertebral column, the vertebral foramina together form the vertebral canal that lodges the spinal cord and its meninges. Through intervertebral foramina, spinal nerves come out.

Gross features of vertebrae vary in different regions.

Cervical vertebrae

Of the 7 vertebrae of the cervical region, first and second vertebrae, C_1 and C_2 (Atlas and Axis) vary much from typical cervical vertebra. C_7 also shows some variations. Others are typical cervical vertebrae.

Body of a typical cervical vertebra is smaller than that in other regions. (Fig. 2.7). Short transverse processes project laterally. It has a foramen transversarium that transmits vertebral artery. Short spine has a bifid end.

Atlas (Fig. 2.8)

1st cervical vertebra. It differs much from a typical cervical vertebra. It has no body, no spine and is a ring shaped bone. Vertebral foramen is bounded anteriorly by a small anterior arch and posteriorly by a larger posterior arch with a posterior tubercle. Laterally bounded by a lateral mass which has articular facets above and below for occipital bone and C_2 vertebra. Prominent transverse process projects laterally from the lateral mass and has foramen transversarium. Anterior arch has a facet on its inner surface for articulation with the dens of C_2.

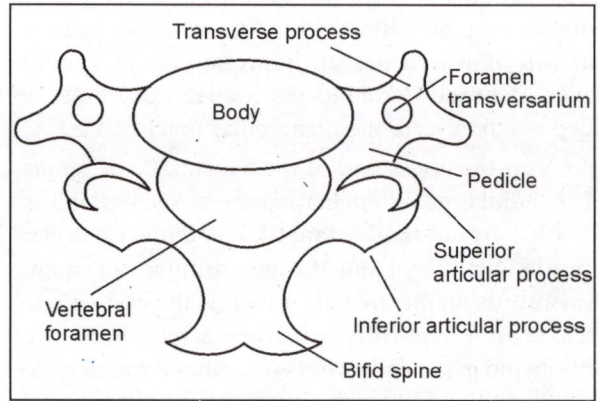

Fig. 2.7: Typical Cervical Vertebra - Seen from above

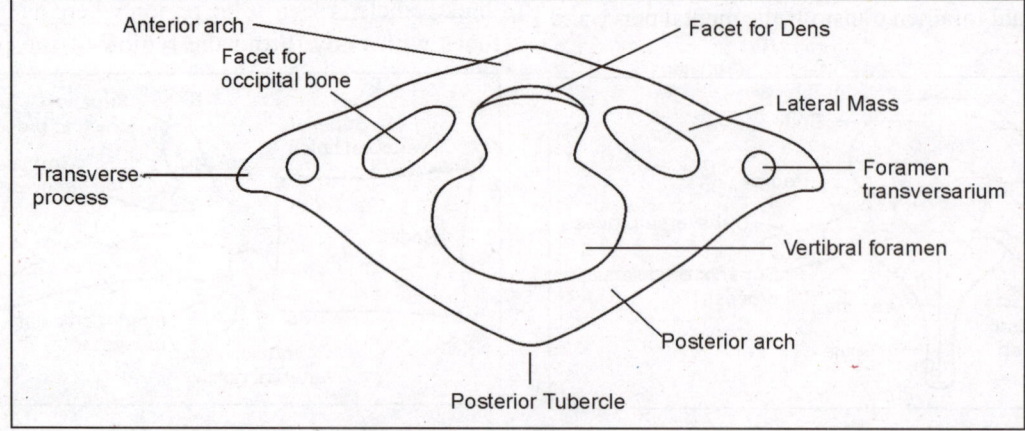

Fig. 2.8: Atlas Vartebra - C1

Axis (Fig. 2.9)

2nd cervical vertebra. It has a body as any other vertebra. From the upper surface of the body, a short strong process projects upwards - dens or odontoid process. It is about 1.5 cm long. To its apex, is attached apical ligament and to the sides two alar ligaments. It articulates with the facet on the anterior arch of atlas forming a pivot type of synovial joint. It represents the body of atlas, which has fused with the body of axis. C_2 has thick laminae and large spine with bifid tip.

3rd to 6th cervical vertebrae have features of typical cervical vertebrae.

7th cervical vertebra C₇ (Fig. 2.10)

Also called vertebra prominens. It has a long horizontal spine which ends in a tubercle which is not bifid. Its foramen transversarium transmits vertebral veins, but not artery.

Thoracic vertebrae (Fig. 2.11)

They are 12 in number

Size of vertebral bodies gradually increase from above downwards and they are cylindrical. Ribs articulate with the bodies and transverse processes of thoracic vertebrae and so have facets for these. Two demi facets near the upper and lower borders of body and a single facet on transverse process are seen. Transverse processes are long and directed posterolaterally. Laminae are short and thick. Spinous process is long and slands downwards. Vertebral foramen is circular.

1st, 9th, 10th, 11th and 12th thoracic vertebrae have some atypical features than typical thoracic vertebra.

T_1 vertebra has a circular upper costal facet on the side of its body to articulate with 1st rib. Its lower demifacet on the side of the body is smaller than other vertebrae. Its spine is longer and horizontal.

T_9 usually has only upper facet on the side of the body. T_{10} and T_{11} have only single circular facet on the side of the body. They don't have facets on the transverse processes.

T_{12} has single circular facet on the middle of the side of body. Its transverse process is short and thick and has a larger body. Similates more a lumbar vertebra.

Lumbar vertebrae (Fig 2.12)

5 in number. Larger than other vertebrae. Body is larger and its tranverse diameter is more (width). They don't bear costal facets. Pedicles are short and spines, thick and quadrangular. Superior articular process faces posteromedially and has a rough mamillary process on its posterior border. Inferior articular process faces anterolaterally. Transverse process is thin and has a small accessory process

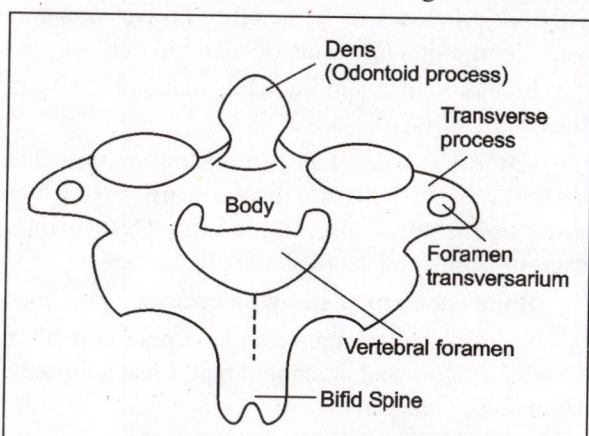

Fig. 2.9: Axis Vertebra - C2

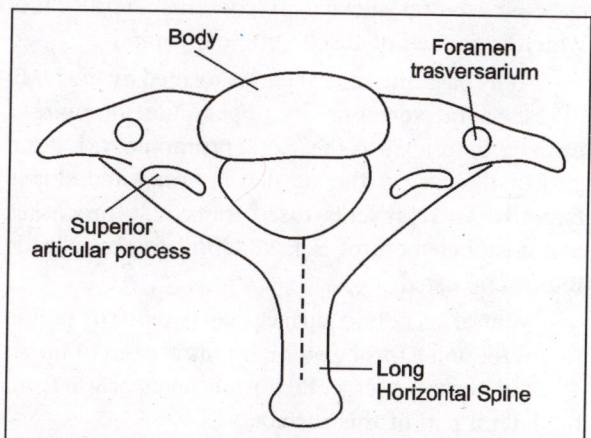

Fig. 2.10: C7 - Vertebra (Vertebra Prominens)

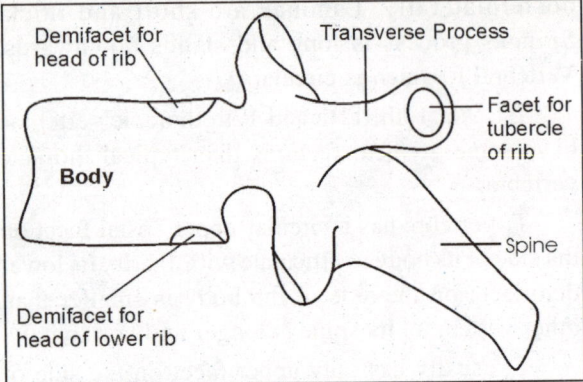

Fig. 2.11: Thoracic Vertebra

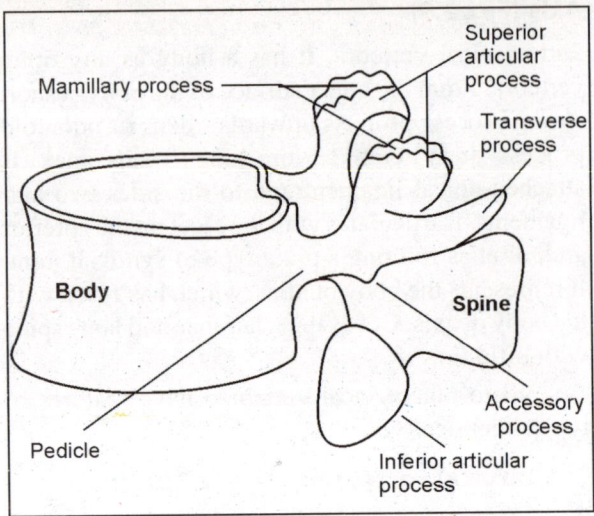

Fig. 2.12: Lumbar Vertebra

near its root on the inferior surface. Vertebral foramen is triangular.

5th lumbar vertebra has the largest body which is deeper in front, to contribute to the lumbosacral angle. It has a prominent and massive transverse process.

Sacrum (Fig. 2.13a & b)

A triangular bone, formed by fusion of 5 vertebrae, forms the posterior wall of bony pelvis. It articulates above at its base with L_5 vertebra, forming lumbosacral angle. Below its blunt apex articulates with coccyx. On its lateral surface, the auricular area articulates with the ilium of hip bone to form sacroiliac joint. It has a convex dorsal surface and a concave ventral surface. It contains sacral canal which is formed of fused vertebral foramina.

At its base, the central part is formed by the body of 1st sacral vertebra. Its upper anterior margin projects anteriorly as the sacral promontory. Lateral part of the base is the ala that is broad and slopes laterally. (It represents fused transverse processes and costal element of S_1). Vertebral foramen leads into sacral canal.

Ventral or pelvic surface has 4 pairs of pelvic sacral foramina through which ventral rami of upper 4 sacral nerves emerge. Piriformis takes origin from the lateral part of this surface.

Dorsal surface is rough due to the presence of a median sacral crest, intermediate and lateral sacral

crests. Median crest formed by fused spinous processes, intermediate crest, by fusion of articular processes and lateral crest by fusion of transverse processes of sacral vertebrae. Between the lateral and intermediate crests, 4 pairs of dorsal sacral foramina transmit dorsal rami of sacral spinal nerves. Lower end of the dorsal surface has an arched opening, sacral hiatus, continous with the sacral canal. It transmits ventral rami of 5th sacral nerve and coccygeal nerve and filum terminale. Inferior articular processes of S_5 vertebra project down as sacral cornu on either side of sacral hiatus.

Erector spinae and multifidus take origin from the dorsal surface.

Lateral surface has the auricular area that articulates with ilium. Remaining part gives attachment to strong ligaments - Sacroiliac, sacrotuberous and sacrospinous ligaments.

Blunt apex articulates with coccyx.

Sacral canal contains cauda equina and filum terminale. Dura and arachnoid mater reach upto the level of S_2 vertebra.

Coccyx (Fig. 2.14)

A small triangular bone, formed by fusion of 3–4

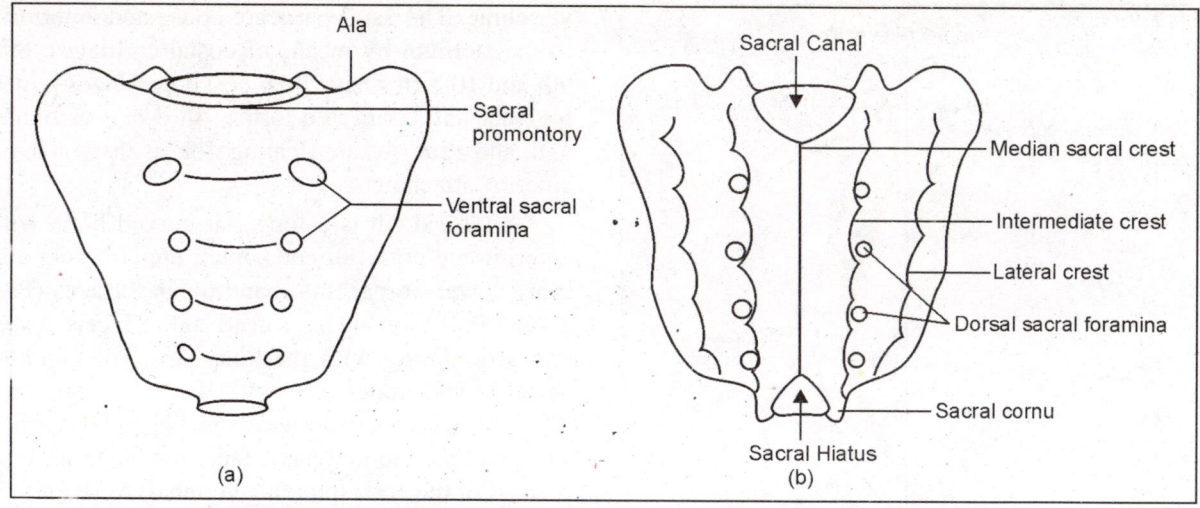

Fig. 2.13: (a) Sacrum - Ventral Surface (b) Sacrum - Dorsal Surface

rudimentary vertebrae. It descends from the apex of sacrum and curves anteriorly.

VERTEBRAL COLUMN AS A WHOLE

Function of vertebral column is to support the trunk and to protect the spinal cord. It is formed of 33 vertebral segments – 7 cervical, 12 thoracic, 5 lumbar, 5 sacral and 4 coccygeal. In male, it is 70cms long and in female, 60 cms long.

The line of gravity of vertebral column descends through dens of axis, anterior to body of T_2, centre

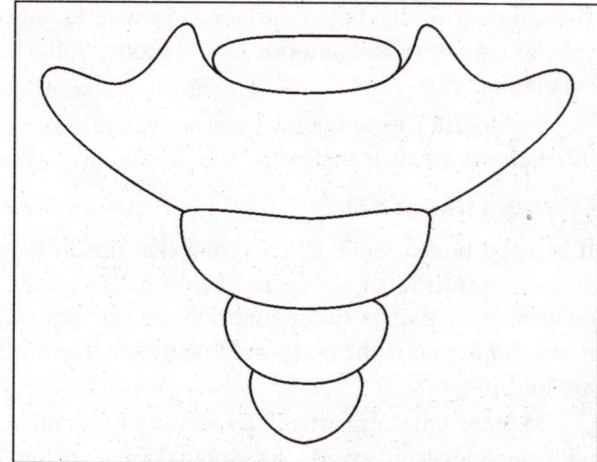

Fig. 2.14: Coccyx

of body of T_{12}, back of body of L_5, to anterior aspect of sacrum.

Curvatures (Fig. 2.15)

There are 4 curvatures in sagital plane – cervical, thoracic, lumbar and pelvic.

In adult, cervical curvature is convex forwards, extends from C_1 to T_2, maximum at level between C_4 and C_5. It is the least prominent of all curvatures.

Thoracic curvature is concave forwards, extends from T_2 to T_{12}. Most prominent at levels of T_6 to T_9. This curvature is formed due to the greater heights of posterior parts of vertebral bodies.

Lumbar curvature is convex forwards, from T_{12} to lumbosacral angle. Most prominent at L_3 level. Formed due to greater heights of anterior parts of vertebral bodies.

Pelvic curvature is concave anteriorly from lumbosacral angle to tip of coccyx, due to concavity of sacrum.

Primary curvatures appear in thoracic and pelvic regions in intrauterine life itself, by 7th to 8th weeks, when the foetus starts movements. Cervical and lumbar curvatures are secondary ones. Cervical curve becomes prominent in postnatal life when the child holds up its head (at 3rd or 4th months).

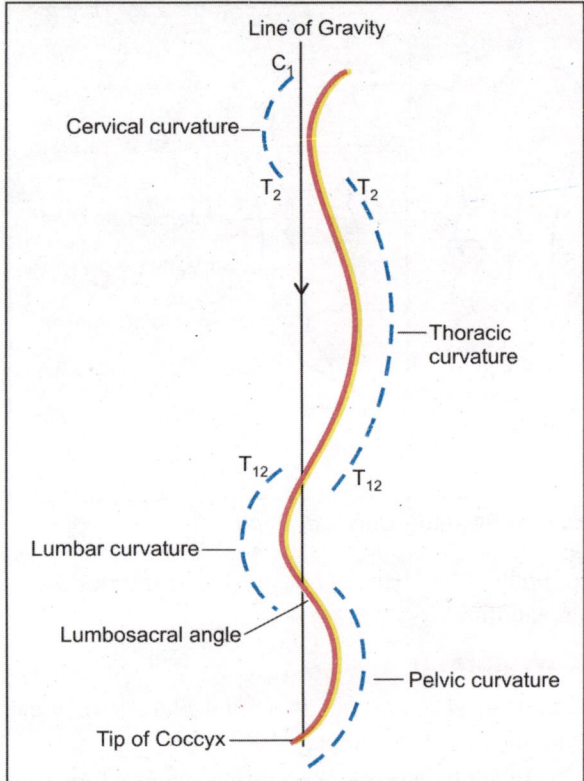

Line of Gravity

Cervical curvature

Thoracic curvature

Lumbar curvature

Lumbosacral angle

Pelvic curvature

Tip of Coccyx

Fig. 2.15: Curvatures of Vertebral Column

Lumbar curve appears when the child begins to walk. (1 to 1.5 years)

Movements

Between adjacent vertebrae, movement is minimum. But the whole vertebral column allows bending. Curvatures help to absorb stress. Effects of thrust from feet due to strong muscular activity as in running and jumping is reduced by intervertebral discs and curvatures.

BONES OF THORACIC WALL

Posteriorly formed of 12 thoracic vertebrae. Sides formed of 12 pairs of ribs and anteriorly in the midline, by the sternum.

Ribs

The 12 pairs of ribs are articulated posteriorly to the bodies and transverse processes of thoracic vertebrae. The 1st 7 pairs are connected anteriorly to the sternum by means of costal cartilages. 8th, 9th and 10th ribs have their costal cartilages joined together and connected to the 7th costal cartilage. 11th and 12th ribs are floating ribs, as they have no anterior attachments.

A typical rib is a long flat curved bone with anterior and posterior ends, blunt upper border and sharp lower border, inner and outer surfaces (Fig. 2.16a). Posterior end has a head, with 2 facets, lower one articulating with the body of corresponding vertebra and upper one, with the upper vertebra. After the head, a narrow neck and then, outer surface shows a tubercle that has a facet for the transverse process of the corresponding vertebra. Anterior to it is the flat shaft, which is bent forwards and slightly twisted. This region is the angle.

Shaft ends anteriorly joining with its cartilage. The lower sharp border has the costal groove on its inner surface, lodging the intercostal nerve and vessels. Spaces between the ribs are intercostal spaces and the borders of the ribs give attachment to intercostal muscles.

Like 11th and 12th ribs, 1st rib also is atypical in that it is short, more curved, with flat upper and lower surfaces and inner and outer borders. (Fig. 2.16 b.) Inner border has a scalene tubercle that gives insertion to scalenus anterior muscle. Behind that, on the upper surface, a groove lodges subclavian artery and anterior to it, a groove lodges subclavian vein.

2nd to 7th ribs are considered as typical ribs as others have atypical features.

Sternum (Fig. 2.17)

It is a flat bone, about 17 cms long that lies in the anterior midline of thoracic skeleton. Its upper quadrangular part is the manubrium sterni. Below it, the major part is the body and lowest small part is xiphoid process.

Manubrium sterni articulates above and laterally with clavicle on either side, by synovial joints, below that, with 1st rib by a primary cartilagenous joint.

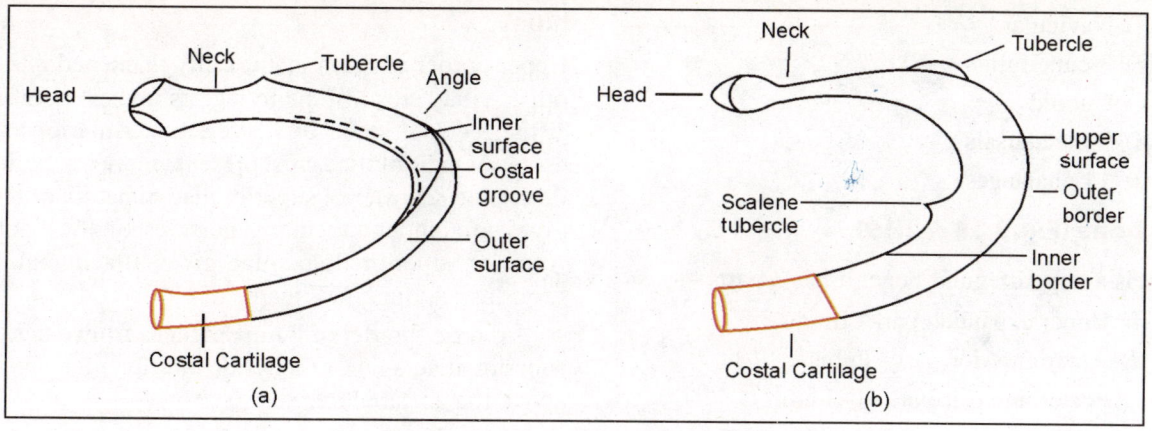

Fig. 2.16: (a) Typical Rib (b) 1st Rib

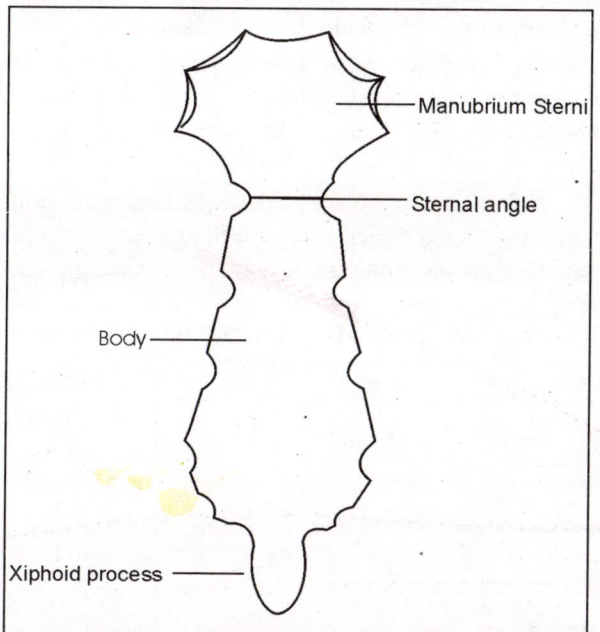

Fig. 2.17: Sternum

Lower border of manubrium joins with body at sternal angle (of Louis), which is at level with lower border of T_4 vertebra. Manubriosternal joint is secondary cartilagenous type. At this level, the lateral border articulates with 2nd costal cartilage, by synovial joint.

Body of sternum, has on its lateral border, facets for articulation with 3rd to 7th costal cartilages.

Lower end articulates with a small xiphoid process by a primary cartilagenous joint.

Thoracic inlet

This is the communication between the thorax and root of neck. Bounded posteriorly by body of T_4 vertebra, laterally by inner border of 1st rib and anteriorly by upper border of manubrium sterni.

Thoracic outlet

Lower part of thorax communicates with abdomen through thoracic outlet, bounded posteriorly by body of T_{12} vertebra, laterally by costal margin, anteriorly by xiphoid process. This is closed by diaphragm.

APPENDICULAR SKELETON

BONES OF LOWER LIMB

Total – 31 bones

　Hip bone

　Femur

　Patella

　Tibia

　Fibula

Tarsal bones

　(i) Calcaneus (Calcanium)

　(ii) Talus

(iii) Navicular

(iv) 3 cuneiforms

(v) Cuboid

(vi) 5 metatarsals

(vii) 14 phalanges

Hip bone (Fig. 2.18 & 2.19)

It is a large irregular bone. It has 3 parts –

1. Upper expanded part - Ilium

2. Anteroinferior part - Pubis

3. Posteroinferior part - Ischium

Lateral surface of the bone shows a deep cup shaped cavity, the acetabulum. The three parts of the bone are joined in the wall of acetabulum. Acetabulum forms the socket for the head of femur at hip joint.

Anteroinferior to acetabulum, hip bone has an oval or triangular opening – obturator foramen.

Hip bones of 2 sides articulate along the anterior midline at pubis to form a cartilagenous joint – pubic symphysis. The 2 hip bones also articulate posteriorly with sacrum at sacroiliac joints. These together form the pelvis.

Ilium

Upper border of ilium is markedly thickened into a ridge – iliac crest. In the living, its highest point is at the level of spine of L_4 vertebra. Anterior and posterior ends of iliac crest present anterior superior iliac spine & posterior superior iliac spine. Iliac crest gives attachment to many muscles of the back. Anterior superior iliac spine gives attachment to sartorius and inguinal ligament.

Anterior border of ilium descends from anterior superior iliac spine to anterior inferior iliac spine, above the acetabulum.

Posterior border descends from the posterior superior iliac spine to posterior border of ischium and shows a deep notch, greater sciatic notch.

The outer surface of ilium is the gluteal surface which presents 3 curved lines – posterior, anterior and inferior gluteal lines. Areas between the lines give origin to the 3 gluteal muscles.

Its inner surface has a smooth and larger anterior part – iliac fossa which gives origin to iliacus muscle and a rough and smaller posterior part – sacropelvic surface. The two parts are separated by a medial border, which descends as arcuate line. The upper

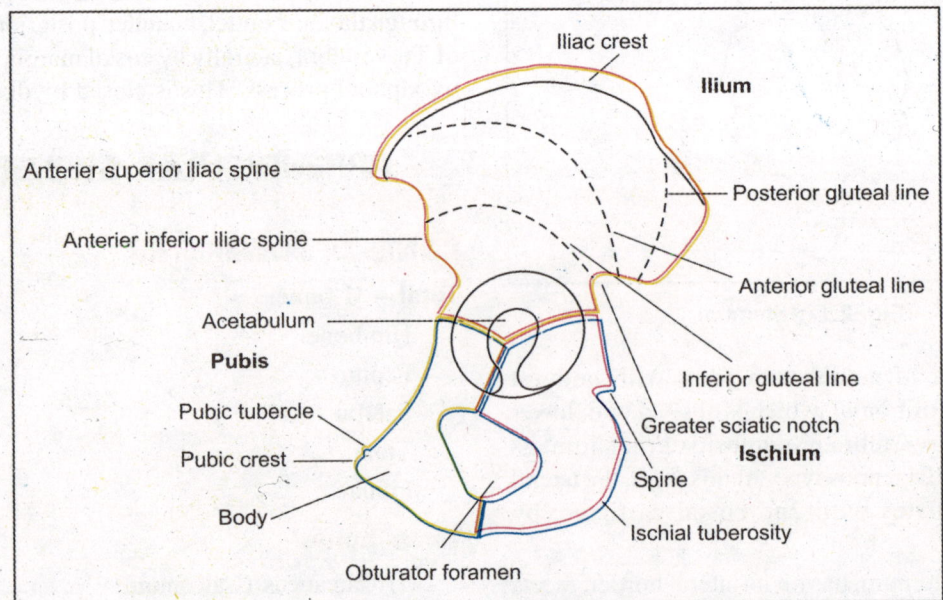

Fig. 2.18: Hip Bone - Outer Surface

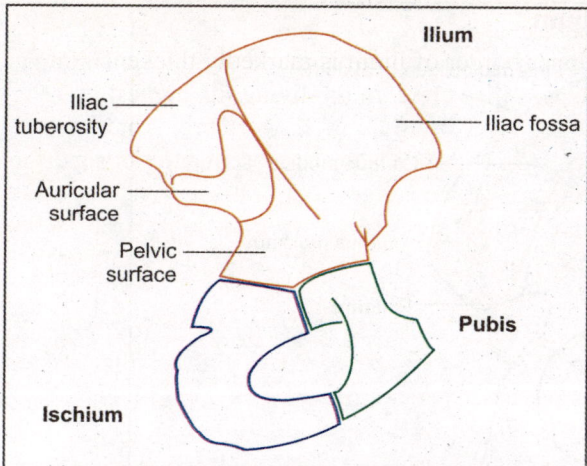

Fig. 2.19: Hip Bone - Inner Surface

part of sacropelvic surface is called iliac tuberosity where strong ligaments of sacroiliac joint are attached. Below that, is the auricular surface which articulates with sacrum. Lower part is the pelvic surface which forms part of true pelvis.

Pubis

Forms the anterior part of hip bone. It has a body, superior ramus and inferior ramus.

Body is flat with anterior, posterior and medial surfaces. Medial surface articulates with opposite pubis at pubic symphysis.

Upper border of the body is the pubic crest at the lateral end of which pubic tubercle is seen. Pubic tubercle gives attachment to the medial end of inguinal ligament.

The superior ramus springs from the upper lateral part of body, runs backwards and laterally to reach the acetabulum. It meets ilium at iliopubic eminence.

The inferior ramus springs from the lower lateral part of the body, passes backwards and laterally to unite with the ramus of ischium to form ischiopubic ramus.

Ischium

It is the lower posterior part of hip bone. Has a body and a ramus. Above, body reaches the acetabulum.

Below, the body gives off the ramus which fuses with the inferior ramus of pubis.

The dorsal surface of body has a large rough ischial tuberosity at its lower part and upper part is continuous with the gluteal surface of ilium.

Ischial tuberosity gives origin to strong muscles of back of thigh. Upper lateral part - semi membranosus, upper medial part - semitendinosus and long head of biceps, lower lateral part - adductor magnus. Lower medial part is covered by fatty tissue and a bursa. This part supports the body in sitting posture.

Posterior border of the body shows a sharp projection – ischial spine. Between ischial spine and ischial tuberosity, is the lesser sciatic notch.

Major muscle attachments to the two surfaces of hip bone are shown in the figures 2.20 & 2.21.

Pelvis (Fig. 2.22)

Composed of the 2 hip bones anteriorly and laterally and sacrum and coccyx, posteriorly. The bones articulate at the pubic symphysis, two sacroiliac joints and sacrococcygeal joint.

Pelvis has two parts

1. Upper – greater pelvis or false pelvis.
2. Lower – lesser pelvis or true pelvis.

This division is made by an oblique plane which passes from sacral promontory to upper margin of pubic symphysis. This is the plane of pelvic inlet. The margins of pelvic inlet form pelvic brim. The true pelvis contains pelvic viscera.

The inferior aperture of the pelvis is the pelvic outlet.

Diameters of pelvis

Diameters of inlet and outlet of pelvis are important in Obstetrics. Certain of them are given below.

1. Anteroposterior diameter of inlet – about 110 mm.
2. Transverse diameter of inlet – about 130 mm.
3. Oblique diameter of inlet – about 125 mm.

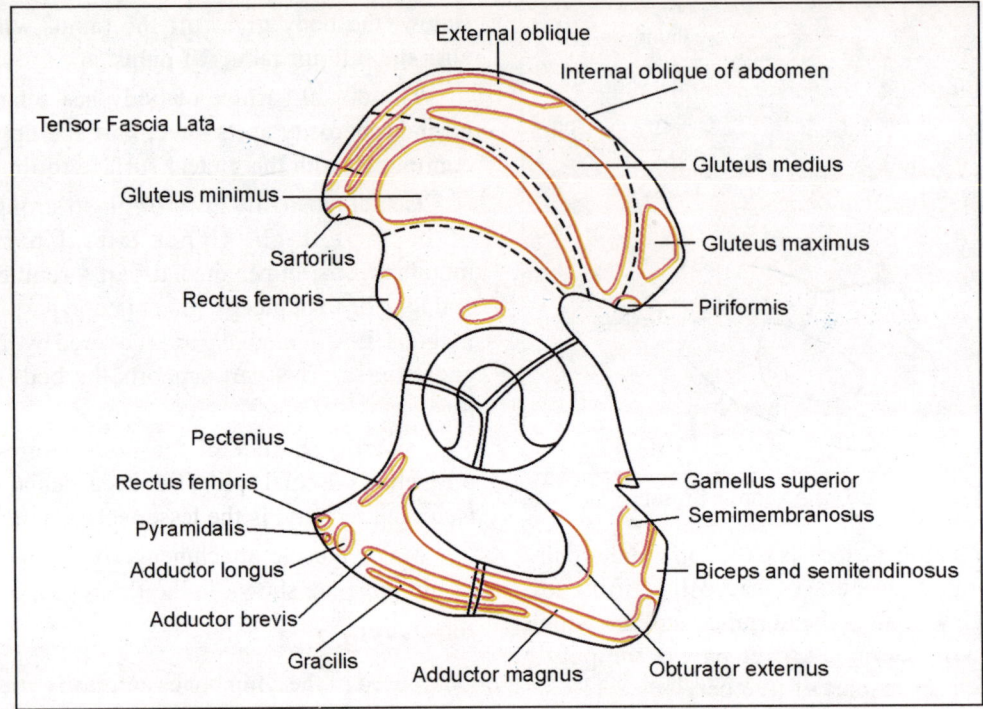

Fig. 2.20: Muscle Attachments on Outer Surface of Hip Bone

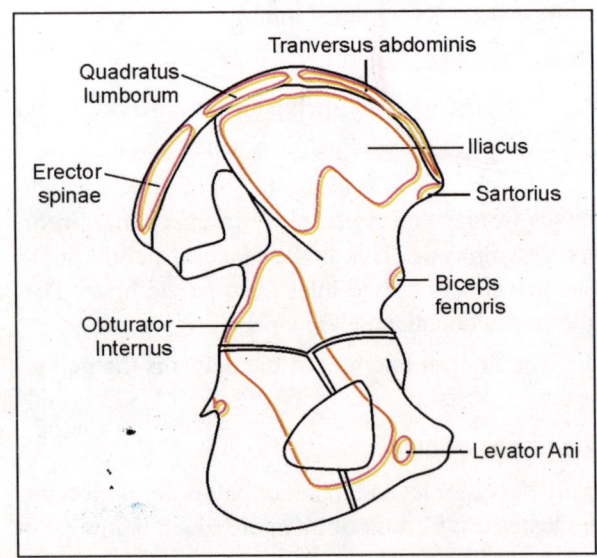

Fig. 2.21: Muscle Attachments on Inner Surface of Hip Bone

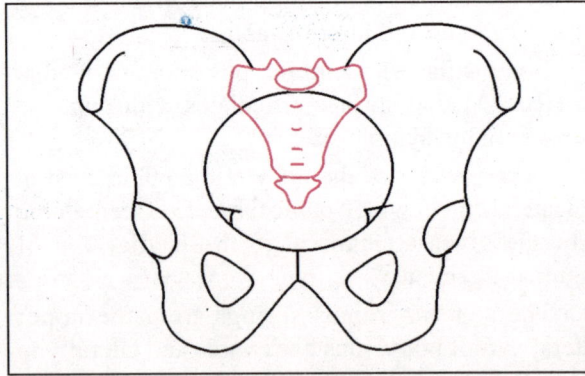

Fig. 2.22: Pelvis

4. Anteroposterior diameter of outlet – about 125 mm.

5. Transverse diameter of outlet – about 110 mm.

6. Oblique diameter of outlet – about 118 mm.

Sex differences in pelvis

1. Subpubic angle is wider in female.
2. Ischiopubic ramus is everted in male.
3. Pelvic inlet diameters are smaller in male.
4. Inlet is heart shaped in male and oval or rounded in female. (Fig. 2.23 a,b)
5. Obturator foramen is oval in male and triangular in female.
6. Greater sciatic notch is wider in female.
7. True pelvis is wide and shallow in female, deep in male.

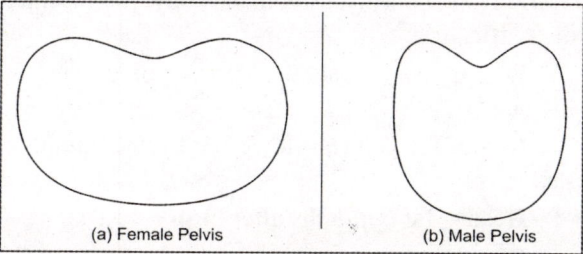

(a) Female Pelvis   (b) Male Pelvis

Fig. 2.23

FEMUR (Fig. 2.24 a, b)

The thigh bone, it is the longest and strongest bone in the body. Has an upper end, shaft and lower end.

Upper end

Upper end has head, neck, greater trochanter and lesser trochanter.

Head: Forms more than half a sphere, articulates with acetabulum to form hip joint. Near its centre head shows a small pit, fovea where the ligament of head of femur is attached.

Neck: About 5 cms long, connects head to shaft. With shaft it makes an angle of about 125°.

Greater trochanter: It is a quadrangular projection from the upper end of the shaft. Greater trochanter has a rough lateral surface, anterior surface, medial surface and an upper border which has an apex and a posterior border. Lower part of medial surface is deeper, trochanteric fossa.

Many muscles are attached to greater trochanter.

1. To lateral surface, gluteus medius.
2. To anterior surface, gluteus minimus.

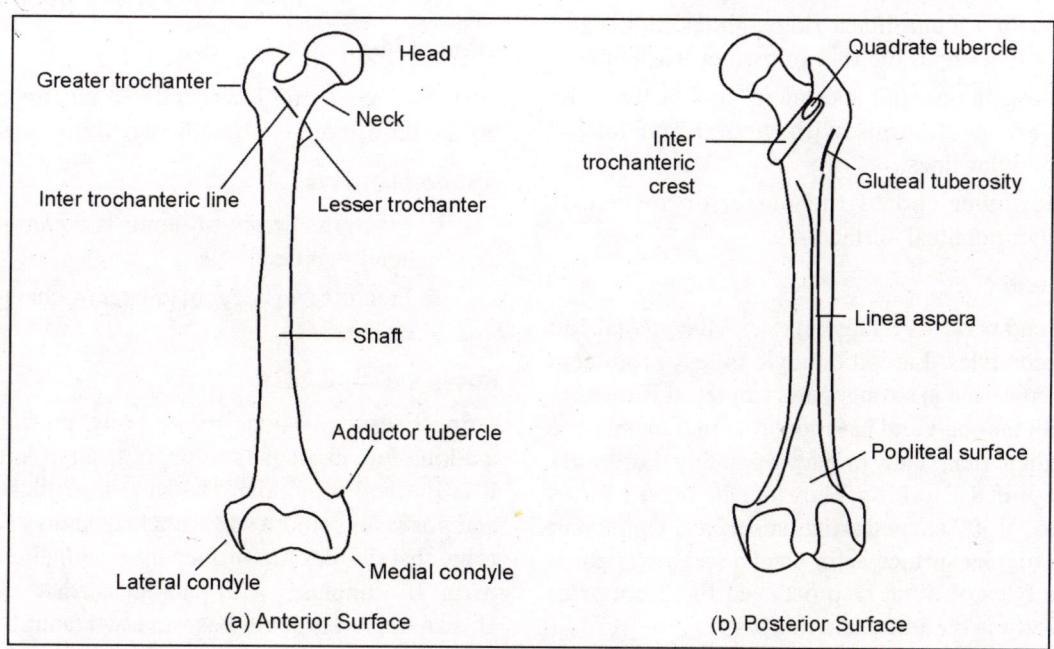

(a) Anterior Surface   (b) Posterior Surface

Fig. 2.24: Femur

3. To apex, piriformis.

4. To medial surface, obturator internus with 2 gamelli.

5. To trochanteric fossa, obturator externus.

Lesser trochanter: It is a smaller conical projection from the medial part of the upper end. Iliacus and psoas major are inserted to it.

Intertrochanteric line is a prominent sharp ridge that runs between greater and lesser trochanters on the anterior surface; where the neck meets the shaft.

Intertrochanteric crest is a rounded ridge which runs between the greater and lesser trochanters on the posterior surface, where the neck meets the shaft. Near its upper end, a quadrate tubercle is seen, to which quadratus femoris is inserted.

Shaft

It is smooth and rounded anteriorly. Posterior surface presents a prominent rough vertical ridge with medial and lateral lips - the linea aspera to which many muscles are attached. Medial lip is continuous above with a rough line, spiral line, which reaches up to the intertrochanteric line. Lateral lip is continuous above, with a rough linear ridge, gluteal tuberosity which reaches upto the root of greater trochanter.

Below, the medial and lateral lips of the linea aspera are continuous with medial and lateral supracondylar lines.

The lower end of the posterior surface is triangular, popliteal surface.

Lower end

Lower end presents 2 large masses - the medial and lateral condyles. Lateral condyle is less prominent than medial, but is stronger and stouter. It is more in line with the shaft and has more role in transmission of weight to tibia. They project separately posteriorly and are united anteriorly. They together have a broad inverted 'V' (^) shaped articular surface. Upper part of the articular surface is for patella and lower parts, for condyles of tibia. Gap between the 2 condyles posteriorly is the intercondylar fossa.

The most prominent point on the medial surface of medial condyle is medial epicondyle. Above it, the upper most part of the surface shows adductor tubercle where tendon of adductor magnus is inserted.

Most prominent point on the lateral surface of lateral condyle is lateral epicondyle. Below it, is a groove – popliteal groove from where popliteus originates.

Attachments of the muscle on femur are shown in the figures 2.25 (a) and (b)

Ossification

Second long bone to ossify in the body. Has 5 centres of ossification.

Primary centre – shaft – 7th week of intra uterine life (i.u.l)

Secondary centre – lower end – 9th month of i.u.l

Head – 1st 6 months after birth

Greater trochanter – 4th year

Lesser trochanter – 13th year

By 16th – 18th years all centres fuse.

Clinical importance

Secondary centre for lower end of femur appears just before birth. So it is of medicolegal importance.

Applied aspects

1. Fracture of neck of femur is common in old aged people.

2. Fracture can occur in greater trochanter, shaft or condyles.

Patella (Fig. 2.26)

Largest sesamoid bone in the body, present in the tendon of quadriceps femoris, in front of knee joint. It is flat and triangular. Has anterior rough surface and posterior smooth surface which shows a vertical ridge that divides the surface into medial and lateral parts. It articulates with patellar surface of femur. Has an upper border or base and two lateral borders.

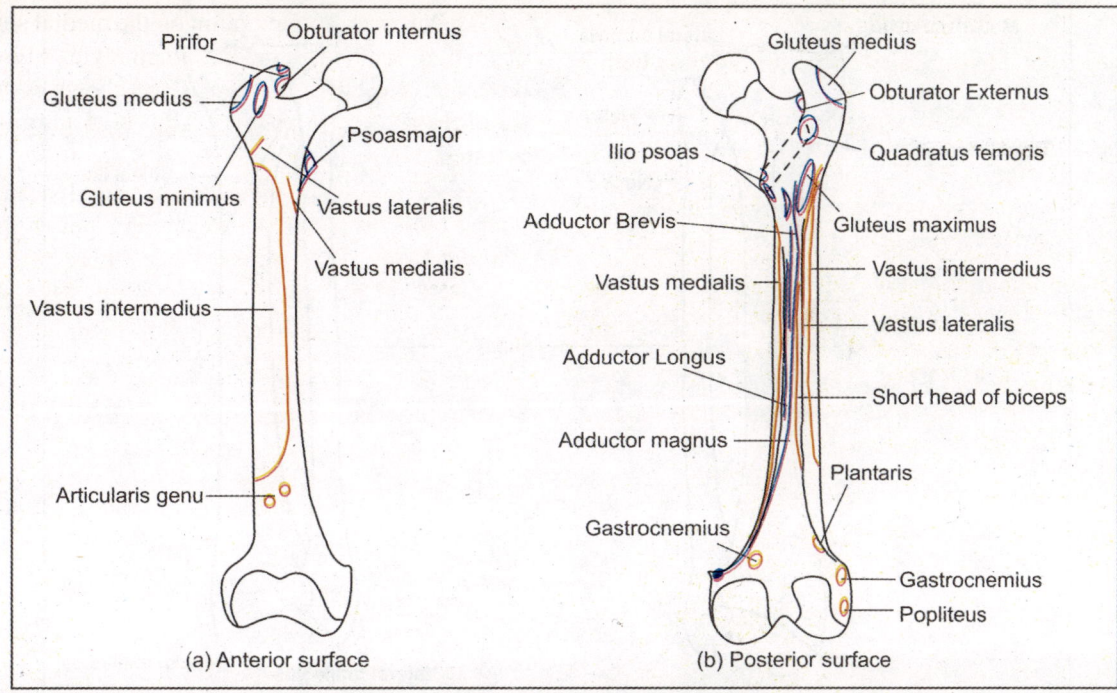

Fig. 2.25: Femur - Muscle Attachments

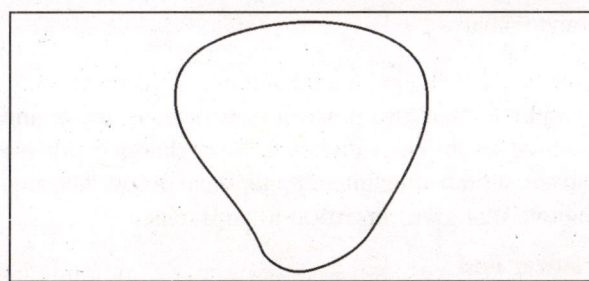

Fig. 2.26: Patella

Apex faces downwards to which ligamentum patellae is attached, which anchors it to tibial tuberosity. To the base and two lateral margins, the tendon of quadriceps femoris is attached. Anterior rough surface gives attachment to some fibers of tenden of quadriceps.

Ossification

Ossifies by several centres which appear in 3rd to 6th year.

Applied aspects

1. Dislocation of patella – usually recurrent.
2. Fracture of patella by direct injury or violent contraction of quadriceps femoris.

TIBIA

Tibia is the medial and stronger of the 2 bones of the leg. (Fig. 2.27 a and b). It has an upper end, shaft and lower end.

Upper end

It is expanded and has 2 masses – medial and lateral condyles. The upper surfaces of the condyles have articular surfaces for the condyles of femur.

Articular surface of medial condyle is larger and oval in shape. Articular surface of lateral condyle is circular in outline. The intercondylar area on the upper surface is rough and presents near its middle, medial and lateral condylar tubercles. In front of the upper end, the tibial tuberosity is seen; its upper part gives attachment to ligamentum patellae.

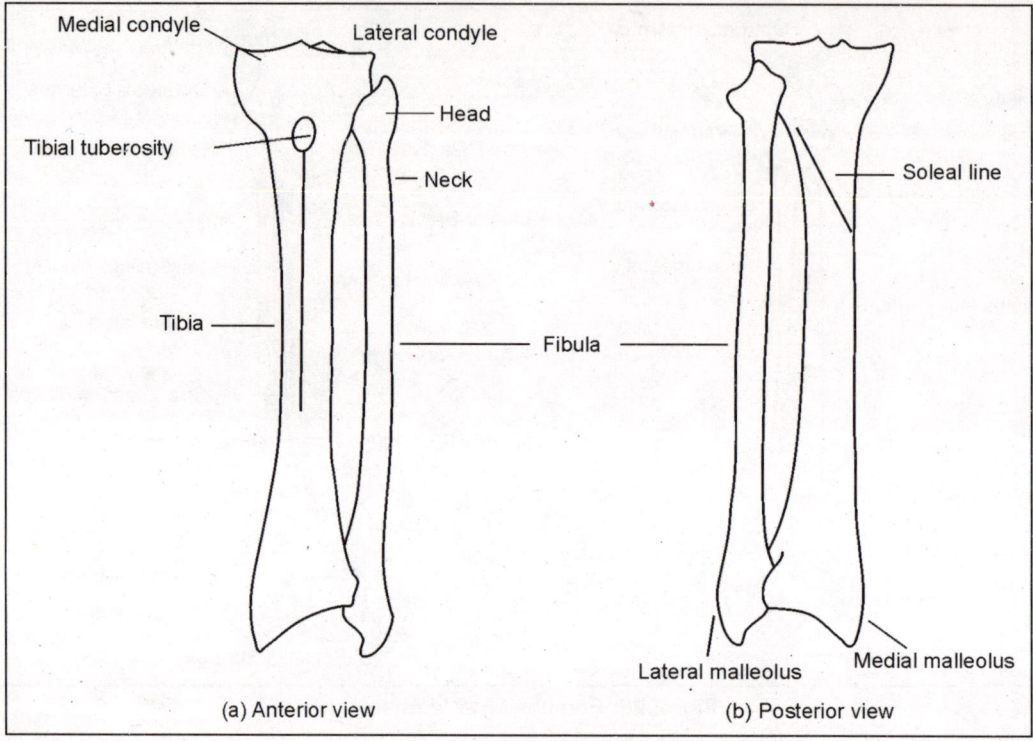

Fig. 2.27: Tibia and Fibula

Posterior surface of the medial condyle presents a rough groove for the insertion of semimembranosus.

Posterolateral part of the lateral condyle has a small circular facet for articulation with fibula.

Along the margins of the upper articular surfaces of the condyles, the medial and lateral menisci are placed. Lateral is more circular and medial one, oval. Their anterior and posterior ends are attached to the intercondylar area as shown in Figure 2.28.

Shaft

It has three surfaces and three borders so that, it is triangular on cross section. Anterior border is subcutaneous and is known as the 'shin'. Lateral border is sharp interosseous border which gives attachment to the interosseous membrane that connects it to fibula. Also it has a medial border.

Medial surface is between anterior and medial borders and is subcutaneous. Lateral surface is between anterior and interosseous borders. Posterior surface is between medial and interosseous borders. Upper end of the posterior surface is broad and shows an oblique ridge, soleal line that gives origin to soleus and attachment to popliteal fascia. The area above that gives insertion to popliteus.

Lower end

Lower end of tibia is slightly expanded and its medial part projects downwards as medial malleolus. Lower part has anterior, medial, lateral, posterior and inferior surfaces. Lateral surface shows a triangular notch to articulate with fibula. Inferior surface articulates with the body of talus. Lateral surface of medial malleolus also has a coma shaped facet to articulate with medial side of talus. Lower border of medial malleolus gives attachment to the deltoid ligament of ankle joint. Dorsum of lower end shows a deep groove for the passage of tibialis posterior tendon.

Muscle attachments are shown in (Fig. 2.29 a,b).

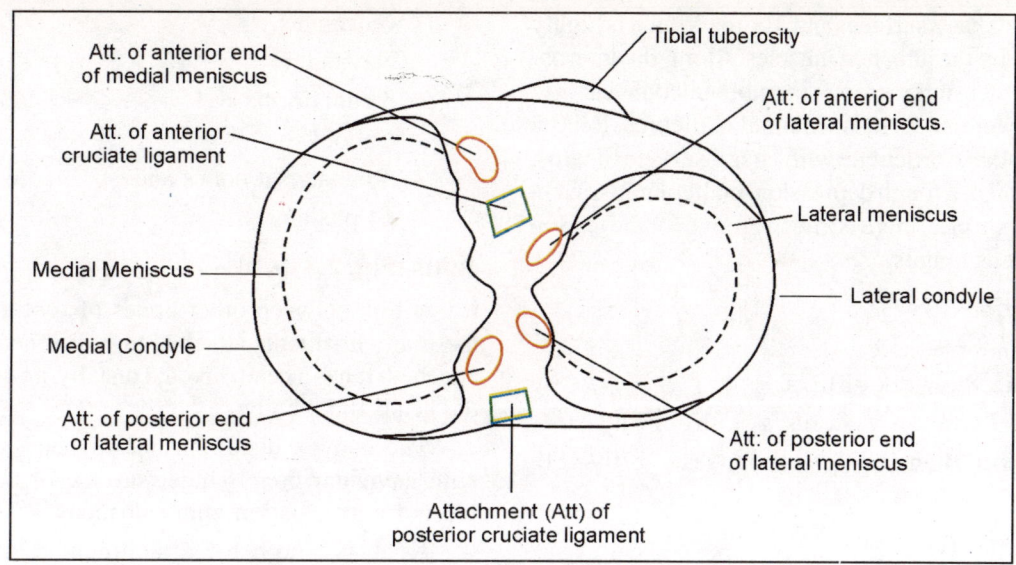

Fig. 2.28: Upper Surface of Tibial Condyles

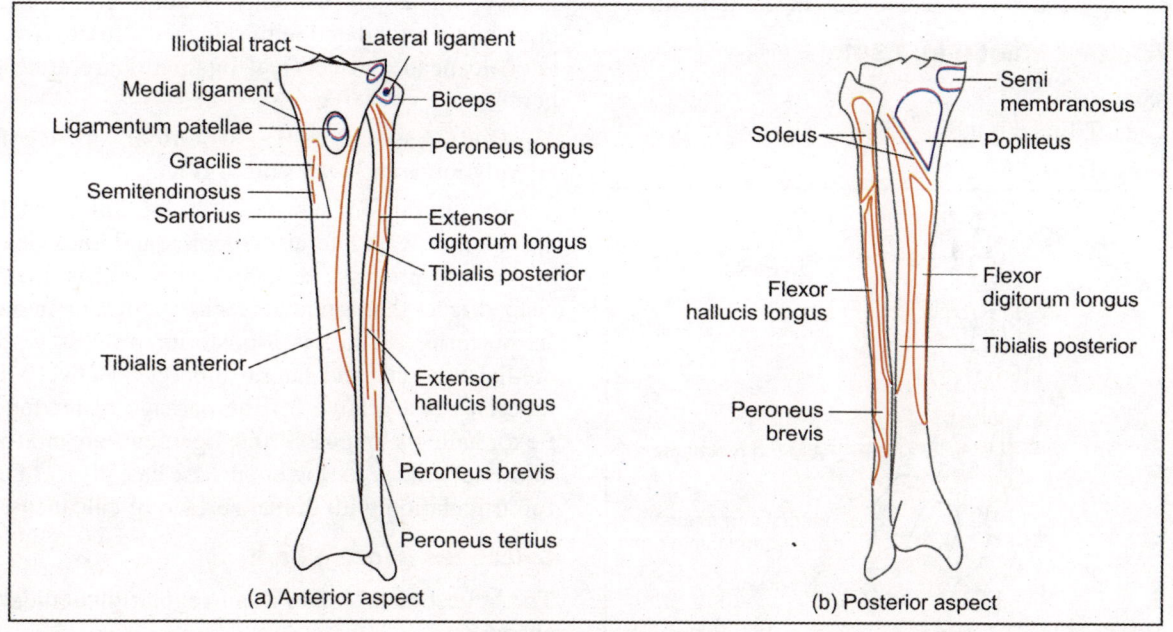

(a) Anterior aspect

(b) Posterior aspect

Fig. 2.29: Tibia and Fibula

Fibula (Fig. 2.27, 2.29)

The slender lateral bone of the leg, has an upper end or head, a shaft and a lower end which forms the lateral malleolus. Just below the head, the narrow part is called neck.

Head has a facet to articulate with lateral tibial condyle. Upper part of the head is the apex to which biceps tendon and lateral ligament of knee joint are attached.

Common peroneal nerve is closely related to the

neck. Shaft has 3 surfaces and 3 borders but it is highly moulded by the attached muscles. Along the interosseous border, interosseous membrane connects it to tibia. Lower end forms the lateral malleolus. It has a medial facet to articulate with lateral surface of talus, and behind it, a rough depression, malleolar fossa. On its dorsal surface, there is a deep groove for the tendon of peroneus longus.

Ossification

Three centres
  Shaft: 8th week of I.U.L.
  Distal end: 1st year, fuses- 15th – 17th years
  Proximal end: 3–4 years, fuses – 17th–18th years

Applied anatomy

Pott's fracture – fracture of both malleoli of lower limb, associated with dislocation of ankle joint.

Skeleton of foot (Fig. 2.30)

It comprises -
  1. 7 Tarsal bones:
    Talus

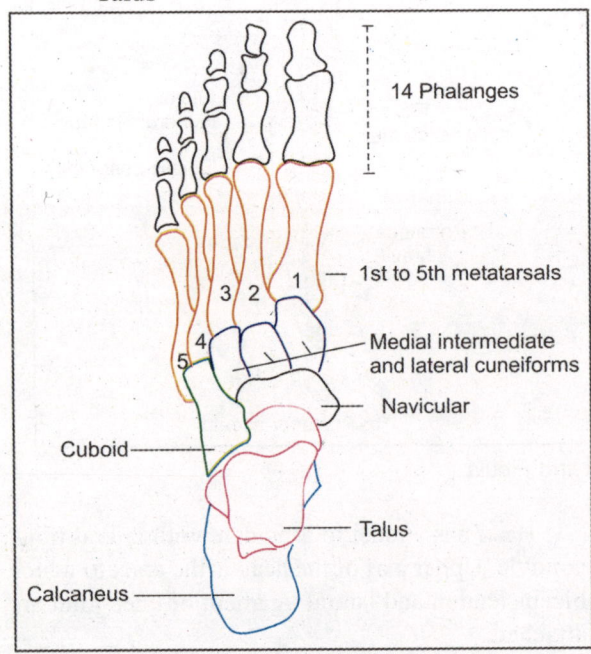

Fig. 2.30: Skeleton of Foot

Calcaneus
Navicular
3 cuneiforms
Cuboid
  2. 5 metatarsal bones and
  3. 14 phalanges.

Talus (Fig. 2.31a,b)

It is a link between other bones of foot and leg. It has many ligaments attached to it. But no muscle is attached. It has a head directed distally, a neck behind the head, and a body.

The convex distal surface of head articulates with navicular bone. Under surface of head has 2 facets for articulation with calcaneus.

Neck is rough for attachment of important ligaments. Lower surface of the neck has a deep groove, sulcus tali that helps to complete the sinus tarsi, when articulated with calcaneus. Interosseous, talocalcanean and cervical ligaments are attached here.

Body has a dorsal – trochlear surface for articulation with lower end of tibia.

Its lateral surface has a triangular facet for articulation with lateral malleolus and ends below in a lateral process. Its medial surface has a coma shaped facet that articulates with medial malleolus. Its posterior surface is a posterior process with a medial tubercle and lateral tubercle. Between the tubercles is a groove for the passage of tendon of flexor hallucis longus. Strong ligaments are attached to the tubercles. Its lower surface has an oval facet for articulation with dorsal surface of calcaneus.

Calcaneus (Fig. 2.32 a,b)

The largest tarsal bone, it is irregularly cuboidal in shape.

Upper surface: Its posterior 1/3 is rough, and slightly concave.

Middle 1/3 carries the posterior facet for body of talus.

Anterior 1/3 has one or 2 facets for head of talus – the middle and anterior.

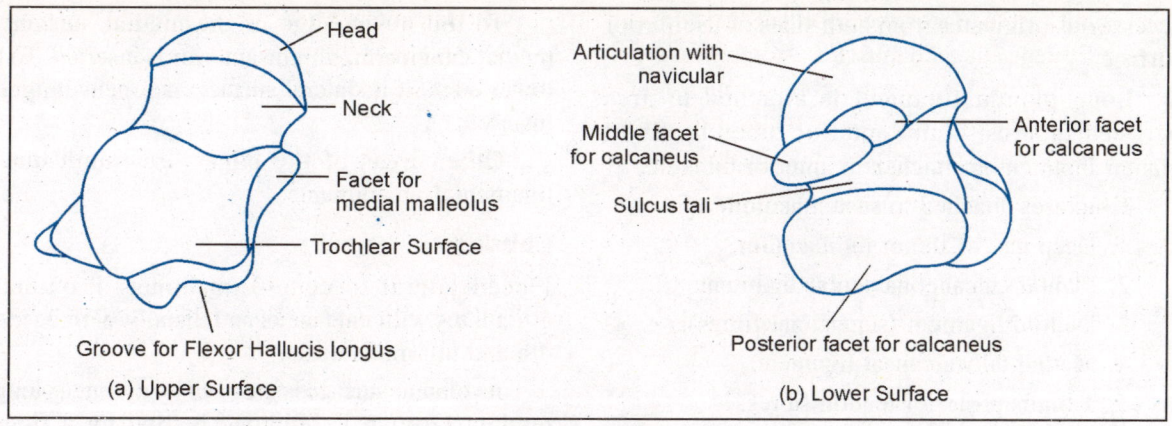

Fig. 2.31: Talus

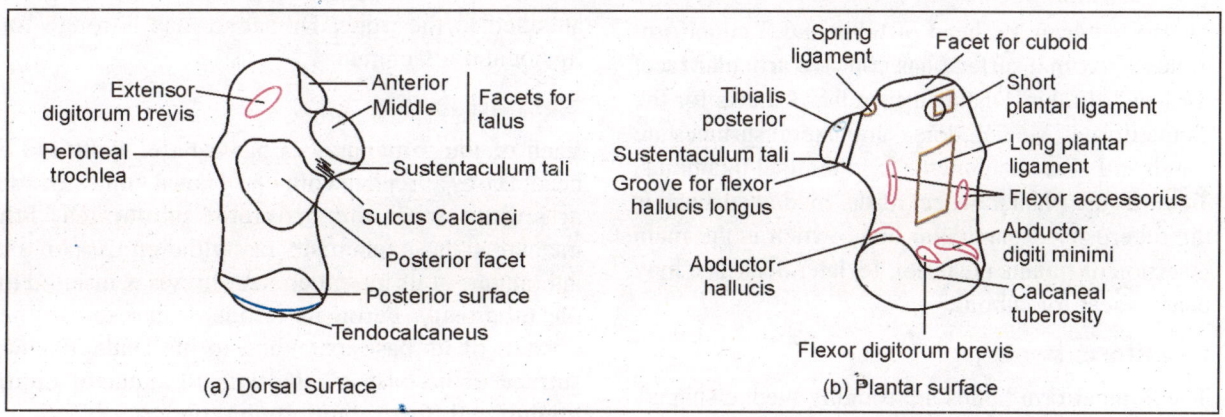

Fig. 2.32: Calcaneus

Middle one is over the sustentaculum tali. Between the posterior and middle facets, a groove is seen, sulcus calcanei – with sulcus tali, it completes sinus tarsi. Anterior surface has articular facet for cuboid.

Posterior surface – has 3 parts. Upper part is related to a bursa and fat. Middle rough part receives the insertion of tendocalcaneus. Lower part is subcutaneous.

Lateral surface is flat. Its anterior part has a tubercle, peroneal trochlea, grooved by tendons of peroneus longus and brevis.

Medial surface is concave. A prominent bony projection – sustentaculum tali is seen from the anterior part of its upper margin. Sustentaculum tali has facet for talus on its upper surface. Tendon of flexor hallucis longus that grooves the posterior surface of talus, grooves the inferior surface of sustantaculum tali. Medial surface of sustentaculum tali is related to the tendon of flexor digitorum longus.

Plantar surface- Its posterior part has the rough calcaneal tuberosity that has medial and lateral processes. Anterior part of this surface has the anterior tubercle.

Anterior part of dorsal surface gives origin to Extensor digitorum brevis. Calcaneal tuberosity and its 2 processes give origin to abductor digiti minimi, abductor hallucis and flexor digitorum brevis and attachment of plantar aponeurosis. Flexor accessorius originates from both sides of its inferior surface.

Long plantar ligament is attached to area between tuberosity and anterior tubercle. Short plantar ligament is attached to anterior tubercle.

Structures attached to sustentaculum tali:

1. Deep part of flexor retinaculum.
2. Plantar calcaneonavicular ligament.
3. Deltoid ligament (superficial fibres).
4. Medial talocalcaneal ligament.
5. Tibialis posterior tendon fibres.

Navicular bone

Placed between the head of talus and 3 cuneiform bones. Proximal surface has concave articular facet for head of talus. Distal surface has 3 facets for the 3 cuneiforms. Medial, dorsal and lateral surfaces are rough and give attachments to intertarsal ligaments. Towards the plantar aspect of the medial surface, is the tuberosity of navicular bone which is the main insertion of tibialis posterior. Its lateral surface may bear a facet for cuboid.

Cuneiform bones

The 3 cuneiform bones are roughly wedge shaped. Medial one is largest. Middle one is smallest. Proximally they articulate with the navicular and distally with the 1st three metatarsal bones. Lateral cuneiform articulates laterally with the cuboid.

To the lower edge of the medial surface of medial cuneiform, tibialis anterior is inserted. To the lower edge of its lateral surface, peroneus longus is inserted.

Other areas of the bones are rough due to ligamental attachments.

Cuboid

Placed lateral to cuneiform bones. Proximally articulates with calcaneus and distally with bases of 4th and 5th metatarsals.

Its plantar surface is grooved by peroneus longus tendon. Groove is bounded behind by a ridge - tuberosity of cuboid. Long plantar ligament is attached to the ridge. Dorsal surface is rough for ligamental attachments.

Metatarsals (Fig. 2.33)

Each of the 5 metatarsals has a base, shaft and a head. Bases articulate witht the 4 tarsal bones. Heads articulate with the proximal phalanges. 5th metatarsal has a tuberosity or styloid process on the lateral part of its base. Peroneus brevis is inserted to the tuberosity. Peroneus tertius is inserted to the dorsum of its base extending to the shaft. Plantar surface of its base gives origin to abductor digiti minimi and flexor digiti minimi brevis.

Applied aspects

Fracture of base of 5th metatarsal is common - usually due to twisting injury.

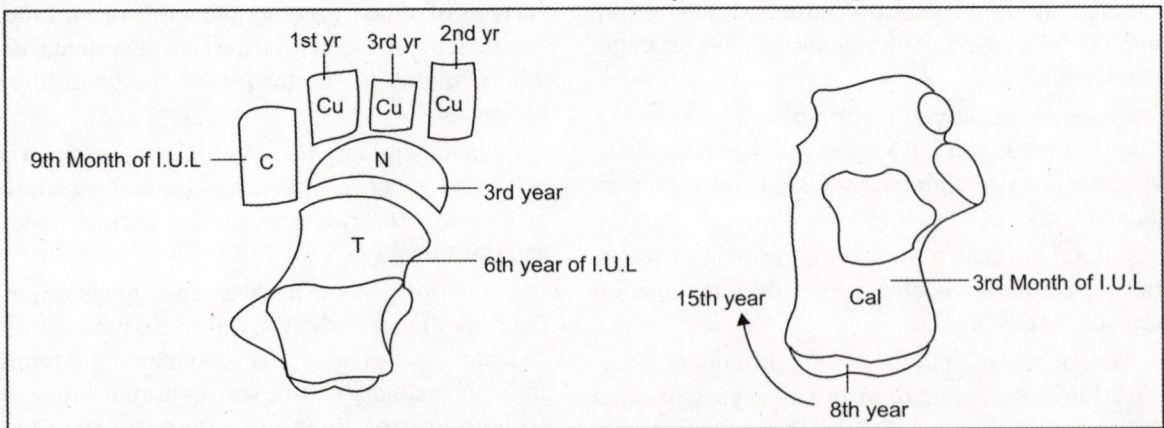

Fig. 2.33: Ossification of Tarsal Bones

Phalanges

2 in big toe and 3 each in other 4 toes. They are shorter than phalanges of hand. The bases of distal phalanges receive insertions of tendons of long flexors and extensors of toes. Bases of middle phalanges receive insertions of short flexors and extensors of the toes.

2nd, 3rd, and 4th proximal phalanges receive insertions of lumbricals and interossei muscles.

BONES OF UPPER LIMB

(32 Bones)

Scapula	
Clavicle	
Humerus	
Ulna	
Radius	carpal bones
Pisiform	
Triquetral	
Lunate	
Scaphoid	
Trapezium	

Trapizoid	
Capitate	carpal bones
Hamate	
5 metacarpals	
14 phalanges	

Scapula (Fig. 2.34)

Flat triangular bone, overlies 2nd to 7th ribs on the dorsum of thorax. It has-

2 surfaces – Dorsal and ventral (costal)

3 borders - Superior, medial and lateral

3 angles - Superior, inferior and lateral

3 processes – Coracoid process, Spine and Acromion

Lateral angle is broad and massive and is known as head of scapula. It has the glenoid cavity which articulates with head of humerus at shoulder joint. Above the glenoid cavity, a small supraglenoid tubercle is seen and below it, a rough infraglenoid tubercle is present. Around the glenoid cavity, a faint neck is seen. **Lateral border** is thick and rough. **Medial border** is thin. **Superior border** is thin and sharp. It shows a suprascapular notch at its lateral end.

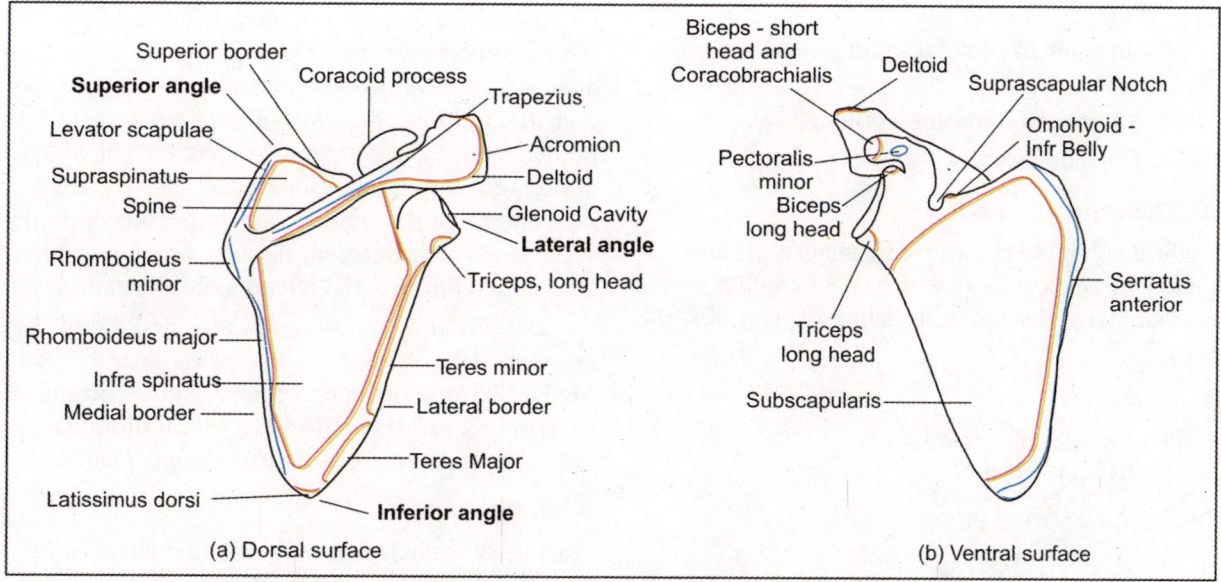

(a) Dorsal surface   (b) Ventral surface

Fig. 2.34: (a) Scapula - Dorsal Surface (b) Scapula - Ventral Surface

Spine of scapula

It is triangular in shape, projects from the dorsal surface, dividing the surface into a smaller upper supraspinous fossa and larger lower infraspinous fossa. Its dorsal border is thick and rough, forms the crest of the spine. Between the spine and the neck, a notch is seen, spinoglenoid notch.

Acromion

A flat bony part projects from the lateral end of spine and curves anteriorly almost at right angles from the spine. Has a upper surface, lateral border medial border and apex. Medial border has a facet for articulation with clavicle.

Coracoid process

Projects from the upper part of the lateral angle or head. Directed laterally and forwards. Supraglenoid tubercle is seen at its root.

Three ligaments are attached to it.

1. Coracoclavicular ligament (having conoid part and trapezoid part) to the dorsal surface.
2. Coraco acromial ligament.
3. Coraco humeral ligament – both to lateral border.

Three muscles are attached to it.

1. Insertion of pectoralis minor – to its anterior surface.
2. Short head of biceps - origin.
3. Coracobrachialis - origin.

Supra scapular notch

It is bridged by the transverse ligament and converts it into a foramen through which suprascapular nerve passes. Above the ligament, suprascapular vessels pass.

Ossification

Scapula ossifies in 8 centres

1 –for body
2 – for coracoid process
2 – for acromion
1 – for medial border
1 – for inferior angle
1 – for glenoid cavity
All fuse by 20th year.

Clavicle (Fig. 2.35)

Clavicle and scapula form the pectoral girdle.

Clavicle, the collar bone has certain peculiarities

1. It is the 1st bone to ossify in the body.
2. It is through out subcutaneous.
3. It is the only long bone placed horizontally.
4. It is the only long bone which has no medullary cavity.
5. It is the only bone having 2 primary centres of ossification.
6. It is the only long bone that develops mostly by intramembranous ossification.
7. It is frequently pierced by cutaneous nerves.

Placed horizontally between manubrium sterni and acromion, it is sinuously curved. Medial end is more rounded than the flat lateral end. Its medial 2/3rd is convex anteriorly and lateral 1/3rd concave anteriorly. Medial end articulates with manubrium sterni and 1st costal cartilage. Lateral end articulates with acromion.

Inferior surface, in its middle 1/3rd, has a groove where subclavius and clavi pectoral fascia are attached. At the junction of the lateral 1/4th with the rest of the bone, inferior surface near posterior border, shows a small conoid tubercle from which, a trapezoid line extends anterolaterally. These give attachment to the conoid and trapezoid parts of coracoclavicular ligament through which weight is transmitted through clavicle to axial skeleton.

Deltoid and trapizeus are attached along the anterior and posterior aspects of its lateral 1/3rd. Medial 2/3rd of its anterior aspect gives origin to part of pectoralis major. Sternocleidomastoid originates from the medial ½ of its upper surface.

Applied aspects

Fracture of clavicle is usually due to indirect forces. Commonest site of fracture is the junction between

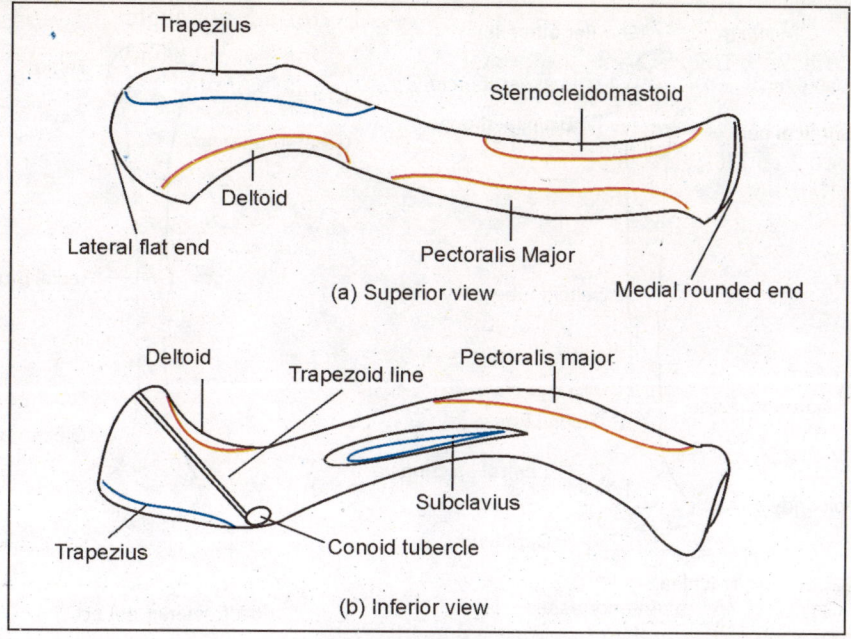

Fig. 2.35: Clavicle

lateral and middle thirds, which is the weakest part of the bone. As the attachment of corococlavicular ligament is lateral to this, weight transmission is affected and shoulder droops.

Ossification

1st bone to ossify.

2 primary centres for shaft - 5th–6th week of i.u.life

One secondary centre for sternal end–around 18 years.

Occassional centre for lateral end

Humerus (Fig. 2.36)

Humerus is the longest bone of the upper limb

It has an upper end, shaft and lower end.

Upper end

Upper end presents a head, neck, greater tubercle and lesser tubercle.

Head: The rounded head is slightly less than ½ a sphere. It articulates with glenoid cavity of scapula at shoulder joint.

Neck: It is a constriction around and adjoining the margin of the head. This is the anatomical neck.

Capsule of shoulder joint is attached to anatomical neck.

Surgical neck – it is the line along which upper end becomes continuous with the shaft. Axillary nerve and posterior circumflex humeral vessels are related here. Fractures are common here, in which case the above structures can be injured.

Lesser Tubercle: Seen on the anterior aspect of upper end. Subscapularis is inserted here.

Greater Tubercle: Projects laterally at the upper end. Supraspinatus, infraspinatus and teres minor are inserted on its posterior aspect, from above, downwards. Anteriorly the sharp margins of greater and lesser tubercles bound the intertubercular sulcus,(bicipital groove) through which the tendon of long head of biceps passes. In its floor, latissimus dorsi is inserted. Along its lateral margin, pectoralis major and medial margin, teres major are inserted.

Shaft

It is somewhat cylindrical. Towards the middle, anterolaterally, the rough deltoid tuberosity is seen, which receives insertion of Deltoid muscle.

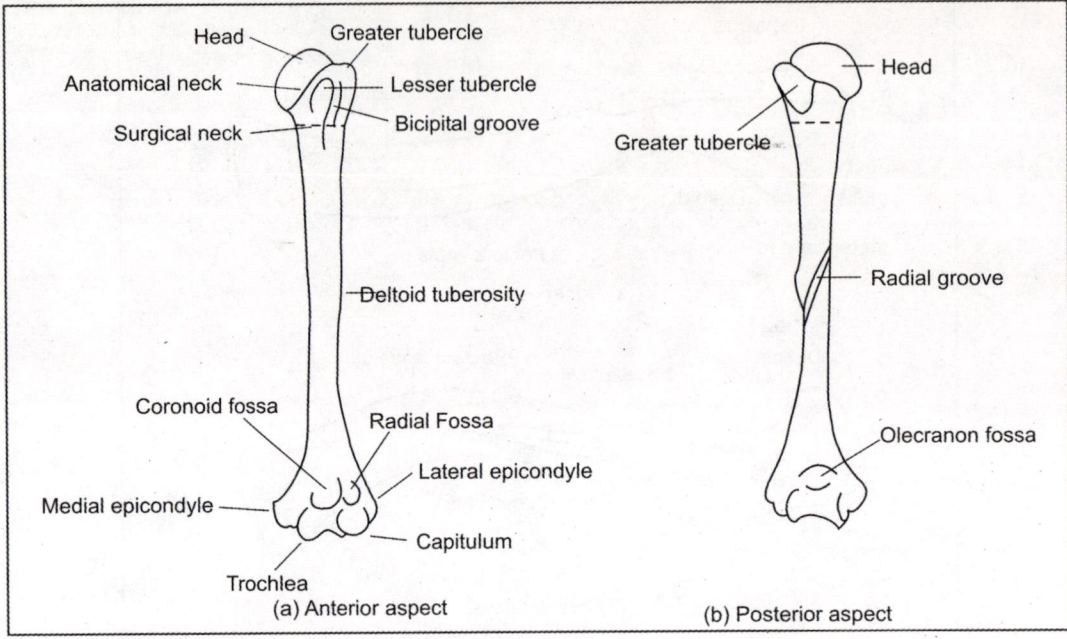

Fig. 2.36: Humerus

At the middle 1/3rd of the shaft, radial groove descends from the posterior, to lateral surface; radial nerve and profounda brachii artery lie there.

Lower end

Lower end has articular and non-articular parts:

Articular parts:

1. Laterally a rounded capitulum which articulates with upper end of radius. It is deficient posteriorly.

2. Medial to capitulum, there is a pulley shaped trochlea. The medial edge of the trochlea is prominent and projects more. This is responsible for the angulation between long axes of upper arm and forearm when forearm is extended and supinated - carrying angle. It articulates with the trochlear notch of ulna.

Non articular parts:

1. Medial to trochlea, there is the medial epicondyle, which is a blunt projection. Ulnar nerve is related to its posterior surface. Anterior surface gives origin to the superficial flexors of forearm. Above it, the medial supra condylar ridge extends up to the shaft as a sharp border.

2. Lateral to capitulum, a less prominent lateral epicondyle is seen, from which, lateral supracondylar ridge extends up. It gives origin to superficial extensors of forearm.

3. Olecranon fossa – A deep hollow on the posterior surface, above the trochlea. Articulates with the olecranon of ulna, in extension of elbow.

4. Coronoid fossa – Seen on the anterior aspect, above the trochlea. Receives the coronoid process of ulna in flexion of elbow.

5. Radial fossa – Smaller one, above the capitulum, receives head of radius in flexion.

Clinical anatomy

Fractures are common at shaft especially at surgical neck. In such a case, axillary nerve can be injured. In fracture of middle of shaft, radial nerve can be injured. Fracture of medial epicondyle can affect ulnar nerve.

Angle of humeral torsion (Fig. 2.37)

In lower animals (mammals), the angle between long axes of the upper and lower articular surfaces make an angle of about 90°. In human, the head of humerus has rotated laterally so that the angle has increased to about 165°. The angle is more in males.

Ossification

Ossifies from eight centres

1. shaft
2. head
3. Greater tubercle
4. Lesser tubercle
5. Capitulum and lateral part of trochlea
6. Medial part of trochlea
7. Medial epicondyle
8. Lateral epicondyle (All fuse by 20th year)

Radius (Fig. 2.39)

The lateral bone of forearm.

Has an upper end, shaft and lower end.

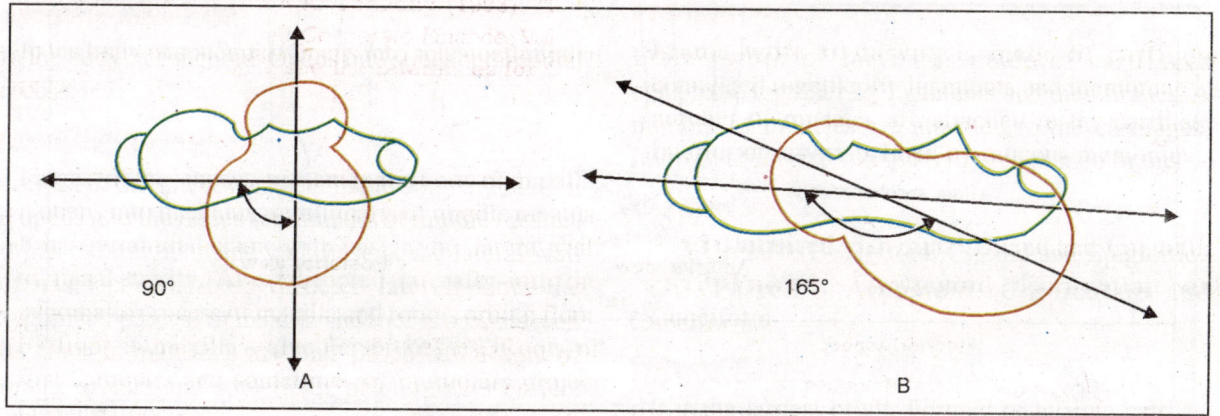

Fig. 2.37: Angle of Humeral Torsion

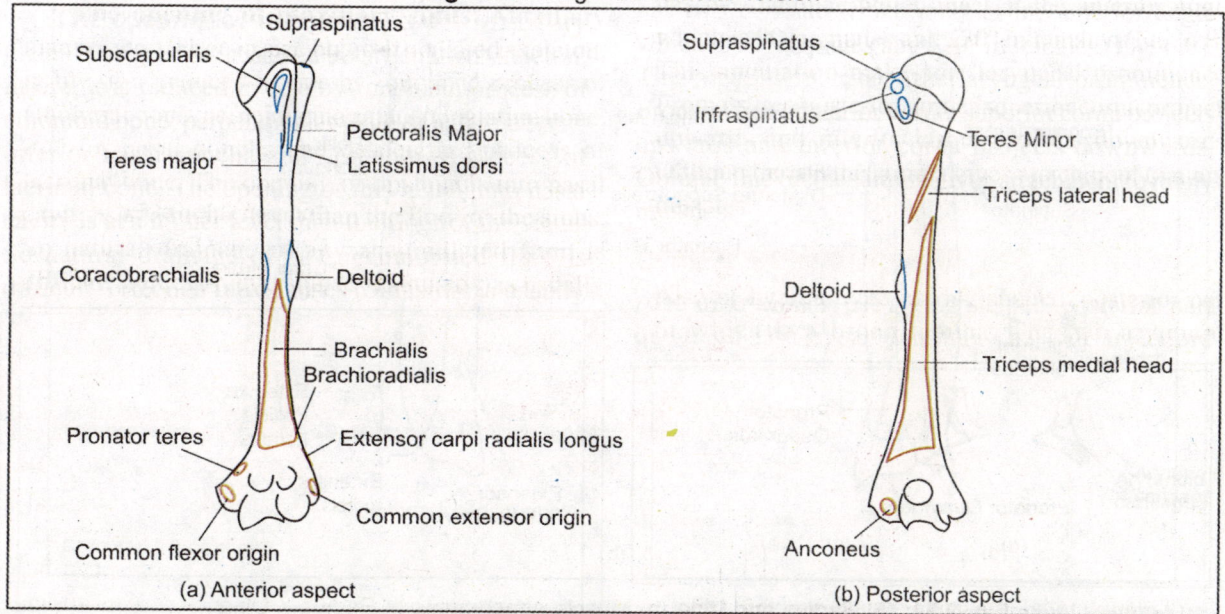

(a) Anterior aspect

(b) Posterior aspect

Fig. 2.38: Muscle Attachments of Humerus

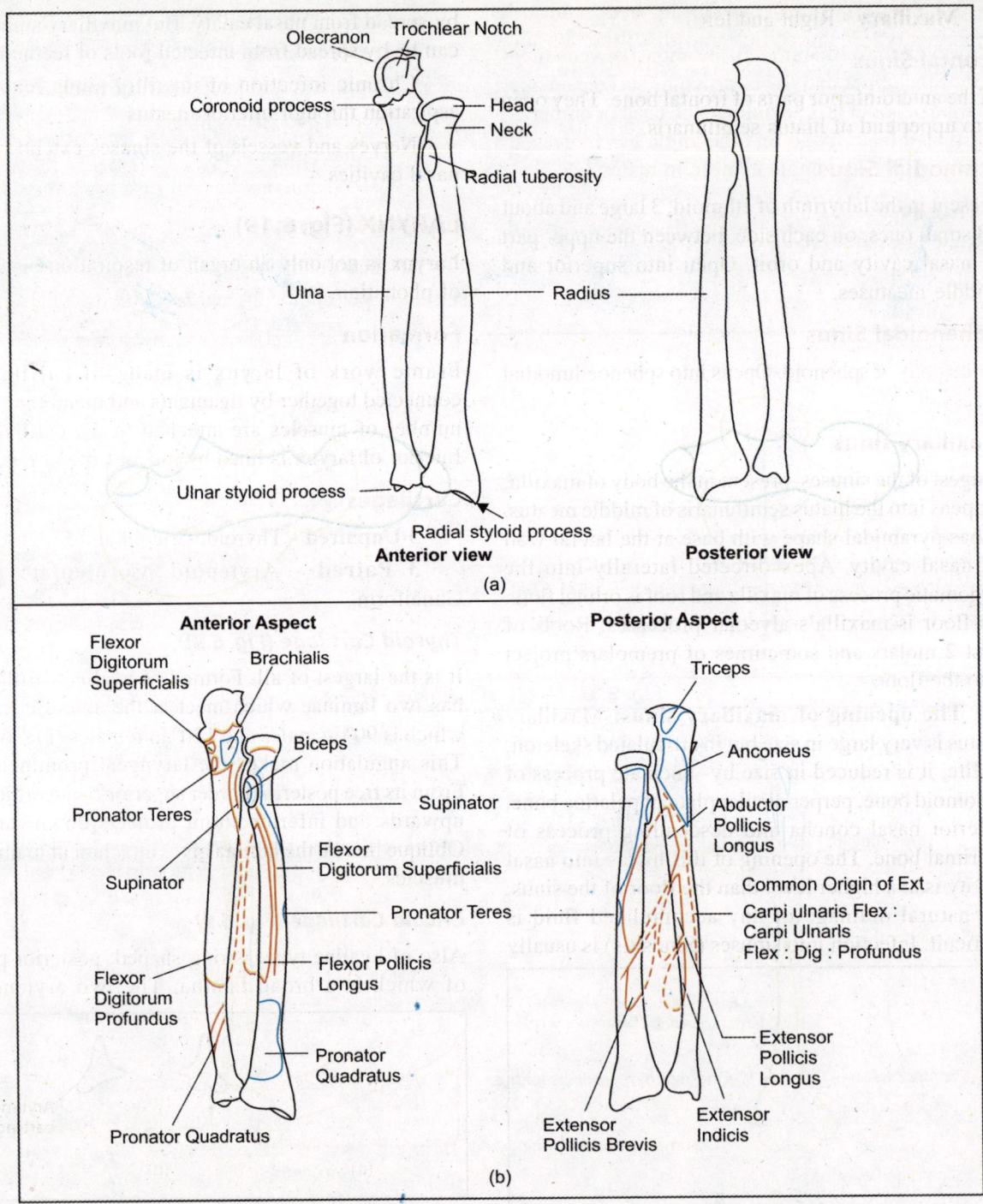

Fig. 2.39: (a) Radius and Ulna (b) Muscle Attachments of Radius & Ulna

Upper end consists of head, neck and radial tuberosity. Head is thick and disc like. Its upper concave surface articulates with capitulum of humerus. Thick margin of the head articulates with radial notch of ulna and is encircled by the anular ligament.

Neck is constricted. Tuberosity is just distal to its medial part. The rough posterior part of the tuberosity gives insertion to tendon of biceps brachii. The oblique line on the shaft starts from the lower end of the tuberosity. Oblique line give origin to flexor digitorum superficialis. Shaft is narrow proximally, slightly expanded distally and has a lateral convexity. Generally it is triangular in section, but only the medial interosseous border is prominent and gives attachment to interosseous membrane. Anterior border is continuous with the oblique line above. Below, it is seen as a sharp crest at the lateral border of anterior surface to which lateral end of extensor retinaculum is attached. Posterior border is not very distinct. Shaft of the radius shows a rough impression on the middle of the lateral convex surface, which gives insertion to pronator teres. Upper part of lateral and posterior surfaces give insertion to supinator.

Lower end of radius is broad, and has wide anterior and posterior surfaces and narrow medial and lateral surfaces. Posterior/dorsal surface of the lower end has a prominent dorsal tubercle which functions as a pulley for the tendon of extensor pollicis longus. (Fig. 2.40)

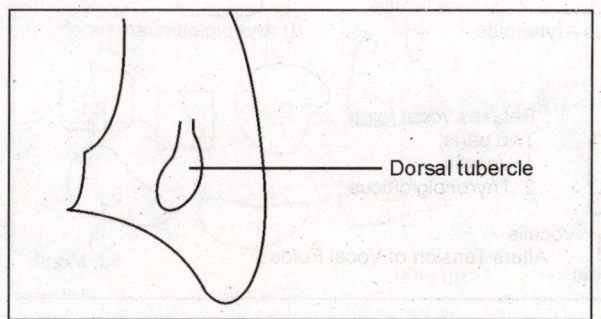

Fig. 2.40: Dorsal Surface of Lower End of Radius

Medial surface articulates with lower end of ulna. Lateral surface projects distally as the radial styloid process.

Distal end of the radius has 2 articular facets on its inferior surface for scaphoid and lunate of carpal bones.

Ossification

Primary centre for shaft at 8th week of i.u. life. One secondary centre for lower end appears at 1st year and joins at 18th year. Secondary centre for upper end appears at 5th year and joins at 16th year.

Ulna (Fig. 2.39)

The medial bone of forearm.

Has an upper end, shaft and lower end.

Upper end has 2 processes – olecranon process and coronoid process and 2 notches – radial notch and trochlear notch.

Olecranon process projects up form the upper end of the bone and its tip is directed anteriorly. Coronoid process is directed anteriorly below the olecranon. The anterior surface of olecranon and upper surface of coronoid process form the trochlear notch that articulates with the trochlea of humerus. The lateral surface of coronoid process shows an articular facet for the head of radius. Below that, there is a triangular area bounded behind by an oblique supinator crest. This area gives origin to supinator. Anterior surface of coronoid process is rough and gives insertion to brachialis.

Upper surface of olecranon gives insertion to triceps. Anconeus is inserted to the lateral surface of olecranon and little below it.

Shaft of ulna has a sharp lateral border and faint anterior and posterior borders, anterior, medial and posterior surfaces. **Muscle attachments of radius and ulna shown in Fig. 2.39(b)**

Lower end of the bone has a small head and styloid process. The inferior surface of head is circular and is separated from the wrist joint by an intra articular disc. Lateral surface of head shows articular facet for head of radius.

Ossification

Primary centre in the shaft – 8th week of i.u. life

Secondary centre for lower end – 5th year, joins with the shaft by 18th year

2 centres for olecranon - 10th year. Joins with shaft at 15th year

Applied anatomy

Colles' fracture: Fracture of lower end of radius, usually lower fragment is displaced back leading into "dinner fork" deformity. Sometimes the distal segment of fracture displaces anteriorly – Smith's fracture or Barton's fracture.

Fracture of shaft of both bones also is common.

Dislocation of elbow is associated with fracture of coronoid process, head of radius, capitulum and medial epicondyle. Radius and ulna will be displaced back.

In children subluxation of head of radius occurs due to a sudden powerful jerk of the hand as in lifting the child by forearm or hand.

Skeleton of hand (Fig. 2.41)

1. Skeleton of wrist - Has 8 small irregular carpal bones, together they form the carpus.
2. Skeleton of the palm is formed by 5 metacarpal bones – They are short long bones.

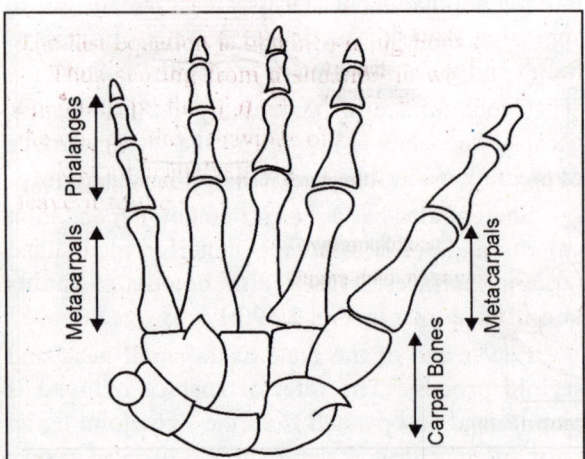

Fig. 2.41: Skeleton of Hand

3. Skeleton of fingers – each finger has 3 phalanges except thumb, which has only 2.

Carpal bones are arranged in two rows. (Fig 2.42.) Proximal from medial to lateral, they are, Pisiform, Triquetral, Lunate, Scaphoid. Distal – from lateral to medial are Trapezium, Trapezoid, Capitate, hamate.

The distal surface of Trapezium is concavoconvex and articulates with base of 1st metacarpal bone and is an example of saddle joint. Carpal bones, with flexor retinaculum form carpal tunnel. Generally inter-carpal joints are plane synovial joints.

Ossification of carpal bones.

1st carpal bone to ossify is capitate and last one is pisiform.

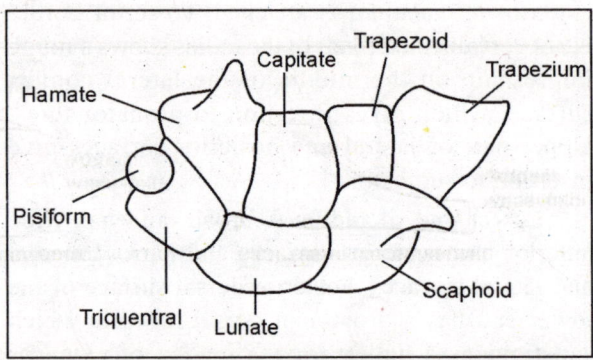

Fig. 2.42: Carpal Bones

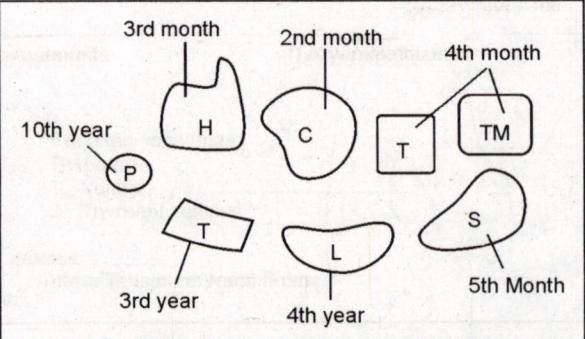

Fig. 2.43: Ossification of Carpal Bones

Single Best Response M.C.Qs

1. Sagital suture is found
   (a) Between frontal and parietal bones
   (b) Between 2 parietal bones
   (c) Between parietal and occipital bone
   (d) Between parietal and temporal bone
2. Following are ossicles of middle ear except
   (a) Vomer   (b) Malleus
   (c) Incus   (d) Stapes
3. Following are correct about C_7 vertebra except
   (a) It is known as vertebra prominens
   (b) It has a long horizontal spine
   (c) Spine ends in a tubercle
   (d) Its foramen transversarium transmits vertebral artery
4. Vertebral level of sternal angle is
   (a) C_7 (b) T_2
   (c) T_4 (d) T_6
5. The muscle that is not attached to ischial tuberosity is
   (a) Semitendinosus
   (b) Semimembranosus
   (c) Short head of Biceps
6. Following are correct about patella except
   (a) It is the largest sesamoid bone
   (b) Present in the tendon of quadriceps femoris
   (c) Ligamentum patellae extends from its apex to tibial tuberosity
   (d) It articulates with femur and tiba at knee joint.
7. Head of Fibula receives insertion of
   (a) Biceps femoris
   (b) Semitendinosus
   (c) Tensor fascia lata
   (d) Sartorius
8. The tarsal bone to which no muscle is attached is
   (a) Calcaneum
   (b) Talus
   (c) Navicular
   (d) Medial cuneiform
9. The Ist bone to ossify in the body is
   (a) Pisiform
   (b) Femur
   (c) Scapula
   (d) Clavicle
10. Humerus is not directly related to
    (a) Ulnar nerve
    (b) Median nerve
    (c) Radial nerve
    (d) Axillary nerve

M.C.Qs - Answers

1. (b), 2. (a), 3. (d), 4. (c), 5. (c), 6. (d), 7. (a), 8. (b), 9. (d), 10. (b)

Short notes

1. Clavicle
2. Scapula
3. Mandible
4. Sternum
5. Differences between male and female pelvis
6. Atlas vertebra
7. Axis vertebra
8. Ist rib
9. Sacrum
10. Typical rib

Essays

I. Describe the Hip bone

II. Describe the vertebral column

3 Muscular System

TYPES OF SKELETAL MUSCLES

Based on the shape of muscles and orientation of the fibres in them, muscles are classified into following types, (Fig. 3.1)

1. *Quadrilateral:* Fibres are parallel and short.
2. *Strap:* Fibres are parallel but long.
3. *Fusiform:* Fibres converge at both ends.
4. *Digastric:* Fusiform muscle bellies with an intervening tendon.
5. *Triangular:* Fibres are oblique to the line of pull.
6. *Bicipital:* Where there are two bellies of origin.
7. *Tricipital:* Where there are three bellies of origin.
8. *Cruciate:* Where the bellies cross each other.
9. *Unipennate:* Fibres arranged as if in a feather, only on one side of the tendon.
10. *Bipennate:* Fibres arranged on both sides of the tendon.
11. *Multipennate:* Fibres arranged among more tendons.
12. *Circumpennate:* Fibres originate from the walls of a boney canal and converge to a central tendon.
13. *Spiral or twisted:* Fibres have a twisted arrangement.

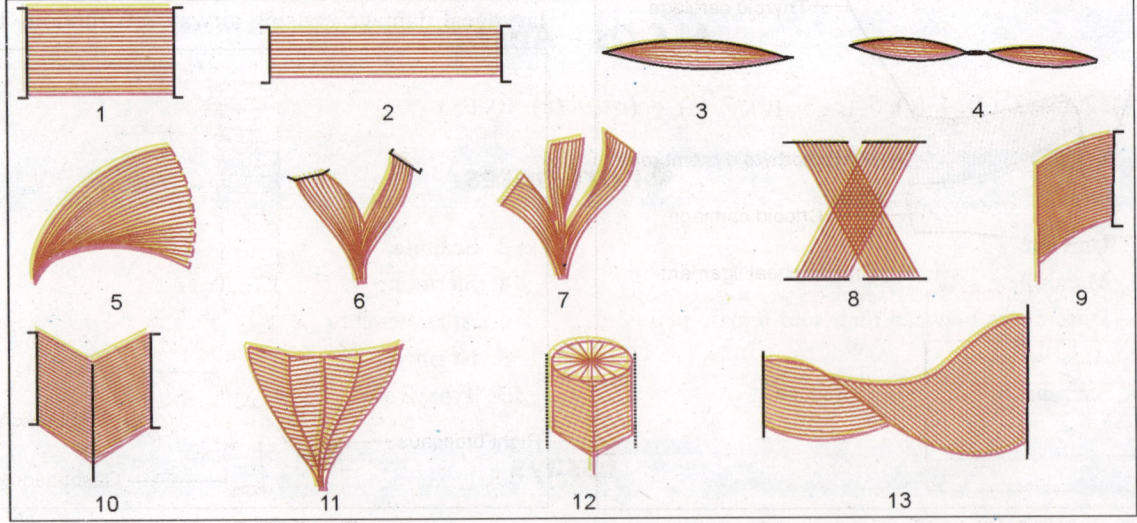

Fig. 3.1 Types of Skeletal Muscles

MUSCLES OF UPPER LIMB

They are of six groups

    I. Muscles that connect upper limb to vertebral column.

  II. Muscles that connect upper limb to thoracic wall.

 III. Muscles of the shoulder region (muscles connecting scapula to humerus)

 IV. Muscles of upper arm.

  V. Muscles of forearm.

 VI. Muscles of hand.

I GROUP

1. Trapezius
2. Latissimus dorsi
3. Levator scapulae
4. Rhomboideus major
5. Rhomboideus minor

1. Trapezius (Fig. 3.2)

A large flat triangular muscle on the back of neck and thorax. Muscles of both sides together form a trapezium.

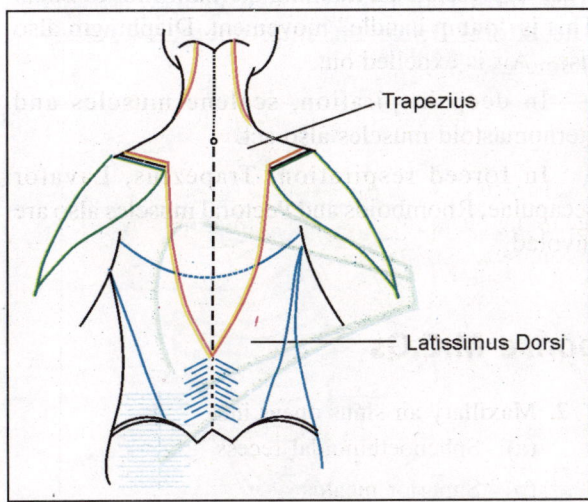

Fig. 3.2

Origin:

1. Medial 1/3rd of the superior nuchal line
2. External occipital protuberance
3. Ligamentum nuchae
4. Spine of 7th cervical vertebrae
5. Spines of all thoracic vertebrae

Insertion:

1. Upper fibers descend to posterior border of lateral 1/3rd of clavicle.
2. Middle fibers pass laterally to the acromion and upper border of spine of scapula.
3. Lower fibers ascend to the medial end of spine of scapula.

Nerve Supply:

1. Accessary nerve (11th cranial nerve).
2. Ventral rami of C_3 & C_4 nerves. (sensory – proprioceptive).

Action:

1. Elevates the scapula.
2. Rotates the scapula so that the upper limb is abducted above the level of horizontal.
3. Retracts the scapula.
4. Both muscles together draws the head back.

2. Latissimus dorsi (Fig. 3.2)

A large flat triangular muscle on the back of lower thoracic & lumbar regions.

Origin:

1. From the spines of lower 6 thoracic vertebrae, deep to trapezius.
2. From thoracolumbar fascia.
3. From posterior part of iliac crest.
4. From lower 3 or 4 ribs.
5. From lower angle of scapula.

Insertion: The muscle fibers are directed laterally, upwards and curves round the lower border of teres major to reach its anterior aspect. There the tendon is inserted into the floor of bicipital groove of humerus.

Nerve supply: Thoracodorsal nerve - from posterior cord of brachial plexus.

Action:

1. Extension, adduction and medial rotation of arm.
2. When the arm is raised and fixed above the head, it pulls the trunk upwards, as when climbing a tree.

3. Levator Scapulae (Fig. 3.3)

Seen at the back and side of neck.

Origin: From transverse processes of upper 4 cervical vertebrae.

Insertion: Into medial border of scapula above the medial end of its spine.

Nerve supply: C_3 and C_4 nerves and dorsal scapular nerve.

Action: Pulls the scapula upwards and medially.

4. Rhomboideus minor (Fig. 3.3)

Origin: From the lower end of ligamentum nuchae and spines of C_7 and T_1 vertebrae.

Insertion: Into a triangular area at the medial end of spine of scapula.

Nerve supply: Dorsal scapular nerve.

Action: Pulls the medial border of scapula upwards and medially.

5. Rhomboideus major (Fig. 3.3)

Origin: From spines of T_2 to T_5 vertebrae

Insertion: Into medial border of scapula below the root of its spine.

Nerve supply: Dorsal scapular nerve.

Action: Pulls the medial border of scapula upwards and medially.

II GROUP

Muscles that connect upper limb to thoracic wall

1. Pectoralis major
2. Pectoralis minor
3. Subclavius
4. Serratus anterior

Pectoralis major and minor and subclavius are the muscles of the pectoral region - the region in the front of thorax.

1. Pectoralis major (Fig 3.4)

Origin:

1. Anterior surface of medial ½ of clavicle.
2. Anterior surface of sternum.
3. 1st to 7th costal cartilages.
4. External oblique aponeurosis.

Insertion: The bilaminar flat tendon is inserted into the lateral lip of the intertubercular sulcus of humerus.

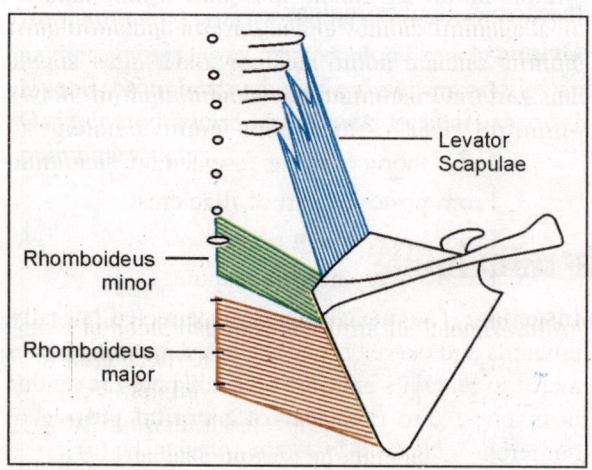

Fig. 3.3

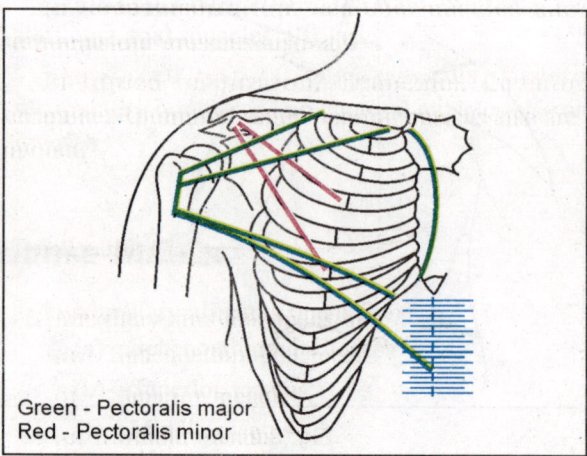

Green - Pectoralis major
Red - Pectoralis minor

Fig. 3.4

Nerve Supply: Medial and Lateral pectoral nerves.

Action: Adduction and medial rotation of upper arm.

2. Pectoralis minor (Fig. 3.4)

Origin: 3rd to 5th ribs near their costal cartilages.

Insertion: Upper surface of coracoid process.

Nerve Supply: Medial & Lateral pectoral nerves.

Action: Pulls the scapula anteriorly and downwards (protraction of scapula).

3. Subclavius

A small triangular muscle

Origin: 1st rib, near its costal cartilage.

Insertion: Under surface of the middle 1/3rd of clavicle.

Nerve supply: Nerve to subclavius from upper trunk of brachial plexus.

Action: Pulls the point of the shoulder & clavicle downwards & forwards.

The breasts (Mammary glands)

Breasts are modified sweat glands in the pectoral region. Present in both sexes, but rudimentary in male, and undergoes major growth and differentiation in females.

In young adult female, breast is hemispherical in shape. Extends between 2nd & 6th ribs in the anterior chest wall from lateral margin of sternum to mid-axillary line

Breast lies in the superficial fascia over the pectoral fascia (Fig 3.5) Between the base of breast & the deep fascia, there is a small space called retromammary space filled with loose connective tissue.

A small part of the gland extends upwards & lateraly into the axilla piercing deep fascia - axillary tail.

Over the centre of the breast the skin shows a darker circular area, the areola. Nipple is a conical projection from the centre of the areola. On to the surface of the nipple about 15–20 lactiferous ducts open through minute orifices.

Structure of the mammary gland

It consists of the glandular tissue with ducts arranged into lobes and lobules, by the loose connective tissue stroma. Glands are tubuloalveolar in type. It also has variable amounts of adipose tissue in the interlobar position. From the upper part, condensation of fibrous tissue run to the skin -

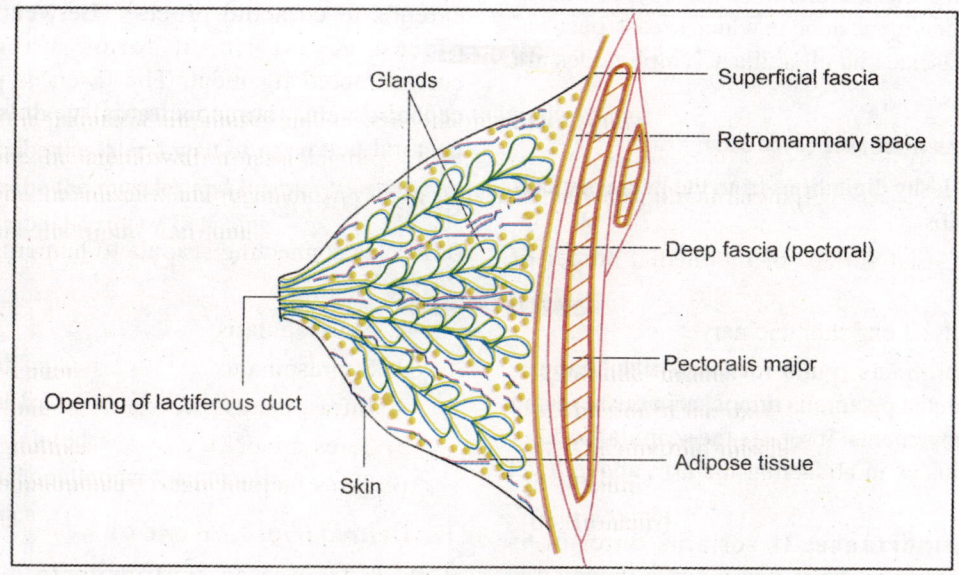

Fig. 3.5

suspensory ligaments of Astley Cooper which are important in the support of breast tissue.

Blood supply: Arteries supplying the gland are:

1. Superior thoracic, pectoral, lateral thoracic and subscapular branches of axillary artery.

2. Perforating branches of internal thoracic and 2nd to 4th intercostal arteries also supply it.

Veins correspond to the arteries

Lymphatic drainage: About 75% of the lymphatics from breast are drained to axillary nodes & remainder to the parasternal nodes.

Generally lymphatics from parenchyma & skin of nipple & areola go to the axillary groups of lymph nodes and some to infraclavicular & intercostal nodes. Lymphatics from the remaining part of the skin mainly go to the parasternal nodes, and some to axillary and supraclavicular nodes. There is overlaping of the area of drainage and a wide ramification of the lymphatics.

CLINICAL ANATOMY

Tumours of breast can be benign or malignant. In malignant tumours, the cancerous cells spread easily to surrounding tissues & lymph nodes expecially axillary nodes. In operation for carcinoma breast, radical mastectomy is done in which breast, pectoral muscles & fasciae and all axillary lymph nodes are removed.

4.   Serratus anterior (Fig. 3.6)

Origin: By fleshy digitations from the lateral aspects of upper 8 ribs.

Insertion: Costal surface of the medial border of scapula.

Nerve supply: Long thoracic nerve.

Action: It protracts (pulls forwards) the scapula, together with the pectoralis minor, as in pushing and punching movements. It rotates the scapula together with trapezius as in abducting the arm above level of head.

Clinical importance: If serratus anterior is paralysed (common cause being nerve injury), the

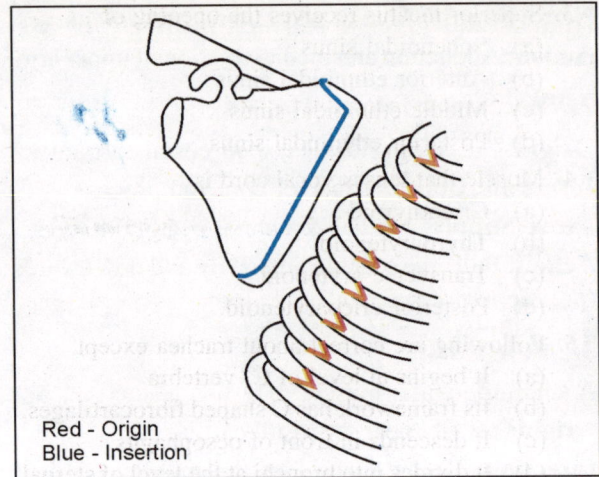

Red - Origin
Blue - Insertion

Fig. 3.6: Serrartus Anterior

medial border of the scapula stands out prominently, when the patient tries to push with his hand - known as "winging" of scapula.

Clavi pectoral fascia: It is a strong sheet of fibrous tissue which extends between pectoralis minor & subclavius and overlies the axillary vessels and nerves. Above it splits to enclose subclavius & below encloses pectoralis minor. Medially it blends with fascia over upper intercostal spaces. Laterally extends to coracoid process. Between coracoid process & 1st rib, it forms a thick band, costocoracoid ligament. The fascia is pierced by cephalic vein, thoracoacromial vessels & lateral pectoral nerve.

III GROUP

0Muscles connecting scapula to humerus:

1. Deltoid
2. Subscapularis
3. Supraspinatus
4. Infraspinatus
5. Teres minor
6. Teres major

1.   Deltoid (Fig. 3.7 a and b)

A thick triangular, multipennate muscle that

surrounds and gives a rounded profile for the shoulder.

Origin: From

(a) Lateral 1/3rd of clavicle.

(b) Lateral border of acromion.

(c) Lower border of crest of scapular spine.

Insertion: Into the deltoid tuberosity of shaft of humerus

Nerve supply: Axillary nerve.

Action: Abduction at shoulder joint. Anterior fibres alone – felxion and medial rotation of arm.

Posterior fibres alone – extension and lateral rotation of arm.

Commonest site chosen for intra muscular injection is on to the middle part of deltoid.

2. Subscapularis (Fig. 3.8)

Origin: From ventral surface of scapula.

Insertion: To the lesser tubercle of humerus.

Nerve supply: Upper and lower subscapular nerves.

Action: Adduction & medial rotation of arm.

3. Supraspinatus (Fig. 3.9)

Origin: From supraspinous fossa of scapula

Insertion: Into the upper facet on the greater tubercle of hemerus.

Nerve supply: Suprascapular nerve.

Action: Initiates abduction of arm.

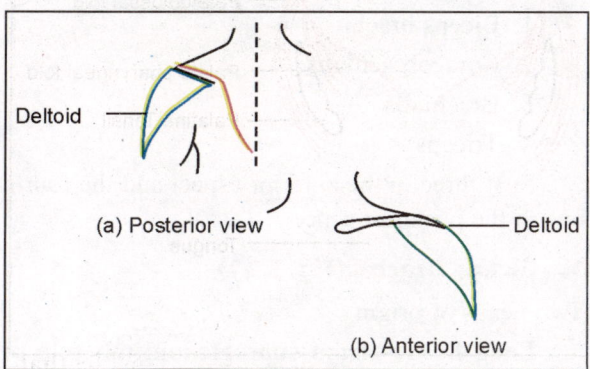

Fig. 3.7: Deltoid

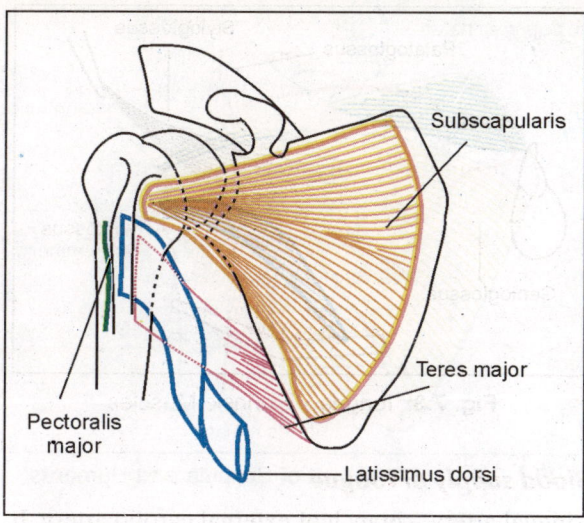

Fig. 3.8: Ventral Aspect of Scapula and Humerus

4. Infraspinatus (Fig. 3.9)

Origin: From infra spinous fossa of seapula.

Insertion: Into the middle facet on the posterior aspect of greater tuburcle of humerus.

Nerve supply: Suprascapular nerve.

Action: Helps abduction and lateral rotation of arm.

5. Teres minor (Fig. 3.9)

Origin: From the upper 2/3rd of the lateral margin of dorsal surface of scapula.

Insertion: On the lower facet of posterior aspect of greater tubercle of humerus.

Nerve supply: Axillary nerve.

Action: Helps abduction & lateral rotation of arm.

Musculotendinous cuff or Rotator cuff: Subscapularis, supraspinatus, infraspinatus and teres minor together form the rotator cuff muscles. These muscles surround the capsule of shoulder joint near their insertion. Their deeper tendinous fibres merge with the capsule of the joint and strengthen it. Also they help to steady the head of humerus on the glenoid cavity. Tendon of supraspinatus passes deep to coracoacromial arch & is separated from it by a subacromial bursa. Infection of the bursa makes initial stage of abduction, painful.

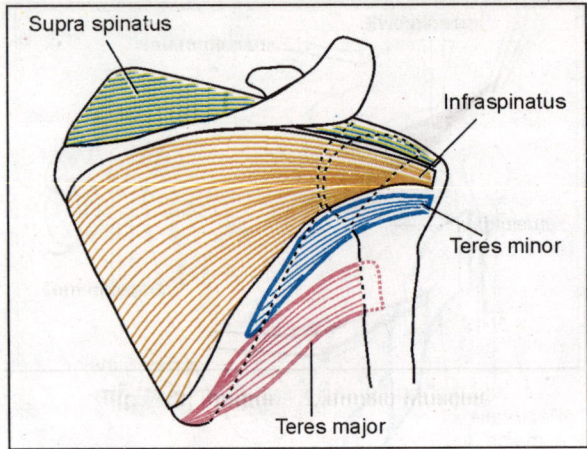

Fig. 3.9: Dorsal aspect of Scapula and Humerus

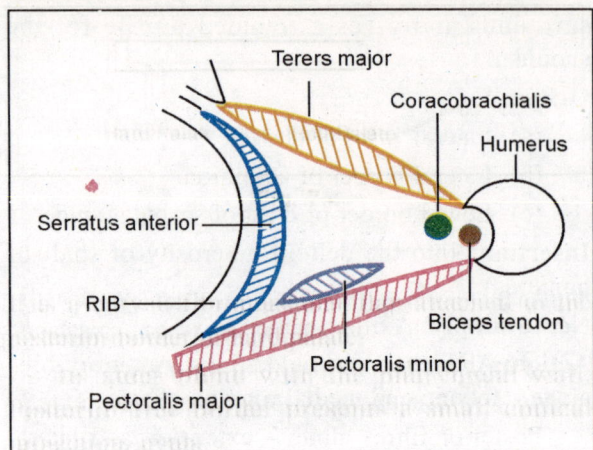

Fig. 3.10: Cross section to show boundaries of left axilla

6.　Teres major (Fig. 3.9)

Origin: From lower 1/3rd of the lateral border of dorsal surface of scapula & its inferior angle.

Insertion: Into medial lip of bicipital groove of humerus.

Nerve supply: Lower subscapular nerve.

Action: Adduction & medial rotation of arm.

Axilla (Arm pit)

Boundaries and contents: Axilla is the region between the upper part of the thorax and upper arm. The nerves and vessels to the upper limb from the root of neck, pass through the axilla.

It is roughly pyramidal in shape, having an apex & base and four walls.

Apex: Bounded by clavicle, outer border of 1st rib and upper border of scapula.

Anterior wall: Formed by pectoralis major, pectoralis minor and subcalvius. Lower border of pectoralis major forms the anterior axillary fold.

Posterior wall: Formed by subscapularis, latissimus dorsi & teres major.

Latissimus dorsi and teres major form posterior axillary fold. (fig 3.8, 3.10)

Medial wall (Fig. 3.10): Formed by upper 4 ribs, their intercostal muscles and upper digitations of serratus anterior.

Lateral wall: It is very narrow. Formed by the intertubercular sulcus of humerus, containing tendons of biceps & coracobrachialis.

Base: Formed by skin & fascia (axillary fascia) stretching between lower borders of pectoralis major and latissimus dorsi.

Contents:

1. Axillary vessels.
2. Lower part of brachial plexus & its major branches.
3. Lymph nodes- Apical group, central group, lateral group, anterior group, posterior group.
4. Axillary tail of the breast.

GROUP IV- MUSCLES OF UPPER ARM

1. Biceps brachii
2. Coracobrachialis
3. Brachialis
4. Triceps

First three in the anterior aspect and the fourth one in the posterior aspect.

1.　Biceps brachii (Fig. 3.11)

Two heads of origin

Long head – from supraglenoid tubercle of scapula.

Short head - from tip of coracoid process of scapula.

Insertion: Both heads join and the common tendon is inserted into the posterior part of radial tuberosity. Also its tendon has an expansion, the bicipital aponeurosis which descends medially over the brachial artery and fuses with deep fascia on medial side of the forearm.

Nerve supply: Musculocutaneous nerve

Actions: It is a powerful supinator of forearm. Also it flexes the elbow. It is a weak flexor of shoulder joint.

2. Coracobrachialis (Fig. 3.11)

Origin: From the tip of coracoid process.

Insertion: Middle of shaft of humerus, on its medial side.

Nerve supply: Musculocutaneous nerve.

Action: Flexion of arm at shoulder joint.

3. Brachialis (Fig. 3.11)

Origin: Anterior aspect of lower half of humerus.

Insertion: Anterior surface of coronoid process of ulna.

Nerve supply: Musculocutaneous nerve. Radial nerve, to the lateral part of the muscle.

Action: Flexion at the elbow.

4. Triceps (Fig. 3.12)

Muscle of the back of the upper arm.

Origin: Has 3 heads of origin

(i) *Long head:* From infraglenoid tubercle of scapula.

(ii) *Lateral head:* From an oblique ridge on the posterior surface of humerus, above spiral groove.

(iii) *Medial head:* From the posterior surface of humerus, below spiral groove.

Insertion: The common tendon is inserted into the upper surface of olecranon process of ulna.

Nerve supply: Radial nerve.

Action: Extension at the elbow joint.

Anatomical spaces around the scapular region (Fig. 3.12)

These are potential intermuscular spaces around shoulder region and upper arm.

1. Quadrangular space

Boundaries:

Above - In front: subscapularis

Behind: teres minor

Below: teres major

Medially: long head of triceps

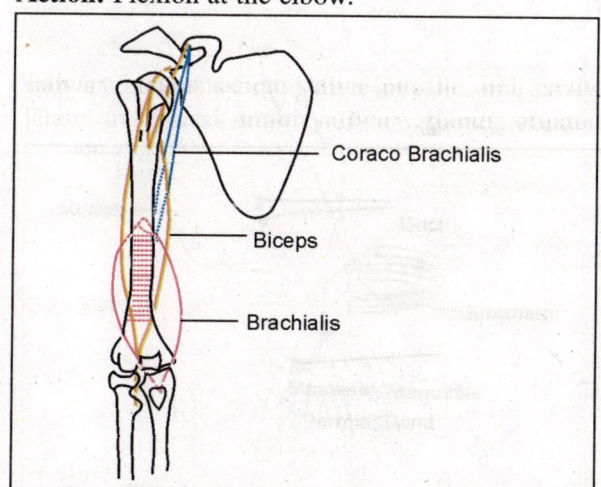

Fig. 3.11: Muscles of Ventral Aspect of Arm

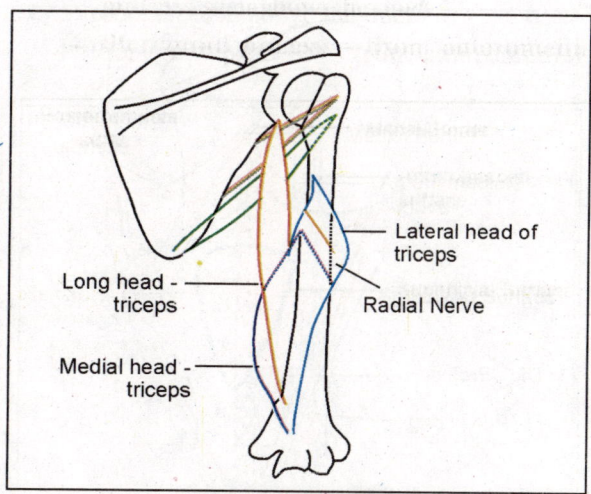

Fig. 3.12: Dorsal Aspect of Arm

Laterally: Surgical neck of humerus

Structures passing through it:

1. Axillary nerve
2. Posterior circumflex humeral vessels.

2. Triangular space

Boundaries:

Above: Teres minor

Below: Teres major

Laterally: Long head of triceps

Structure passing through it:

Circumflex scapular artery

V GROUP - MUSCLES OF FOREARM

I. Muscles of front of forearm (Flexor compartment muscles)

(a) Superficial group of muscles.

1. Ponator teres
2. Flexor carpi radialis
3. Palmaris longus
4. Flexor carpi ulnaris
5. Flexor Digitorum Superficialis

(b) Deep group of muscles

1. Flexor digitorum profundus

2. Flexor pollicis longus
3. Pronator quadratus

(a) Superficial group (Fig. 3.14)

Muscles of this group have a common origin from the medial epicondyle of humerus (by common flexor tendon) and they have additional sites of origin also.

1. PRONATOR TERES

Origin: has two heads of origin.

(i) Humeral head from medial epicondyle & supracondylar ridge.

(ii) Ulnar head from medial side of coronoid process. (Fig 3.13).

Insertion: Lateral surface of the middle of the shaft of radius.

Nerve supply: Median nerve.

Action: Pronation of forearm. It is a weak flexor at elbow.

2. FLEXOR CARPI RADIALIS

Origin: From medial epicondyle of humerus through common flexor origin.

Insertion: Into the base of 2nd metacarpal bone.

Nerve supply: Median nerve.

Action: Flexion & abduction at wrist.

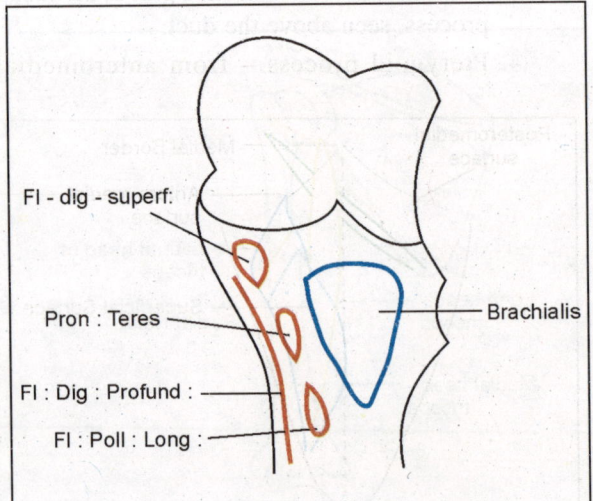

Fig. 3.13: Coronoid Process - Ventral Aspect

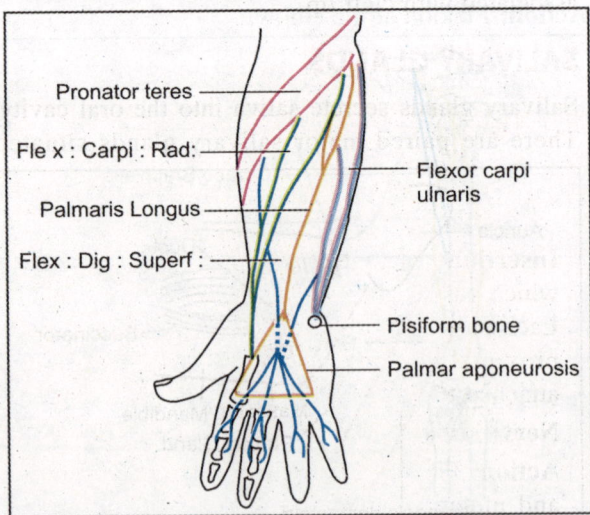

Fig. 3.14: Forearm - Superficial Flexors

Clinical importance: Radial artery lies just lateral to its tendon near the wrist, and radial pulse is felt here.

3. PALMARIS LONGUS: (Often it is absent)

Origin: From medial epicondyle of humerus.

Insertion: On to the flexor retinaculum and palmar aponeurosis.

Nerve supply: Median nerve

Action: Flexion at wrist

4. FLEXOR CARPI ULNARIS

Origin: Two heads of origin

   (i) Humeral head – from medial epicondyle of humerus.

   (ii) Ulnar head – from medial side of olecranon process & posterior border of ulna, through an aponeurosis.

Insertion: Into pisiform bone, which is sesamoid bone in its tendon.

Nerve supply: Ulnar nerve

Action: Flexion & adduction at wrist.

5. FLEXOR DIGITORUM SUPERFICIALIS

Origin: Two heads of origin

   (i) Humeroulnar head – from medial epicondyle of humerus, from the ulnar collateral ligament of elbow joint and from medial margin of coronoid process of ulna.

   (ii) Radial head – from an oblique line on the anterior surface of radius, above its middle. Median nerve and ulnar artery pass between the 2 heads.

Insertion: Near the wrist, it gives off 4 tendons, which pass to the hand deep to flexor retinaculum. Each passes into the medial 4 fingers. Against the proximal phalanx, each splits into two and are attached to the sides of the middle phalanx.

Nerve supply: Median nerve

Action: Flexion of proximal interphalangeal joints and metacarpophalangeal joints of the medial 4 fingers and flexion of wrist.

(B) Deep group (Fig. 3.15)

1. Flexor digitorum profundus
2. Flexor poillicis longus
3. Pronator quadratus

1. FLEXOR DIGITORUM PROFUNDUS

Has an extensive origin from -

   (a) Upper 3/4th of anterior surface of ulna.

   (b) Upper 3/4th of medial surface of ulna extending to coronoid process.

   (c) Upper 3/4th of posterior border of ulna through an aponeurosis.

   (d) From anterior surface of interosseous membrane.

(Its origin covers the anterior, medial & posterior aspects of upper 3/4th of ulna).

Insertion: It divides into 4 tendons which pass deep to flexor retinaculum and go to the medial 4 fingers. Each passes between the 2 slips of tendon of flexor digitorum superficialis and gets inserted into base of distal phalanx. The 4 lumbrical muscles are attached to the tendons in the palm.

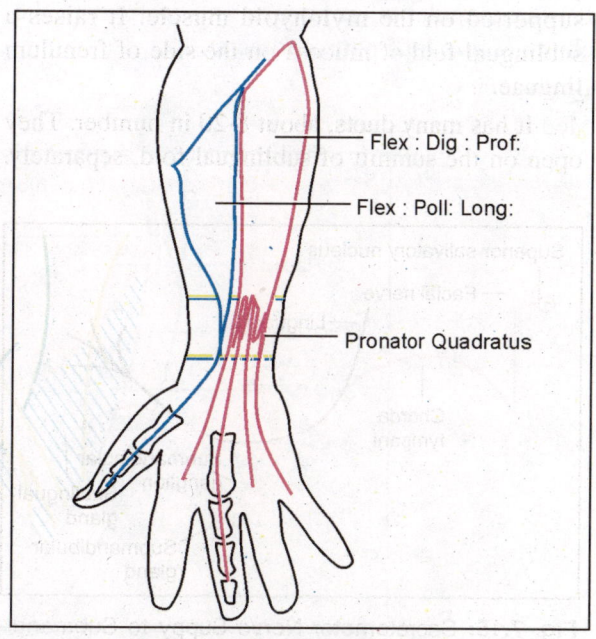

Fig. 3.15: Forearm - Deep Flexors

Nerve supply: Medial part – ulnar nerve

Lateral part: Median nerve, through anterior interosseous branch.

Action: Flexion of distal & proximal interphalangeal joints, meta-carpophalangeal joints and wrist.

2. FLEXOR POLLLICIS LONGUS

Origin: From the middle 2/4th of the anterior surface of radius and interosseous membrane.

Insertion: Base of distal phalanx of thumb.

Nerve supply: Median nerve through anterior interosseous branch.

Action: Flexon of phalanges of thumb.

3. PRONATOR QUADRATUS

Origin: From an oblique line on the lower 1/4th of anterior surface of ulna.

Insertion: Into the lower 1/4th of the anterior surface of radius.

Nerve supply: Anterior interosseous nerve.

Action: Pronation of forearm.

Cubital fossa (Fig. 3.16)

It is a triangular intermuscular area in front of the elbow & proximal part of forearm.

Boundaries:

Medial – Pronator teres

Lateral – Brachioradialis

Base - An imaginary line between the 2 epicondyles of humerus. Lateral and medial boundaries meet at the apex.

Floor – Above brachialis & below supinator.

Roof – Skin and fascia with the median cubital vein.

Contents:

1. Median nerve
2. Brachial artery divides into radial & ulnar arteries.
3. Tendon of biceps going to insertion at radial tuberosity.
4. Bicipital aponeurosis.
5. Radial nerve & its deep branch.

Flexor retinaculum (Fig. 3.20 a, b)

In the proximal part of the hand in front of the carpal bones, the deep fascia of forearm is thickened to form a fibrous band, the flexor retinaculum.

Attachments:

Medially to pisiform bone and hook of hamate.

Laterally to tubercles of scaphoid and trapezium.

    The retinaculum bridges the space in front of carpal bones & converts it into a tunnel - carpal tunnel. The flexor tendons of forearm along with the median nerve, pass deep to the retinaculum, to

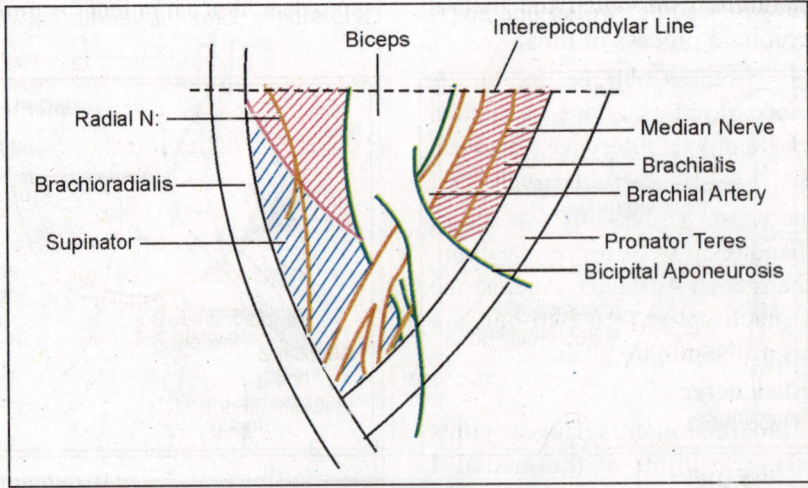

Fig. 3.16: Cubital Fossa

the hand. Ulnar nerve & vessels pass superficial to the retinaculum.

Carpal tunnel syndrome

There is usually compression of median nerve in the carpal tunnel, due to synovitis of accompanying tendons. There will be waisting of thenar muscles and altered sensation on thenar eminence and lateral 3 ½ fingers.

II. Muscles of the back of forearm (Extensor compartment muscles)

(a) Superficial muscles (Fig. 3.17)

1. Brachioradialis
2. Extensor carpi radialis longus
3. Extensor carpi radialis brevis
4. Extensor digitorum
5. Extensor digiti minimi
6. Extensor carpi ulnaris
7. Anconeus

(b) Deep muscles (Fig. 3.18, 19)

1. Abductor pollicis longus
2. Extensor pollicis brevis
3. Extensor pollicis longus
4. Extensor indicis
5. Supinator

The first two are seen along the lateral aspect of forearm.

(a) Superficial muscles

The first three of this group – brachioradialis, extensor carpi radialis longus & brevis are seen on the anterolateral aspect of the forearm.

1. Brachioradialis

Origin: From upper 2/3rd of lateral supracondylar ridge of humerus and the lateral intermuscular septum.

Insertion: Into the lateral side of lower end of radius above styloid process.

Nerve supply: Radial nerve.

Action: It is a flexor of the elbow joint and is most active when the forearm is in midprone position.

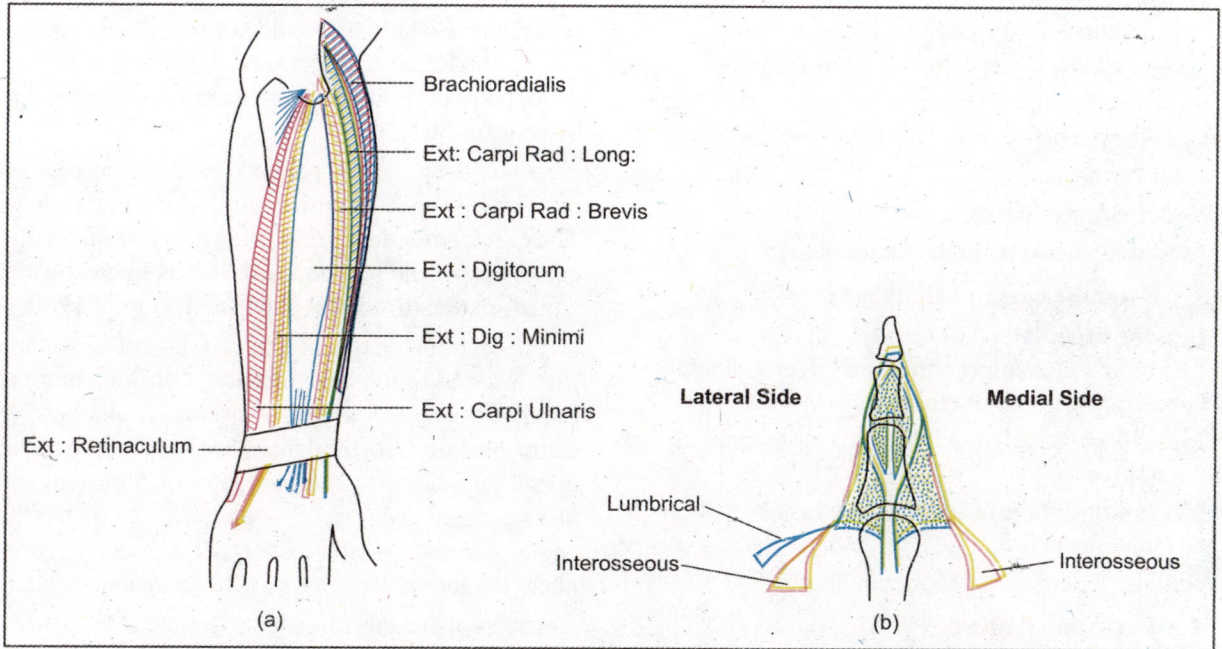

Fig. 3.17: (a) Superficial Extensors of Forearm (b) Extensor Digital Expansion

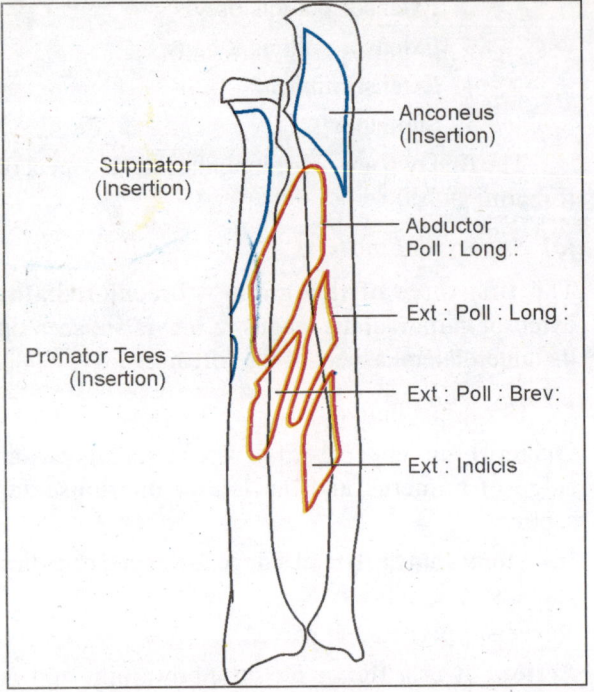

Fig. 3.18: Origins of Deep Extensors of Forearm

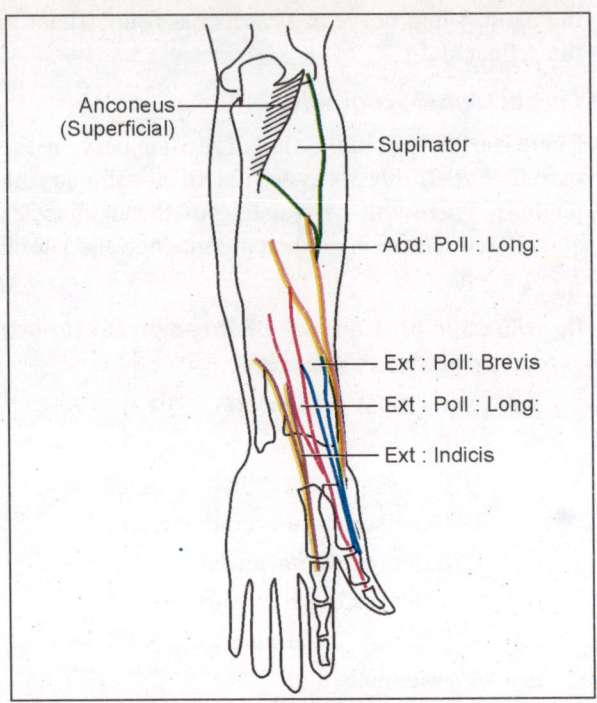

Fig. 3.19: Deep Extensors of Forearm

2. Extensor carpi radialis longus

Origin: From lower 1/3rd of lateral supracondylar ridge of humerus and lateral intermuscular septum.

Insertion: Into the base of 2nd metacarpal, on its dorsal surface.

Nerve supply: Radial nerve

Action: Extension and abduction at wrist.

3. Extensor carpi radialis brevis

Origin: From lateral epicondyle of humerus (by a common extensor tendon) and from the radial collateral ligament of elbow joint.

Insertion: Base of 3rd metacarpal bone on its dorsum.

Nerve supply: Posterior interosseous nerve (branch of radial nerve).

Action: Extension & abduction at wrist.

4. Extensor digitorum

Origin: Lateral epicondyle of humerus – common extensor origin.

Insertion: Distally the tendon of the muscle divides into 4, one for each finger other than the thumb. On the dorsum of hand, the 4 tendons are interconnected by thin fibrous bands.

Over the proximal phalanx, each tendon divides into 3 slips - one intermediate & 2 collateral ones. They get embedded in a triangular aponeurotic expansion of the tendon itself, that is known as the dorsal- extensor- digital expansion. (Fig. 3.17 b)

In each finger, the intermediate slip of the tendon gets inserted to the base of middle phalanx and the 2 collateral slips join to get inserted to the base of distal phalanx. To the lateral angle of the base of dorsal digital expansion, one lumbrical muscle and one interosseous muscle get attached. To its medial angle, one interosseous alone gets attached. These make the lateral margins of the expansion, thick.

Nerve supply: Posterior interosseous nerve.

Action: Extension of wrist joint, metacarpo-phalangeal, and interphalangeal joints of fingers.

5. Extensor digiti minimi

Origin: Common extensor origin from lateral epicondyle of humerus.

Insertion: Its tendon joins the tendon of extensor digitorum for the little finger and is inserted through dorsal digital expansion, to bases of middle & distal phalanges.

Nerve supply: Posterior interosseous nerve.

Action: Extension of wrist, and little finger.

6. Extensor carpi ulnaris

Origin: From lateral epicondyle, through common extensor origin and also from the posterior border of ulna through an aponeurosis common for flexor digitorum profundus and flexor carpi ulnaris.

Insertion: Medial side of base of 5th metacarpal bone.

Nerve supply: Posterior interosseous nerve.

Action: Extension at wrist and adduction of the hand.

7. Anconeus

A triangular muscle.

Origin: From lateral epicondyle of humerus, by a separate tendon.

Insertion: To the lateral side of olecranon process and upper 1/4th of posterior surface of ulna.

Nerve supply: Nerve to anconeus, from radial nerve

Action: It is a weak extensor of elbow joint.

Tendons of the muscles of the extensor compartment (other than brachioradialis) pass deep to extensor retinaculum to reach the dorsum of hand.

(b) Deep muscles (Fig. 3.18, 3.19)

1. Abductor pollicis longus

Origin: From posterior surfaces of ulna and radius below the insertion of Anconeus & supinator and from the intervening interosseous membrane.

Insertion: To the base of 1st metacarpal bone on its lateral side and to trapezium.

Nerve supply: Posterior interosseous nerve.

Action: Abduction & extension of thumb.

2. Extensor pollicis brevis

Origin: From posterior surface of radius and from interosseous membrane (below the origin of abductor pollicis longus).

Insertion: Base of proximal phalanx of thumb.

Nerve supply: Posterior interosseous nerve.

Action: Extension of thumb.

3. Extensor pollicis longus

Origin: From posterior surface of ulna & interosseous membrane below the origin of abductor pollicis longus.

Insertion: Base of distal phalanx of thumb.

Nerve supply: Posterior interosseous nerve

Action: Extension of thumb

Anatomical snuff box: When the thumb is fully extended, a triangular depression is seen on the dorsum of wrist, laterally. This is known as anatomical snuff box. Bounded laterally by tendons of Abductor pollicis longus & extensor pollicis breivis and medially by tendon of extensor pollicis longus. In its floor, lie the styloid process of radius, scaphoid, Trapezium & base of 1st metacarpal bone. The fossa is crossed by radial artery.

4. Extensor indicis

Origin: From posterior surface of ulna & the interosseous membrane, below the origin of extensor pollicis longus.

Insertion: Its tendon goes along with that of extensor digitorum for index finger and joins the extensor expansion.

Nerve supply: Posterior interosseous nerve.

Action: Extension of index finger and wrist.

5. Supinator

Origin: From the following parts:
- Lateral epicondyle of humerus.
- Radial collateral ligament of elbow joint.
- Annular ligament of superior radioulnar joint.
- Supinator crest of ulna & area in front of it.

Insertion: The muscle wraps, round the upper 1/3rd of radius to get inserted to the posterior, lateral and anterior surfaces of upper 1/3rd of radius.

Nerve supply: Deep branch of radial nerve.

Action: Supination of forearm.

Extensor retinaculum (Fig. 3.20 c, d)

It is a fibrous band seen obliquely at the back of wrist. Formed of thickening of deep fascia, it is about 2.5 cms broad, and holds the extensor tendons in position.

Attachments: Laterally to the lower end of anterior border of radius. Medially to the pisiform and triquetral bones and styloid process of ulna. Deep to it, tendons are arranged in six compartments.

Palmar aponeurosis (Fig. 3.21)

It is a triangular band of thickened deep fascia at the central part of palm. Triangular in shape, apex directed proximally where tendon of palmaris longus is attached. Distal border is the base. It divides into 4 slips at the base of each finger. Each slip further divides into two and go deep to get attached to the deep transverse metacarpal ligament. Through the gap between the slips, flexor tendons pass to the fingers. From the lateral borders of the aponeurosis, their fascial covering extend over the thenar and hypothenar muscles.

It overlies and protects the deeper lying vessels, nerves, tendons and muscles. Earlier it was customary to describe potential fascial spaces in the

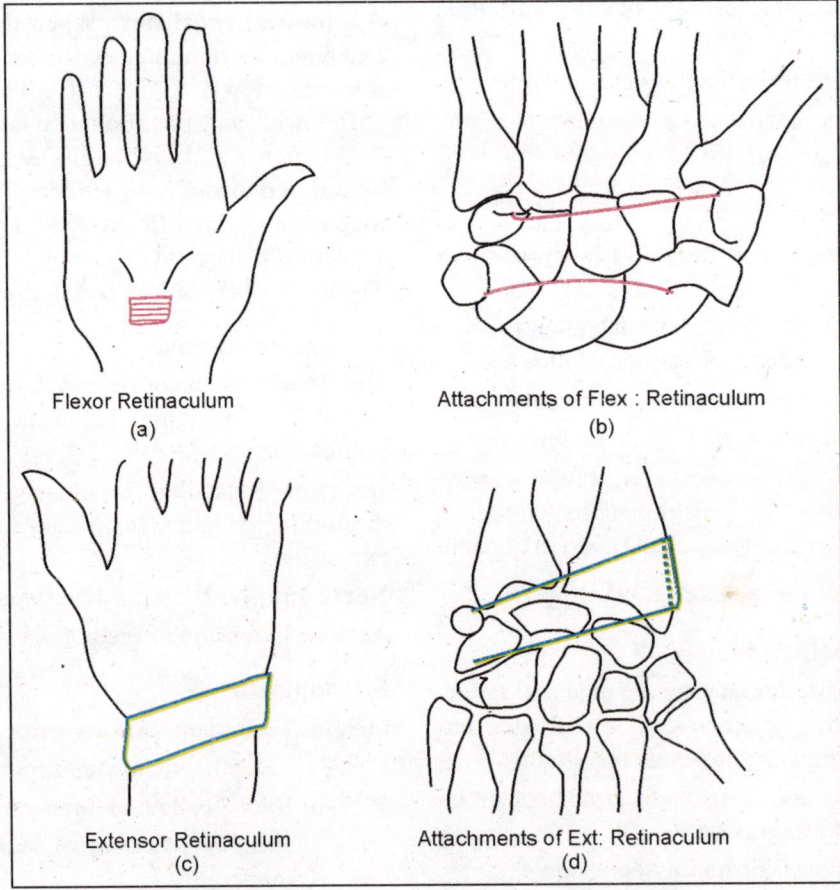

Flexor Retinaculum
(a)

Attachments of Flex : Retinaculum
(b)

Extensor Retinaculum
(c)

Attachments of Ext: Retinaculum
(d)

Fig. 3.20: Flexor and extensor retinacula.

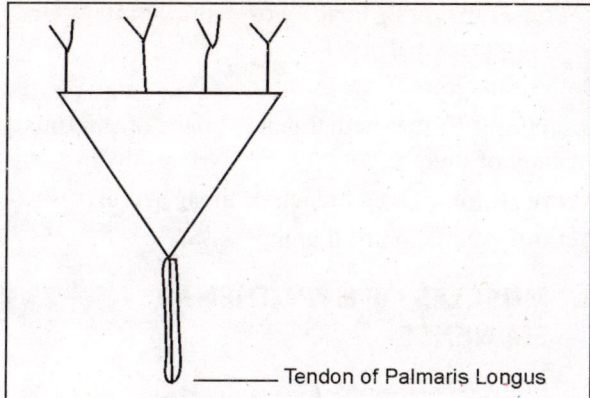

Fig. 3.21: Palmar Aponeurosis

palm deep to the aponeurosis which are of clinical significance. But it is difficult to define margins of such palmar spaces. So the present concept is to know the structures in the palm deep to the aponeurosis and not to deliniate the boundaries of such potential spaces.

MUSCLES OF HAND

Three groups

I. Muscles that act on the thumb (Fig. 3.22)

They are:

1. Abductor pollicis brevis
2. Flexor pollicis brevis
3. Opponens pollicis
4. Adductor pollicis

First 3 of these form thenar eminence.

II. Muscles that act on the little finger (Fig. 3.22)

They are:

1. Abductor digiti minimi brevis
2. Flexor digiti minimi
3. Opponens digiti minimi

These together with palmaris brevis, form the hypothenar eminence.

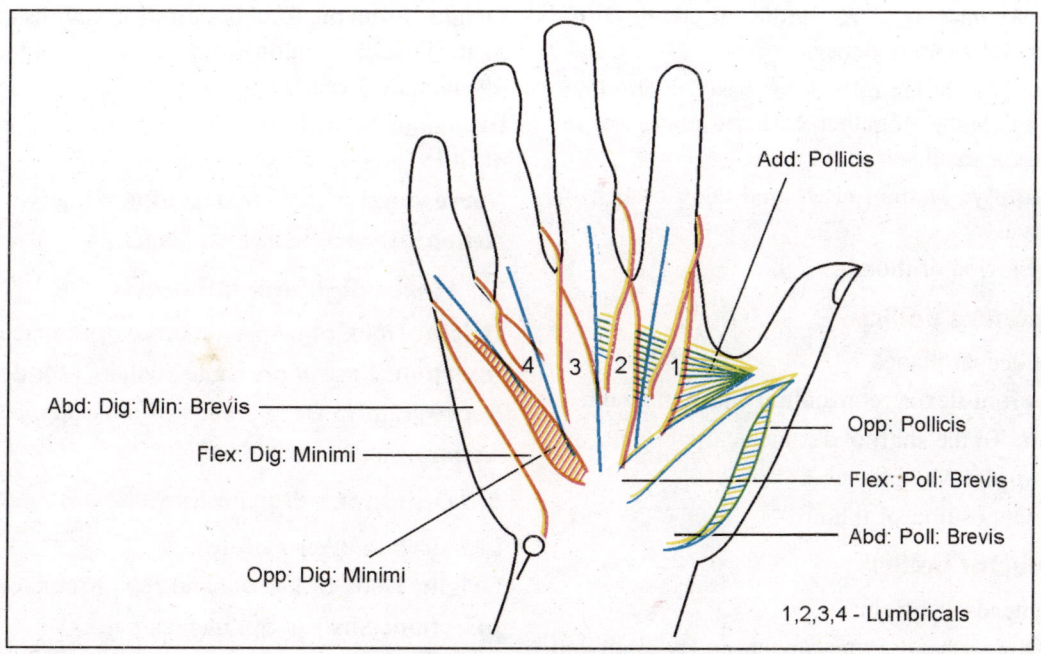

Fig. 3.22: Muscles of Hand

III. Muscles that act on other fingers. They are interossei and lumbricals

1. 4 palmar interossei
2. 4 dorsal interossei
3. 4 lumbricals

I. THENAR MUSCLES AND ADDUCTOR OF THUMB

All the 3 muscles of thenar eminence take origin from flexor retinaculum and adjacent carpal bones.

1. Abductor pollicis brevis

Lies laterally in the thenar eminence.

Origin: From flexor relinaculum and from tubercles of scaphoid and trapezium.

Insertion: Lateral side of base of proximal phalanx of thumb.

Action: Abduction of thumb.

Nerve supply: Median nerve.

2. Flexor pollicis brevis

Lies medial to abductor.

Origin: From flexor retinaculum, trapezium, trapezoid and capitate bones.

Insertion: To the lateral side of base of proximal phalanx of thumb, together with the abductor. Its tendon has a small sesamoid bone.

Nerve supply: Median nerve and deep branch of ulnar nerve.

Action: Flexion of thumb.

3. Opponens pollicis

Lies in a deeper plane.

Origin: From flexor retinaculum and trapezium.

Insertion: To the shaft of 1st metacarpal bone.

Nerve supply: Median nerve

Action: Opposition of thumb

4. Adductor pollicis

Has two heads of origin:

1. Oblique head: From capitate and bases of 2nd and 3rd metacarpals.

2. Transverse head: From the shaft of 3rd metacarpal.

Both heads join.

Insertion: To the medial side of base of proximal phalanx of thumb.

Nerve supply: Deep branch of ulnar nerve.

Action: Adduction of thumb.

II. MUSCLES OF HYPOTHENAR EMINENCE

1. Palmaris brevis

It is a subcutaneous muscle of quadrangular shape, lies beneath the skin of hypothenar eminence.

Origin: From flexor retinaculum and palmar aponeurosis.

Insertion: Skin of medial border of palm.

Nerve supply: Superficial branch of ulnar nerve.

Action: Wrinkles the skin of hypothenar eminence and helps to have a better grip.

2. Abductor digiti minimi

Origin: From pisiform bone and structures attached to it. That is, tendon of flexor carpi ulnaris and pisohamate ligament.

Insertion: Medial side of base of proximal phalanx of little finger.

Nerve supply: Deep branch of ulnar nerve.

Action: Abduction of little finger.

3. Flexor digiti minimi brevis

Origin: Hook of hamate and flexor retinaculum.

Insertion: Base of proximal phalanx of little finger.

Nerve supply: Deep branch of ulnar nerve.

Action: Flexion of little finger.

4. Opponens digiti minimi

Lies deep to other muscles.

Origin: Hook of hamate and flexor retinaculum.

Insertion: Shaft of 5th metacarpal.

Nerve supply: Deep branch of ulnar nerve.

Action: Brings the little finger in opposition with thumb.

III. INTEROSSEI AND LUMBRICALS (Fig. 3.23,24,25)

There are 4 dorsal and 4 palmar interossei. They occupy spaces between metacarpal bones – hence the name.

There are 4 lumbricals attached to the 4 tendons of flexor digitorum profundus.

1. Interossei

(a) Palmar

Origin: 1st one originates from the medial side of base of 1st metacarpal bone. 2nd, 3rd and 4th, from the anterior surfaces of the shafts of the corresponding metacarpals.

Insertion: 1st and 2nd, to the medial sides of bases of proximal phalanges. 3rd and 4th to the lateral sides of bases of proximal phalanges. Their insertions reach the dorsal digital expansion.

(b) Dorsal

Origin: The 4 dorsal interossei originate from the adjacent sides of metacarpal bones – 1st - from 1st and 2nd bones, 2nd -from 2nd and 3rd bones, 3rd - from 3rd and 4th bones and 4th - form the 4th and 5th bones.

Insertion: 1st and 2nd are inserted to the lateral sides of bases of proximal phalanges. 2nd and 3rd are inserted to the medial sides of bases of 3rd and 4th phalanges. Also they reach the extensor expansion

Nerve supply: Deep branch of ulnar nerve.

Action: Palmar interossei adduct the fingers and dorsal interossei abduct the fingers. They also help in flexion of metacarpo phalangeal joints.

2. Lumbricals:

4 in number. Originate from the four tendons of flexor digitorum profundus.

Inserted to the lateral side of corresponding extensor expansion.

Nerve Supply:

1st and 2nd – median nerve.

3rd and 4th – deep branch of ulnar nerve.

Action: They flex the metacarpophalangeal joints and extend the interphalangeal joints.

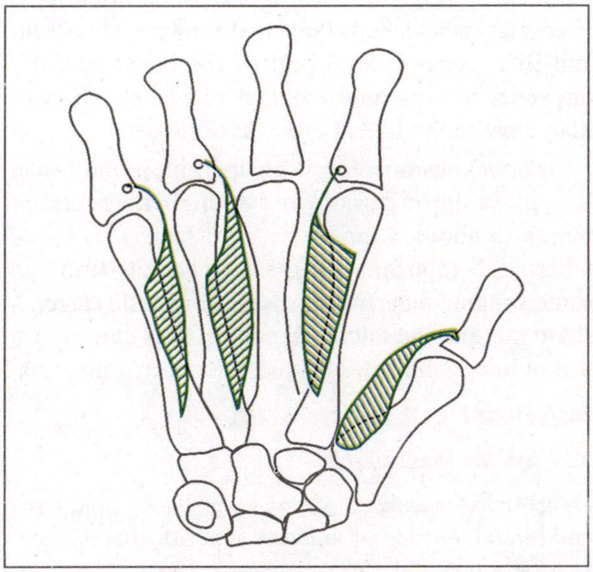

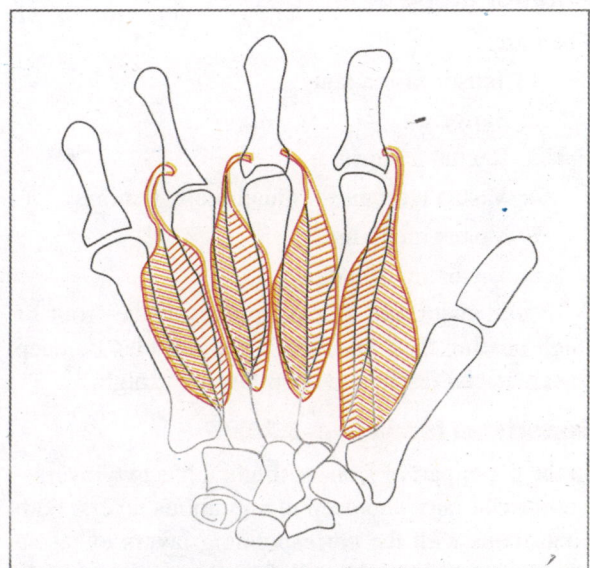

Fig. 3.23: Palmar Interossei

Fig. 3.24: Dorsal Interossei

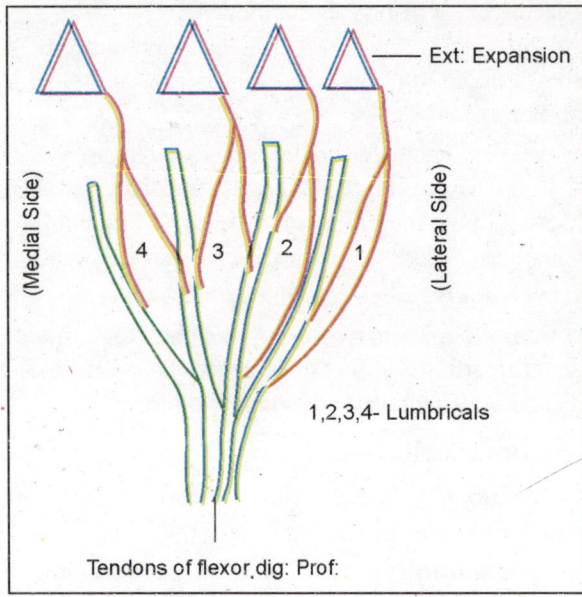

Fig. 3.25: Attachments of Lumbricals

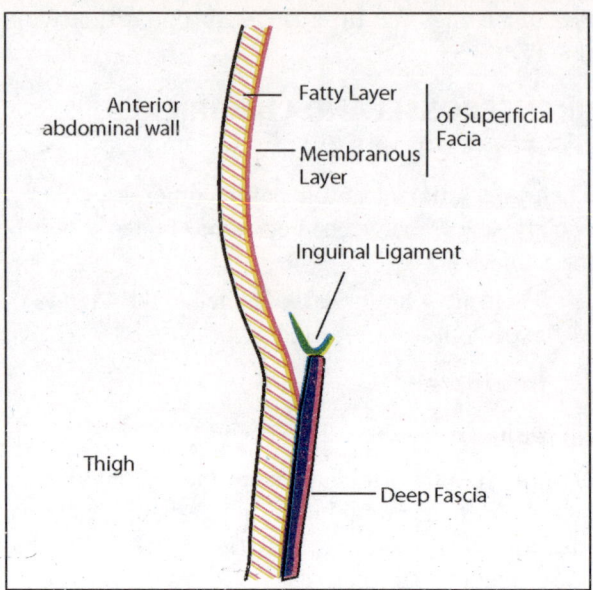

Fig. 3.26: Fascia of Thigh

MUSCLES OF LOWER LIMB

MUSCLES OF THE THIGH

Anterior group of muscles

They are,

1. Tensor fascia lata
2. Sartorius
3. Rectus femoris
4. Vastus lateralis   Quadriceps femoris
5. Vastus medialis
6. Vastus intermedius

Psoas major and iliacus appear on the front of thigh nearing their insertions. The muscles lie deep to superficial fascia and deep fascia of thigh.

Superficial fascia (Fig. 3.26)

In the upper part of front of thigh, it has two layers – Superficial fatty and deep membranous layers, both continuous with the corresponding layers of fascia of anterior abdominal wall. The deep membranous layer fuses with the deep fascia below the inguinal ligament and the superficial layer continues down the thigh.

Deep fascia (Fig. 3.26)

Deep fascia of thigh is thin posteriorly and thick on the front of thigh where it is known as fascia lata. Fascia lata is attached above to the inguinal ligament and iliac crest. Lateral part of the fascia is more thickened to form iliotibial tract which extends from iliac crest to the lateral condyle of tibia.

Saphenous opening is an aperture in the fascia lata, in the upper part of front of thigh, the centre of which is about 3 cm below and lateral to pubic tubercle. It transmits the great saphenous vein and some smaller superficial vessels. (Fig. 3.27) It has a sharp margin, the falciform margin. It is closed by a pad of loose connective tissue, the cribriform fascia.

Muscles (Fig. 3.28 and 3.29)

1. Tensor fascia lata

Origin: From outer 5 cm of outer lip of iliac crest and lateral surface of anterior superior iliac spine.

Insertion: Muscle extends down to about upper 1/3rd of thigh and is inserted into iliotibial tract.

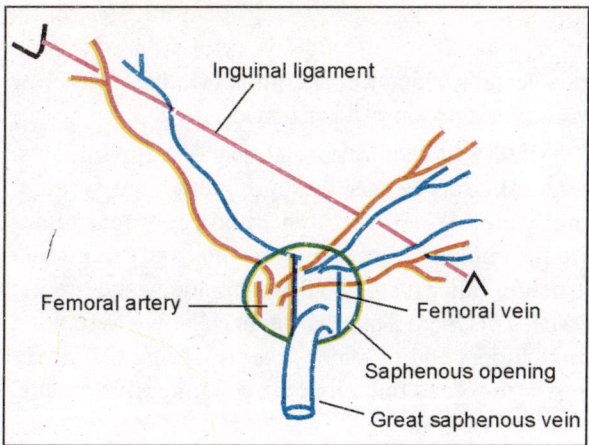

Fig. 3.27: Saphenous Opening

Nerve supply: Superior gluteal nerve

Actions:

1. Extension and lateral rotation at knee joint.
2. Abduction and medial rotation at hip joint.
3. Stabilises the pelvis on femur and femur on tibia in upright posture.

2. Sartorius

It is a narrow strap like muscle and is the longest muscle in the body.

Origin: Anterior superior iliac spine.

Insertion: Upper part of medial surface of tibia.

Nerve supply: Femoral nerve.

Actions:

1. Flexion at knee joint
2. Flexion, abduction and lateral rotation at hip joint.

3. Quadriceps femoris (Fig. 3.29)

The four constituents of this muscle – rectus femoris, vastus medialis, lateralis and intermedius – they cover the front and sides of the femur. Together they constitute a single tendon which is inserted into the upper border of patella and through ligamentum patellae, to the tibial tuberosity. Supplied by femoral nerve. Quadriceps femoris is the great extensor at knee joint. Rectus femoris flexes the thigh at hip joint also.

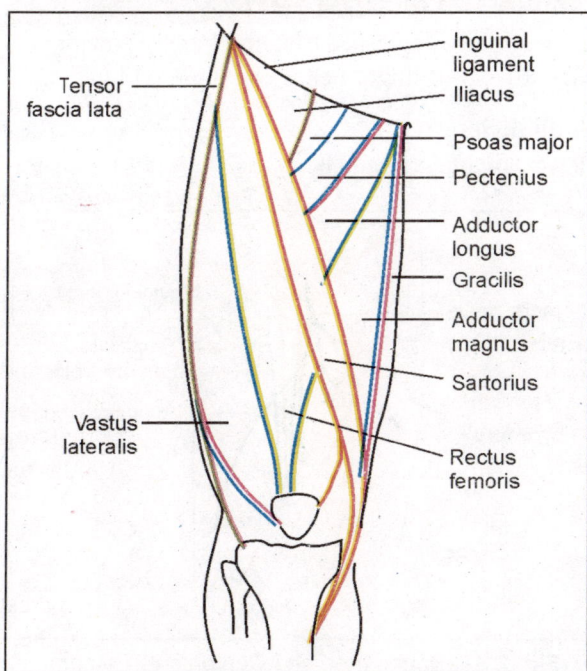

Fig. 3.28: Muscles of Front of Thigh

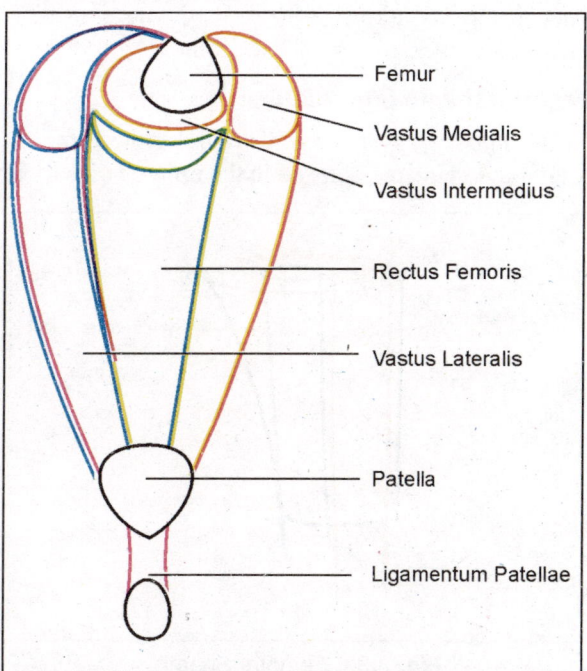

Fig. 3.29: C.S. of thigh to show quadriceps femoris

Origin of individual muscle:

Rectus femoris

Two heads of origin

1. Straight head from anterior inferior iliac spine.
2. Reflected head from just above acetabulum.

Vastus medialis

1. Intertrochanteric line – lower part
2. Medial lip of linea aspera.

Vastus lateralis

1. Upper part of intertrochanteric line.
2. Lateral lip of linea aspera.

Vastus intermedius

Lies deep to rectus femoris. Originates from.

1. Anterior surface of shaft of femur.
2. Lateral surface of shaft of femur.

Articularis genu is a small muscle considered as a detached part of vastus intermedius. It originates from lower part of anterior surface of shaft of femur and inserted into a fold of synovial membrane of knee joint. Its action is to pull up the synovial membrane in extension of knee joint.

Femoral sheath (Fig. 3.30)

In the upper part of femoral triangle, the femoral artery and vein are enclosed in the upper 3 cms by a funnel shaped fascial covering- Femoral sheath. Its anterior wall is formed by extension of fascia transversalis of anterior abdominal wall and posterior wall by extension of fascia iliaca.

Cavity of femoral sheath has 3 compartments. Femoral artery passes through lateral compartment and femoral vein through middle compartment. Medial compartment does not contain any important structure other than 2 or 3 lymph nodes and areolar tissue. This medial compartment is known as femoral canal, upper end of which is femoral ring that opens into abdomen, but closed by connective tissue, femoral septum.

Clinical importance: Femoral canal is a week region below the abdominal wall. In conditions of sustained stress in abdomen as in chronic cough etc. there is a chance of protrusion of abdominal contents - peritonium, small intestine etc through the femoral ring into canal – Femoral hernia. Presents as a soft swelling below inguinal ligament. More common in females due to wider pelvis.

Femoral triangle (Fig. 3.31)

It is a slightly depressed triangular area in the upper part of front of thigh, below the inguinal ligament.

Boundaries:

Base – Inguinal ligament

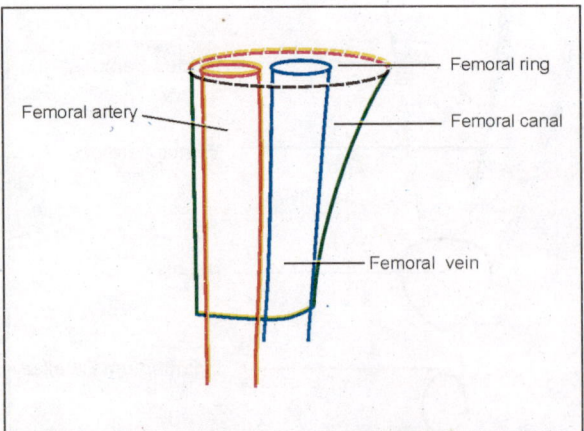

Fig. 3.30: Femoral Sheath

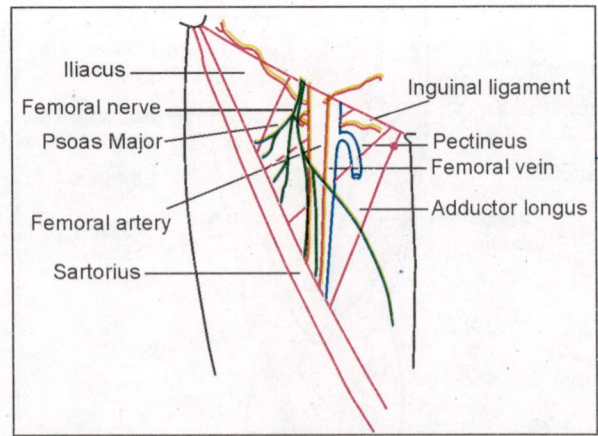

Fig. 3.31: Boundaries and Contents of Femoral Triangle

Laterally – Sartorius

Medially – Medial border of adductor longus.

Apex – The medial and lateral borders meet and is continuous with adductor canal.

Roof – Fascia of thigh with superficial inguinal lymph nodes and superficial branches of the vessels and nerves.

Floor – From lateral to medial, the iliopsoas, pectineus and adductor longus.

Contents:

1. Femoral nerve and branches.
2. Femoral artery and vein inside femoral sheath.
3. Deep inguinal lymph nodes.
4. Branches of femoral artery.
5. Great saphenous vein.

Adductor canal (subsartorial canal) (Fig. 3.32)

It is an intermuscular aponeurotic tunnel located on the medial part of the middle 1/3rd of thigh extending from the apex of the femoral triangle to the opening in the adductor magnus. On section it is triangular in shape.

Boundaries:

Laterally – Vastus medialis

Posteriorly – Adductor longus in the upper part and adductor magnus in the lower part.

Anteromedially – A strong aponeurosis that stretches between lateral and posterior walls.

Over the aponeurosis, sartorius is placed.

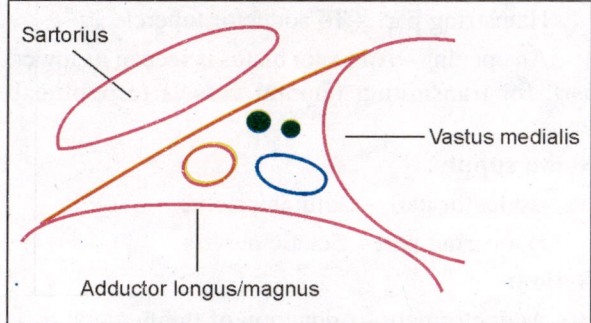

Fig. 3.32: C.S. of adductor canal

Contents:

1. Femoral artery,
2. Femoral vein,
3. Saphenous nerve and
4. Nerve to vastus medialis.

Medial Group of Muscles (Fig. 3.33 – 3.35)

Muscles of the medial side of thigh are generally known as adductors of thigh. They are,

1. Gracilis,
2. Pectineus,
3. Adductor longus,
4. Adductor brevis,
5. Adductor magnus.

1. Gracilis

It is a narrow flat muscle.

Origin: Medial margin of pubic arch.

Insertion: Upper part of medial surface of tibia.

Nerve supply: Obturator nerve.

Actions: Flexion of leg at knee joint, adduction of thigh at hip joint.

2. Pectineus

Origin: Superior ramus of pubis.

Insertion: On the posterior aspect of femur, to a line between lesser trochanter and linea aspera.

Nerve supply: Femoral nerve and obturator nerve.

Action: Adduction and flexion of thigh.

3. Adductor longus

Origin: From the front of body of pubis below and medial to pubic tubercle.

Insertion: Middle 1/3rd of linea aspera.

Nerve supply: Anterior division of obturator nerve.

Action: Adduction and flexion of thigh.

4. Adductor brevis

Lies deep to pectineus and adductor longus.

Origin: Body and inferior ramus of pubis.

Insertion: Upper part of linea aspera.

Nerve supply: Obturator nerve.

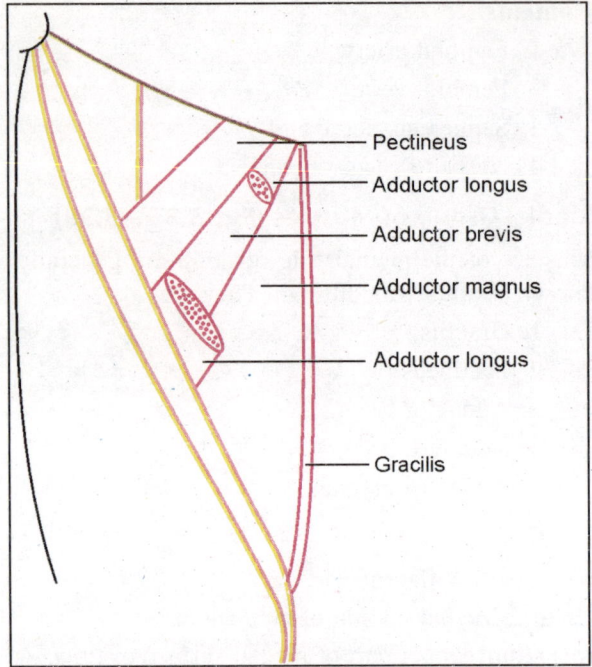

Fig. 3.33: Medial group of thigh muscles

- Pectineus
- Adductor longus
- Adductor brevis
- Adductor magnus
- Adductor longus
- Gracilis

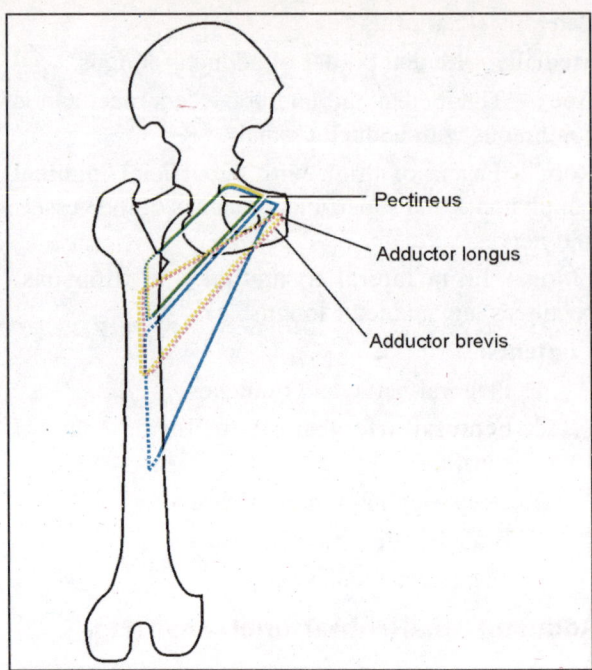

Fig. 3.34

- Pectineus
- Adductor longus
- Adductor brevis

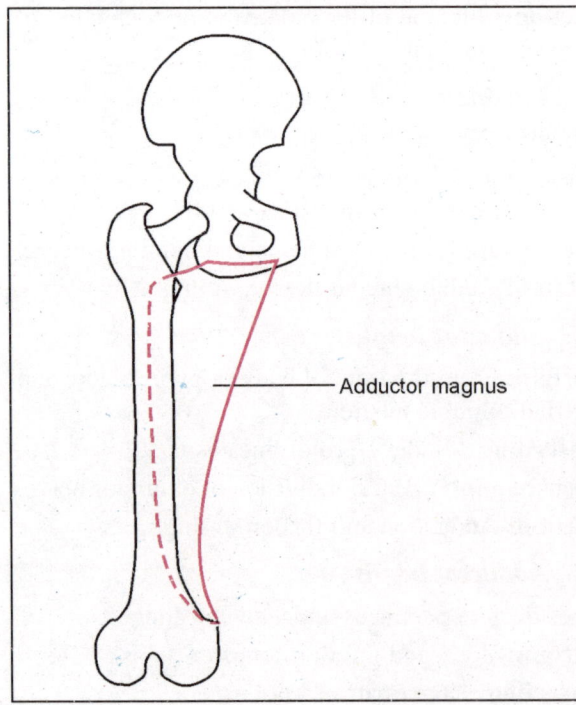

Fig. 3.35: Adductor magnus

- Adductor magnus

Action: Adduction and lateral rotation of thigh.

5. Adductor magnus

A large triangular muscle, has an adductor part and hamstring part.

Origin: Adductor part- From lower part of inferior pubic ramus and ischial ramus.

Hamstring part- From ischial tuberosity.

Insertion: Adductor part along the linea aspera upto medial supracondylar line.

Hamstring part – To adductor tubercle.

An opening – Adductor hiatus is seen in its lower part, for transmiting femoral vessels to popliteal fossa.

Nerve supply:

Adductor part – Obturator nerve

Hamstring part – Sciatic nerve

Action:

Adductor part – Adduction of thigh

Hamstring part – Extension of thigh

POSTERIOR GROUP OF MUSCLES (Fig. 3.36)

They are

1. Biceps femoris
2. Semitendinosus
3. Semimembranosus

Known as hamstring muscles. They act at both hip and knee joints – Extension of thigh and flexion of knee.

1. Biceps femoris – Two heads of origin

Origin: Long head, from the ischeal tuberosity together with semitendinosus. Short head, from the lateral lip of linea aspera and lateral supracondylar ridge.

Insertion: The common tendon is inserted into the head of fibula.

Nerve supply:

Long head – Tibial part of sciatic nerve.

Short head – Common peroneal part of sciatic nerve

Action: Flexion at knee joint and extension at hip joint.

2. Semitendinosus

Origin: Ischial tuberosity.

Insertion: It has a long tendon, inserted on to the upper part of medial surface of tibia.

Nerve supply: Tibial part of sciatic nerve.

Action: Flexion of leg at knee joint and extension of thigh at hip joint.

3. Semimembranosus

Origin: Ischial tuberosity.

Insertion: Posteromedial part of the medial condyle of tibia.

Nerve supply: Tibial part of sciatic nerve.

Action: Flexion at knee joint and extension at hip joint.

Muscles of Gluteal Region (Fig. 3.36, 37, 38, 39)

1. Gluteus maximus
2. Gluteus medius
3. Gluteus minimus
4. Piriformis
5. Obturator internus
6. Obturator externus

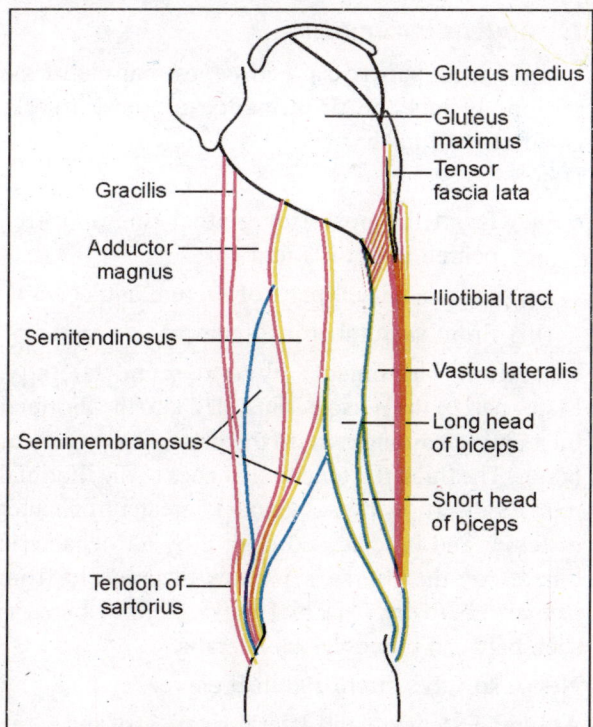

Fig. 3.36: Muscles of Back of Thigh

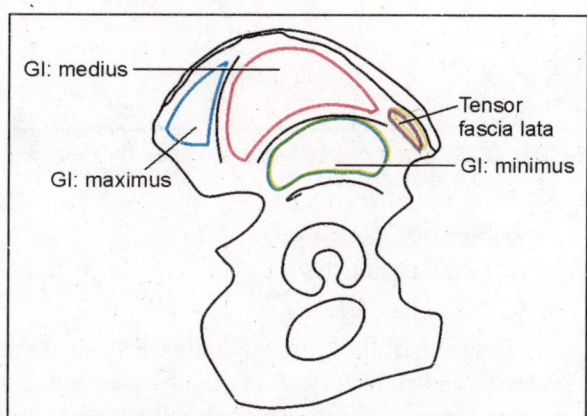

Fig. 3.37: Origin of Gluteal Muscles

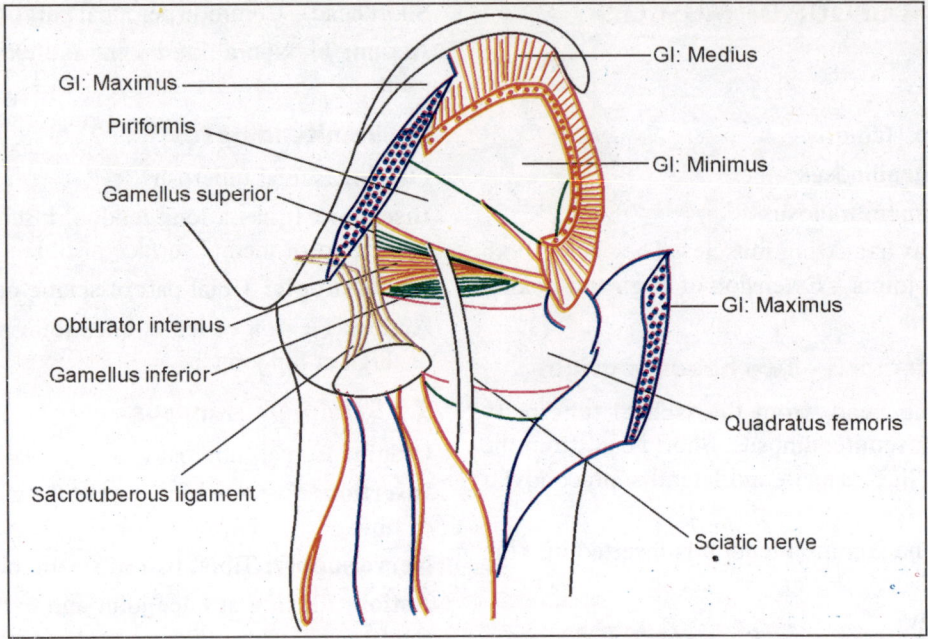

Fig. 3.38: Deep Muscles of Gluteal region

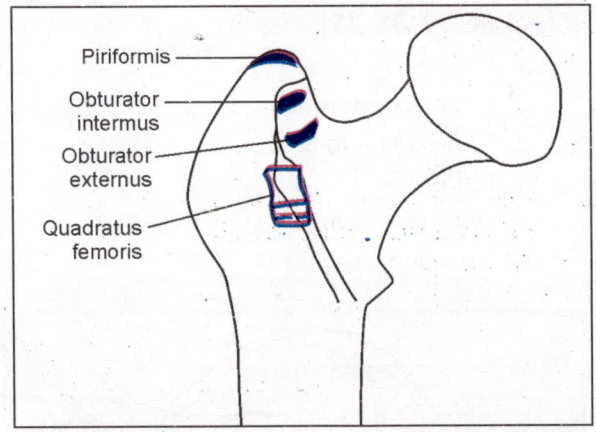

Fig. 3.39: Insertions of Deep Muscles on Femur

7. Superior gamellus
8. Inferior gamellus
9. Quadratus femoris

First three of these are large muscles and act as extensors and abductors of thigh, others are smaller muscles, deep to the larger ones and act as lateral rotators of thigh.

1. Gluteus maximus

It is the most superficial and largest muscle of the region. Froms the prominence of the buttock. Quadrelateral in shape.

Origin:

(i) From the posterior gluteal line and area behind it on the ilium.

(ii) From adjacent parts of sacrum and coccyx.

(iii) From sacrotuberous ligament.

Insertion: The muscle fibers descend laterally. Major part of the muscle is inserted into the iliotibial tract and remaining part, to the gluteal tuberosity of femur. The thick flat tendon that goes to the iliotibial tract for insertion, passes lateral to greater trochanter of femur and is separated from it by a trochanteric bursa. Another bursa separates the muscle from ischial tuberosity – Ischial bursa. A third bursa is seen between it and vastus lateralis.

Nerve supply: Inferior gluteal nerve.

Action: Extension and lateral rotation of hip joint. Its upper fibers abduct the thigh at hip joint. Through iliotibial tract it stabilises femur on tibia. Active in walking and climbing stairs.

2. Gluteus medius

A fan shaped thick muscle, Partly covered by gluteus maximus.

Origin: From the outer surface of ilium between anterior and posterior gluteal lines.

Insertion: Lateral surface of greater trochanter.

Nerve supply: Superior gluteal nerve.

Action: Abduction and medial rotation of thigh at hip joint.

3. Gluteus minimus

It is also a fan shaped muscle deep to gluteus medius.

Origin: From outer surface of ilium between inferior and anterior gluteal lines.

Insertion: Anterior border of greater trochanter.

Nerve supply: Superior gluteal nerve.

Action: Abduction and medial rotation of thigh at hip joint.

The three gluteal muscles act to steady the pelvis on lower limb while walking or running. Gluteus medius and minimus support the trunk upright when the foot of the opposite side is off the ground. When these two muscles are paralised, if the patient stands on the affected side's limb, the pelvis sinks to that side- Trendelenberg's sign positive. The patient will have a lurching gait.

4. Piriformis

Origin: From anterior surface of sacrum by three digitations, within the pelvis. Emerges into the gluteal region through greater sciatic foramen.

Insertion: Upper border of greater trochanter.

Nerve supply: Branches from S1 and S2 nerves.

Action: Lateral rotation and abduction of thigh.

5. Obturator internus

Origin: From the pelvic surface of obturator membrane and bone around it. Muscle comes out of pelvis to the gluteal region through lesser sciatic foramen.

Insertion: Its tendon is joined by tendons of gamellus superior and inferior and gets inserted on the upper part of medial surface of greater trochanter (inferior to the insertion of piriformis).

Nerve supply: Nerve to obturator internus – from sacral plexus.

Action: Lateral rotation of thigh at hip joint.

6. Gamellus superior

Origin: From the outer surface of ischial spine.

Insertion: Into tendon of Obturator internus.

Nerve supply: Nerve to obturator internus.

Action: Lateral rotation of thigh.

7. Gamellus inferior

Origin: From upper border of ischial tuberosity.

Insertion: Into tendon of obturator internus.

Nerve supply: Nerve to quadratus femoris.

Action: Lateral rotation of thigh at hip joint.

8. Quadratus femoris

Origin: From lateral border of ischial tuberosity.

Insertion: Into quadrate tubercle.

Nerve supply: Nerve to quadratus femoris, from sacral plexus.

Action: Lateral rotation of thigh.

9. Obturator externus (Fig. 3.40)

Deeply placed muscle.

Origin: From outer surface of obturator membrane and adjacent bony margin.

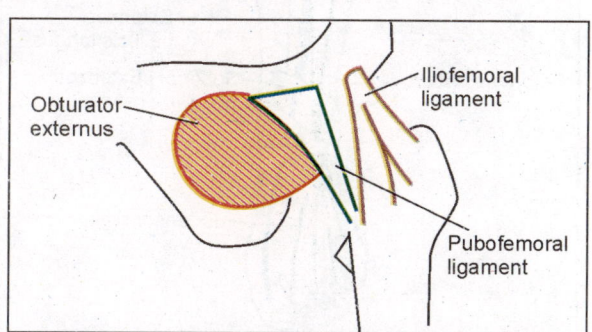

Fig. 3.40: Obturator Externus (Anterior View)

Insertion: The muscle and its tendon spirals back and laterally beneath and then behind the hip joint to get inserted to trochanteric fossa.

Nerve supply: Obturator nerve.

Action: Lateral rotation of thigh.

MUSCLES OF THE LEG

1. Anterior group- Extensor muscles, Produce dorsiflexion of foot. (Extension)
2. Posterior group – Flexors, produce plantar flexion of foot. (Flexion)
3. Lateral group – Peroneal muscles, produce evertion of foot.

ANTERIOR GROUP OF MUSCLES (Fig. 3.41)

They are in the anterior compartment of leg. Muscles are:

1. Tibialis anterior
2. Extensor digitorum longus
3. Extensor hallucis longus

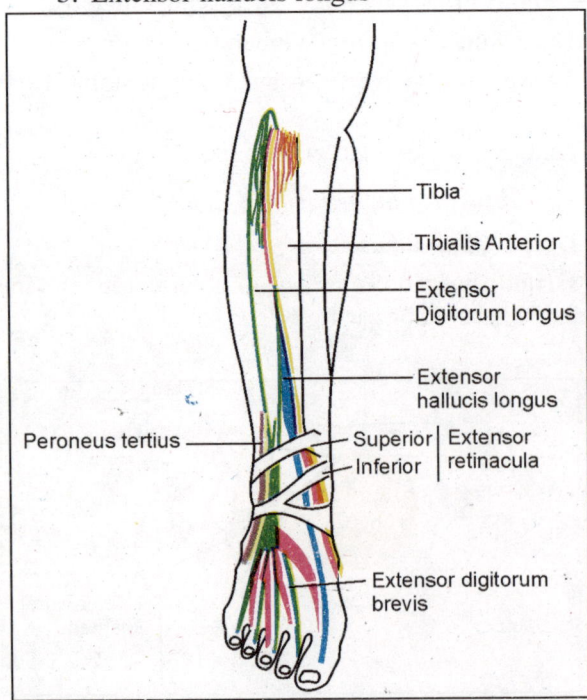

Fig. 3.41: Anterior Compartment of Leg - Muscles

4. Peroneus tertius

Deep peroneal nerve and anterior tibial artery supply the structures in the anterior compartment of leg.

1. Tibialis anterior

Origin: From upper 2/3rd of lateral surface of tibia and interosseous membrane.

Insertion: Medial side of medial cuneiform bone and adjacent part of first metatarsal.

Nerve supply: Deep peroneal nerve.

Action: Dorsiflexion (extension) of foot at ankle and inversion of foot at subtalar joints.

2. Extensor digitorum longus

Origin: From upper 2/3rd of anterior surface of fibula and interosseous membrane.

Insertion: The tendon of the muscle passes deep to extensor retinacula and divides into four slips on the dorsum of foot, going to lateral four toes. Over the proximal phalanx, each tendon expands into a triangular extensor expansion. Within the expansion the central part of tendon goes to get inserted to base of middle phalanx. Two lateral parts of the tendon converge to the base of distal phalanx.

Nerve supply: Deep peroneal nerve.

Action: Extension of toes and dorsiflexion of foot.

3. Extensor hallucis longus

Lies between tibialis anterior and extensor digitorum longus.

Origin: From the middle 1/3rd of medial surface of fibula and interosseous membrane.

Insertion: Tendon passes deep to extensor retinacula and gets inserted to base of distal phalanx of big toe.

Nerve supply: Deep peroneal nerve.

Action: Extension of big toe and extension of ankle.

4. Peroneus tertius

It is a part of extensor digitorum longus. Although it is an evertor of foot, it is seen in the anterior extensor compartment

Origin: Lower 1/3rd of anterior surface of fibula and interosseous membrane.

Insertion: Medial side of dorsum of base of fifth metatarsal.

Nerve supply: Deep peroneal nerve.

Action: Evertion and extension of foot.

LATERAL GROUP OF MUSCLES (FIG. 3.42)

They are the peroneal muscles – Peróneus longus and brevis.

1. Peroneus longus

Origin: From the upper 2/3rd of lateral surface of fibula.

Insertion: Its tendon descends behind the lateral malleolus, in a groove, deep to the superior peroneal retinaculum, together with the tendon of peroneus brevis. Then it passes forwards deep to inferior peroneal retinaculum, crosses the lateral border of cuboid and goes to its under surface in a groove. It

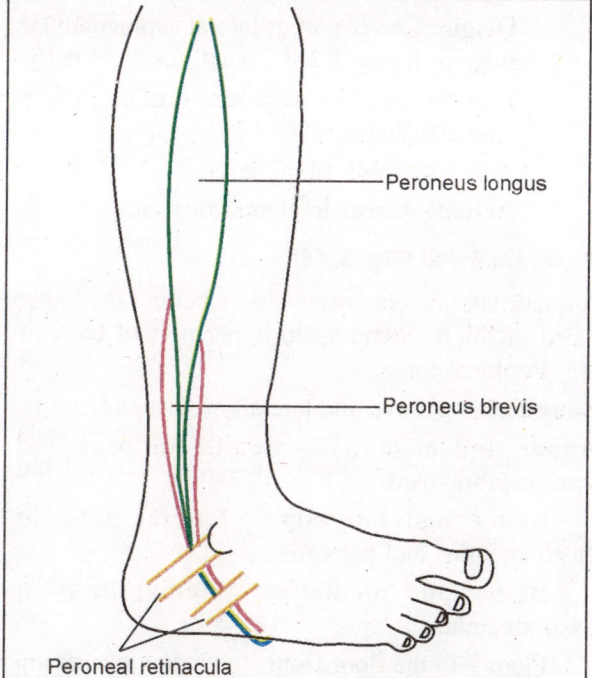

Peroneus longus

Peroneus brevis

Peroneal retinacula

Fig. 3.42: Lateral compartment Muscles - Leg

crosses the sole obliquely and gets inserted on to the base of 1st metatarsal and medial cuneiform on their lateral sides.

Nerve supply: Superficial peroneal nerve.

Action: Eversion of foot and plantar flexion. It has a key role in maintaining the lateral longitudinal arch of foot.

2. Peroneus brevis

Origin: From the lower 2/3rd of lateral surface of fibula.

Insertion: Tendon passes behind the lateral malleolus deep to peroneal retinacula. Gets inserted into tubercle on the base of 5th metatarsal bone.

Nerve supply: Superficial peroneal nerve.

Action: Eversion and plantar flexion of foot.

Superficial peroneal nerve is the nerve of lateral compartment of leg. Branches of the peroneal artery of posterior compartment reach the lateral compartment.

MUSCLES OF POSTERIOR COMPARTMENT (Fig. 3.43 a,b)

They are arranged in two groups.- Superficial and deep, separated by a deep transverse fascia.

1. Superficial group

Muscles are
   (i) Gastrocnemius
   (ii) Soleus
   (iii) Plantaris

2. Deep group

Muscles are
   (i) Popliteus
   (ii) Flexor hallucis longus
   (iii) Flexor digitorum longus
   (iv) Tibialis posterior

Posterior tibial artery is the artery of posterior compartment and tibial nerve is the nerve of the compartment.

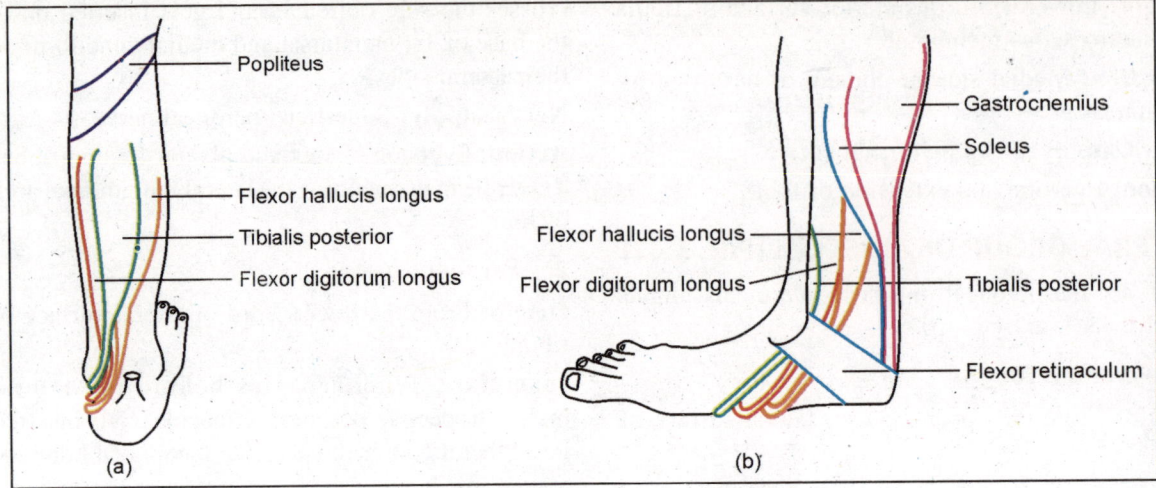

Fig. 3.43: Muscles of Posterior Compartment

1. Superficial muscles

(i) Gastrocnemius: Most superficial of the group.

Origin: Two heads of origin

Lateral head – From the lateral surface of lateral condyle of femur.

Medial head – From the posterior surface of medial condyle of femur.

Both heads arise also from the adjacent parts of capsule of knee joint.

Insertion: The two heads join to form a strong tendon, the tendocalcaneus which is common for all the three superficial muscles. Tendocalcaneus or Achilles tendon is the strongest and thickest tendon in the body. About 15 cm long, is attached to the middle of the posterior surface of calcaneus.

Nerve supply: Tibial nerve

Action: Plantar flexion of foot at ankle joint. It also flexes the knee joint.

(ii) Soleus: Lies deep to gastrocnemius.

Origin: From the soleal line of tibia and upper 1/4th of posterior surface of fibula.

Insertion: Its tendon joins the anterior aspect of tendocalcaneus.

Nerve supply: Tibial nerve

Action: Plantar flexion

(iii) Plantaris

Sometimes the muscle is absent.

Origin: Lower part of lateral supracondylar ridge of femur. It has a small fusiform belly.

Insertion: Its slender tendon joins tendocalcaneus.

Nerve supply: Tibial nerve

Action: Assists in plantar flexion.

Popliteal fossa (Fig. 3.44)

A quadrilateral depression is seen behind the lower 1/3rd of thigh extending to upper part of back of leg- Popliteal fossa.

Boundaries: Above and laterally – biceps femoris

Above and medially – Semitendinosus and semimembranosus.

Below and laterally – Lateral head of gastrocnemius and plantaris.

Below and medially – Medial head of gastrocnemius.

Floor – In the floor from above downwards are – popliteal surface of femur, capsule of knee joint and popliteus muscle.

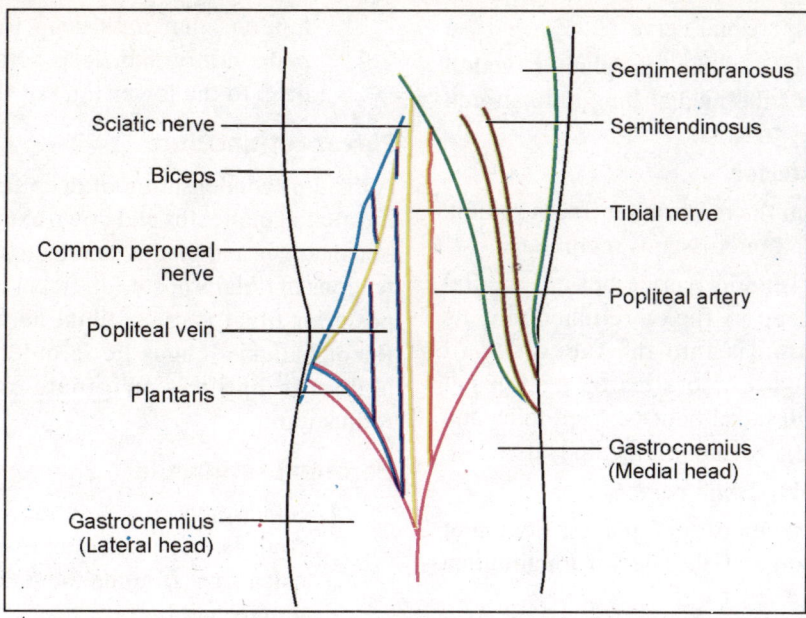

Fig. 3.44: Popliteal Fossa

Contents:

1. Popliteal artery, most anteriorly.
2. Genicular branches of popliteal artery.
3. Popliteal vein behind the artery.
4. Common peroneal nerve discends laterally.
5. Tibial nerve discends vertically.

2. Deep muscles (Fig. 3.43 a,b)

(i) **Popliteus –** Seen in the Popliteal fossa.

Origin: Lateral surface of lateral condyle of femur, inside the knee joint.

Insertion: From within the capsule of knee joint, it comes out through the opening in the lower posterior part of capsule and is inserted to the posterior surface of tibia above soleal line. Within the joint, it separates the lateral meniscus from the lateral ligament of knee joint.

Nerve supply: Nerve to popliteus from tibial nerve.

Action: Lateral rotation of femur on tibia at the initial stage of flexion of knee from extended position – unlocking muscle.

(ii) **Flexor digitorum longus**

Origin: From the medial part of posterior surface of tibia below soleal line.

Insertion: Tendon passes behind the medial malleolus deep to flexor retinaculum and enters the sole. The tendon divides into four tendons that go to the lateral four toes and get inserted to the bases of distal phalanges.

Nerve supply: Tibial nerve

Action: Flexion of toes, Plantar flexion of foot and helps to maintain longitudinal arches of foot.

(iii) **Flexor hallucis longus**

Origin: Lower 2/3rd of posterior surface of fibula.

Insertion: The tendon passes behind the medial malleolus deep to flexor retinaculum. Goes to sole by passing below the sustentaculum tali. In the sole, it gives a slip to the tendon of flexor digitorum longus. Tendon gets inserted to the base of distal phalanx of big toe.

Nerve supply: Tibial nerve

Action: Flexion of big toe, plantar flexion and maintains the medial longitudinal arch of foot.

(iv) **Tibialis posterior**

Origin: From the posterior surfaces of tibia and fibula and interosseous membrane

Insertion: Tendon passes behind medial malleolus deep to flexor retinaculum. Its main insertion is into the tuberosity of navicular bone. Also slips of tendon get inserted to all tarsal bones except talus and bases of 2nd, 3rd and 4th metatarsals.

Nerve supply: Tibial nerve

Action: Invertion of foot, plantar flexion of foot and maintains the medial longitudinal arch of foot

RETINACULA AROUND ANKLE (Fig. 3.41, 42, 43b)

Around the region of ankle, the tendons of the muscles are held down by localized thickenings of deep fascia called retinacula. They are superior and inferior extensor retinacula, flexor retinaculum and peroneal retinacula.

Extensor retinacula

1. **Superior extensor retinaculum**

   Seen just above the front of ankle joint. Laterally attached to the distal end of anterior border of fibula, medially to the anterior border of tibia. It holds down the extensor tendons and peroneus tertius tendon. Anterior tibial artery and deep peroneal nerve pass deep to it.

2. **Inferior extensor retinaculum**

   It is a Y shaped band. Stem of Y is attached laterally to the upper surface of calcaneus. The upper limb of Y is attached to the medial malleolus and lower limb reaches the plantar aponeurosis. The stem and the upper limb of the retinaculum form loops around the tendons that pass deep to them. Dorsalis pedis artery and deep peroneal nerve pass deep to the lower limb of the retinaculum.

Flexor retinaculum

A band of condensation of deep fascia. Attached to the medial malleolus and down to the medial process of calcaneus and plantar aponeurosis. Deep to it, the tendons of tibialis posterior, flexor digitorum longus, posterior tibial vessels, tibial nerve and tendon of flexor hallucis longus lie in order. Many fibers of abductor hallucis originate from the flexor retinaculum.

Peroneal retinacula

1. Superior peroneal retinaculum – Stretches from lateral malleolus to lateral surface of calcaneus, It holds the tendons of peroneus longus and brevis.

2. Inferior peroneal retinaculum – Attached to lateral surface of calcaneus. It holds both the tendons of peroneus longus and brevis.

MUSCLE ON THE DORSUM OF FOOT (Fig. 3.41)

Extensor digitorum brevis

It is a thin muscle.

Origin: From the upper surface of anterior part of calcaneus.

Insertion: The muscle is directed anteriorly and medially and divides into four tendons. Most medial one is called extensor hallucis brevis, gets inserted to the base of proximal phalanx of big toe. Other three tendons go to join the long extensor tendons, to the 2nd, 3rd and 4th toes.

Nerve supply: Deep peroneal nerve.

Action: Extension of the first four toes.

MUSCLES OF THE SOLE

The deep fascia of the sole that covers the muscles is thickened to form plantar aponeurosis.

PLANTAR APONEUROSIS

It is very thick and strong and overlies the flexor digitorum brevis. From its lateral borders, thinner fascia extend over the abductor muscles of big toe and little toe. It is triangular in shape. Apex is attached behind on to the medial process of calcaneal tuberosity. Traced anteriorly it becomes broader. At the bases of the toes, the base of aponeurosis divides into five slips, one for each toe.

At the level of the heads of metatarsals, each slip divides into two. They diverge around the flexor tendons of the toes and fuse with them and also get attached to the deep transverse metatarsal ligaments. Some superficial fibres from each of the five slips pass to get attached to the skin.

Function of plantar aponeurosis is to give firm anchorage to the superficial skin and to protect deeper lying structures. It has a major role in maintaining the longitudinal arches of foot.

Muscles

Muscles of the sole are arranged in four layers.

First layer — Abductor hallucis
Abductor digiti minimi
Flexor digitorum brevis

Second layer — Tendon of flexor digitorum longus
Tendon of flexor hallucis longus
Flexor accessorius
Lumbricals

Third layer — Flexor hallucis brevis
Flexor digiti minimi brevis
Adductor hallucis

Fourth layer — Tendon of tibialis posterior
Tendon of peroneus longus
Interossei

1st layer of muscles (Fig. 3.45)

1. Abductor hallucis

Origin: From the medial tubercle of calcaneus and from flexor retinaculum.

Insertion: Medial side of the base of proximal phalanx of big toe.

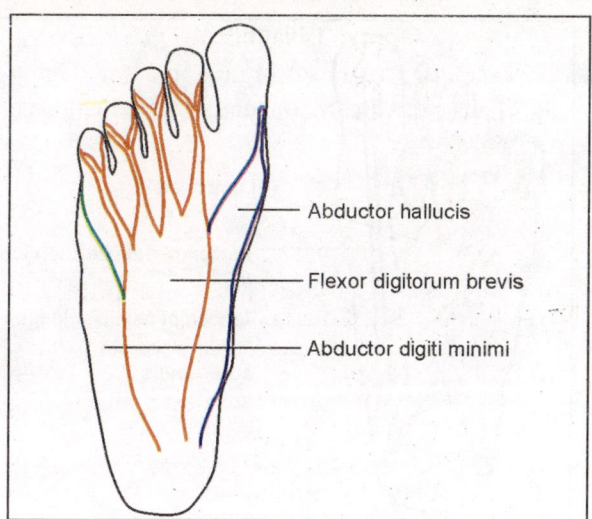

Fig. 3.45: Sole - 1st Layer of Muscles

Nerve supply: Medial plantar nerve

Action: Abduction and flexion of big toe. Helps to maintain medial longitudinal arch of foot.

2. Flexor digitorum brevis

Origin: Medial tubercle of calcaneus.

Insertion: It has four tendons for the lateral four toes. Each tendon divides into two slips between which tendon of flexor digitorum longus passes. The two slips unite, again divides into two slips which get attached to the sides of middle phalanx.

Nerve supply: Medial plantar nerve

Action: Flexion of the lateral four toes and also maintains the medial and lateral longitudinal arches of foot.

3. Abductor digiti minimi

Origin: From the medial and lateral tubercles of calcaneus.

Insertion: Into the lateral side of the base of the proximal phalanx of little toe.

Nerve supply: Lateral plantar nerve

2nd layer of muscles (Fig. 3.46)

1. Flexor digitorum accessorius

Origin: From the medial and lateral sides of calcaneus.

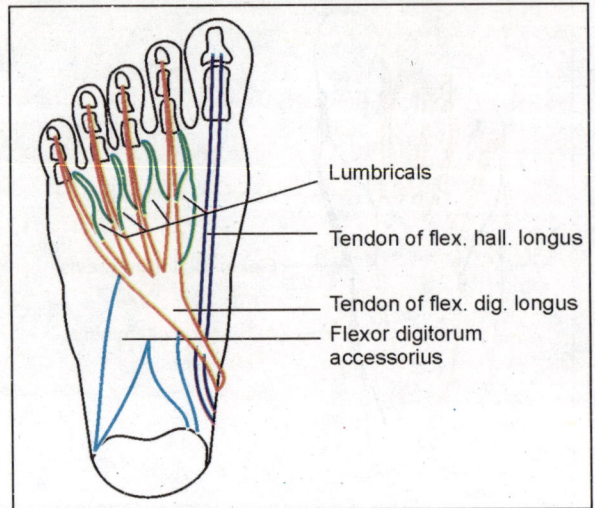

Fig. 3.46: Sole - 2nd Layer of Muscles

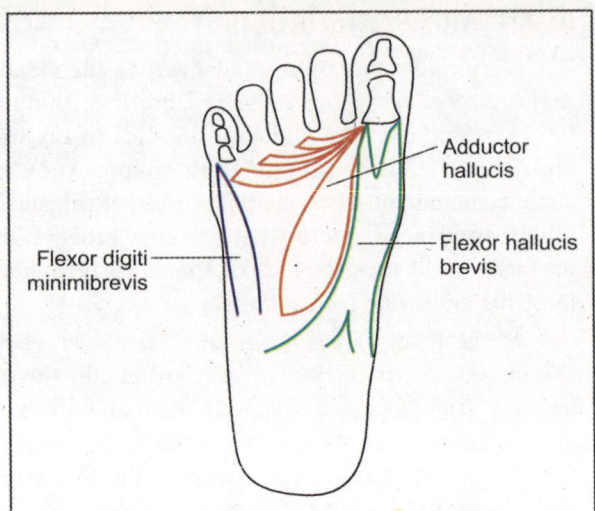

Fig. 3.47: Sole - 3rd Layer of Muscles

Insertion: Into the tendon of flexor digitorum longus.

Nerve supply: Lateral plantar nerve.

Action: It straightens the oblique pull of flexor digitorum longus.

2. Lumbricals

The four slender muscles.

Origin: From the tendons of flexor digitorum longus

Insertion: The slender tendon curves round the medial side of the metatarsophalangeal joint. Gets inserted to the base of proximal phalanx and to the medial side of dorsal digital expansion.

Nerve supply: 1st lumbrical, by medial plantar nerve and lateral 3 lumbricals, by lateral plantar nerve.

Action: Extend the toes at interphalangeal joints.

3. Tendon of flexor digitorum longus

4. Tendon of flexor hallucis longus

(their details discussed earlier)

Muscles of 3rd layer (Fig. 3.47)

1. Flexor hallucis brevis

Origin: From the cuboid and lateral cuneiform bones.

Insertion: The muscle divides into 2 bellies. Tendon of medial belly joins with that of abductor hallucis

and is inserted to the medial side of base of proximal phalanx. Tendon of lateral belly joins with that of abductor hallucis and is inserted to the lateral side of base of proximal phalanx of big toe. A sesamoid bone may be present in each tendon near insertion.

Nerve supply: Medial plantar nerve.

Action: Flexion of big toe.

2. Adductor hallucis

Origin: It has two heads of origin.

Oblique head – From bases of 2nd, 3rd and 4th metatarsals.

Transverse head – From the plantar metatarso-phalangeal ligaments of 3rd, 4th and 5th toes and also from the deep transverse metatarsal ligaments.

Insertion: The combined tendon is inserted into the lateral side of base of proximal phalanx of big toe together with the tendon of flexor hallucis brevis.

Nerve supply: Deep branch of lateral plantar nerve.

Action: Helps flexion of big toe. Also maintains transverse arch of foot.

3. Flexor digiti minimi brevis

Origin: Base of 5th metatarsal bone.

Insertion: It is inserted into lateral side of base of proximal phalanx of little toe.

Nerve supply: Lateral plantar nerve.

Action: Flexion of little toe.

4th layer of muscles

1. Tendon of tibialis posterior

It goes behind medial malleolus and beneath plantar calcaneonavicular ligament to the sole towards its extensive insertion.

2. Tendon of peroneus longus

As this tendon goes to its insertion, it goes deep to long plantar ligament, in a groove.

3. Interrossei (Fig. 3.48)

Dorsal interossei: Four in number. Seen between the metatarsal bones. They are bipennate muscles arising from the sides of adjacent metatarsal bones. The first one gets inserted to the medial side of the proximal phalanx and others to the lateral sides of the bases of proximal phalanges of the four toes. Also they are attached to dorsal digital expansion.

Plantar interossei: Three in number. Unipennate muscles seen on the deep surfaces of the intermetatarsal spaces. They arise from the medial sides of the lateral three metatarsals and are inserted to the medial sides of the bases of proximal phalanges and also to dorsal digital expansion of latral three toes.

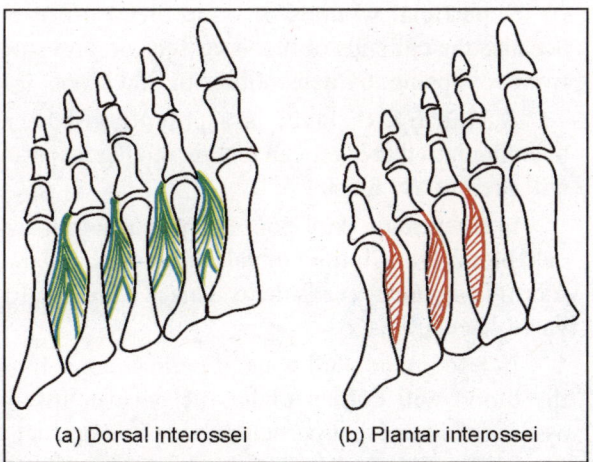

(a) Dorsal interossei   (b) Plantar interossei

Fig. 3.48: (a)Dorsal interossei (b) Plantar interossei

Nerve supply: All interossei except lateral ones are supplied by deep branch of lateral plantar nerve. The lateral most interossei are supplied by superficial branch of lateral plantar nerve.

Action: The plantar interossei adduct the toes and dorsal interossei abduct the toes. They help in maintaining the transverse arches of foot.

MUSCLES OF HEAD

1. Muscles of cranium
2. Muscles of face
3. Ocular and extraocular muscles
4. Muscles of tongue
5. Muscles of palate
6. Masticatory muscles
7. Muscles of middle ear
8. Muscles of pharynx
9. Muscles of larynx

4,5,7,8 and 9 will be discussed with the corresponding organs.

1. Muscles of cranium (Fig. 3.49)

Occipitofrontalis

This is the only muscle of the cranium, contained in the soft tissue over the cranium, the scalp.

Scalp

It has 5 layers and covers the hair bearing area of cranium and extends over the forehead upto upper eye lids. The layers are:

1. Skin – Generally thick and hair bearing.
2. Connective tissue layer – Formed of dense fibrous tissue. In this layer, nerves and vessels of scalp run.
3. Aponeurotic layer – This layer consists of the muscle of cranium, the occipitofrontalis, which has a frontal part – frontalis and occipital part, occipitalis, both connected by the common tendon, flattened into the aponeurosis – epicranial aponeurosis.

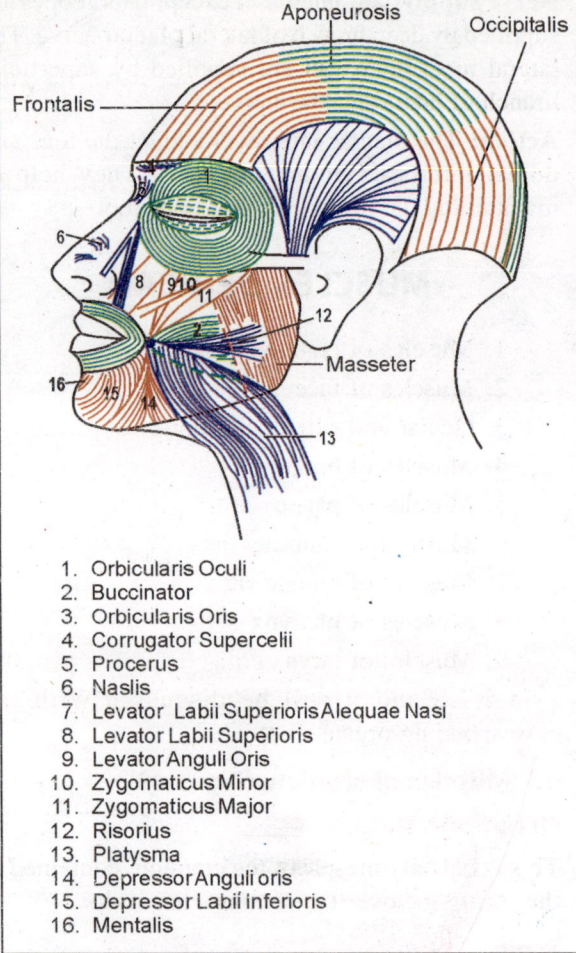

1. Orbicularis Oculi
2. Buccinator
3. Orbicularis Oris
4. Corrugator Supercelii
5. Procerus
6. Naslis
7. Levator Labii Superioris Alequae Nasi
8. Levator Labii Superioris
9. Levator Anguli Oris
10. Zygomaticus Minor
11. Zygomaticus Major
12. Risorius
13. Platysma
14. Depressor Anguli oris
15. Depressor Labii inferioris
16. Mentalis

Fig. 3.49: Muscles of face and scalp

Frontalis: A thin flat muscle, has no bony attachment, seen on the forehead. Anteriorly, below its fibres merge with the superficial fascia of eye brow and orbicularis oculi fibres of upper lid. Above and posteriorly attached to the aponeurosis.

Occipitalis: Arises behind from the lateral 2/3rds of superior nuchal line of occipital bone. Between the muscles of both sides there is a triangular gap filled with aponeurosis. Above, the flat muscle bellies are attached to the aponeurosis.

Nerve supply: Both bellies supplied by branches of facial nerve.

Action: Frontalis produces horizontal wrinkles on forehead. Occipitalis has no specific action in human.

4. Loose connective tissue layer -- It is formed of loose areolar tissue and acts as a potential space. First three layers act as a single unit and move along the plane of fourth layer. In scalping, the first three layers get avulsed through the plane of fourth layer. Fluid or blood can spread in this layer. Emissary veins have a longer course through this layer. They connect superficial veins of scalp to intracranial venous sinuses. So any infection from the outer layers can spread through emissary veins to fourth layer because these veins are very thin walled. Due to these reasons, this layer is known as dangerous layer of scalp.

5. Pericranium – Periosteum of skull. Loosely attached to the bone surface but firmly anchored along sutural lines.

Applied anatomy

Because skin of scalp is hairy, chances of sebaceous glands getting infected is common leading to abscess formation.

Superficial wounds of scalp bleed profusely because the cut ends of blood vessels are prevented from collapsing, by dense fibres of 2nd layer

As the fourth layer is a potential space, a bleeding into that layer can remain undiagnosed and will present as "black eye".

In fracture of skull bones, if periostium is also cut, blood from intracrannial veins ooze out into fourth layer and spreads there. This is called "safety valve haematoma".

In fracture of skull bone, if periosteum is intact the blood will collect under the periosteum and assume shape of that particular bone and present as a swelling. This is called "cephal-haematoma".

Sensory nerve supply: to scalp is from branches of trigeminal nerve and cervical plexus.

Arterial supply: from branches of ophthalmic artery and external carotid artery.

2. Muscles of face (Fig. 3.49)

Muscles of the face are known as muscles of facial expression. They are all supplied by branches of facial nerve and are inserted into the skin. Position of various muscles are shown in fig 3.49. Major muscles of face are described here.

Orbicularis oculi (Fig. 3.50 a b c)

It is the muscle around the eye lids. Has three parts-

(a) Palpebral part – confined to the lids.

(b) Orbital part – around the orbital margin

(c) Lacrimal part – related to lacrimal sac

(a) Palpebral part –

Origin: From the medial palpebral ligament. Fibres pass over the lids laterally. The upper and lower fibres decussate to form lateral palpebral raphe.

(b) Orbital part --

Origin: From the medial palpebral ligament, from frontal process of maxilla and from the nasal part of frontal bone. The fibres encircle the orbital margin without any lateral attachment. Some fibres get attached to the skin.

(c) Lacrimal part –

A small part lies behind the lacrimal sac.

Origin: From the crest of lacrimal bone and lacrimal fascia. Fibres run laterally and merge with palpebral part.

Nerve supply: Temporal and zygomatic branches of facial nerve.

Action:

Palpebral part – Gentle (mild) closure of lids.

Orbital part – Tight closure of lids.

Lacrimal part – Pulls the lids medially, dilates the lacrimal sac and thus helps drainage of tear into the sac.

Buccinator (Fig. 3.51)

Muscle of cheek

Origin:

1. From outer surface of maxilla just above the molar teeth.

2. From outer surface of mandible just below molar teeth.

3. From pterygomandibular raphe.

Insertion: Fibres are directed towards the angle of mouth. About 1cm lateral to the angle, uppermost fibres pass to the upper lip, lowermost fibers pass to the lower lip. Middle fibres intersect. Lower of them

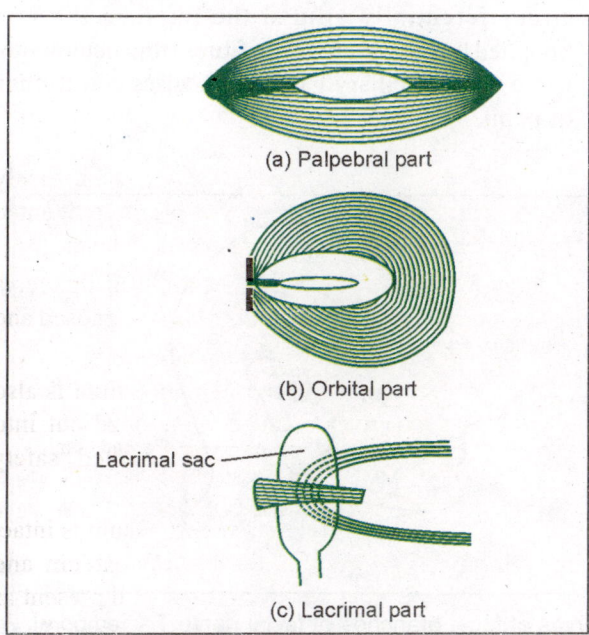

Fig. 3.50: Orbicularis Oculi

(a) Palpebral part

(b) Orbital part

Lacrimal sac

(c) Lacrimal part

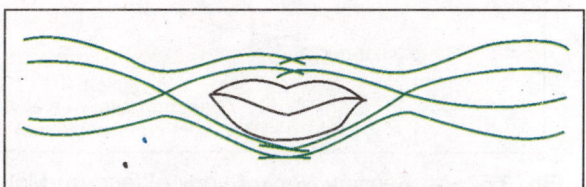

Fig. 3.51: Insertion of Buccinator

pass to the upper lip and upper of them, to the lower lip. Thus buccinator contributes most of the bulk of oribicularis oris.

The region where the middle set of fibres decussate is known as modiolus – a fibromuscular nodule. Many of the muscles around lip converge to modiolus.

Relations: Covered by buccopharyngeal fascia and buccal pad of fat. Parotid duct pierces it. Facial artery and vein cross it obliquely. Certain branches of facial nerve lie on it.

Action: Compresses the cheek against teeth, thus prevents accumulation of food in the vestibule of mouth while chewing. It is active while blowing and whistling.

Orbicularis oris

A sphincter muscle around oral orifice. It has three types of fibres in it.

1. Major bulk is formed of other muscles converging to the lips, main contribution being from buccinator.
2. Intrinsic muscle fibres of the lips – run from the skin to mucous membrane of lips.
3. Upper and lower incisive muscles originate from the mandible and maxilla near incisor teeth and go to the lips.

Action: It is a sphincter muscle, helps to close the mouth.

Nerve supply to face (Fig. 3.52 a, b)

Motor nerve of face is facial nerve, the VII cranial nerve.

Sensory nerve supply to face is from various branches of trigeminal nerve. A small region near the angle of jaw, below auricle is supplied by branch of cervical plexus. Refer diagrams.

OCULAR AND EXTRAOCULAR MUSCLES (MUSCLES OF ORBIT)

Ocular muscles

1. Ciliaris

A small circular mass of smooth muscle contained in the ciliary body of the eye ball. Concerned with accommodation of lens. Supplied by para-sympathetic fibres from oculomotor nerve. (Through ciliary ganglion)

2. Sphincter pupillae (Fig. 3.53)

A thin stratum of smooth muscle fibres arranged circumferentially around the pupil in the iris. Supplied by parasympathetic fibres from oculomotor nerve through ciliary ganglion. Causes constriction of pupil.

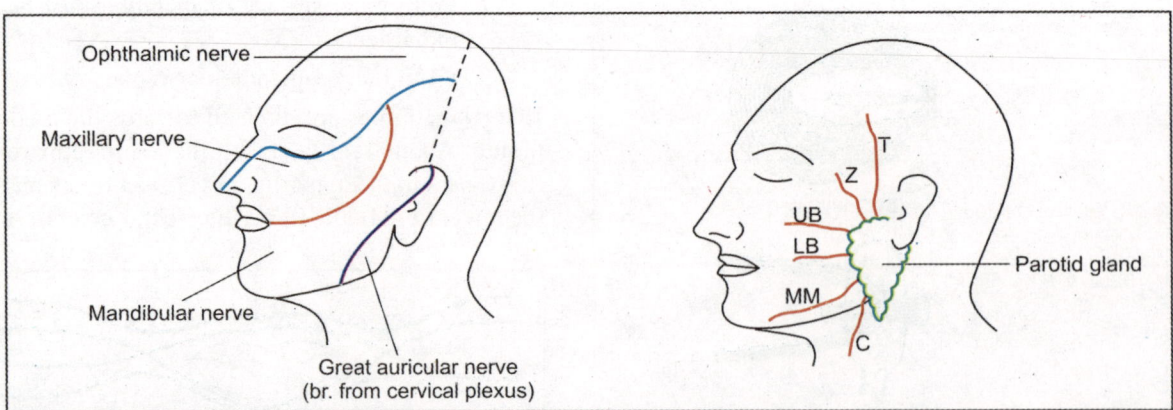

Fig. 3.52: (a) Sensory Nerve Suppy of face (b) Motor nerves of face, branches of facial nerve T - Temporal, Z - Zygomatic, UB - Upper Buccal, LB - Lower Buccal, MM - Marginal Mandibular, C - Cervical

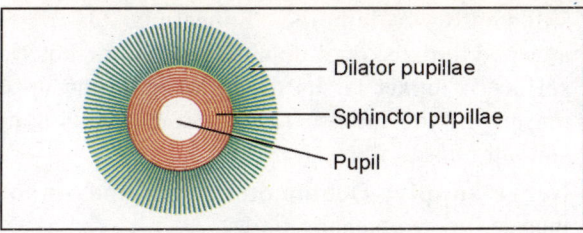

Fig. 3.53

3.   Dilator pupillae (Fig. 3.53)

A thin layer of smooth muscle fibres arranged radially in the iris, peripheral to the sphinctor. Causes dilatation of pupil. Supplied by sympathetic nerve fibres from the superior cervical sympathetic ganglion.

MUSCLES OF THE ORBIT

Extraocular muscles

They are:

  (a) 4 recti muscles –
    1. Superior rectus (SR)
    2. Inferior rectus (IR)
    3. Medial rectus (MR)
    4. Lateral rectus (LR)

  (b) 2 Oblique muscles –
    1. Superior oblique (SO)
    2. Inferior oblique (IO)

    These 4 + 2 = 6 muscles are attached to the eye ball and move the eye ball.

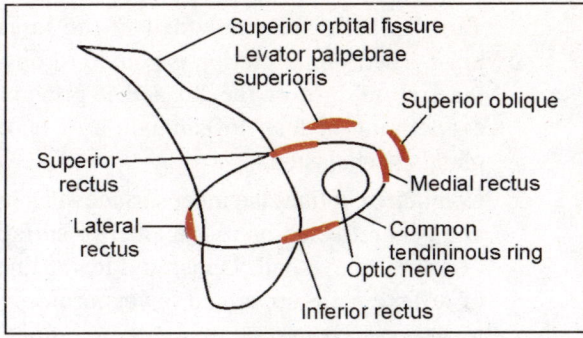

Fig. 3.54

(c) Levator palpebrae superioris (LPS)– Elevates the upper lid.

(d) Smooth muscles –
    1. Superior tarsal muscle
    2. Inferior tarsal muscle
    3. Orbitalis

(a) Recti muscles (Fig. 3.54, 3.55)

Origin: The 4 recti muscles take origin from a common tendinous ring at the back of orbit. The ring surrounds the optic canal and crosses superior orbital fissure.

Insertion: The recti muscles run forwards and surround the eye ball to get inserted into the sclera about 6 mm behind the cornea, but in front of the equator of eye ball, on the respective sides.

(b) Oblique Muscles

The **superior oblique** originates from the body of sphenoid, above and medial to the tendinous ring. The muscle runs forwards and ends in a tendon which passes through the trochlea attached to the frontal bone at its roof near the anterior margin of orbit. From the pulley the tendon passes back and laterally and gets inserted on to the sclera deep to the superior rectus, behind the equator.

Inferior oblique originates from the anterior, medial part of floor of orbit. It winds round the eye ball by passing first laterally and then upwards. Gets

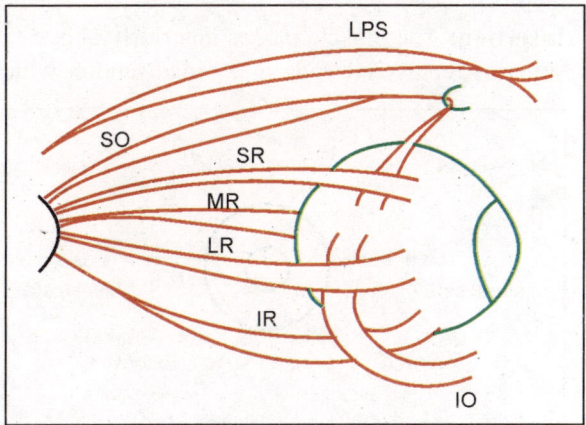

Fig. 3.55: Extra Ocular Muscles

inserted into the sclera deep to lateral rectus behind the equator.

Nerve supply:

Superior oblique – Trochlear nerve

Lateral rectus – Abducent nerve

Superior rectus, Inferior rectus, Medial rectus, Inferior oblique – Oculomotor nerve

Actions of recti and oblique muscles (Fig. 3.56)

Medial rectus – Turns the eye ball medially.

Lateral rectus – Turns the eye ball laterally.

Superior rectus – Turns the eye ball upwards and medially.

Inferior rectus – Turns the eye ball downwards and medially.

Superior oblique – turns the eye ball downwards and laterally.

Inferior oblique – Turns the eye ball upwards and laterally.

Also superior rectus and superior oblique muscles cause intorsion of eye ball. Inferior rectus and inferior oblique cause extorsion of eye ball.

(c) Levator palpebrae superioris

It does not act on the eye ball but on the upper lid.

Origin: From the lesser wing of sphenoid above the optic canal.

Insertion: The muscle passes anteriorly above the superior rectus and ends in a broad tendon which splits into two lamellae. Superficial layer gets attached to the skin of upper lid and to the anterior surface of upper tarsus. Deep layer, to the upper margin of the tarsus. This layer contains some smooth muscle fibres.

Nerve supply: Oculomotor nerve and smooth muscle, by sympathetic fibres.

Action: Raises the upper lid to open the eye.

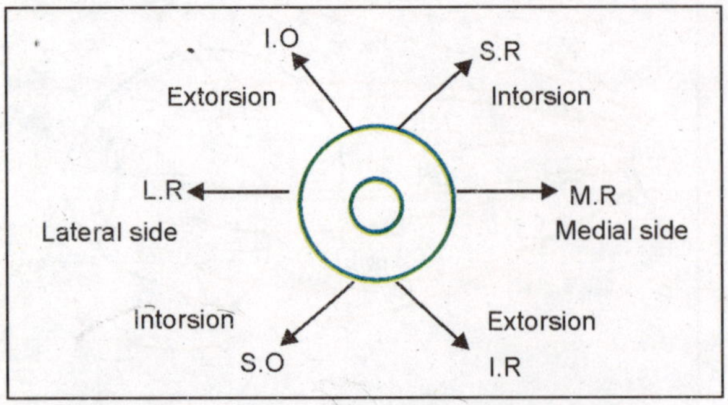

Fig. 3.56: Actions of Extra Ocular Muscles

EYE LIDS AND LACRIMAL APPARATUS

Eye lids (Fig. 3.57a)

Upper and lower eye lids, when closed, protect the anterior surface of eye ball. Space between the lids is palpebral fissure.

From outer to inner, the layers of eye lid are –

1. Skin – very thin
2. Subcutaneous tissue – A thin layer of loose connective tissue.
3. Muscle layer – Palpebral part of orbicularis oculi.
4. Orbital septum – Extension from periosteum of orbital margin, attached to tarsus.
5. Tarsus – The skeleton of the lid, a plate of dense connective tissue. Fibres of tendon of levator palpebrae superioris are attached to its anterior surface near upper border. Along with the tendon, superior tarsal muscle (smooth muscle) is attached to the tarsus.

   Tarsal glands are embedded in the tarsal plate. Their oily secretion is poured through the free margin of the lid and it prevents evaporation of tear. Inflammation of tarsal glands is chalasion.
6. Conjuctiva. It lines the inner surface of tarsus and gets reflected on to the anterior surface of sclera of eye ball. Upper and lower lines of reflexion are upper and lower fornices.

   Eye lashes are present along the lid margin.

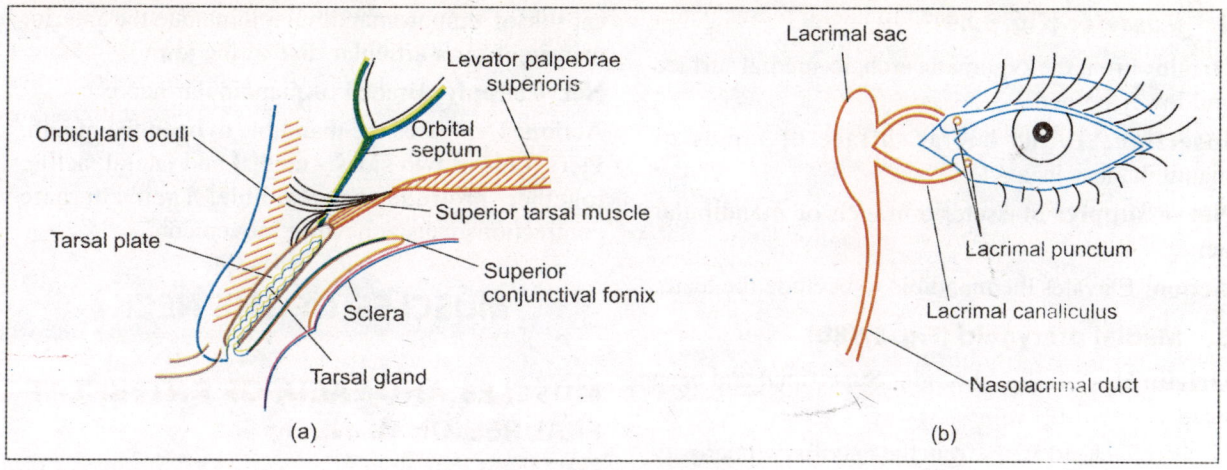

Fig. 3.57: Upper eye lid

Sebaceous and sweat glands are present related to them. Inflammation of these glands is stye.

LACRIMAL APPARATUS (Fig. 3.57b)

Consists of – Lacrimal gland, Lacrimal canaliculi, Lacrimal sac and Nasolacrimal duct.

Lacrimal gland

Secretes watery lacrimal fluid (tear). It has 2 parts, palpebral and orbital, as it curves round the flat tendon of levator palpebrae superioris. Upper part is orbital part and lower, palpebral part.

Tear is poured into lateral part of superior fornix through 6 ducts. It spreads to medial angle of eye by blinking of lids.

Nerve supply – Parasympathetic fibres – Post ganglionic from pteryopalatine ganglion.

Canaliculi

The canaliculi open through lacrimal punctum at the medial lid margins. Tear is drained through the punctum into canaliculi which open together into lacrimal sac.

Lacrimal sac

Placed in the lacrimal fossa on the medial orbital wall.

Nasolacrimal duct

It is the continuation of lower part of lacrimal sac. It opens into the inferior meatus of nasal cavity. Tear is drained from lacrimal sac by the duct.

MASTICATORY MUSCLES

They are,

  Temporalis
  Masseter
  Medial pterygoid
  Lateral pterygoid

1. Temporalis (Fig. 3.58a)

Origin: From the temporal fossa and from the inner surface of the temporal fascia covering the muscle.

Insertion: The fan shaped muscle converges into a tendon that passes deep to zygomatic arch and gets inserted into the coronoid process of mandible except on its lateral surface.

Nerve supply: Branches from mandibular nerve- deep temporal nerves.

Action: The muscle elevates the mandible, its posterior horizontal fibres retract the protruded mandible.

2. Masseter (Fig. 3.49)

Origin: From the zygomatic arch, its medial surface and lower border.

Insertion: To the lateral surface of ramus of mandible,near its angle.

Nerve supply: Masseteric branch of mandibular nerve.

Action: Elevates the mandible to occlude the teeth.

3. Medial pterygoid (Fig. 3.58b)

Origin: Has 2 heads of origin- Superficial and deep heads.

Superficial head arises from the maxillary tuberosity and deep head from the medial surface of lateral pterygoid plate.

Insertion:

Muscle is inserted into the medial surface of the angle and ramus of mandible.

Nerve supply: Branch from the mandibular nerve.

Action: Medial pterygoid elevates the mandible.

4. Lateral pterygoid (Fig. 3.58b)

Origin: Has 2 heads of origin – upper and lower.

Upper head - from the infratemporal crest of the greater wing of sphenoid bone and Lower head- from the lateral surface of the lateral pterygoid plate.

Insertion: The muscle is inserted into the pterygoid fovea of the neck of mandible and through the capsule of temporomandibular joint, into the anterior margin of intra articular disc of the joint.

Nerve supply: Branch of mandibular nerve

Action: Depresses the mandible to open the mouth. Pterygoids of two sides - medial and lateral, acting together, protrude the mandible. Their alternate contractions cause chewing movements.

MUSCLES OF THE NECK

MUSCLES AND FACIA OF ANTEROLATERAL REGION OF NECK

Many of this group of are covered or enclosed by the deep fascia of neck – the deep cervical fascia.

Superficial fascia of neck is very thin and contains the thin platysma muscle.

Deep cervical fascia

It has 3 layers.

1. **General investing layer** - completely encircles the neck and splits to enclose Trapezius and sternocleidomastoid muscles. Behind it is attached to the ligamentum nuchae. Above its attachment extends from external occipital protuberance along the superior nuchal line, mastoid process, lower border of mandible and body of hyoid bone. At the lower border of mandible, it splits to

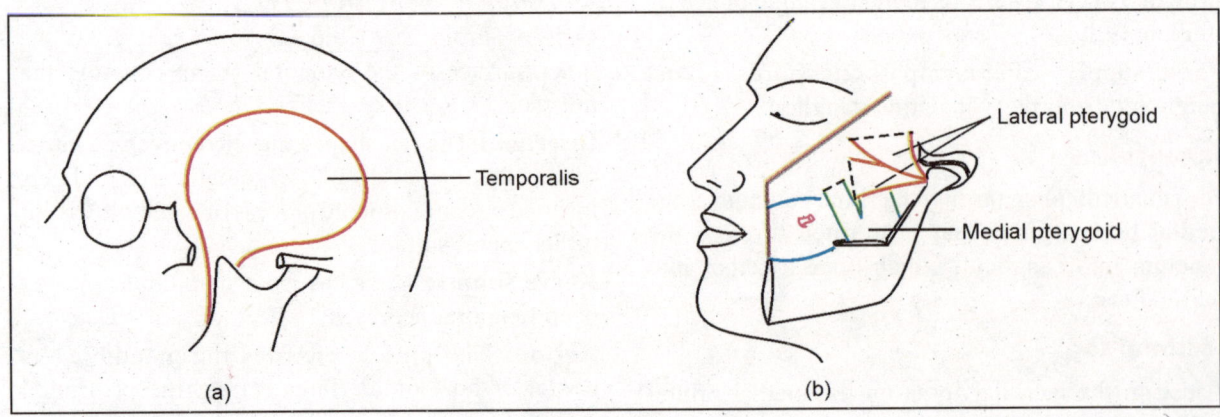

(a)   (b)

(Fig. 3.58a)

enclose the submandibular salivary gland and parotid gland. Between the angle of mandible and styloid process, it condenses into stylomandibular ligament.

Below it is attached to the acromion, clavicle and manubrium sterni. Above manubrium, the layer splits to enclose a small suprasternal space.

2. **Pretracheal layer** – This thin layer forms a complete covering to thyroid gland and is attached to the thyroid and cricoid cartilages. So the gland moves up and down in swallowing.

3. **Prevertebral layer** – This layer covers the prevertebral muscles. Above attached to base of skull. Below extends to thorax and blends with anterior longitudinal ligament of vertebral column. Anterior to it, the pharynx is separated from the layer by a space, retropharyngeal space.

A. SUPERFICIAL AND LATERAL MUSCLES OF NECK

1. Platysma
2. Sternocleidomastoid
3. Trapezius

Platysma (Fig. 3.49)

Lies in the superficial fascia of neck.

Origin: From the deep fascia covering the upper parts of deltoid and pectoralis major. Muscle crosses clavicle and passes obliquely upwards.

Insertion: Anterior fibres interlace with fibres of opposite side. Majority of fibres get attached to the lower border of mandible. Most posterior fibres reach the angle of mouth and merge with the superficial muscles there.

Nerve supply: Cervical branch of facial nerve

Action: Causes wrinkles on the neck, depresses the angle of mouth and lower lip.

Sternocleidomastoid (Fig. 3.59)

Origin: Sternal head arises from the upper part of anterior surface of manubrium sterni.

Clavicular head, from the medial 1/3rd of clavicle.

Insertion: The 2 heads join and the muscle passes upwards to get inserted on to the lateral surface of the mastoid process and lateral part of superior nuchal line.

Nerve supply: Spinal part of accessory nerve and ventral rami of C_2 and C_3 nerves which are proprioceptive.

Action: When the muscle of one side contracts, it

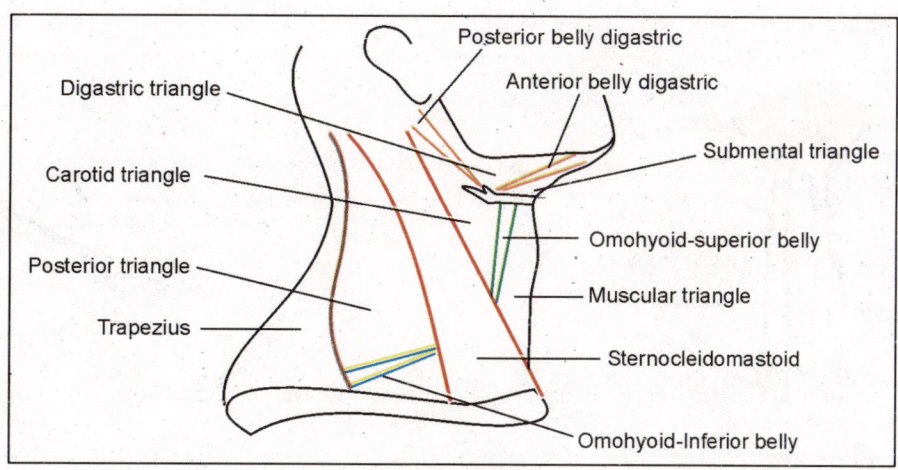

Fig. 3.59

tilts the head to the shoulder of that side. When both side mucles contract together, flex the cervical part of vertebral column.

Trapezius (Fig. 3.59)

Described along with muscles of upper limb.

B. SUPRAHYOID MUSCLES OF NECK (Fig. 3.60 a, b)

They are:

1. Digastric
2. Stylohyoid
3. Mylohyoid
4. Geniohyoid

Digastric

It lies below the body of mandible and has 2 fleshy bellies united by an intermediate tendon.

Origin: Anterior belly arises from the digastric fossa of mandible and is directed down towards the hyoid bone. Posterior belly arises from the medial surface of mastoid process of temporal bone (mastoid notch). It is directed downwards and forwards to the hyoid bone. Both bellies are united by the intermediate tendon which is held in position connected to the junction of greater horn and body of hyoid bone by a fibrous loop.

Nerve supply: Anterior belly, by mylohyoid branch of mandibular nerve.

Posterior belly, by branch of facial nerve.

Action: Depresses the mandible and elevates hyoid bone.

Stylohyoid

Origin: From the styoid process near its base.

Insertion: To the hyoid bone at the junction of greater horn and body. (here it is pierced by the tendon of digastric)

Nerve supply: Branch of facial nerve

Action: Elevates the hyoid bone.

Mylohyoid

A flat triangular muscle. Muscles of both sides meet in the median raphe and forms the floor of mouth.

Origin: From the mylohyoid line on medial surface of mandible.

Insertion: Fibres are directed downwards and forwards. Most posterior fibres get inserted to the body of mandible. Remainig major parts of the muscles of 2 sides end in a median raphe that extends from symphysis menti to hyoid bone.

Nerve supply: Mylohyoid branch of mandibular nerve.

Action: Elevates the floor of mouth in deglutition.

Geniohyoid

A narrow muscle, seen above the mylohyoid, each on either side of midline.

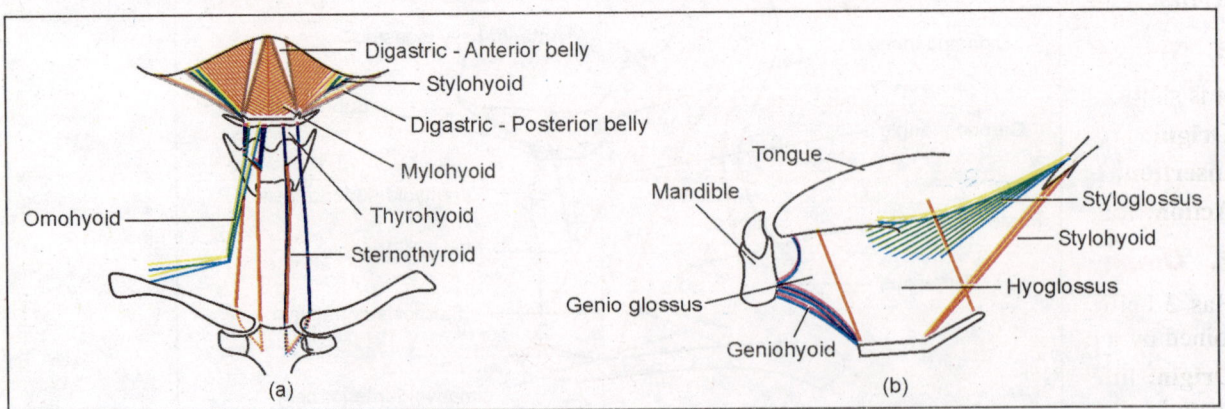

Fig. 3.60

Origin: Inferior mental spine behind the symphysis menti.

Insertion: Body of hyoid bone

Nerve supply: C_1 nerve through hypoglossal nerve.

Action: Elevates hyoid bone or depresses mandible.

C. INFRAHYOID MUSCLES (Fig. 3.60 A)

1. Sternohyoid
2. Sternothyroid
3. Thyrohyoid
4. Omohyoid

Generally these muscles are narrow and long hence known as strap muscles. All eccept thyrohyoid are supplied by branches of ansa cervicalis. Thyrohyoid is supplied by a branch from C_1 nerve through hypoglossal nerve.

1. Sternohyoid

Origin: From behind the upper end of manubrium sterni and medial end of clavicle.

Insertion: Into the lower border of body of hyoid bone.

Action: Depresses hyoid bone in deglutition.

2. Sternothyroid

Origin: From behind the upper part of manubrium sterni and medial end of first costal cartilage.

Insertion: Into the oblique line of thyroid cartilage.

Action: Pulls the larynx downwards.

3. Thyrohyoid

It is shorter than others and quadrilateral in shape.

Origin: From oblique line of thyroid cartilage.

Insertion: Into the greater horn of hyoid bone.

Action: Raises the larynx

4. Omohyoid

Has 2 bellies. – Superior and inferior, which are joined by a common tendon.

Origin: Inferior belly arises from upper border of scapula. It passes forwards in the lower part of posterior triangle of neck and ends in the

intermediate tendon behind sternomastoid. The tendon is held in position by a fibrous band connected to clavicle.

Superior belly arises from the common tendon and passes upwards.

Insertion: Superior belly is inserted into the body of hyoid bone.

Action: Omohyoid depresses hyoid bone.

D. ANTERIOR VERTEBRAL MUSCLES (Fig. 3.61)

1. Longus colli
2. Longus capitis
3. Rectus capitis anterior
4. Rectus capitis lateralis

1. Longus colli

Its fibres extend in front of the bodies and transverse processes of cervical and upper three thoracic vertebrae.

Nerve supply: Ventral rami of C_2 to C_6 nerves.

Action: Flexes the neck

2. Longus capitis

Extends from anterior tubercles of transverse

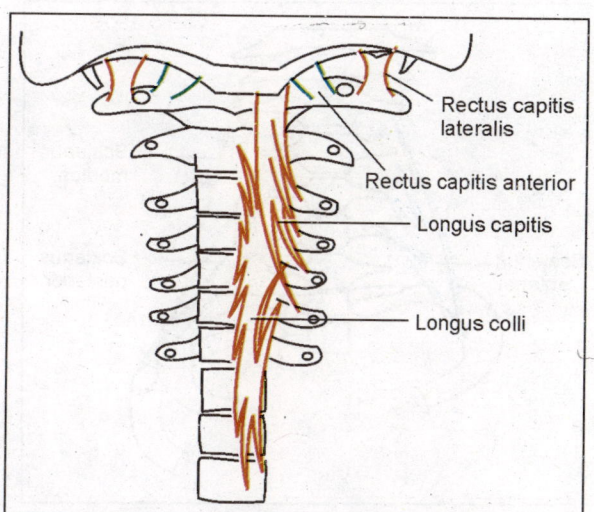

Fig. 3.61: Anterior Vertebral Muscles

processes of C_3 to C_6 vertebrae to the basilar part of occipital bone.

Nerve supply: Ventral rami of C_1 to C_3 nerves

Action: Flexes the head

3. Rectus capitis anterior

Extends from anterior surface of lateral mass of atlas to basilar part of occipital bone.

Nerve supply: Ventral rami of C_1 and C_2 nerves.

Action: Flexes the head

4. Rectus capitis lateralis

Extends from transverse process of atlas to jugular process of occipital bone.

Nerve supply: Ventral rami of C_1 and C_2 nerves.

Action: Bends the head to its side.

E. LATERAL VERTEBRAL MUSCLES (Fig. 3.62)

1. Scalenus anterior
2. Scalenus medius
3. Scalenus posterior

1. Scalenus anterior

Origin: From anterior tubercles of transverse processes of C_3 to C_6 vertebrae.

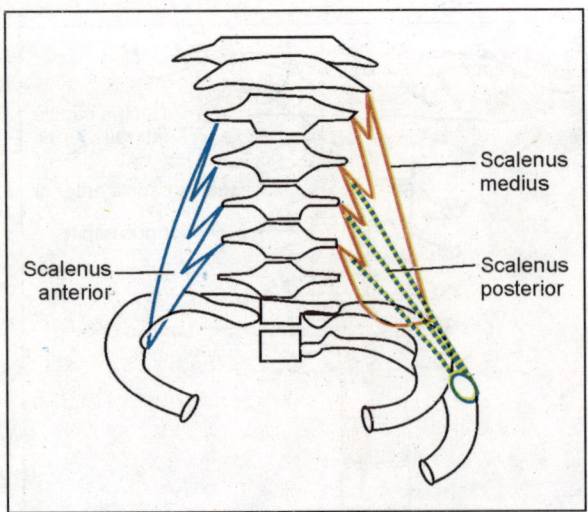

Fig. 3.62: Lateral Vertebral Muscles

Insertion: Into scalene tubercle of first rib

Nerve supply: Ventral rami of C_4 to C_6 nerves

Action: Bends the neck forwards and laterally.

2. Scalenus medius

Origin: From transverse process of axis and from posterior tubercles of transverse processes of C_3 to C_7 vertebrae.

Insertion: Upper surface of first rib behind the groove for subclavian artery.

3. Scalenus posterior

Origin: From the posterior tubercles of transverse processes of C_4 to C_6 vertebrae.

Insertion: Outer surface of second rib behind its middle.

Nerve supply: Ventral rami of C_6 to C_8 nerves.

Action: Bends the neck to its side.

TRIANGLES OF NECK (Fig. 3.59)

For the purpose of description, the region of neck is divided into different triangles by certain muscles.

The sternomastoid muscle divides the anetrolateral part of neck into anterior and posterior triangles. Anterior triangle is further divided into smaller triangles.

The triangles are,

1. Posterior triangle

2. Anterior triangles-

    (a) Submental triangle

    (b) Digastric triangle

    (c) Carotid triangle

    (d) Muscular triangle

3. In the posterior part of upper part of neck deep to the muscles, there is the **suboccipital triangle**.

1. Posterior triangle (Fig. 3.63 a, b)

Boundaries:

Anteriorly – Posterior border of sternomastoid

Posteriorly – Anterior border of trapezius

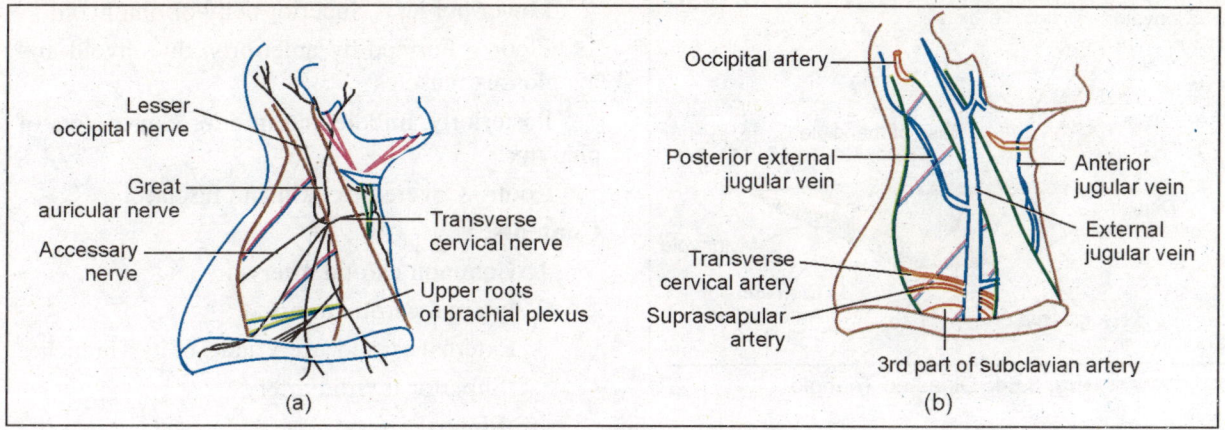

Fig. 3.63: Posterior Triangle

Base – Middle 1/3rd of clavicle

Floor – In the floor the following muscles are seen from above downwards – Semispinalis capitis, Splenius capitis, Levator scapulae, Scalenus medius and scalenus anterior – all covered by prevertebral layer of cervical fascia.

Roof – General investing layer of cervical fascia, superficial fascia and skin.

Lower part of the triangle is crossed obliquely by the inferior belly of omohyoid muscle dividing the posterior triangle into upper larger occipital triangle and lower smaller supraclavicular triangle. (Fig. 3.59)

Contents:

A. **Nerves**
   1. Spinal accessory nerve
   2. Lesser occipital nerve
   3. Great auricular nerve   } Branches of cervical plexus
   4. Transverse nerve of neck
   5. Supraclavicular nerves
   6. Upper roots of brachial plexus

B. **Arteries**
   1. Third part of subclavian artery
   2. Suprascapular artery
   3. Transverse cervical artery
   4. Part of occipital artery

C. **Veins**
   External jugular vein and its tributaries

D. **Lymph nodes**

ANTERIOR TRIANGLES

1. Submental triangle (Fig. 3.59)

Boundaries:

Sides – Anterior bellies of digastric muscle

Base – Body of hyoid bone

Floor – Mylohyoid muscle

Roof – Skin and fasciae

Contents - Lymph nodes and beginning of anterior jugular vein.

2. Digastric triangle (Fig. 3.64)

Boundaries:

Above – (Base) – Lower border of mandible.

Sides – Anterior belly of digastric anteriorly.

Posterior belly of digastric and stylohyoid muscle posteriorly.

Floor – Mylohyoid and hyoglossus muscles

Roof – Skin and fasciae

Contents - Anterior part has –

Submandibular salivary gland,

Facial artery,

Facial vein,

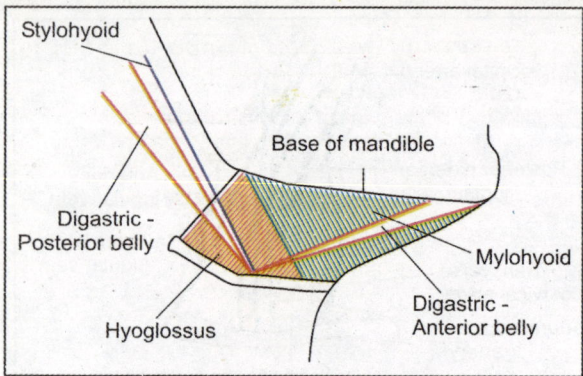

Fig. 3.64: Digastric Triangle

Lymph nodes,

Hypoglossal nerve,

Mylohyoid nerve and vessels,

Posterior part has –

Carotid sheath and contents,

Stylopharyngeus,

Glossopharyngeal nerve.

3. Carotid triangle (Fig. 3.65, 66)

Boundaries:

Posterior border – Anterior margin of sternomastoid.

Upper border – Posterior belly of digastric

Lower border – Superior belly of omohyoid.

Floor – Formed by anteriorly, thyrohyoid and hyoglossus muscles

Posteriorly, middle and inferior constrictors of pharynx.

Roof – Covered by skin and fasciae.

Contents:

1. Common carotid artery
2. Internal carotid artery
3. External carotid artery and 5 of its 8 branches
   -Superior thyroid artery
   -Lingual artery
   -Facial artery
   -Ascending pharyngeal artery
   -Occipital artery
4. Internal jugular vein
5. Vagus nerve with its superior laryngeal branch.
6. Hypoglossal nerve
7. Ansa cervicalis
8. Cervical part of sympathetic trunk.
9. Part of spinal accessory nerve, near its upper part.
10. Cervical lymph nodes.

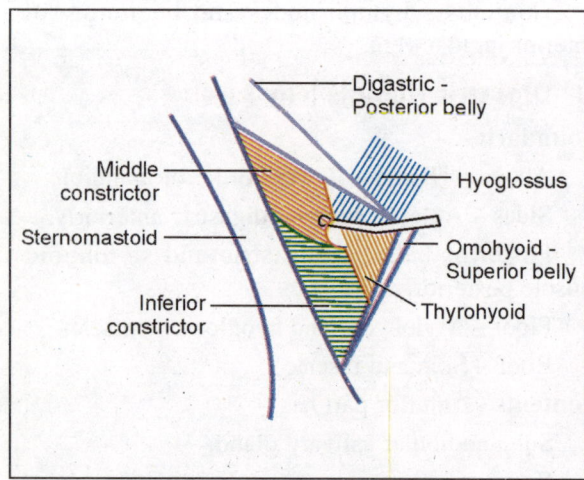

Fig. 3.65: Carotid Triangle

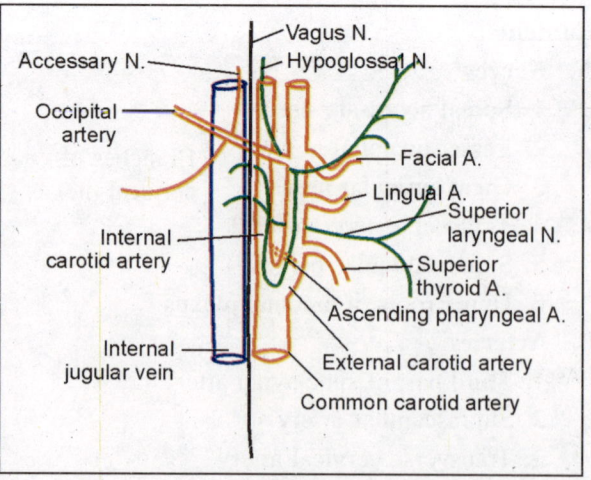

Fig. 3.66

CAROTID SHEATH (Fig. 3.67)

Of the contents of carotid triangle, common carotid artery below and internal carotid artery above, internal jugular vein and vagus nerve are ensheathed by a fascial covering – carotid sheath, derived from the three layers of deep cervical fascia. Anterior to it lies the nerve loop, ansa cervicalis. Behind it, the sheath is related to sympathetic trunk.

Ansa cervicalis (Fig. 3.68)

A nerve loop in the carotid triangle, formed by a descending limb, branching from the hypoglossal nerve but they are fibres from C_1 spinal nerve. Loop is completed by union with ascending limb, derived from C_2 and C_3 nerve fibres. Branches of ansa supply the infrahyoid muscles.

4. Muscular triangle (Fig. 3.59)

Boundaries:

Posteroinferior side – Sternomastoid

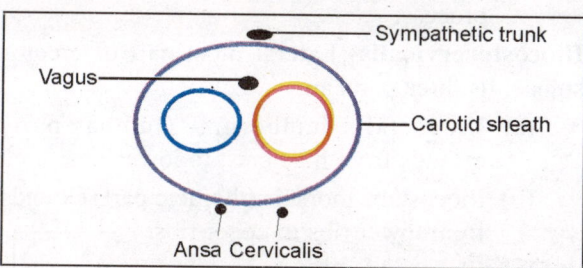

Fig. 3.67: C. S. of Carotid Sheath

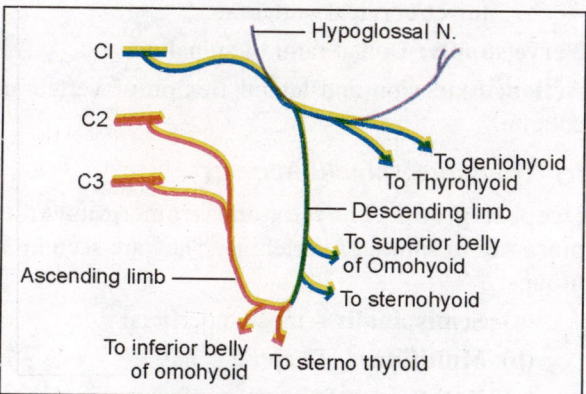

Fig. 3.68: Ansa Cervicalis

Posterosuperior side – Superior belly of omohyoid.

Medial side – Anterior midline of neck.

Floor – Sternothyroid and Sternohyoid muscles.

Contents – Infrahyoid strap muscles .

Suboccipital triangle is described with suboccipital muscles.

MUSCLES OF TRUNK

1. Deep muscles of the back
2. Suboccipital muscles
3. Muscles of the thorax
4. Muscles of the abdomen
5. Muscles of the pelvis
6. Muscles of the Perineum

1. Deep muscles of back

Generally these muscles control the movements of vertebral column. They are arranged in three layers on the side of the vertebral column.

From superficial to deep they are,

(a) Splenius muscles. (Fig. 3.69)

1. **Splenius cervicis:** Extends from upper thoracic spines ($T_3 - T_6$) to upper cervical transverse processes ($C_1 - C_3$).
2. **Splenius capitis:** From spines of C_7 to T_3 and lower half of ligamentum nuchae, to the

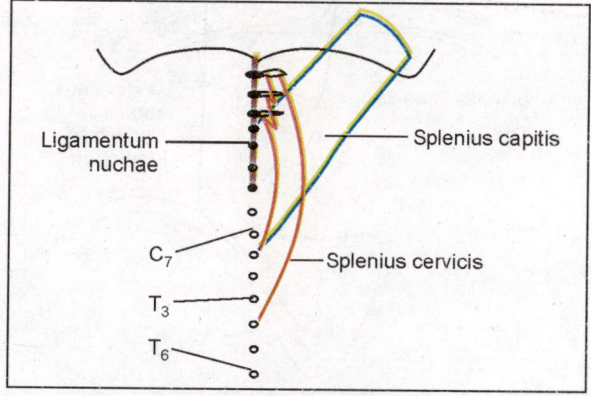

Fig. 3.69

mastoid process and occipital bone below lateral part of superior nuchal line.

Nerve supply: Dorsal rami of cervical nerves.

Action: Head is pulled back.

(b) Erector spinae (Fig- 3.70)

Deep to splenius muscles. A strong vertical muscle, extends from back of sacrum and illum to the skull. Laterally extends from the spines of vertebrae to the angles of ribs.

It has three parts

1. Medialmost part – Spinalis
2. Intermediate part – Longissimus
3. Lateral part – Iliocostalis

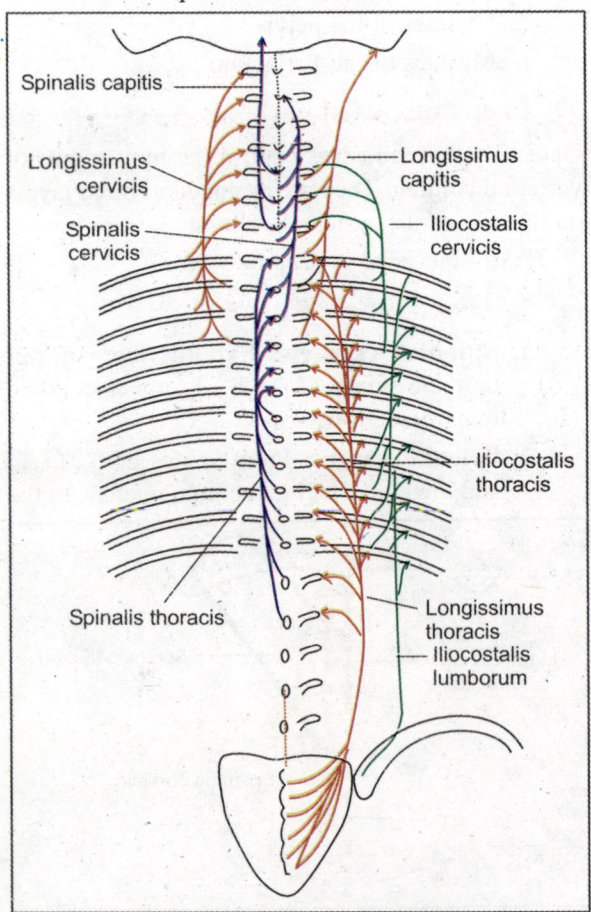

Fig. 3.70: Parts of Erector Spinae

Origin: Erector spinae originates from the back of the sacrum (median and lateral sacral crests) from the back of iliac crest and from the spines of lumbar vertebrae.

From the origin, as the muscle ascends up, the three parts are identified.

Spinalis – Extends from spines to spines of the vertebrae. (Spinalis thoracis, Spinalis cervicis and Spinalis capitis)

Longissimus – Main part of the muscle

(a) *Longissimus thoracis* – Extends from sacrum to transverse processes of lumbar and thoracic vertebrae and to ribs.

(b) *Longissimus cervicis* – Extends from transverse processes of upper thoracic vertebrae and upper ribs, to the transverse processes of cervical vertebrae.

(c) *Longissimus capitis* – extends from transverse processes of upper thoracic and lower cervical vertebrae to the mastoid process.

Iliocostocervicalis- Lateral most part of erector spinae. Its three parts are-

(a) Iliocostalis lumborum- (lumbar part) extends from iliac crest to lower ribs.

(b) Iliocostalis thoracis (thoracic part) extends from lower ribs to upper ribs.

(c) Iliocostalis cervicis (cervical Part) extends from upper ribs to transverse processes of lower cervical vertebrae.

Nerve supply: Dorsal rami of spinal nerves.

Action: Extension and lateral flexion of vertebral column.

(c) Transversospinalis Muscles

Deepest group. They extend from transverse processes to spines of vertebrae. They are seen in 3 groups:

(a) **Semispinalis** – most superficial

(b) **Multifidus** – Deep

(c) **Rotatores** – Deepest

(a) SEMISPINALIS

(i) Semispinalis thoracis – From transverse processes of lower thoracic vertebrae to spines of upper thoracic vertebrae.

(ii) Semispinalis cervicis- From upper thoracic transverse processes to cervical spines.

(iii) Semispinalis capitis – From transverse processes of upper thoracic and 7th cervical vertebrae and from articular processes of C_4, C_5, C_6 vertebrae. Inserted to occipital bone between superior and inferior nuchal lines.

Nerve supply: Dorsal rami of thoracic and cervical spinal nerves.

Action: Extend the head.

(b) MULTIFIDUS

Small muscles, present throughout the length of vertebral column. Spans 2-4 vertebrae. From transverse processes to spines. Best developed in lumbar region.

(c) ROTATORES

From transverse processes to spines of the higher vertebrae. Well developed in thoracic region. They also extend throughout the length of vertebral column.

Actions: All these muscles extend and rotate vertebral column.

Apart from these, there are smaller deeper muscles which run between adjacent spines and adjacent transverse processes - Interspinales and intertransversarii.

2. Subocipital muscles

Small muscles seen in the uppermost part of back of neck deep to semispinalis capitis.

1. Rectus capitis posterior minor
2. Rectus capitis posterior major
3. Obliquus capitis inferior
4. Obliquus capitis superior

1 and 2 extendthe head at atlanto occipital joint. 3 and 4 cause rotation of head at atlanto axial joints. 2, 3 and 4 form boundries of suboccipital triangle.

Rectus capitis posterior minor

Origin: Tubercle of posterior arch of atlas.

Insertion: Area on occipital bone below inferior. nuchal line – on medial part.

Rectus capitis posterior major

Origin: Spine of axis

Insertion: Lateral part of the occipital bone below inferior nuchal line.

Obliquus inferior

Origin: Spine of axis

Insertion: Transverse process of atlas.

Obliquus superior

Origin: Transverse process of atlas

Insertion: Lateral part of area between superior and inferior nuchal lines.

Nerve supply: All are supplied by dorsal ramus of C_1 nerve.

Subocipital triangle (Fig. 3.71)

Present deep in the upper part of back of neck below the occipital bone deep to semispinalis capitis.

Boundaries:

Superomedially – Rectus capitis posterior major.

Superolaterally – Obliquus capitis superior.

Inferiorly – Obliquus capitis inferior.

Roof – Semispinalis capitis.

Floor – Posterior arch of atlas and posterior atlanto occipital membrane.

Contents:

1. 3rd part of vertebral artery.
2. Suboccipital nerve – Dorsal ramus of C_1 (supplies subocipital muscles).
3. greater occipital nerve crosses the triangle.
4. suboccipital venous plexus.

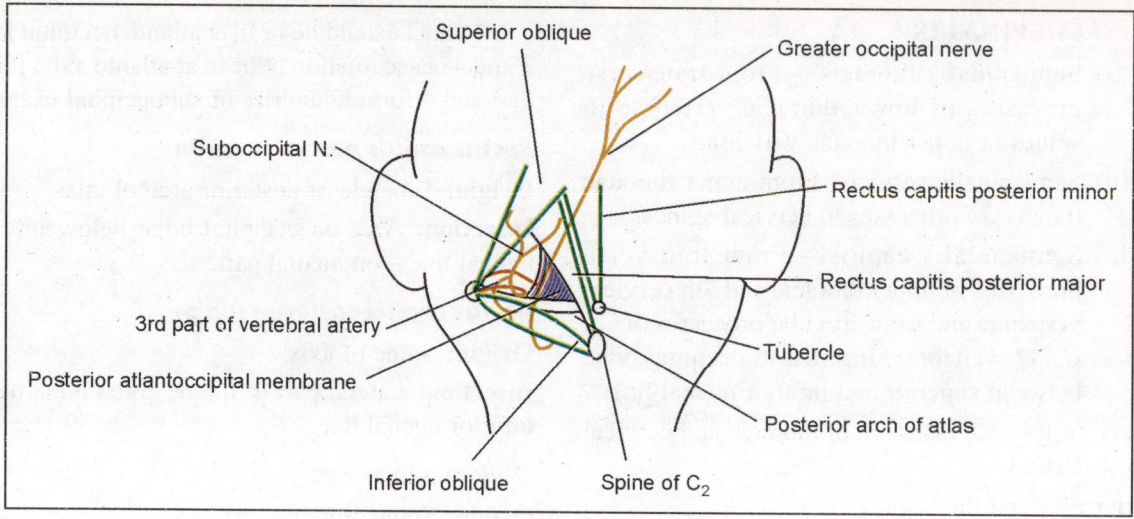

Fig. 3.71: Suboccipital Triangle

MUSCLES OF THORAX

They include:

1. Muscles that interconnect the adjacents ribs – Intercostales
2. Muscles that connect sternum to ribs – Sternocostalis
3. Muscles that connect several ribs – Subcostales
4. Muscles that connect ribs to vertebrae – Levetores costorum, Seratus posterior superior and Serratus posterior inferior
5. Diaphragm

Intercostal muscles are seen in the intercostal spaces (Fig. 3.72, 3.73, 3.74)

1. Extrernal intercostals

Outermost muscle. Extends from the lower border of a upper rib to the upper border of the next lower rib. Fibers directed downwards and medially. Muscle fibers are replaced by external intercostal membrane from the level of costochondral junction, to the sternal margin.

2. Internal intercostals

Deeper to external intercostals. Extends from costal groove of an upper rib to the upper border of next lower rib. Fibres directed downwards and laterally. Posteriorly behind the angle of rib, it is replaced by internal intercostal membrane.

3. Intercostalis intimi

Attached to the inner surfaces of adjacent ribs. Prominent only in the lateral (middle) 2/4th of the lower intercostal spaces.

Sternocostalis (Transversus thoracis)

Seen anteriorly behind the sternum and adjacent costal cartilages. Arises from the inner surface of lower 1/3rd of sternum near its margin. The muscle ascends as separate slips and extend laterally to get inserted from 2nd to 6th costal cartilages near their lateral ends. (Fig. 3.74)

Subcostales

Well developed only in the lower part of the posterior spaces. Extends from the inner surface of one rib near its angle to the inner surface of 2nd and 3rd rib below.

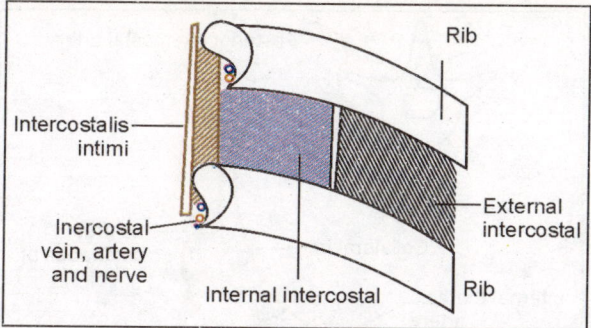

Fig. 3.72

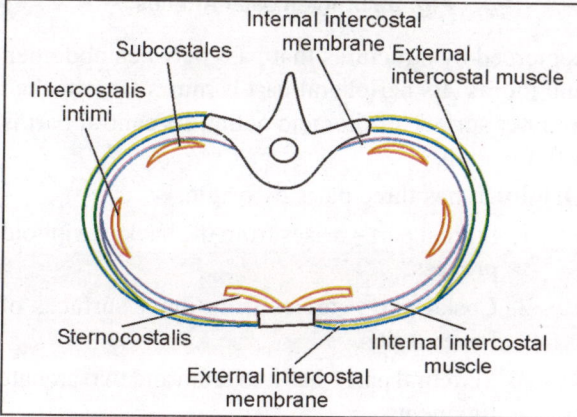

Fig. 3.73

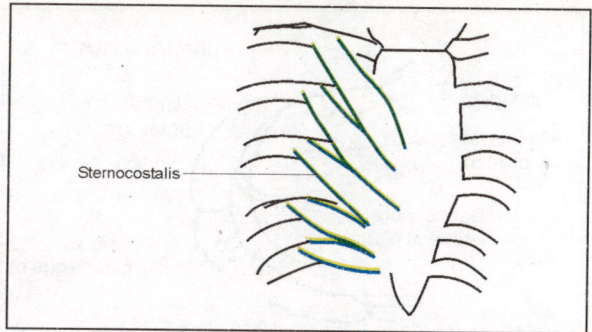

Fig. 3.74

Action: Intercostal muscles form a firm elastic support to the intercostal spaces and help in movements of respiration.

Nerve supply: Intercostal nerves.

Intercostal spaces (Fig. 3.72)

Spaces between ribs are called intercostal spaces

Contents:

1. ntercostal muscles
   - External intercostals
   - Internal intercostals
   - Intercostalis intimi
   - Subcostales
   - Sternocostalis
2. Intercostal nerve

3. Intercostal vessels

(Of the contents, muscles are described earlier)

Intercostal nerves (Fig. 3.75)

They are ventral rami of the 12 thoracic spinal nerves. Upper 11 pairs seen in the intercostal spaces, through the lower part of costal groove. Lowest one is below the 12th rib and is called subcostal nerve. Of the 12 nerves 3rd, 4th, 5th and 6th are restricted to the supply of thoracic region only. So they are the typical intercostal nerves. Others Supply the region of upper limb and abdomen also. Branches are as shown in the diagram.

Intercostal arteries (Fig. 3.76)

Each intercostal space contains a large posterior intercostal artery and 2 smaller anterior intercostal arteries.Their branches supply the muscles, skin, mammary gland etc.

Posterior intercostal arteries of upper two spaces are branches of superior intercostal artery, a branch of costocervical trunk from subclavian artery. Arteries in the lower spaces are direct branches from descending thoracic aorta. The posterior intercostal artery runs in the costal groove together with vein and nerve. It gives a collateral branch that runs parallel to it in the lower part of the intercostal space.

Anterior intercostal arteries are branches of internal thoracic artery and musculophrenic artery. They run in the upper and lover parts of the space and anastamose with posterior intercostal arteries.

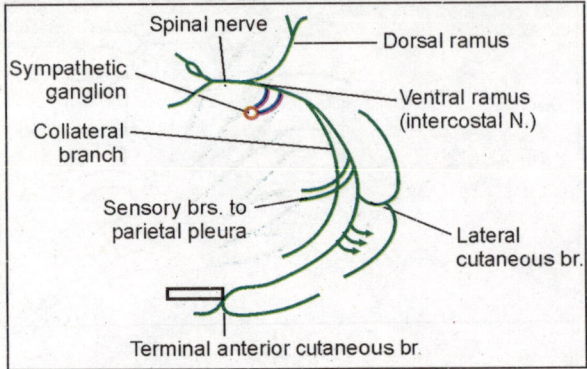

Fig. 3.75: Intercostal Nerve

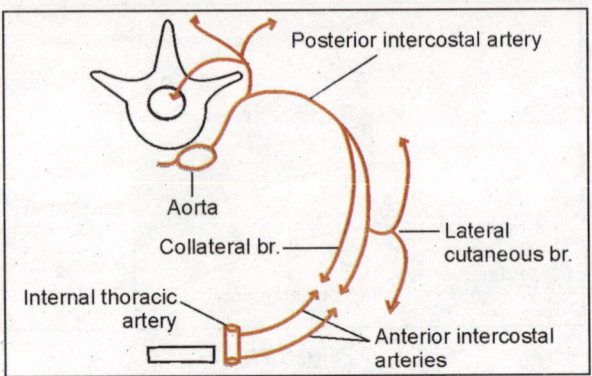

Fig. 3.76: Intercostal Arteries

Intercostal veins

Posterior intercostal veins drain into azygos vein and anterior ones into internal thoracic vein.

Levatores costorum

They are short strong muscles on either side of the vertebral column, 12 in number. Arise from the tips of transverse processes of C_1 to T_{11} vertebrae. Each is inserted to the rib below, lateral to the tubercle.

Supplied by the dorsal rami of the spinal nerves.

Action: Elevate the ribs

Serratus posterior superior

An inconstant muscle. Extends as 4 – 6 digitations from lower cervical and upper thoracic spines, downwards and laterally to the outer surfaces of 2nd to 4th or 6th rib.

Supplied by 2nd to 5th intercostal nerves.

Action: Elevates ribs

Serratus posterior inferior

Similar to the superior one, arising by 4 or 5 digitations from lower thoracic and upper lumbar spines. Go upwards and laterally to get attached to outer surfaces of lower 4 ribs.

Action: Depresses ribs

Supplied by lower 4 spinal nerves.

Diaphragm (Fig. 3.77 a, b)

It is the primary muscle of respiration, a dome shaped musculotendinous septum, at the thoracic outlet. It

is pierced by structures that pass between abdomen and thorax. Its peripheral part is muscular, attached to inner surface of thoracic outlet. Its central part is a flat tendon.

Origin: It has three parts by origin.

1. Sternal part – arises from the back of xiphoid process.
2. Costal part – arises from inner surfaces of lower 6 ribs.
3. Vertebral part – has two crura and two arcuate ligaments.

Crura are tendinous origins. Right crus arises from sides of first three lumbar vertebral bodies. Left crus arises from the sides of first two lumbar vertebral bodies.

Arcuate ligaments:

Medial - arches from the side of L_2 vertebra to the tip of L_1 transverse process.

Lateral – arches from the tip of L_1 transverse process to the lower border of 12th rib.

Medial arcuate ligament overlies psoas major muscle and lateral one overlies quadratus lumborum on each side.

Median arcuate ligament – fibres from the upper parts of two crura arch in front of T_{12} body.

Insertion: From these peripheral attachments, the muscular fibres converge into a flat aponeurotic central tendon, which is shaped as if having three leaves.

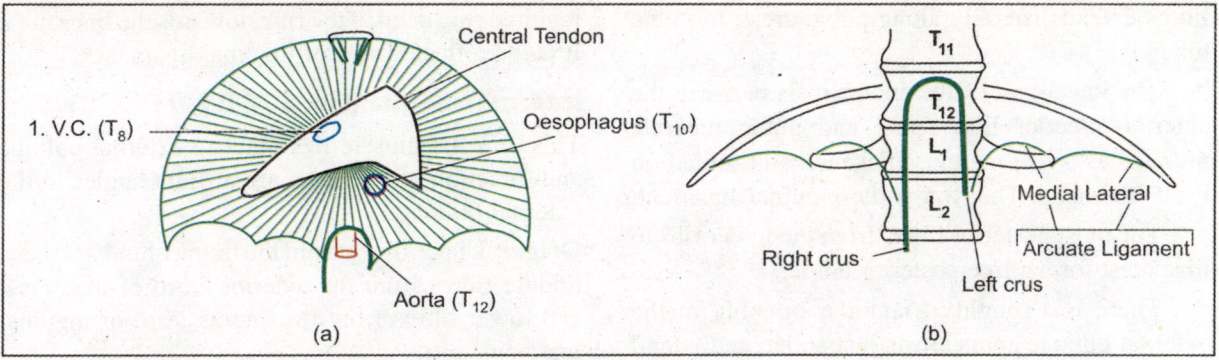

Fig. 3.77: Diaphragm

Openings (Apertures) in the diaphragm:

Three major openings:

1. Aortic opening- behind median arcuate ligament at T_{12} level. Transmits aorta, azygos vein, thoracic duct and sympathetic trunk.

2. Oesophageal opening – slightly to the left of midline, at level with T_{10} vertebra. Through it Vagus nerve also passes.

3. Vena caval opening – for inferior vena cava, at level with T_8 vertebra. Through it, right phrenic nerve also comes down.

Nerve supply:

Motor – Phrenic nerve ($C_{3,4,5}$)

Sensory – pheripheral part form lower 6 intercostal nerves. Central part from phrenic nerve.

Major relations:

Above – pleura and pericardium.

Below – Liver, Stomach, kidneys, suprarenals and spleen.

Action: Muscle of respiration. It is active during abdominal straining as in defecation.

MUSCLES OF ABDOMEN

Two groups

1. Anterolateral group
2. Posterior group

Anterolateral group

Consists of three large flat muscles, a long vertical muscle and a small triangular muscle. These muscles constitute the anterior abdominal wall. They are:

1. External oblique ⎫
2. Internal oblique   ⎬ flat
3. Tranversus abdominis ⎭
4. Rectus abdominis – vertical
5. Pyramidalis – small triangular

Outside, the muscles are covered by skin and superficial fascia. There is no deep fascia. On the inner surface, lined by a thin fascia – fascia transversalis. Superficial fascia has two layers- a superficial fatty layer (fascia of Camper) and a deep membranous layer (fascia of Scarpa).

External oblique abdominis (Fig. 3.78 a)

Most superficial of the 3 flat muscles.

Origin: From the outer surfaces of lower 8 ribs. The muscle is directed downwards and medially.

Insertion: Fibres from the lower 2 or 3 ribs run vertically downwards and get inserted to the outer lip of iliac crest. The remaining upper muscle fibres which are directed downwards and medially get converted into an aponeurosis. The aponeurosis of both sides decussate along the vertical midline from xiphoid process to pubic symphysis forming a midline raphe – linea alba. Lower attachment of these fibres extends laterally along pubic crest, to pubic tubercle.

The lower part of the aponeurosis between the anterior superior iliac spine and pubic tubercle presents as a free margin, thickened and folded on itself internally. This forms the inguinal ligament.

The most posterior fibres from the lower ribs to iliac crest form a free posterior border.

There is a roughly triangular opening in the external oblique aponeurosis just above and lateral to the pubic crest. This is the superficial inguinal ring.

Inguinal ligament (Poupart's ligament) (Fig. 3.79)

It is a thick band of fibrous tissue formed of lower end of external oblique aponeurosis. Extends between pubic tubercle and anterior superior iliac spine. As it is folded upon itself, It has a grooved upper surface which forms floor of inguinal canal.

At the medial end of the inguinal ligament, it extends along the pecten pubis for a short distance. This, the medial end of the inguinal ligament and a free curved lateral margin form the triangular lacunar ligament. Some fibres of the lacunar ligament extend along the pectineal line and is called pectineal ligament. (Cooper's ligament)

Some fibres of the inguinal ligament get reflected from the medial margin of superficial inguinal ring deep to the ring, towards the linea alba. It is the reflected part of inguinal ligament.

Internal oblique (Fig. 3.78 b,80)

This thin flat muscle lies inner to external oblique and direction of its fibres are at right angles to the external oblique.

Origin: Upper fibres from the thoracolumbar fascia, middle fibres from the anterior 2/3rd of iliac crest and lower fibres from the lateral 2/3rd of inguinal ligament.

Insertion: Generally fibres are directed upward and medially. Fibers from thoracolumbar fascia and posterior part of iliac crest get inserted to lower 3 or 4 ribs.

Fibres from anterior part of iliac crest and lateral part of inguinal ligament spread out into an aponeurosis. The superiorly directed fibers get attached to the costal margin – 7th to 9th costal cartilages and Xiphoid process. The succeeding fibres are directed to linea alba.

Fibres from middle part of inguinal ligament pass medially and arch upwards over the inguinal canal, then directed downwards and medially behind the canal. Here the fibres have become tendinous and join with the tendon of transversus abdominis to form the conjoint tendon which is attached to the pubic crest. Thus the lower fibres of internal oblique form parts of the anterior wall, roof and posterior wall of inguinal canal.

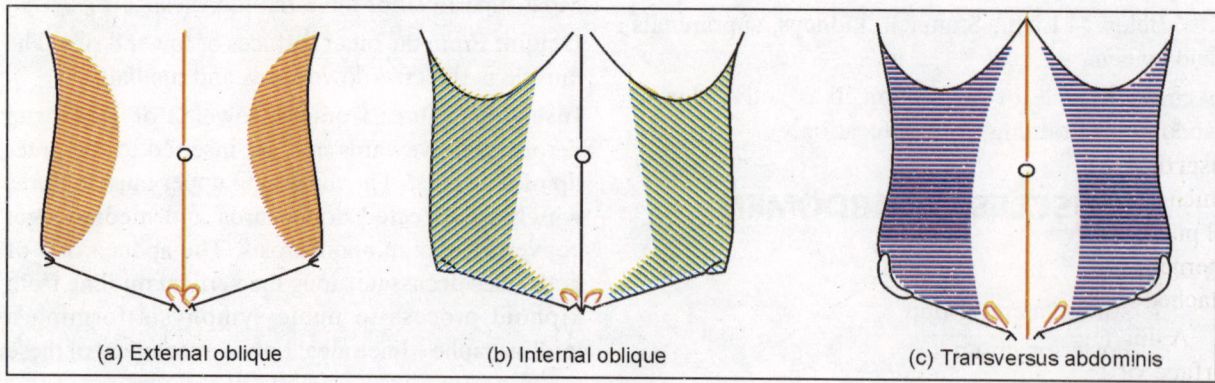

(a) External oblique   (b) Internal oblique   (c) Transversus abdominis

Fig. 3.78

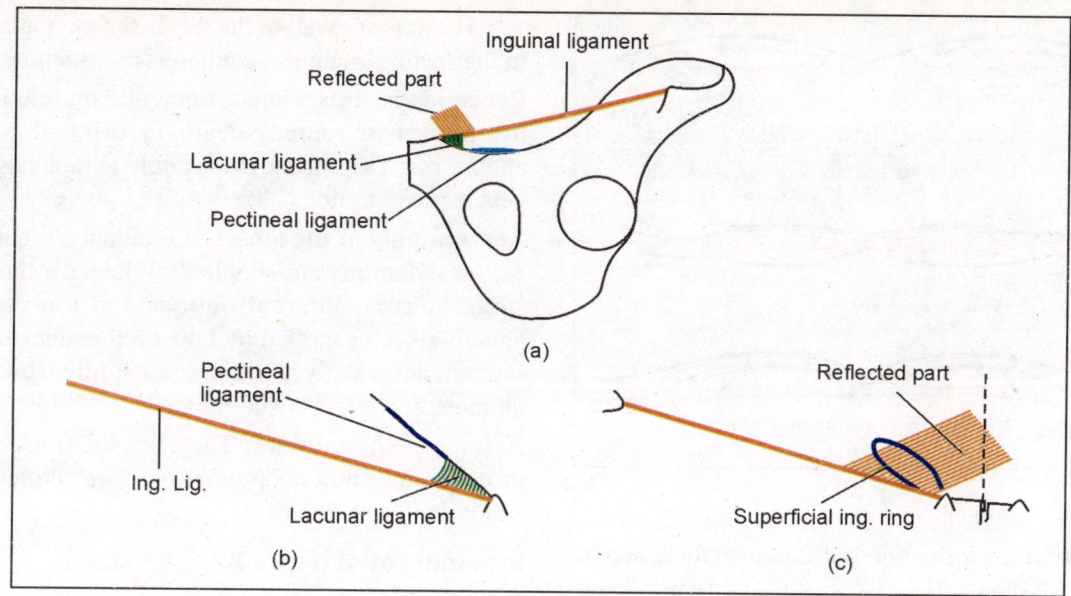

Fig. 3.79: Inguinal ligament

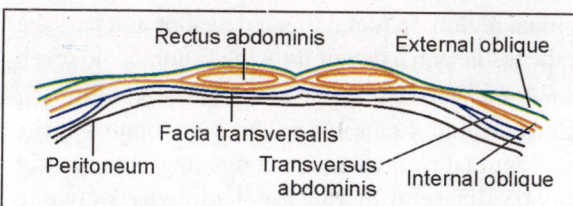

Fig. 3.80: C.S. anterior abdominal wall

Transversus abdominis (Fig. 3.78c, 80)

Innermost muscle. Fibres run horizontally.

Origin:

1. Inner surfaces of the lower 6 costal cartilages.
2. Thoracolumbar fascia.
3. Anterior 2/3rd of iliac crest.
4. Lateral 1/3rd of inguinal ligament.

Insertion: Muscle fibres change into an aponeurosis which is inserted into linea alba from xiphoid process till pubic symphysis. The lowest fibres join those of internal oblique to form conjoint tendon which is attached to the pubic crest.

A thin layer of connective tissue lines the inner surface of transversus abdominis. This is fascia transversalis.

Rectus abdominis (Fig. 3.80)

It is a vertical muscle on either side of the linea alba.

Origin: 2 heads of origin.

1. from the front of pubic symphysis.
2. from the pubic crest.

Muscle ascends and is inserted into the 5th, 6th and 7th costal cartilages. Its lateral margin is seen as linea semilunaris which extends from tip of 9th costal cartilage to pubic tubercle.

The muscle is interrupted at 3 sites by 3 cross bands – tendinous intersections – one at the level of umbilicus, one at level of xiphoid process and the 3rd between 1st and 2nd.

Rectus sheath (Fig. 3.81)

Rectus abdominis is enclosed in an aponeurotic sheath – rectus sheath, derived from the aponeurosis of the 3 flat muscles.

Contents:

Rectus abdominis

Pyramidalis muscle

Superior and inferior epigastric vessels

Ventral rami of lower 6 thoracic nerves

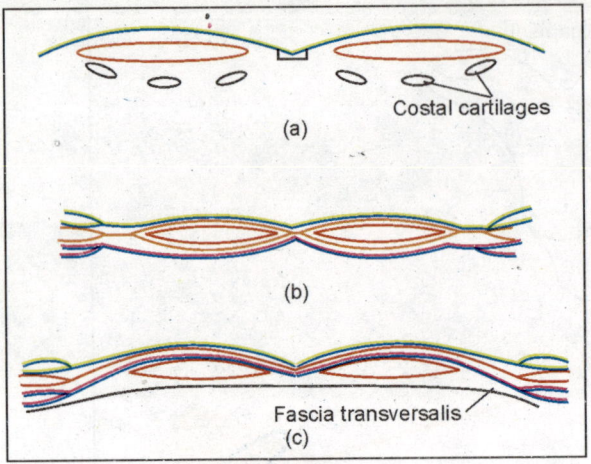

Fig. 3.81

Formation: Its formation is different at three levels.

1. Above the level of costal margin-the rectus abdominis lies directly over the costal cartilages, so the posterior wall of the sheath is formed of cartilage. Its anterior wall is formed of external oblique aponeurosis.

2. Between the levels of costal margin and anterior superior iliac spine, the internal oblique aponeurosis splits to enclose the muscle. Anteriorly and posteriorly the layer is reinforced by external oblique aponeurosis and transversus abdominis aponeurosis.

3. Below the level of anterior superior iliac spine and upto the pubis, aponeuroses of all the three flat muscles pass anterior to the muscle to form the anterior wall of the sheath. Posterior wall is deficient and muscle rests on fascia transversalis.

4. At the level where the posterior wall of rectus sheath also passes into the anterior wall, the posterior wall leaves a free slightly curved lower border behind the muscle, this is **arcuate line.**

Between the two recti, along the midline a vertical line is seen from xiphoid process, to pubis. This is linea alba and is formed by the intersection of the aponeuroses of both sides.

The anterior wall of the rectus sheath is attached to the rectus, along the tendinous intersections.

Pyramidalis: It is a small triangular muscle in the lower part of rectus sheath in front of rectus abdominis. Originates from pubic symphysis and gets inserted to linea alba.

Nerve supply of the muscles: External oblique and rectus abdominis are supplied by lower 6 thoracic spinal nerves. Internal oblique and transversus abdominis are supplied by lower 6 thoracic and 1st lumbar nerves. Pyramidalis is supplied by 12th thoracic nerve (subcostal nerve).

Actions of the muscles: They flex the trunk. Help in increasing intra abdominal pressure. Protect the abdominal structures.

Inguinal canal (Fig. 3.82, 3.83a,b,c,)

It is an oblique passage in the lower part of the anterior abdominal wall, on either side, in the inguinal region. In foetal life, it develops as a passage for the testis which develops in the abdomen, to reach the scrotal sac.

Extent: About 4 cms long. The canal begins at the deep inguinal ring which is an opening in the fascia transversalis seen at the level midway between anterior superior iliac spine and pubic symphysis, half inch above inguinal ligament.

The canal inclines medially, above and parallel to the inguinal ligament and ends at the superficial inguinal ring which is a triangular opening in the external oblique aponeurosis just above and lateral to pubic crest (Fig 3.82)

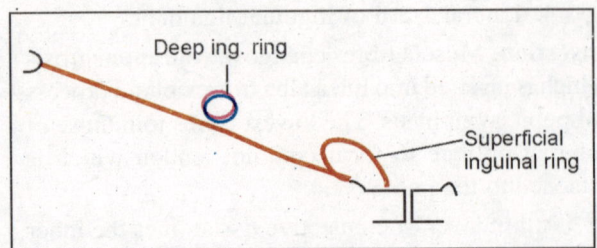

Fig. 3.82

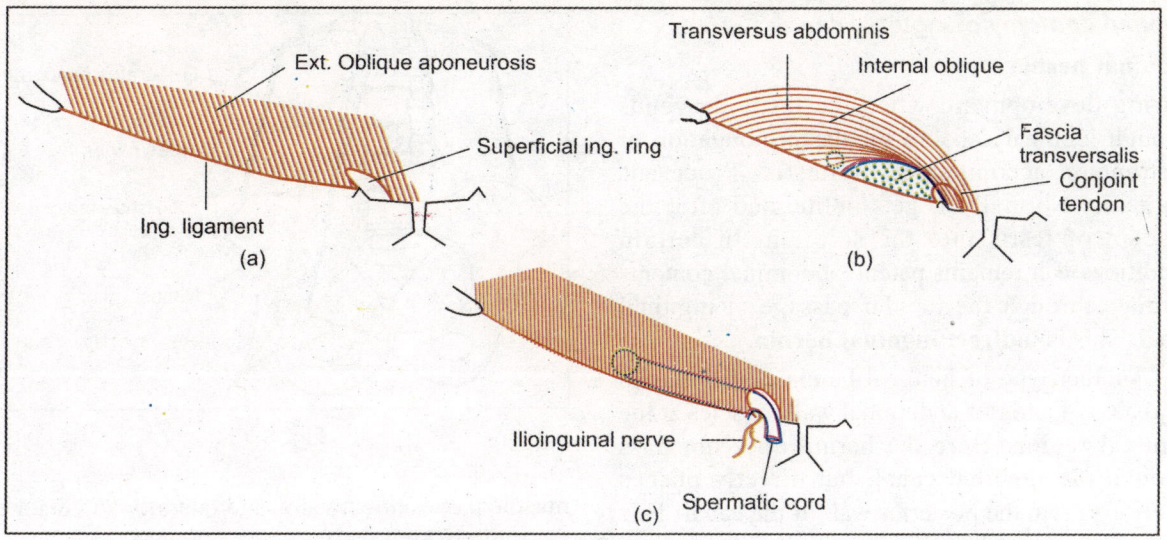

Fig. 3.83: Inguinal Canal

Boundaries:

Floor – The upper grooved surface of inguinal ligament.

Roof – Formed by the lowest arching fibres of internal oblique. Lowest fibres of tranversus abdominis also join to form the roof.

Anterior wall – External oblique aponeurosis throughout its extent, reinforced by fleshy fibres of origin of internal oblique in the lateral 1/3rd.

Posterior wall – Formed by the fascia transversalis along its entire length and reinforced on its medial 1/3rd by conjoint tendon.

Contents: Inguinal canal transmits spermatic cord in male and round ligament in female with ilioinguinal nerve.

Spermatic cord (Fig. 3.84)

Passes through the inguinal canal.
Structures in the cord:

1. Ductus deferens (Vas deferens)
2. Artery to the vas
3. Testicular artery
4. Artery to cremaster muscle
5. Testicular veins

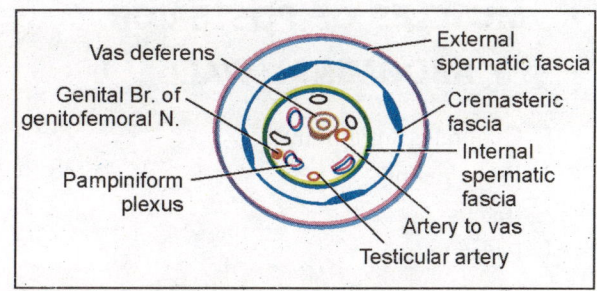

Fig. 3.84: Coverings and Contents - Spermatic Cord (Cross Section)

6. Genital branch of genitofemoral nerve
7. Lymph vessels

The contents of spermatic cord are covered by-

1. Internal spermatic fascia- A prolongation of fascia transversalis as the cord passes out of the deep ring.
2. Cremasteric fascia- Extends from the internal oblique muscle. This fascia contains cremaster muscle, embedded in it.
3. External spermatic fascia – Prolongation from the external oblique aponeurosis from the margin of superficial inguinal ring.

Applied anatomy of inguinal canal:

Inguinal hernia

During development, when the testis descends through inguinal canal, a tubular prolongation of peritoneum accompanies the testis- Processus vaginalis. Normally it gets obliterated after the descent of testis into the scrotum. In certain conditions if it remains patent, abdominal contents herniate through the tubular passage at inguinal canal. This is **indirect inguinal hernia**.

Another type of inguinal hernia occurs due to weakness of anterior abdominal wall muscles at the inguinal region. Here the hernia does not pass through the inguinal canal, but directly pushes anteriorly from the posterior wall of the canal. This is **direct inguinal hernia**.

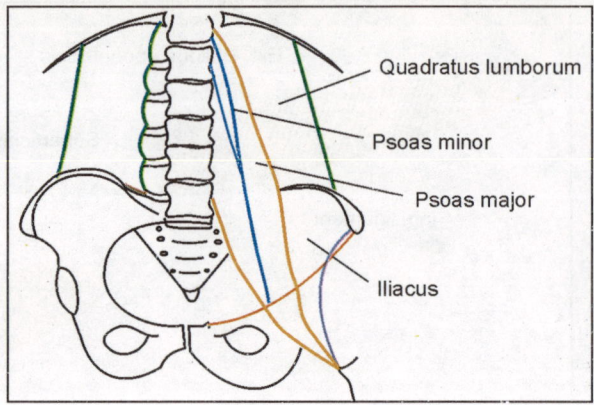

Fig. 3.85

MUSCLES OF POSTERIOR ABDOMINAL WALL

1. Quadratus lumborum
2. Psoas major
3. Iliacus
4. Psoas minor

Psoas major and iliacus partially belong to the lower limb also, as their insertions reach the femur.

1. Quadratus lumborum (Fig. 3.85)

A flat quadrilateral muscle, on either side of vertebral column enclosed in the thoracolumbar fascia.

Origin: From iliolumbar ligament and adjoining 5 cms of iliac crest.

Insertion: To the medial half of 12th rib and tips of transverse processes of L_1 to L_5 vertebrae.

Nerve supply: Ventral rami of T_{12} to L_4 nerves.

Action: Fixes the 12th rib, thus helps in respiration. Causes lateral flexion of vertebral column.

2. Psoas major (Fig. 3.85)

Origin: From the transverse processes, bodies and intervertebral discs of all lumbar vertebrae. The muscle passes downwards and laterally and reaches the thigh behind the inguinal ligament.

Insertion: Into the lesser trochanter of femur together with iliacus.

Nerve supply: Ventral rami of L_1 to L_3.

Action: Flexion of thigh at hip.

3. Iliacus (Fig.3.85)

Origin: From the upper 2/3rd of iliac fossa and inner lip of iliac crest. Descends lateral to psoas major.

Insertion: Lesser trochanter of femur with psoas. major as ilio-psoas.

Nerve supply: From femoral nerve

Action: Flexion of thigh

4. Psoas minor (Fig. 3.85)

It is an inconstant muscle. Originates from bodies of T_{12} and L1. Lies on anterior surface of psoas major. Inserted on to the pectineal line and ilio pubic eminence.

Nerve supply: L_1 nerve

Action: A weak flexor of trunk

THORACOLUMBAR FASCIA (Fig. 3.86)

The fascia has three layers that cover the muscles of posterior abdominal wall and deep muscles of back.

Posterior layer is attached to lumbar and sacral spines, covers erector spinae of back. Middle layer

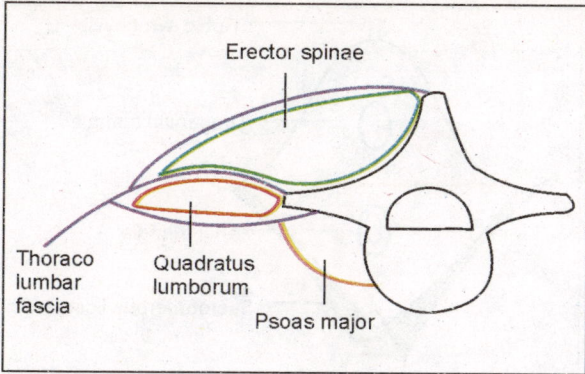

Fig. 3.86

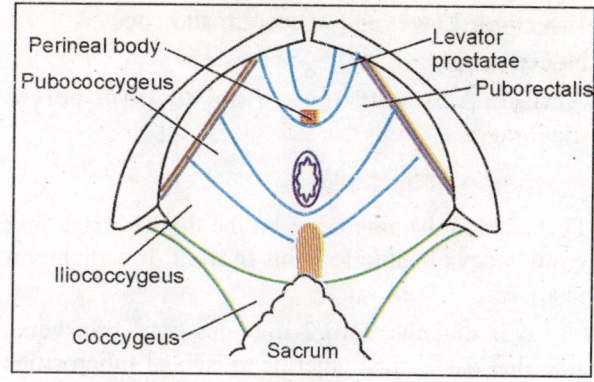

Fig. 3.87

is attached to tips of transverse processes of lumbar vertebrae and separates quadratus lumborum from erector spinae.

Anterior layer is attached to anterior surfaces of transverse processes of lumbar vertebrae. Quadratus lumborum is seen between anterior and middle layers.

The three layers fuse laterally to form a single layer of fascia from which internal oblique and transverusus abdominis muscles take origin.

MUSCLES OF PELVIS

Four muscles originate from within the pelvis (Fig. 3.87)

1. Piriformis
2. Obturator internus
3. Levator ani
4. Coccygeus

Of these, piriformis passes out through greater sciatic foramen and obturator internus through lesser sciatic foramen to the gluteal region and are included in the group of muscles of lower limb.

Levator ani and coccygeus of both sides form the **pelvic diaphram** that forms support of pelvic viscera (pelvic floor).

Levator ani

Origin: It has a linear origin from

1. Back of body of pubis
2. Obturator fascia, by a tendinous arch
3. Spine of ischium

From the extensive origin, fibres are directed downwards and medially towards insertion. Based on insertion, 4 parts are described for levator ani.

1. Levator prostatae in male or sphincter vaginae in female.

   Formed of anterior fibres which form a sling around prostate or vagina and is inserted into perineal body, a fibromuscular mass in front of anal canal. This part supports the prostate or constricts the vagina and stabilizes perineal body.

2. Puborectalis

   Forms a sling around anorectal junction.

3. Pubococcygeus

   The intermediate fibres pass posteriorly to get inserted into anococcygeal body, a fibrous mass behind anal canal.

4. Iliococcygeus

   Posterior fibres go to get inserted into coccyx and anococcygeal body.

Nerve supply: Perineal branch of S4 nerve and perineal branch of pudendal nerve.

Coccygeus

Origin: Ischial spine

Insertion: Lower end of sacrum and coccyx.

Nerve supply: S_4 and S_5 nerves.

Action: Acts with levator ani to form pelvic diaphragm.

Perineum (Fig. 3.88)

Perineum is the area between the thighs, extending from coccyx behind to pubis in front. It is diamond shaped.

It is divisible into 2 triangles by a transverse line that passes just anterior to ischeal tuberosities and anal orifice. Posterior one is anal triangle and anterior one is urogenital triangle.

Muscles of perineum and spaces related to them (Perineal spaces or pouches) (Fig 3.89 a b)

Urogenital triangle is the space between the 2 ischiopubic rami. Across this triangular space, three membranes are attached, one over the other, with 2 intervening spaces.

The layers are,

1. Superior fascia of urogenital diaphragm. This is continuous with the obturator fascia of lateral pelvic wall.
2. Inferior fascia of urogenital diaphragm. It is otherwise known as perineal membrane.. The first 2 layers enclose a space, the deep perineal pouch.

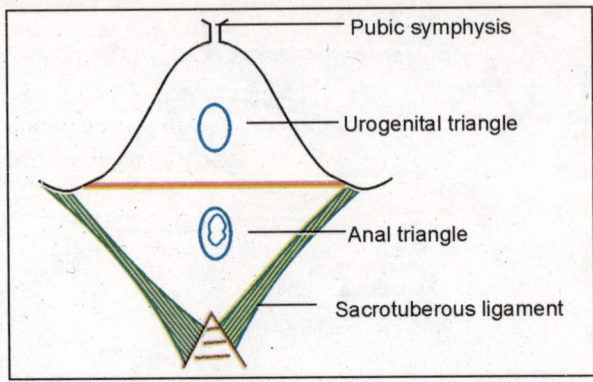

Fig. 3.88

3. Outermost layer is the membranous layer of superficial fascia. The 2nd and 3rd layers enclose the superficial perineal pouch.

The three layers are fused together, along their posterior margins, thus closing the spaces between them posteriorly.

Deep perineal pouch (Fig. 3.89b, 3.90)

It is the space between the superior fascia of urogenital diaphragm and perineal membrane.

Muscles (Fig. 3.90)

1. Sphinctor urethrae

It stretches between the 2 ischiopubic rami, pierced by urethra in male and urethra and vagina in female.

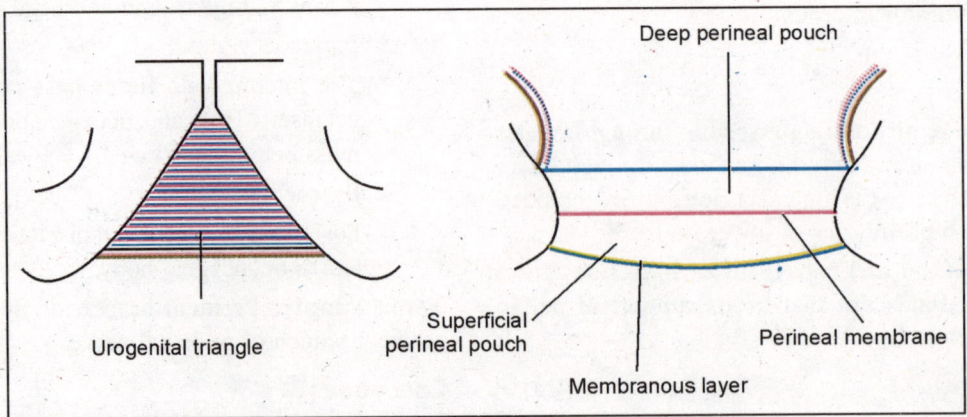

Fig. 3.89

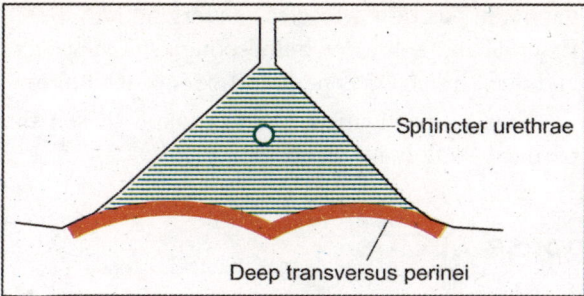

Fig. 3.90

2. Deep transversus perinei

Attached laterally to the ischial ramus and medially converges to the perineal body.

Apart from the 2 muscles, the deep perineal pouch also contains,

1. Bulbourethral glands. Their ducts go to superficial pouch and enter the urethra there.
2. Perineal branch of pudental nerve.
3. Dorsal nerve of penis.
4. Internal pudental vessels.

Boundaries and contents of deep perineal pouch constitute the **urogenital diaphragm.**

Superficial perineal pouch (Fig. 3.89.b, 3.91)

It is the space between perineal membrane and membranous layer of superficial fascia.

Muscles in this space are-

1. Bulbospongiosus.

Arises from perineal body and encircles the bulb of penis in male and bulb of clitoris in female.

Action: Helps to empty the urethra.

2. Ischiocavernosus.

Covers crus of penis. Originates from ischial tuberosity and ischial ramus. Ends on the under surface of crus.

Action: Maintains penile erection.

3. Superficial transversus perinei.

A narrow muscle, originates from ischial tuberosity and is inserted to perineal body.

Nerve supply: All three muscles are supplied by perineal branch of pudental nerve.

Apart from muscles, the superficial perineal pouch contains root of penis consisting of bulb and 2 crura. In the female, root of clitoris.

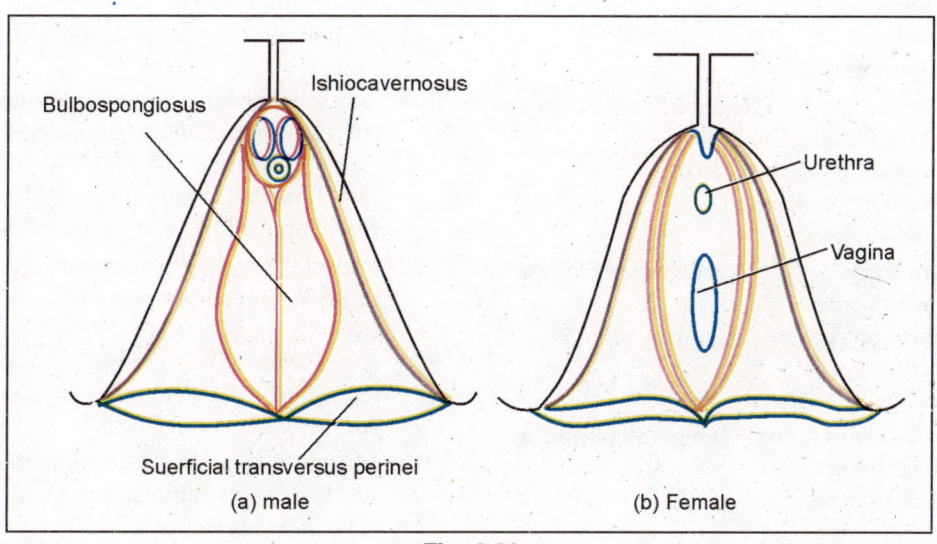

Fig. 3.90

Perineal body

It is the central tendon of perineum. A fibromuscular mass, seen in the midline between anal and urogenital triangles. Many muscles converge and get attached to it. So it has a role in keeping rectum and vagina in position. Muscles converging into it are – External anal sphincter, bulbospongiosus, superficial and deep transversus perinei, fibers of levator ani.

During parturition, care is taken to see that perineal body is not damaged.

Single Best Response M.C.Qs

1. Latissimus dorsi is inserted into
   - (a) Lesser tubercle of humerus
   - (b) Lateral lip of bicipital groove
   - (c) Medial lip of bicipital groove
   - (d) Floor of bicipital groove
2. Following are mucles of pectoral region except
   - (a) Pectoralis minor
   - (b) Pectoralis major
   - (c) Serratus anterior
   - (d) Subclavius
3. Muscle that is not a member of Rotator cuff is
   - (a) Teres major
   - (b) Supraspinatus
   - (c) Infraspinatus
   - (d) Subcapularis
4. Muscle that is inserted to the front of coronoid process of ulna is
   - (a) Biceps
   - (b) Triceps
   - (c) Brachialis
   - (d) Coracobrachialis
5. Following are the deep flexors of forearm except
   - (a) Flexor Pollicis Longus
   - (b) Flexor Digitorum profundus
   - (c) Pronator quadratus
   - (d) Pronator teres.
6. Structure that is not a content of cubital fossa is
   - (a) Radial nerve
   - (b) Ulnar nerve
   - (c) Median nerve
   - (d) Tendon of Biceps
7. Nerve affected in Carpal Tunnel Syndrome is
   - (a) Ulnar nerve
   - (b) Median nerve
   - (c) Radial nerve
   - (d) Deep branch of ulnar nerve

8. Following are correct about lumbricals except
   - (a) They originate from tendons of flexor digitorum superficialis
   - (b) They are inserted to lateral side of extensor expansion
   - (c) Ist and 2nd are supplied by median nerve
   - (d) 3rd and 4th are supplied by deep branch of ulnar nerve
9. Muscle that is not a component of quadriceps femoris is
   - (a) Vastus lateralis
   - (b) Vastus medialis
   - (c) Vastus intermedius
   - (d) Biceps femoris
10. Femoral canal contains
    - (a) Femoral vein
    - (b) Femoral artery
    - (c) Lymph nodes
    - (d) Femoral nerve
11. Following are correct about gluteus maximus except
    - (a) It is the largest muscle of gluteal region.
    - (b) Major part of it is inserted into gluteal tuberosity.
    - (c) It extends hip joint.
    - (d) Supplied by inferior gluteal nerve.
12. Muscle that is not a component of deep muscles of posterior compartment of leg is
    - (a) Plantaris
    - (b) Flexor hallucis longus
    - (c) Flexor digitorum longus
    - (d) Tibialis posterior
13. Muscle that prevents accumulation of food in vestibule of mouth while chewing is
    - (a) Orbicularis oris
    - (b) Masseter

(c) Buccinator
(d) Temporalis

14. Muscle that turns eye ball downwards and laterally is
(a) Superior oblique
(b) Inferior oblique

(c) Superior rectus
(d) Inferior rectus

15. Inguinal ligament is a part of
(a) Fascia lata of thigh
(b) External oblique aponeurosis
(c) Internal oblique aponeurosis
(d) Transversus abdominis aponeurosis

Essays

I. Describe the extent, deep relations, structure, blood supply, lymphatic drainage and clinical aspects of mammary gland.

II. Describe the boundaries and enumerate the contents of Axilla.

III. Describe the boundaries and contents of cubital fossa.

IV. Describe the boundaries and contents of femoral triangle.

V. Name the muscles of thenar eminence and describe them.

VI. Name of muscles of anterior compartment of leg and describe them.

VII. Name the muscles of lateral compartment of leg and describe them.

VIII. Describe the muscles of mastication.

IX. Describe the boundaries and contents of posterior triangle.

X. Give the subdivisions of anterior triangle and describe carotid triangle.

XI. Describe the structures of intercostal space.

XII. Describe the Diaphragm.

XIII. Describe the Rectus sheath.

XIV. Describe the extra ocular muscles.

XV. Describe the rotator cuff muscles.

M.C.Qs - Answers

1. (d), 2. (c), 3. (a), 4. (c), 5. (d), 6. (b), 7. (b), 8. (a), 9. (d), 10. (c), 11. (b), 12. (a), 13. (c), 14. (a), 15. (b)

Short notes

1. Trapezius
2. Intermuscular spaces of scapular region
3. Pectoralis major
4. Supinator
5. Flexor retinaculum
6. Adductor pollicis
7. Extensor retinaculum
8. Palmar aponeurosis
9. Anatomical snuff box
10. Fascia lata
11. Interossei and lumbricals
12. Tensor fascia lata
13. Adductor canal
14. Adductor magnus
15. Hamstring muscles
16. Retinacula around ankle
17. Popliteal fossa
18. Flexor accessorius
19. Orbicularis occuli
20. Buccinator
21. Orbicularis oris
22. Sternocleidomastoid

23. Digastric muscle
24. Omohyoid
25. Scalenus anterior
26. Carotid sheath
27. Ansa cervicalis
28. Inguinal ligament
29. Inguinal canal
30. Spermatic cord
31. Levator ani
32. Perineal pouches
33. Levator palpebrae superioris
34. Femoral sheath
35. Popliteus

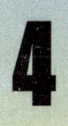

4   Joints of the Body

Study of joints of body is arthrology.

JOINTS OF UPPER LIMB

SHOULDER JOINT

Shoulder joint is a synovial joint of ball and socket variety.

Articular Parts

Medially (proximally) – shallow glenoid cavity of scapula.

Laterally (distally) – Spheroidal head of humerus. Both the articular surfaces are covered by hyaline cartilage

The glenoid cavity is a very shallow cup which cannot accommodate the rounded head of humerus except a small portion. The concavity of the glenoid cavity is deepened by a fibrocartilagenous rim- the glenoid labrum, along its margin.

Capsule and ligaments

Capsule is thin and lax allowing freedom of movements at the joint. It is strengthened by fibres from the tendons of the surrounding muscles.

Attached medially to margin of glenoid cavity outside the glenoid labrum. Laterally attached along the anatomical neck of humerus, but below and medially the line of attachment descends along the shaft of humerus for one cm. Here it is very lax. Lined by synovial membrane.

Ligaments

1. Glenohumeral ligaments (Intrinsic) (Fig. 4.1a)

   They are three in number – superior, middle and inferior, seen on the anterior aspect of capsule, visible better on its deep surface.

   Superior one – Extends from upper part of glenoid margin, to the upper part of neck of humerus.

   Middle one – From anterior margin of glenoid cavity to the lesser tubercle.

   Inferior one – From the lower part of glenoid margin to the lower part of neck of humerus.

2. Coracohumeral ligament. (Extrinsic) (Fig. 4.1b)

   A thick band from the root of coracoid process to the upper part of front of greater tubercle. Merges with the capsule.

3. Transverse humeral ligament. (extrinsic)

   Stretches between the lips of intertubercular sulcus of humerus; converts it into a canal for passage of tendon of long head of biceps from within the joint cavity. Merges with the lower part of anterior aspect of capsule.

4. Coraco acromial ligament (Accessary/ Extrinsic).

A strong triangular ligament. Apex attached to the acromion and base to the lateral border of coracoid process. Forms an arch over the capsule of the joint and protects it.

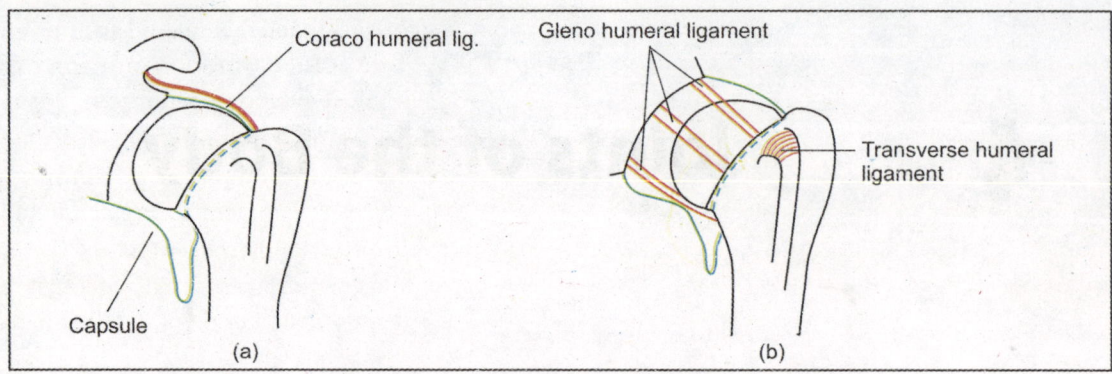

Fig. 4.1: Shoulder Joint

Muscles related: (Fig. 4.2)

Anteriorly - Subscapularis

Posteriorly –Infraspinatus & Teres minor

Above— Supraspinatus

Below — Long head of triceps.

Deltoid covers the joint in front, behind and laterally.

Tendons of subscapularis, supraspinatus, Infraspinatus and Teres minor are very closely related to the joint capsule near their insertions. Fibres from them merge with the capsule and help to stabilise the joint which is otherwise unstable due to the non-congruence of the articular parts and lax joint capsule. These four muscles together form a **rotator cuff** for reinforcing and supporting the capsule.

Bursae

1. Subscapular bursa deep to subscapularis tendon. Communicates with the joint cavity through an opening.

2. Infraspinatus bursa deep to infraspinatus. Frequently communicates with the joint cavity.

3. Subacromial bursa.Deep to deltoid, extends under acromion and coracoacromial ligament, separates them from supraspinatus.

4. Subcoracoid bursa- Between capsule and coracoid process.

Nerve supply

Axillary Nerve, Suprascapular Nerve and Lateral Pectoral Nerve.

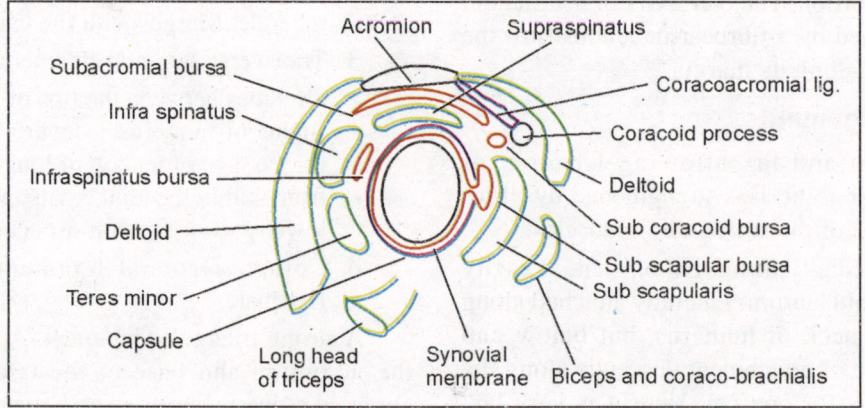

Fig.: 4.2: Relations of Shoulder Joint

Blood supply

Anterior and posterior circumflex humeral vessels,
Circumflex scapular vessels,
Supra scapular vessels.

Movements and muscles causing them

1. Flexion - Anterior fibres of deltoid,
   Clavicular fibres of pectoralis major,
   Biceps, Coracobrachialis
2. Extension - Posterior fibres of Deltoid, Teres Major.
3. Abduction - Initiated by supraspinatus (to upto horizontal (90degrees).
   (Abduction from 90 degrees upto 180° is possible, but it does not occur at shoulder joint but is due to rotation of scapula.)
4. Adduction - Pectoralis Major and Latissimus Dorsi
5. Medial rotation - Pectoralis major,
   Anterior fibres of deltoid, Latissimus Dorsi, Teres major, Subscapularis
6. Lateral rotation - Deltoid (posterior fibres), Infraspinatus, Teres minor
7. Circumduction - Is a combination of all other movements.

Clinical aspects

1. Dislocation: Due to the instability of the joint and laxity of capsule, shoulder joint is frequently dislocated. Dislocation occurs anteroinferiorly, where the capsule is least protected by muscles.
2. Osteoarthritis and rheumatoid arthritis affect the joint. In chronic condition, joint replacement surgery is indicated.
3. Supraspinatus tendinitis. Usually occurs secondary to subacromial bursits and presents as severe pain during abduction.
4. In chronic conditions of supraspinatus tendinitis, supraspinatus tendon gets calcified or ruptures. Patient complaints of inability to initiate abduction.

ELBOW JOINT

Type – A compound synovial joint of hinge variety. (Fig 4.3, 4.4)

Includes 2 articulations

1. Humeroulnar
2. Humeroradial

Articular parts

Trochlea of humerus articulates with trochlear notch of ulna. Capitulum of humerus articulates with head of radius. They are lined by hyaline cartilage.

Capsule and ligaments

Capsule is attached above – in front, to the medial epicondyle and upper margins of coronoid and radial fossae. Behind, along the trochlear margin, margin of olecranon fossa and over the capitulum.

Below – Along the margins of coronoid and olecranon processes and to the anular ligament around head of radius.

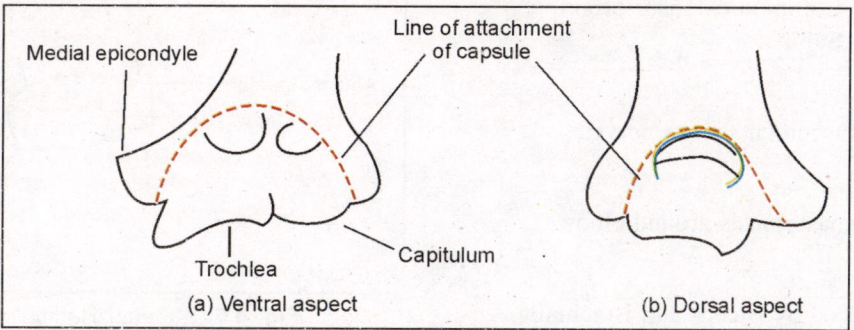

Medial epicondyle • Line of attachment of capsule • Capitulum • Trochlea • (a) Ventral aspect • (b) Dorsal aspect

Fig.: 4.3: Lower end of Humerus in Elbow Joint

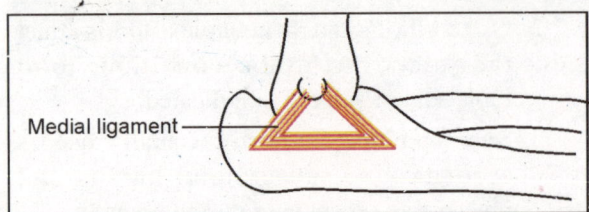

Fig. 4.4

Inner surface of the capsule and the 3 fossae are lined by synovial membrane. In the 3 fossae and between the radius and ulna, synovial membrane makes folds which cover pads of fat.

Ligaments

1. Medial ligament (Fig 4.4)-Ulnar collateral ligament – It is a triangular band with anterior, posterior and inferior thick bands and a middle thin part.
2. Lateral (radial collateral) ligament – Extends from lateral epicondyle to anular ligament.
3. Anterior and posterior ligaments strengthen the capsule in front and behind.

Relations

Anteriorly –   Brachialis,
                 Tendon of biceps,
                 Median nerve,
                 Brachial artery.
Posteriorly –   Triceps,
                 Anconeus.
Medially –   Common flexor origin,
                 Ulnar nerve.
Laterally –   Common extensor origin,
                 Supinator.

Nerve supply

Radial nerve, Musculocutaneous nerve.

Blood supply

Branches from anastomosis around elbow

Movements

Flexion – Produced by Biceps and Brachialis

Extension – Produced by Triceps and anconeus

Applied anatmy

Posterior dislocation,

Fracture of coronoid process,

Subluxation of head of radius.

RADIO ULNAR JOINTS

Superior, middle and inferior joints

1. Superior radioulnar joint (Fig 4.5, 4.6)

Type – Synovial joint of pivot type

Articular parts

   (a) Circumference of head of radius.

   (b) Radial notch of ulna and anular ligament.

The bony parts and inner surface of the anular ligament are lined by hyaline cartilage.

Capsule

It encloses the joint and is continuous above with that of elbow joint. Lined by synovial membrane.

Ligaments

1. Anular Ligament – It is a strong band, encircles the radial head and holds it against radial notch of ulna. Attached to the anterior and posterior edges of the radial notch and forms a circle with it.

2. Quadrate ligament – A small fibrous band stretches from neck of radius to ulna below radial notch.

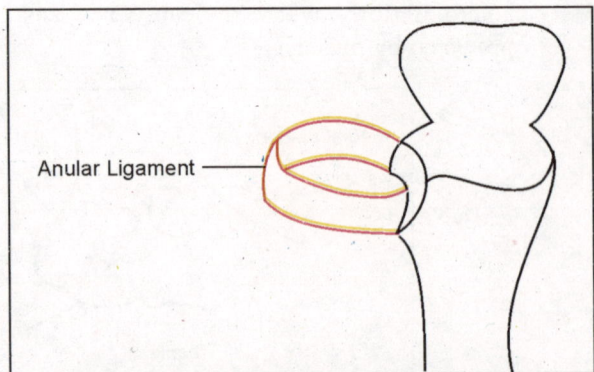

Fig. 4.5: Superior Radioulnar Joint

Relations

Anteriorly – Supinator

Posteriorly – Anconeus

Movements

1. Pronation – Pronator teres and Pronator quadratus.
2. Supination – Supinator, Biceps brachii.

Nerve supply

Ulnar, Median, Radial and Musculocutaneous nerves.

2. Middle radioulnar joint (Fig 4.6)

It is a fibrous joint of syndesmosis variety.

The interosseus borders of radius and ulna are joined by a band of fibrous tissue – Interosseous membrane. Fibres of interosseous membrane are directed downwards and medially from the radius to ulna. Above the upper border of the membrane, the posterior interosseous artery goes posteriorly. Near its lower end, a small opening is seen for the passage of anterior interosseous artery posteriorly. Deep muscles of forearm are attached to it anteriorly and posteriorly.

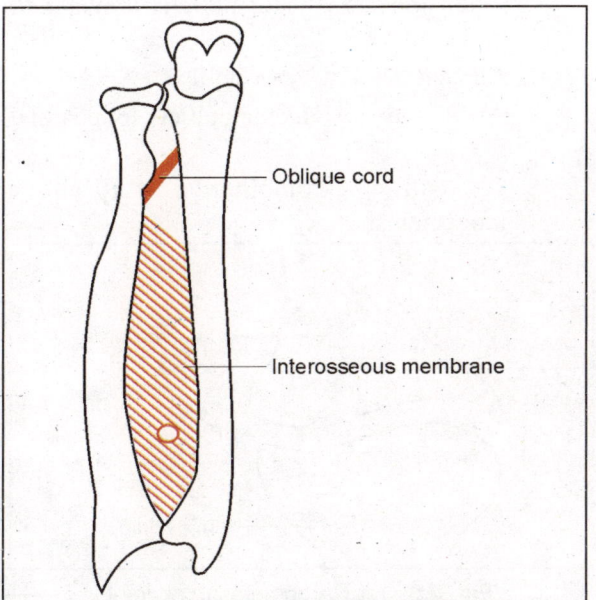

Fig. 4.6: Middle Radioulnar Joint

Oblique cord is a small additional fibrous band connecting radius and ulna. It extends from tuberosity of ulna to below the radial tuberosity.

Movements

Pronation and supination – same group of muscles as in superior joint.

3. Distal radioulnar joint

Type – Synovial joint of pivot variety.

Articular parts – Head of ulna and ulnar notch of radius.

The bones are enclosed by the fibrous capsule, lined by synovial membrane.

Articular disc – There is an articular fibrocartilagenous disc of triangular shape. Attached to the ulnar styloid process and lower edge of ulnar notch. Its distal surface is part of radiocarpal joint.

Movements – Pronation and supination

PRONATION AND SUPINATION

Pronation – Radius moves obliquely across the ulna, proximal end of radius remains lateral and distal end becomes medial to ulna. Interosseous membrane gets spiralised. Hand moves with radius caused by pronator teres and pronator quadratus.

Supination – Radius returns to the lateral position, interosseous membrane is despiralised.

Caused by Biceps and supinator.

Axis of the movement passes through centre of head of radius and apex of articular disc.

WRIST JOINT (Fig 4.7)

Type – Synovial, Ellipsoidal variety.

Articular parts

Proximal – Distal end of radius and articular disc. These form a concave surface.

Distal – Upper surfaces of Triquetral, Lunate and scaphoid. These together form a convex surface.

Bony parts are covered by hyaline cartilage.

Capsule – Encloses the joint. Lined by synovial membrane.

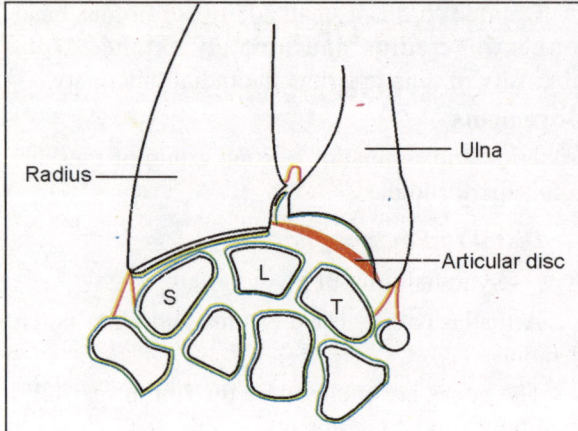

Fig. 4.7: Wrist Joint

Ligaments

1. Palmar radiocarpal
2. Palmar ulnocarpal
3. Dorsal radiocarpal
4. Lateral ligament
5. Medial ligament

1. **Palmar radiocarpal -** Extends from lower border of radius to the 3 carpal bones.
2. **Palmar ulnocarpal -** From styloid process of ulna and articular disc to Triquetral and Lunate.
3. **Dorsal radiocarpal -** Thin, from radial end to dorsal surfaces of Triqurtal, Lunate and Scaphoid bones.
4. **Lateral ligament -** From radial styloid process to Scaphoid and Trapezium.
5. **Medial ligament –** From ulnar styloid process to pisiform and triquetral.

Arteries and nerves – Both interosseous nerves and arteries.

Movements:

Flexion – Flexors
Extension - Extensors
Abduction – Flexor Carpi radialis
Adduction - Flexor Capri ulnaris.

Intercarpal joints

They are small synovial joints – plane type. Connected by interosseous ligaments and dorsal and ventral ligaments

First carpo metacarpal joint (Fig 4.8)

Type – Synovial, Saddle variety.

Articular parts:

Base of 1st Metacarpal and Trapezium
Lined by hyaline cartilage

Capsule:

It is thick but loose. Attached around the margins of articular parts. Lined by synovial membrane. Ligaments support the capsule on all sides.

Relations:

Anterior – Thenar muscles
Posterior – Extensor tendons of thumb
Lateral – Abductor pollicis longus tendon
Medial – 1st dorsal interosseous and radial artery

Movements:

1. Flexion – Flexor pollicis brevis and opponens pollicis.
2. Extension – Extensor pollicis longus and brevis.
3. Adduction – Adductor pollicis.
4. Abduction – Abductor pollicis longus and brevis.
5. Opposition – Combination of all above movements.

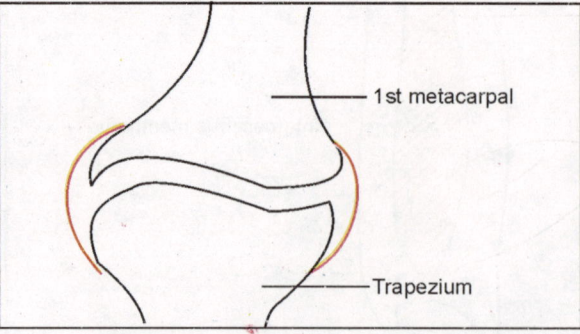

Fig. 4.8: 1st Carpometacarpal Joint

Other small joints of hand

2nd to 5th carpometacarpal joints and inter carpal joints are plane synovial joints where a small amount of gliding movement is possible.

Metacarpophalangeal joints are synovial joints of condylar variety. Movements possible are flexion, extension, abduction and adduction.

Interphalangeal joints are synovial joints of hinge variety where flexion and extension are possible.

STERNOCLAVICULAR JOINT (Fig. 4.9)

It is a synovial joint of saddle variety. Articulation is between sternal end of clavicle and manubrium sterni, also it is connected to first costal cartilage.

Articular surfaces are covered by a capsule and a fibrocartilagenous disc completely divides the joint cavity into two compartments. Capsule is lined by synovial membrane. Anterior and posterior sternoclavicular ligaments strengthen the capsule.

Supplied by supraclavicular nerve and the nerve to subclavius. Elevation depression, forward and backward movements are possible at the joint.

ACROMIOCLAVICULAR JOINT

Joint between lateral end of clavicle and acromion of scapula. A synovial joint of plane variety. Capsule is supported by superior and inferior ligaments. Coracoclavicular ligament is a strong accessory ligament. Gliding movements take place at the joint.

JOINTS OF PELVIS AND LOWER LIMB

SACROILIAC JOINT (Fig. 4.10)

It is the articulation between lateral articular surface of sacrum and auricular surface of ilium.

Type

Synovial joint, usually described as plane variety. But in adults, the 2 articular surfaces are markedly irregular. The irregularities restrict movements at the joint and help to strengthen the joint in transmitting weight of the body from vertebral column, to lower limbs.

Both surfaces are covered by cartilage.

Capsule:

Attached along the margins of the articular surfaces.

Ligaments:

1. Ventral sacroiliac ligament – Seen as a thickening of the anterior fibres of the capsule.
2. Interosseous sacroiliac ligament – It is a strong bond of union between the two bones, stretching between the rough parts, posterosuperior to the two articular surfaces.

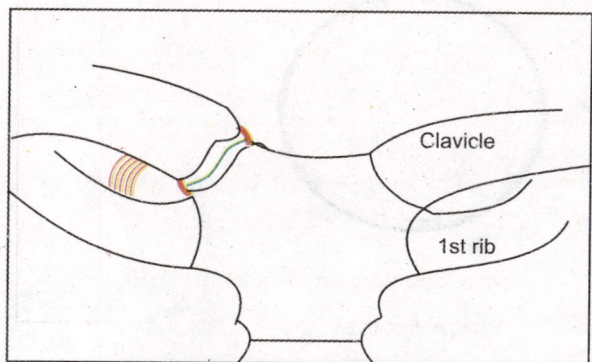

Fig. 4.9: Sternoclavicular Joint

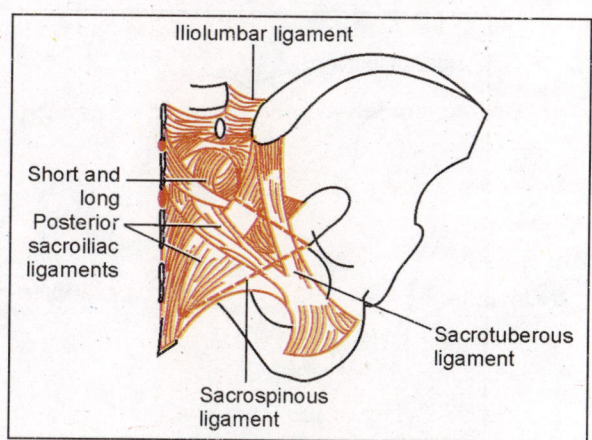

Fig. 4.10: Sacroiliac Joint

3. Short and long posterior sacroiliac ligaments – Seen covering the dorsal aspects of interosseous ligaments. Stretch between sacral crest to posterior superior iliac spine and adjacent part of internal lip of iliac crest.

There are three other ligaments associated with the sacroiliac joint. They are -

1. Iliolumbar ligament – From transverse process of L_5 to internal lip of iliac crest.
2. Sacrotuberous ligament – Partially blended with posterior sacroiliac ligaments. Extends from posterior superior iliac spine to the medial margin of ischial tuberosity. Its medial margin is attached to the lateral margins of sacrum and coccyx.
3. Sacrospinous ligament – Extends from lateral margin of sacrum and coccyx to ischeal spine, seen anterior to sacrotuberous ligament.

Movements

Anteroposterior rotation occurs at the sacroiliac joint, around a transverse axis, the movement is involved in flexion and extension of trunk.

Pubic symphysis

A secondary cartilaginous joint between bodies of pubis along midline.

Pubic surfaces covered by hyaline cartilage and intervened by fibrocartilage.

A superior pubic ligament connects the pubic tubercles.

An arcuate pubic ligament connects the lower surfaces of the 2 bones forming the pubic arch.

Joint is strengthened anteriorly by interlacing collagen fibres.

Movements – Slight rotatory movements associated with movements at sacroiliac and hip joints. Some seperation is possible during parturition in female.

HIP JOINT

Joint between acetabulum of hip bone and head of femur.

It has to support the weight of body and has to transmit forces during walking and running. So the joint has to be strong and stable. Strength and stability are obtained at the expense of limitation of movements.

Type – Synovial joint of ball and socket variety.

Articular parts (Fig. 4.11 a and b)

Rounded head of femur articulates with the cup shaped acetabulum of hip bone.

The actual articular area in acetabulum is a horse shoe shaped part. The nonarticular depression at the centre is acetabuluar fossa and deficiency below it is acetabular notch. The cavity of acetabulum is

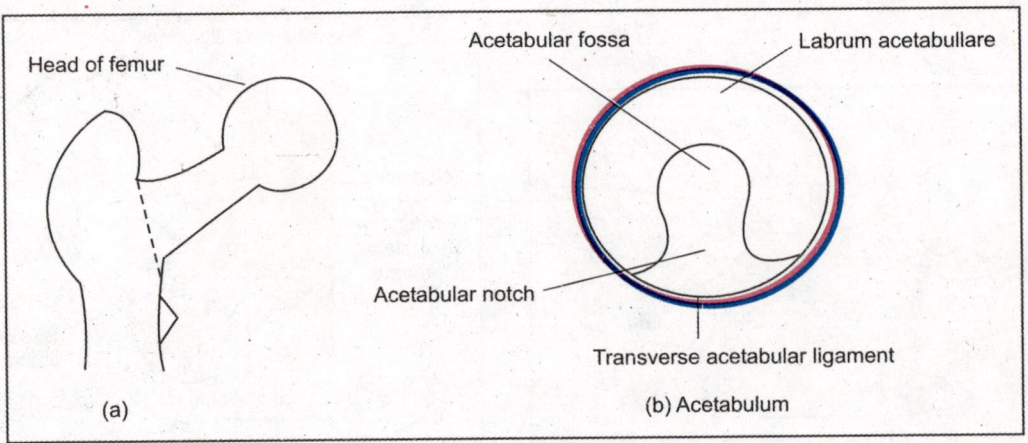

Fig. 4.11: Hip Joint

deepened by a rim of fibrocartilage along its margin- the labrum acetabulare - Where the labrum bridges acetabular notch, it forms the transverse acetabular ligament.

Head of femur is more than ½ a sphere. Its apex is marked by a pit, the fovea.

Both articular parts are covered by hyaline cartilage.

Capsule

Strong fibrous capsule covers the joint.

Medially-attached along the margin of acetabulum.

Laterally

On the anterior surface, along the inter-trochanteric line of femur and on posterior surface, along the middle of neck of femur. Above and below, to the base of neck.

Capsule consists of more longitudinal fibres and some circular fibres. Some longitudinal fibres attached to the intertrochanteric line are reflected back along the neck upto head, accompanied by blood vessels, which supply neck and head of femur.

Inner circular fibres of capsule form zona orbicularis.

Ligaments (Fig.4.12, and 4.13)

Capsule is strengthened by 3 ligaments

1. **Iliofemoral ligament.** It is the strongest ligament in the body.

An inverted Y shaped one. Stem attached above, to the anterior inferior iliac spine. 2 limbs attached to the upper and lower ends of intertrochanteric line. The ligament limits extension of joint while standing.

2. **Pubofemoral ligament:** A triangular ligament. Base attached to the superior pubic ramus. Apex attached to the lower end of intertrochanteric line. Limits extension and abduction.

3. **Ischiofemoral ligament:** Spiral in shape. Extends from the body of ischium posteriorly to the greater trochanter. This also limits extension.

4. **Transverse acetabular ligament:**

5. Ligament of head of femur. A flat triangular band, lies inside the joint. Apex of the ligament attached to a pit on the head of femur (fovea) and base to the transverse ligament.

Opening in the capsule

An opening is present in front, below iliofemoral and pubofemoral ligaments. Through this, synovial membrane protrudes and forms a bursa deep to psoas major – Psoas bursa.

Synovial membrane

Lines the interior of capsule, nonarticular parts of bones and the ligament of head of femur. It covers a pad of fat in acetabular fossa.

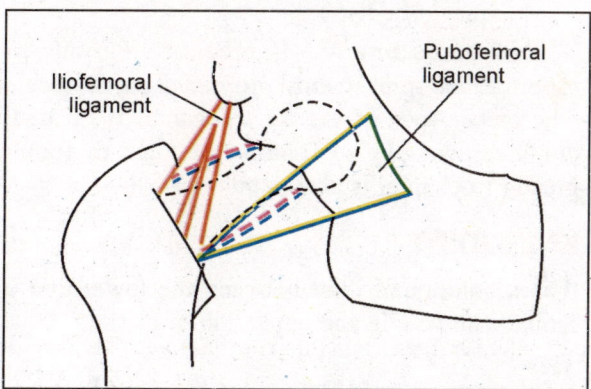

Fig. 4.12

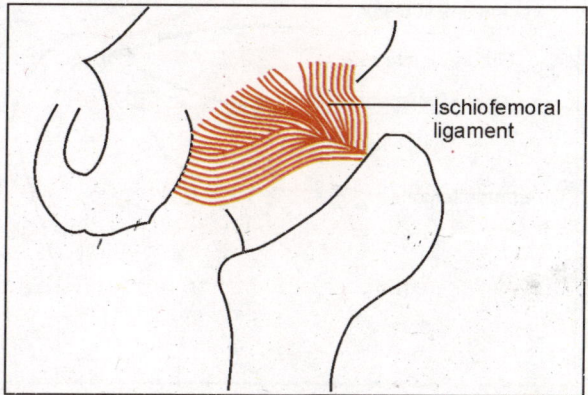

Fig. 4.13

Relations

Anteriorly – Pectineus, iliopsoas, straight head of rectus femoris – from medial to lateral.

Posteriorly – Obturator externus tendon and over that, Quadratus femoris, Obturator internus with 2 Gamelli and Piriformis – from below upwards. (Fig. 4.14)

Superiorly – Reflected head of rectus femoris and Gluteus minimus.

Inferiorly – Obturator externus – curving to posterior aspect.

Movements

Flexion – Iliopsoas, assisted by rectus femoris and pectineus.

Extension – Gluteus maximus and Hamstrings.

Abduction – Gluteus medius and Minimus, helped by Tensor fascia lata and Sartorius.

Adduction – Adductors, helped by gracilis and pectineus.

Lateral rotation – Piriformis, Obturator internus and Gamelli, Obturator externus and Quadratus femoris.

Medial rotation – Tensor fascia lata, helped by anterior fibres of Gluteus medius and minimus.

Circumduction – Combination of the above movements.

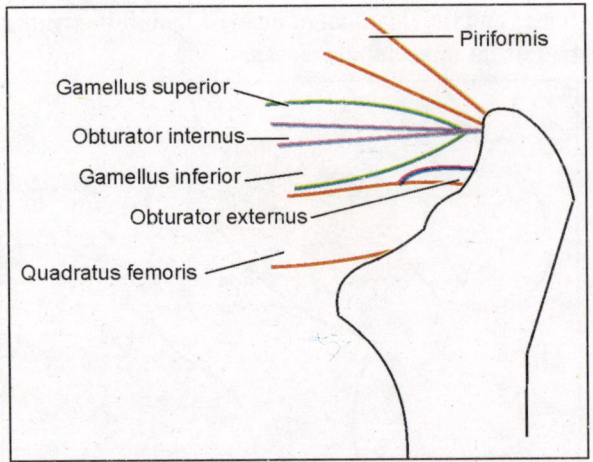

Fig. 4.14: Posterior Relations of Hip Joint

Gamellus superior
Obturator internus
Gamellus inferior
Obturator externus
Quadratus femoris
Piriformis

Nerve supply

Femoral nerve, obturator nerve, nerve to quadratus femoris.

Arterial supply

Obturator, medial circumflex femoral and both gluteal arteries.

Applied aspects

Dislocation of hip joint is very rare because it is very stable, strong and supported by strong ligaments and muscles.

1. Congenital dislocation – Due to failure of development of upper lip of acetabulum, head of femur gets dislocated to gluteal surface of ilium.
2. Traumatic dislocation – Rare, but if occurs, in posterior direction.
3. Osteoarthritis is common is adults.

   Trendelenburg's Sign: Stability of hip joint when a person stands on one leg when other leg is off the ground depends on -
   (a) Gluteus medius and minimus function normally.
   (b) Head of femur is in normal position.
   (c) Neck of femur is intact.

   If any of these factors is defective, the other side hip sinks down from horizontal – Trendelenburg's sign is positive.
4. Fracture of neck of femur is usually due to transmitted stress.

   Nelaton's line – A line connecting anterior superior iliac spine to most prominent part of ischial tuberosity. Apex of greater trochanter is on it. In displacement due to fracture of neck of femur, greater trochanter is above the line.

KNEE JOINT

It is a compound joint between the lower end of femur with patella and upper end of tibia.

Type:

It is a synovial joint of condylar variety and also a

modified hinge joint. Between femur and tibia, it is synovial condylar joint and between femur and patella, it is synovial, gliding joint.

The joint cavity is divided partially into upper and lower compartments by the presence of 2 cartilagenous menisci.

Articular parts (Fig 4.15 a, b, c and d)

Upper:

1. Rounded condyles of femur articulate with tibia.
2. A concave patellar surface on the lower end of anterior surface of femur articulates with patella.

Lower – Upper surfaces of the condyles of tibia, articulate with femoral condyles. Tibial surfaces are slightly concave. Shape of medial condylar surface is oval and lateral is circular.

Patella – Its posterior articular surface is convex. All articular surfaces are covered by hyaline cartilage.

Capsule

Fibrous capsule is weak and partially deficient. Above and below, it is attached beyond the articular surfaces.

In front, it is deficient and completely replaced by, the lower end of tendon of quadriceps femoris, patella and the ligamentum patellae.

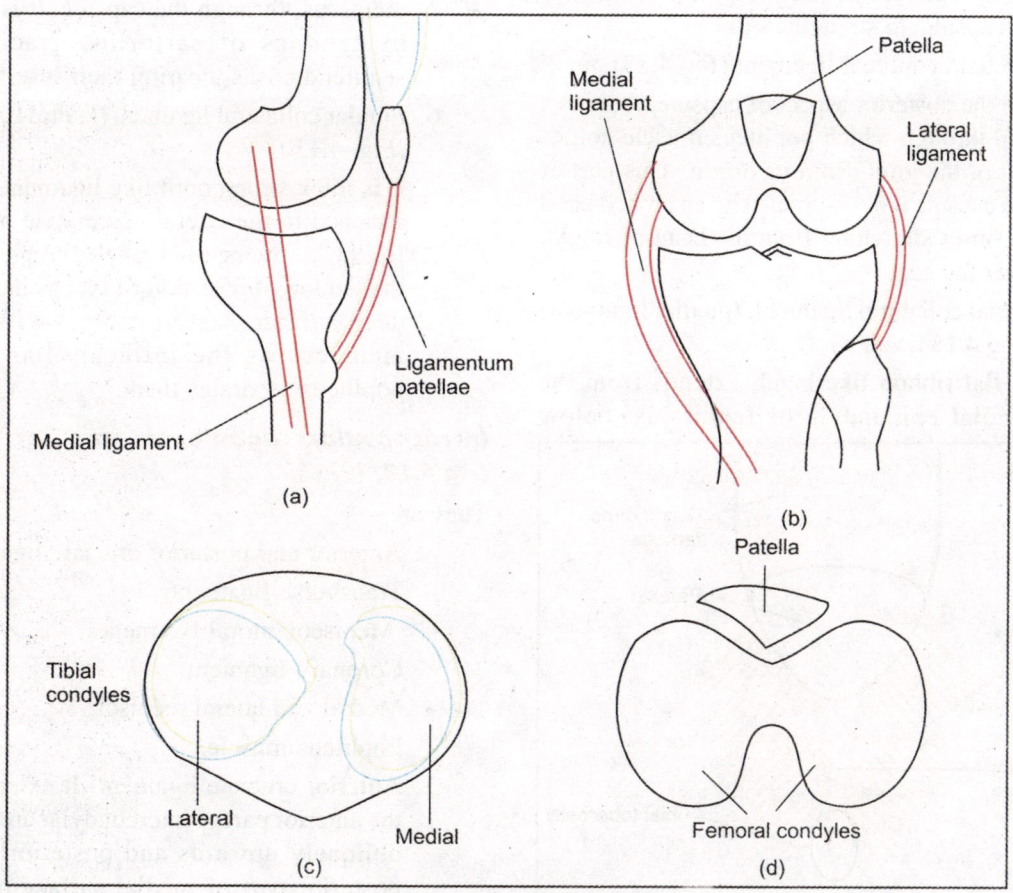

Fig. 4.15: Knee Joint

Ligaments – Extracapsular

1. **Ligamentum patellae. (Fig 4.16)**

   The tendon of quadriceps femoris is attached to the upper ½ of the margin of patella. Its superficial fibres continue over patella and at its apex, forms ligamentum patellae which is attached to tibial tuberosity.

2. **Patellar retinacula (Fig 4.16)**

   On either side of patella, there is fibrous expansion from the quadriceps tendon over the capsule, to strengthen the capsule anteriorly on either side.

3. **Oblique popliteal ligament (Fig 4.17)**

   A fibrous expansion from tendon of semimembranous, on the posterior surface of capsule, to strengthen it.

4. **Arcuate popliteal ligament (Fig 4.17)**

   On the posterior aspect of capsule, there is a gap through which popliteus muscle comes out of the joint, from its origin. This part of the capsule is strengthened by an arched band of fibres stretching from the head of fibula, over the gap.

5. **Tibial collateral ligament. (medial ligament) (Fig 4.15 a and b)**

   A flat ribbon like band, extends from the medial epicondyle of femur just below

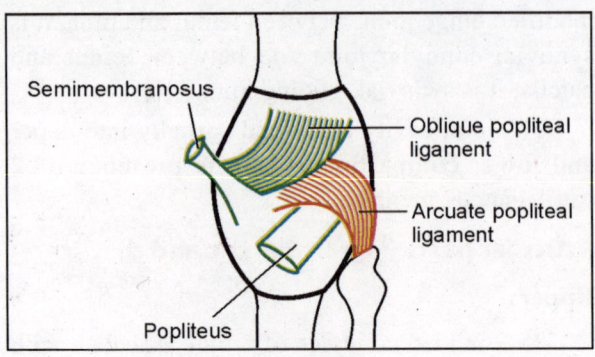

Fig. 4.17

adductor tubercle, to the upper end of medial surface of shaft of tibia. Its deep surface is firmly attached to the outer margin of medial meniscus, through the capsule. It is crossed by tendons of sartorius, gracilis and semitendinosus, nearing their insertions.

6. **Fibular collateral ligament (lateral Ligament) (Fig. 4.15b)**

   It is thick strong cord like ligament. Above, attached to the lateral epicondyle of femur. Below, to the head of fibula, where it splits the tendon of insertion of biceps muscle. Its deep surface has no contact with lateral meniscus as the intracapsular part of popliteus separates them.

Intracapsular ligaments and structures (Fig 4.18, 19)

They are –

- Anterior and posterior cruciate ligaments.
- Transverse ligament.
- Meniscofemoral ligament
- Coronary ligament
- Medial and lateral menisci
- Popliteus muscle.

1. Anterior cruciate ligament- It extends from the anterior part of intercondylar area of tibia obliquely upwards and posteriorly to the posterior part of medial surface of lateral femoral condyle.

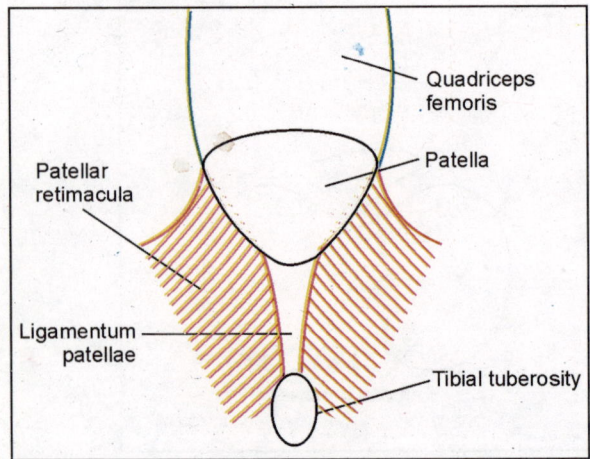

Fig. 4.16

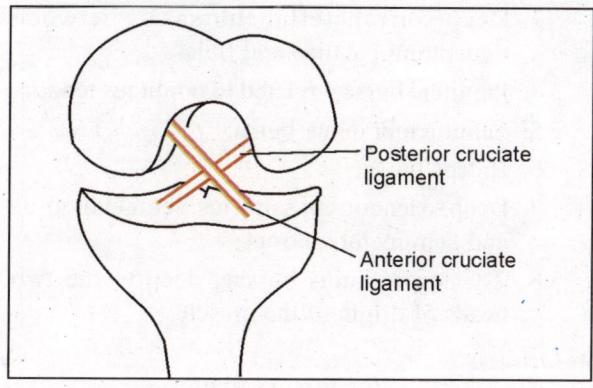

Fig. 4.18

2. Posterior crutiate ligament. – Extends from the posterior part of intercondylar area to the anterior part of lateral surface of medial femoral condyle. The 2 cruciate ligaments cross each other and they function as a strong bond of union of the two bones - femur and tibia. They are more taut in extention of joint.

3. Menisci (Fig 4.19) (semilunar cartilages) – They are C shaped fibrocartilagenous bands on the upper surfaces of tibial condyles. They are triangular in cross section and attached along their outer margins, to the inner surface of fibrous capsule. They function to deepen

the concavity of tibial articular surfaces and also as cushions between tibial and femoral condyles.

Medial meniscus: More oval in shape. Its anterior narrow end is attached to the intercondylar area of tibia, anterior to the attachment of anterior cruciate ligament. Posterior end attached to intercondylar area, anterior to the attachment of posterior cruciate ligament. The outer margin of the meniscus is attached to the deep surface of medial ligament, through the capsule.

Lateral meniscus: More circular in shape. Its ends are attached to the intercondylar area, close to each other. Its outer margin is separated from the capsule at the region where the tendon of origin of popliteus crosses it down. Also a few fibres of politeus are attached to it.

4. Coronary ligaments – Some short fibres of the capsule connect the periphery of the menisci to the tibial condyles.

5. Meniscofemoral ligament – Posterior part of the lateral meniscus, close to its attachment, sends a strong band, the posterior meniscofemoral ligament, behind the

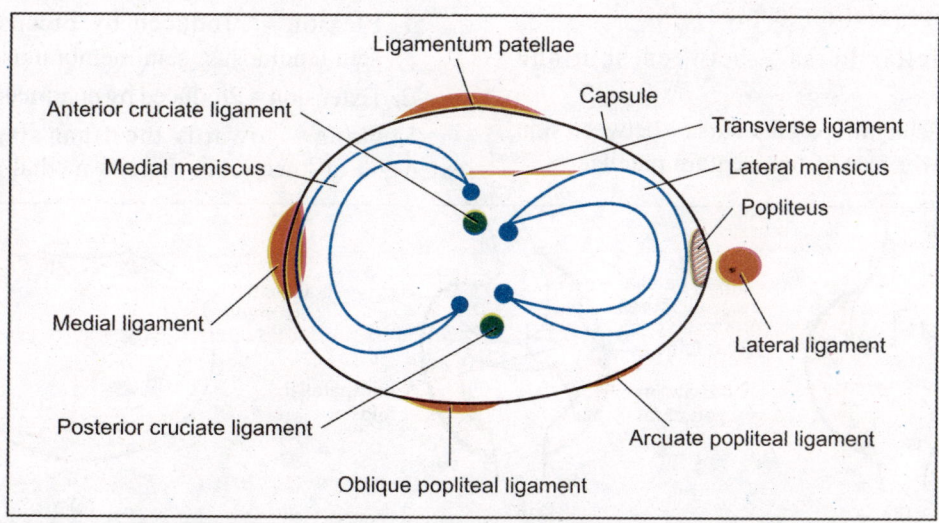

Fig. 4.19: Interior of Knee Joint -Upper Surface of Tibial Condyles

posterior cruciate ligament, to the medial condyle of femur.

6. Transverse ligament – Anterior end of medial meniscus is connected to the anterior margin of lateral meniscus by this ligament.

Synovial membrane (Fig. 4.20 a, b, c)

Lines the inner surface of capsule and is attached to the margins of articular surfaces and to the peripheral edges of semilunar cartilages.

From the upper border of patella, the upward extension of the membrane deep to quadriceps, for about 4 cms - is called suprapatellar bursa. To the upper edge of this fold, a small muscle, (part of vastus intermedius) articularis genu is attached.

Below the patella, synovial membrane descends, deep to the infra patellar pad of fat. There is a posterior extension of the membrane from this part, as two folds, alar folds, deep into the cavity of the joint. The two layers of the folds join posteriorly to form infrapatellar fold, which is attached to the intercondylar area of femur.

From the posterior part of the capsule, synovial membrane turns forwards to enclose the two cruciate ligaments which are thus intracapsular, but extrasynovial.

Other Bursae in relation to knee joint

1. Prepatellar bursa – between skin and patella.
2. Superficial infrapatellar bursa – between skin and lower part of ligamentum patellae.

3. Deep infrapatellar bursa – between ligmentum patellae and tibia.
4. Popliteal bursa – related to popliteus tendon.
5. Semimembranous bursa.
6. Biceps bursa.
7. Deep to tendons of sartorius, semitendinosus and semimembranosus.
8. 2 Gastrocnemius bursae, deep to the two heads of origin of the muscle.

Relations:

Anteriorly - quadriceps tendon and its expansion.

Posteriorly – popliteal fossa and contents.

Medially – sartorius, gracilis, semitendinosus tendons.

Laterally – Biceps tendon.

Nerve supply:

Femoral, obturator, tibial, and common peroneal nerves.

Blood supply:

Branches from an arterial anastamosis around knee joint supply the joint.

Movements:

1. Flexion – produced by biceps femoris, semitendinosus, semimembranosus.
2. Extension – Produced by quadriceps femoris.

Locking – towards the final stage of full extension of knee joint, there is medial rotation of

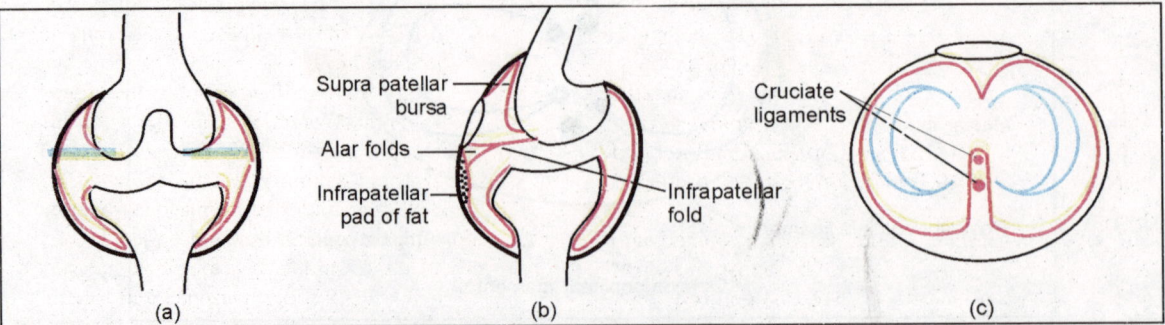

Fig. 4.20: Synovial Membrane

femoral condyles over tibia. Then all the major ligaments of the joint get tightened, the joint becomes a rigid structure. This medial rotation of femur is called screw home movement and joint is in the locked position.

To initiate flexion, the locked knee is to be unlocked. That is femur is to be laterally rotated and this is done by popliteus, the unlocking muscle.

Applied anatomy:

1. Capsule, collateral ligaments or cruciate ligaments can be torn when excess forcible movements take place at the knee joint.

2. Injury to menisci is common. In sudden unexpected forcible movements at knee causing rotation of the condyles, more frequently the medial meniscus gets caught between the condyles. It tears along its length – bucket handle tear. This occurs for medial meniscus because it is attached to the medial ligament and cannot slip away. But lateral meniscus is saved due to its attachment to the popliteus which can pull it out when such forcible movements take place.

ANKLE JOINT

Joint between the lower ends of tibia and fibula and upper surface of talus.

Type: Synovial, hinge variety

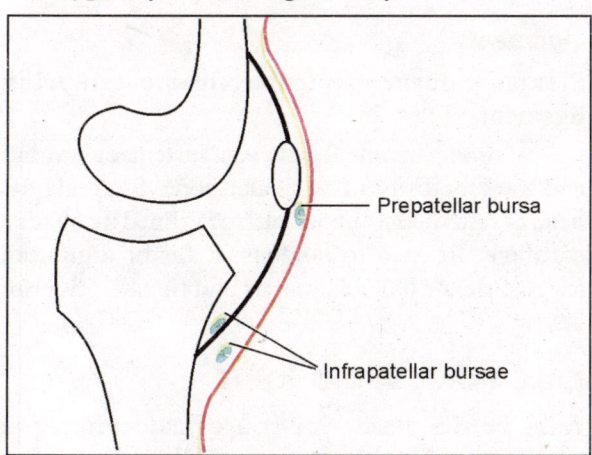

Fig. 4.21: Bursae

Articular parts

1. Superior trochlear surface of talus articulates with lower end of tibia.

2. Medial side of talus has a comma shaped articular facet to articulate with the inner surface of medial malleolus of tibia.

3. Lateral side of talus has a triangular area to articulate with the inner surface of lateral malleolus of fibula.

Posteriorly the upper articular parts get a contribution from the inferior transverse tibiofibular ligament.

Articular surfaces are covered by hyaline cartilage.

Capsule – attached around the margins of articular bones.

Ligaments – (Fig 4.22 & 23)

1. **Medial or Deltoid ligament**

   A very strong triangular ligament, apex attached to tip of medial malleolus. Base attached to the medial surface of talus, tuberosity of navicular bone, to spring ligament and to sustentaculum tali of calcanius.

2. **Lateral ligament**

   It has 3 bands. Anterior talo fibular, posterior talo fibular, and Calcaneo fibular bands.

   Synovial membrane - lines the interior of capsule.

Nerve supply

Tibial and deep peroneal nerves

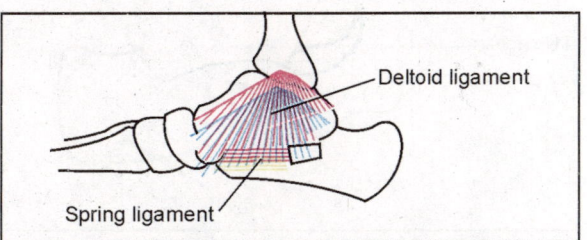

Fig. 4.22: Ankle Joint - Deltoid Ligament

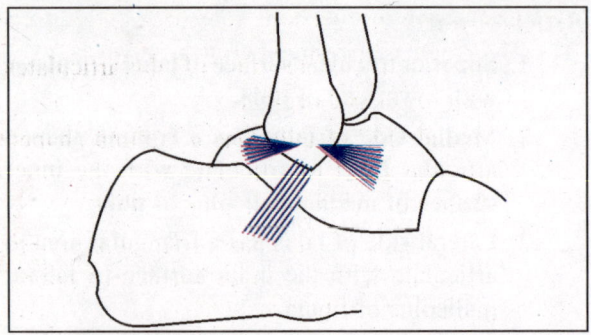

Fig. 4.23: Ankle Joint - Lateral Ligament

Arteries

Peroneal artery and anterior tibial artery

Movements

1. Dorsiflexion – produced by tibialis anterior and extensors.
2. Plantar flexion – produced by posterior compartment muscles.

Applied aspects

Sprain of ankle is usually due to tear or stretching of lateral ligament and less commonly of medial ligament.

Subtalar and Midtarsal joints (Fig 4.24)

I. There are two joints between talus and calcaneus
   1. A posterior one between under surface of talus and upper surface of calcaneus – Subtalar joint.
   2. Between under surface of talus and upper surface of sustentaculum tali. This is

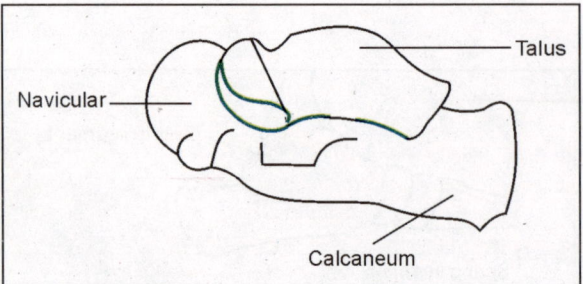

Fig. 4.24: Subtalar and Midtarsal Joints

continuous anteriorly with talonavicular joint and hence together called talocalcaneonavicular joint.

II. There is a joint between anterior aspect of calcaneus and cuboid bone – calcaneiocuboid joint.

Talocalcaneonavicular and Calcaneocuboidal joints are together known as midtarsal or transverse tarsal joints.

1. SUBTALAR JOINT

Between undersurface of body of talus and upper surface of calcaneus, both covered by hyaline cartilage. It is plane synovial in type. Capsule attached along margins of articular parts and lined by synovial membrane.

Ligaments are:
1. Medial and lateral talocalcanian ligaments.
2. Interosseous talocalcanean ligament in the sinus tarsi.
3. Cervical ligament between neck of talus and calcaneus.

2. TALOCALCANEONAVICULAR JOINT

It is the joint between head of talus with upper surface of sustentaculum tali and with posterior concave surface of navicular bone. It is synovial in type and has an incomplete capsule, lined by synovial membrane.

Ligaments

Plantar calcaneonavicular ligament (**spring ligament**) (Fig 4.25)

A strong ligament between sustentaculum tali and the tuberosity of navicular bone. Supports the head of talus and its upper surface is lined by hyaline cartilage. Related to tendons of flexor digitorum longus, flexor hallucis longus and tibialis posterior below.

CALCANEOCUBOID JOINT

Joint between anterior end of calcanium and posterior surface of cuboid, both lined by hyaline

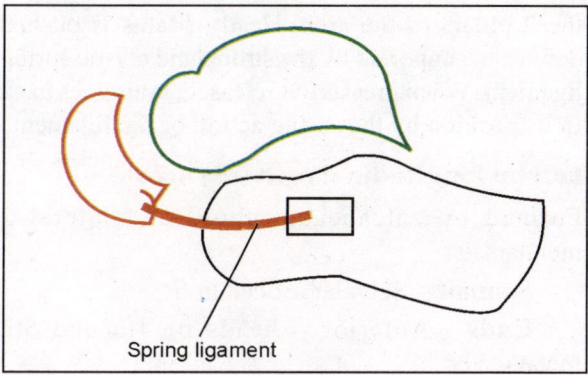

Fig. 4.25

cartilage. It is synovial joint of plane type. Capsule encloses the bony parts, lined by synovial membrane.

Ligaments

Strong ligaments strengthen the joint.

1. **Bifurcated ligament**

   A -Y- shaped ligament, stem attached to the upper surface of calcaneus and two limbs attached to upper surfaces of cuboid and navicular bones.

2. **Long plantar ligament**

   Attached behind to the under surface of calcaneus and in front, to under surfaces of cuboid and bases of 3rd to 5th metatarsals. Deep to it, peroneus longus tendon goes towards insertion.

3. **Short plantar ligament**

   Broad and short ligament, deep to the long plantar ligament. Stretches between anterior part of calcaneus and cuboid bone, on the under surface.

Movements:

At subtalar and midtarsal joints, inversion and eversion of foot take place.

Inversion: In inversion,sole of foot is turned medially. Muscles Causing inversion are tibialis anterior, tibialis posterior and extensor Hallucis longus.

Eversion: In eversion, sole of foot is turned lateraly Produced by three peroneal muscles.

ARCHES OF FOOT

Skeleton of foot in human is constructed in an arched form.

Entire body weight is supported by feet and during weight bearing and jumping, extra strain is taken by the feet. To meet this requirement, and to function efficiently the foot is shaped into an elastic arched structure by its bones, ligaments and muscles.

There are two longitudinal arches and a series of transverse arches.

LONGITUDINAL ARCHES

Medial – More arched

Lateral – Low lying

Medial longitudinal arch (Fig 4.26)

Formed by calcaneus, talus, navicular, 3 cuneiforms and 3 metatarsals

Ends:

Posterior – medial tuberosity of calcaneus.

Anterior – heads of first three metatarsals.

Summit: Superior surface of talus.

Pillars: Posterior pillar is strong and less oblique. Formed by medial part of calcaneus. Anterior pillar is weaker, more oblique and longer. Formed by talus, navicular, three cuneiforms and three metatarsals.

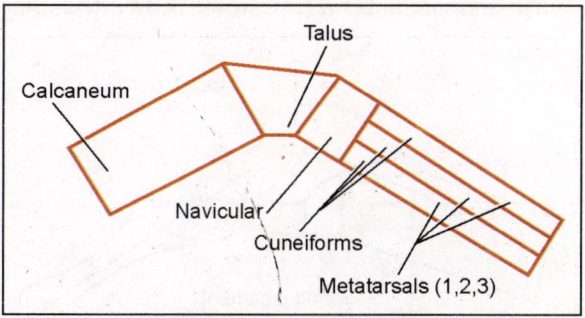

Fig. 4.26: Medial Longitudinal Arch

Factors that maintain the arch:

1. **Shape of bones:**

    Articulating surfaces of the bones of foot are not flat, but curved to maintain the arched form.

2. **Ligaments (intersegmental ties):**

    (a) Ligaments that pass from bone to bone in the long axis of plantar surface of foot.

    (b) Plantar calcaneonavicular ligament (spring ligament) – between sustentaculum tali and tuberosity of navicular bone. It supports head of talus. Due to its elasticity it is the main ligamentous support of medial longitudinal arch.

3. **Bow-string arrangement:**

    Structures that connect both ends of the arch. They are-

    (a) Medial part of plantar aponeurosis.

    (b) Abductor hallucis.

    (c) Medial part of flexor digitorum brevis.

    (d) Flexor hallusis brevis.

4. **Sling support arrangement**

    Supporting the arch from above.

    This includes -

    (a) tibialis posterior

    (b) Tibialis anterior

    (c) Flexor digitorum longus

    (d) Flexor hallucis longus

Mechanism of the medial arch (Fig 4.27)

When pressure falls on talus, force is diverted along the 2 pillars of the arch. Head of talus is pushed down and supported by the strong and elastic spring ligament. When pressure is released, talus goes back to its position by the spring action of the ligament.

Lateral longitudinal arch (Fig 4.28)

Formed by calcaneus, cuboid and lateral 2 metatarsals.

   Summit – Subtalar articulation

   Ends - Anterior – heads of 4th and 5th metatarsals.

   Posterior – Lateral tuberosity of calcaneus.

   Pillars -Posterior – Lateral part of calcaneus

       Anterior – Cuboid and lateral 2 metatarsals.

Factors that maintain the arch

1. Shape of bones

2. Intersegmental ties (ligaments)

    (a) Short ligaments that connect the bones in long axis.

    (b) Long plantar ligament (Fig 4.29)

    (c) Short plantar ligament.

3. Bow-string arrangement

    Formed by-

    (a) Lateral part of plantar aponeurosis.

    (b) Lateral part of flexor digitorum brevis.

    (c) Abductor digiti minimi.

    (d) Flexor digiti minimi.

4. Sling support arrangement

    Formed by -

    (a) Peroneus longus

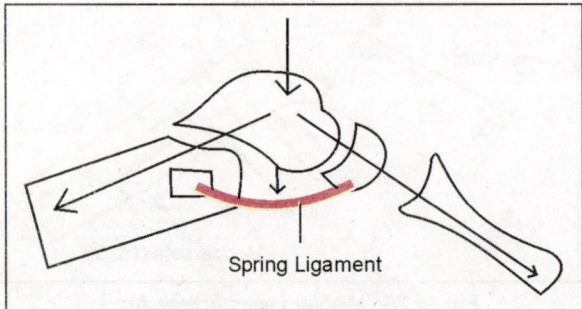

Fig. 4.27

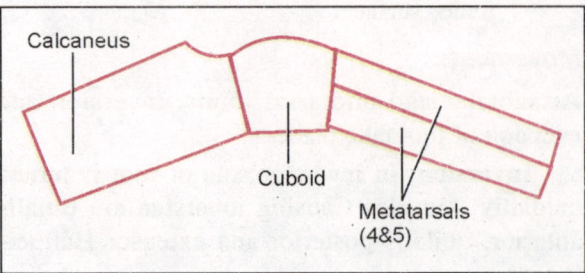

Fig. 4.28: Lateral Longitudinal Arch

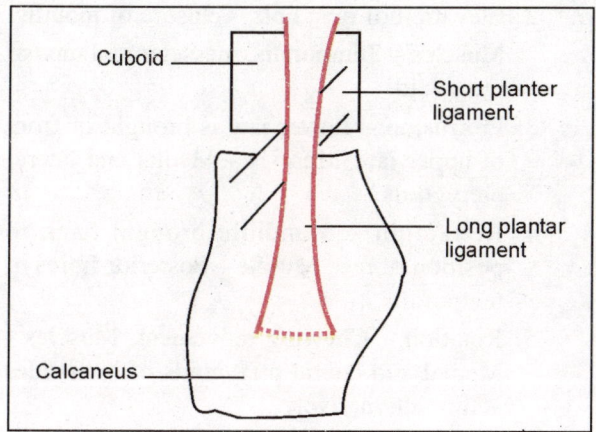

Fig. 4.29

(b) Peroneus brevis

(c) Peroneus tertius

Transverse arch

In front, formed by bodies of metatarsals and behind by cuneiforms and cuboid. In each foot, only ½ the transverse arch is formed and they become a complete arch when both feet are kept close together. (Fig. 4.30)

Factors that maintain the arches

1. Boney configuration
2. Intersegmental ties -
   (a) Interosseous ligaments – Transverse plantar ligament.
   (b) Dorsal interossei muscles bunch up all metatarsals.
3. Bow – string arrangement – by adductor hallucis
4. Sling support arrangement -
   (a) Peroneus longus tendon.
   (b) Tibialis posterior tendon.

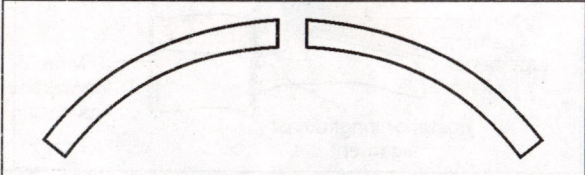

Fig. 4.30: Transverse Arch

Applied anatomy

1. Pes planus – Flat foot
   Medial longitudinal arch is collapsed or depressed. Ligaments get permanently stretched.
2. Pes cavus – claw foot

Medial longitudinal arch is unduely high – usually due to imbalance of muscles resulting from diseases like polyomyelitis.

MAJOR JOINTS OF HEAD AND TRUNK

TEMPOROMANDIBULAR JOINT – JAW JOINT

It is the joint between the mandible and temporal bone.

Type – Synovial joint of bicondylar variety.

Articular parts (Fig 4.31)

Above – mandibular fossa and articular tubercle of temporal bone.

Below – Condyle or head of madible

Both surfaces are covered by fibrocartilage. An oval **articular disc** divides the joint cavity into upper and lower compartments.

Capsule

Above attached to the margin of mandibular fossa and articular tubercle.

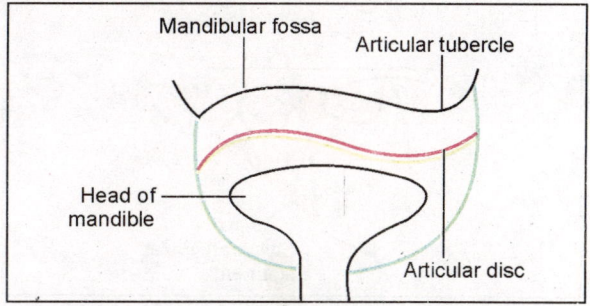

Fig. 4.31

Below, to the neck of mandible. The margin of the intra articular disc is attached to the inner surface of fibrous capsule.

Ligaments (Fig.4.32)

1. Lateral ligament or temporomandibular ligament. This is the only true ligament that strengthens the capsule. The triangular ligament extends from the tubercle at the root of zygoma to the neck of mandible. This ligament prevents posterior displacement of the condyle of mandible. Two accessary ligaments are also present-

   (i) Stylomandibular ligament – from styloid process to angle of mandible.-condensed part of general investing layer of cervical fascia.

   (ii) Sphenomandibular ligament – from spine of sphenoid to lingula of mandible-Remnant of 2nd arch cartilage.

Nerve supply

Masseteric nerve and auriculotemporal nerve – branches of mandibular nerve.

Arteries

Superficial temporal artery and maxillary artery.

Movements

1. Depression of mandible – opening of mouth. Muscles involved in this movement are – Lateral pterygoids assisted by digastric, mylohyoid and geniohyoid.

2. Elevation of mandible – closure of mouth. Muscles – Temporalis, masseter and medial pterygoid.

3. Protrusion – Lower jaw is brought in front of upper jaw. Muscles – Medial and lateral pterygoids.

4. Retraction – Mandible brought back to position of rest. Muscle – Posterior fibres of temporalis.

5. Rotation – Chewing movement. Muscles - Medial and lateral pterygoids of both sides acting alternatively.

Applied aspects

Dislocation of the head of mandible anteriorly into infratemporal fossa. This happens consequent to a sudden muscle spasm when the mouth is widely opened.

Damage to the intra articular disc causes an audible click in movements of the joint.

JOINTS OF THE VERTEBRAL COLUMN

1. Joints between vertebral bodies (Fig.4.33)

Bodies of vertebrae are joined together by:

1. Anterior longitudinal ligament.
2. Posterior longitudinal ligament.
3. Intervertebral disc.

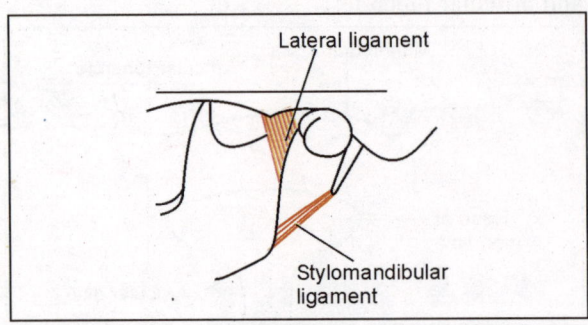

Fig. 4.32

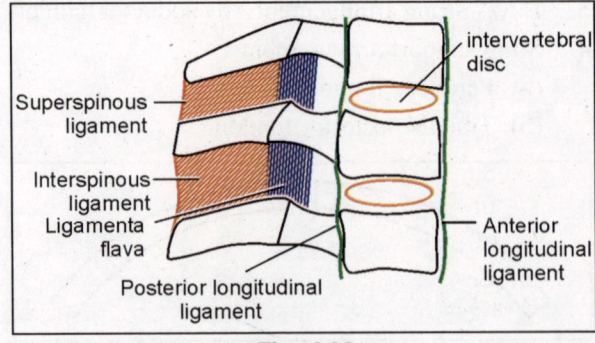

Fig. 4.33

Anterior longitudinal ligament is a strong fibrous band extending from the base of occipital bone to the sacrum, on the anterior surfaces of the vertebrae. Its upper part between the occipital bone and anterior arch of atlas is called anterior atlanto occipital membrane.

Posterior longitudinal ligament is seen on the posterior surfaces of the bodies of vertebrae and extends from the body of axis, below to the sacrum. Its upper end continues as membrana tectoria from the body of C_2, behind the dens, to get attached to the upper surface of body of occipital bone, in front of foramen magnum.

Intervertebral discs are placed between bodies of vertebrae from axis to sacrum. Its shape corresponds to the shape of the vertebral bodies. Its major peripheral part is formed of fibrocartilage – anulus fibrosus and central part formed of soft thick gelatinous material, nucleus pulposus, which contains some remnant cells of notochord.

Applied aspects

With advancing age, there can be degenerative changes in the disc. Leads to herniation/ prolapse of nucleus pulposus of disc; in posterolateral direction, can compress the spinal nerve roots.

2. Joints in the vertebral arches (Fig.4.33)

1. Joints between articular processes – plane synovial variety.
2. Joints between laminae – Laminae of adjacent vertebrae are connected by flat ligamenta flava formed of mainly yellow elastic tissue. They restrict excessive flexion of vertebrae.
3. Interspinous ligaments connect spines of adjacent vertebrae.
4. Supraspinous ligament – It is a strong thick fibrous ligament connecting the tips of spines of 7th cervical vertebra to the sacrum.
5. Ligamentum nuchae is thick and fibroelastic ligament extending from tip of C_7 to external occipital protuberance – continuous with supra spinous ligament.
6. Intertransverse ligaments connect the transverse processes of vertebrae.

3. Atlanto axial joints (Fig. 4. 34)

These are three in number. Lateral 2 are between the lateral mass of atlas and superior facet of axis. The 3rd one is median, between the dens of axis and anterior arch of atlas.

The lateral atlanto axial joints are plane synovial joints with thin capsule and supporting ligaments.

The median atlanto axial joint is between dens of axis and a ring formed by anterior arch of atlas and transverse ligament of atlas. It is a synovial pivot type of joint. Transverse ligament of atlas is a thick strong fibrous band, attached to a small tubercle on the medial aspect of lateral mass of atlas. It is broader at its middle and there on its anterior aspect, articular cartilage is present to articulate with dens.

As the transverse ligament crosses the dens, a band of fibres go up to get attached to the base of occipital bone between the attachments of apical ligament and membrana tectoria. Another band descends to get attached to the back of axis. The transverse ligament and the 2 bands together form cruciform (cruciate) ligament of atlas. (Fig 4.36) Transverse ligament is the main factor that retains the dens in position.

Movements possible at the three atlanto axial joints is rotation of atlas (and skull) on axis.

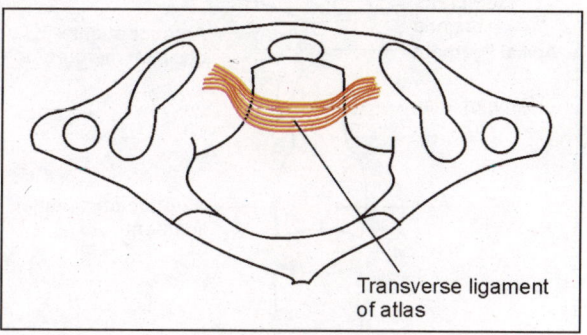

Transverse ligament of atlas

Fig. 4.34

4. Joints between vertebral column and skull (Fig. 4.35)

Atlanto occipital joints – Between the condyle of occipital bone and the superior articular facet on lateral mass of atlas on each side. It is a synovial joint of ellipsoid variety with a capsule. The anterior atlanto occipital membrane, a continuation of anterior longitudinal ligament from the tubercle on the anterior arch of atlas, strengthens the capsule.

Another broad membrane, posterior atlantoocci-pital membrane extends up from the posterior arch of atlas to the posterior margin of the foramen magnum.

Movements at atlanto occipital joints is nodding movements of head.

Ligaments between axis and occipital bones:

1. Membrana tectoria – It is the upward continuation of posterior longitudinal ligament. Extends from the back of body of axis, up to get attached to the upper surface of the basilar part of occipital bone, in front of foramen magnum.

2. Apical ligament – Extends from the tip of dens to the anterior margin of foramen magnum. [It may contain remains of notochord in it.]

3. Alar ligaments – They are strong fibrous cords, arise from the 2 sides of upper part of dens, pass obliquely upwards and laterally to get attached to the medial side of condyles of occipital bone.

Applied anatomy

Rupture of transverse ligament of atlas and thus dislocation of dens of axis causes injury to spinal cord. This is the cause of death in hanging.

5. Joints of vertebrae with ribs

1. Joints of the heads of ribs with thoracic vertebral bodies.

   Heads of typical ribs articulate with adjacent margins of bodies of vertebrae and intervertebral disc. 1st, 10th, 11th and 12th ribs articulate with body of only one vertebra. They are synovial joints.

2. Joints of tubercles of ribs with transverse processes of vertebrae. They are also synovial joints.

STERNOCOSTAL JOINTS

Anterior ends of ribs are cartilagenous - costal cartilage.

1st costal cartilage articulates with manubrium sterni by a primary cartilagenous joint. Other costal cartilages join with sternum by synovial joints.

Manubriosternal joint

It is a symphysis, but in later life, it undergoes synostosis.

Xiphisternal joint also is a symphysis which undergoes synostosis later in life.

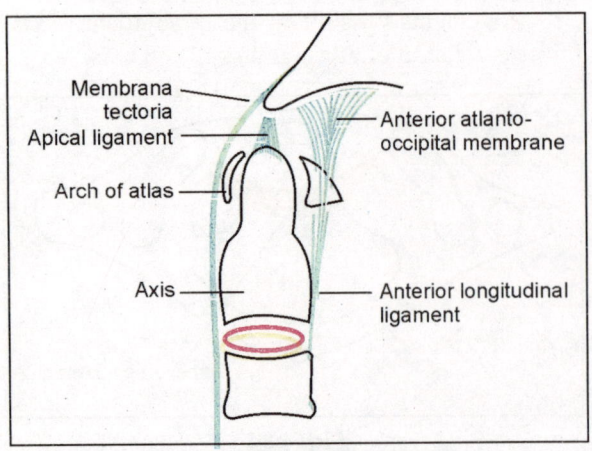

Fig. 4.35

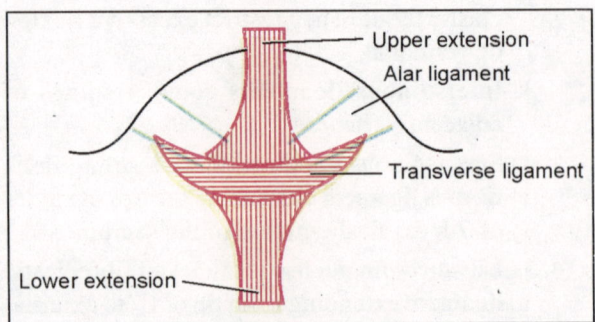

Fig. 4.36: Cruciate Ligament

Single Best Response M.C.Qs

1. Muscle that is not closely related to shoulder joint is
   (a) Supraspinatus
   (b) Infraspinatus
   (c) Subscapularis
   (d) Pectoralis major

2. Muscle that initiates abduction at shoulder joint is
   (a) Supraspinatus
   (b) Infraspinatus
   (c) Deltoid
   (d) Trapezius

3. Pronation and supination take place at
   (a) Shoulder joint
   (b) Elbow joint
   (c) Radioulnar joints
   (d) Wrist joint.

4. Strongest ligament in the body is
   (a) Coracoacromial ligament
   (b) Sacrotuberous ligament
   (c) Iliofemoral ligament
   (d) Spring ligament

5. Medial ligament of knee joint is overlapped by following tendons
   (a) Sartorius
   (b) Gracilis
   (c) Semitendinosus
   (d) Semimembranosus

6. Plantar calcaneonavicular joint is otherwise known as
   (a) Deltoid ligament
   (b) Spring ligament
   (c) Cruciate ligament
   (d) Long plantar ligament

7. The muscle that depresses mandible at temporamandibular joint is
   (a) Temporalis
   (b) Masseter
   (c) Medial pterygoid
   (d) Lateral pterygoid

8. Median atlanto axial joint is
   (a) Ellipsoid joint
   (b) Condylar joint
   (c) Hinge joint
   (d) Pivot joint

9. Extension at hip joint is produced by
   (a) Gluteus Maximus
   (b) Gluteus Medius
   (c) Gluteus Minimus
   (d) Iliopsoas

10. Following are intracapsular structures in knee joint except
    (a) Popliteus
    (b) Cruciate ligaments
    (c) Menisci
    (d) Arcuate popliteal ligament.

M.C.Qs - Answers

1. (d), 2. (a), 3. (c), 4. (c), 5. (d), 6. (b), 7. (d), 8. (d), 9. (a), 10. (d)

Essays

1. Describe the shoulder joint in detail. Discuss its clinical aspects.
2. Describe the Elbow joint
3. Define pronation and supination and describe the joints at which these movements take place.
4. Describe the Hip joint in detail. Discuss the applied aspects.
5. Describe the knee joint under following headings.
   (a) Articular parts & Type
   (b) Capsule and extracapsular ligaments
   (c) Intracapsular structures
   (d) Synovial membrane and bursae related
   (e) Movements and muscles causing them
   (f) Nerve supply

(g) Applied aspects.

6. Describe the arches of foot. Discuss the factors maintaining them and applied aspects.

7. Describe the Temporomandibular joint in detail. Discuss the movements and muscles causing them. Mention applied aspects.

Short Notes

1. Wrist joint
2. Ist carpometacarpal joint.
3. Sternoclavicular joint
4. Sacroiliac joint
5. Ligamentum patellae
6. Ankle joint
7. Inversion and evertion
8. Subtalar joints
9. Spring ligament
10. Atlanto axial joints

5 Cardiovascular System

Cardiovascular system consists of heart and a great number of tubular structures – blood vessels. Vessels that lead away from the heart carry oxygenated blood to all parts of the body; they are arteries. The deoxygenated blood from various parts of the body is returned to the heart by vessels called veins.

Heart, enclosed in the pericardium is situated in the thoracic cavity in the middle mediastinum between the lungs.

Mediastinum (Fig. 5.1a & 5.1b)

The median partition in the thorax between the two lungs is the mediastinum. Mediastinum is divided into upper and lower parts by a plane passing through lower border of T_4 vertebra and sternal angle.

The upper part is called superior mediastinum. Trachea and oesophagus descend through it. Arch of aorta and some other large vessels also are seen in it.

Lower part of mediastinum is divided into an anterior narrow – anterior mediastinum (thymus being its only major content), middle larger part – middle mediastinum (occupied by heart) and the part posterior to it is the posterior mediastinum through which aorta and oesophagus descend.

Applied anatomy

1. Mediastinal shift – secondary to pneumothorax.
2. Mediastinal masses – may be tumors or enlarged lymph nodes.
3. Aortic aneurysm

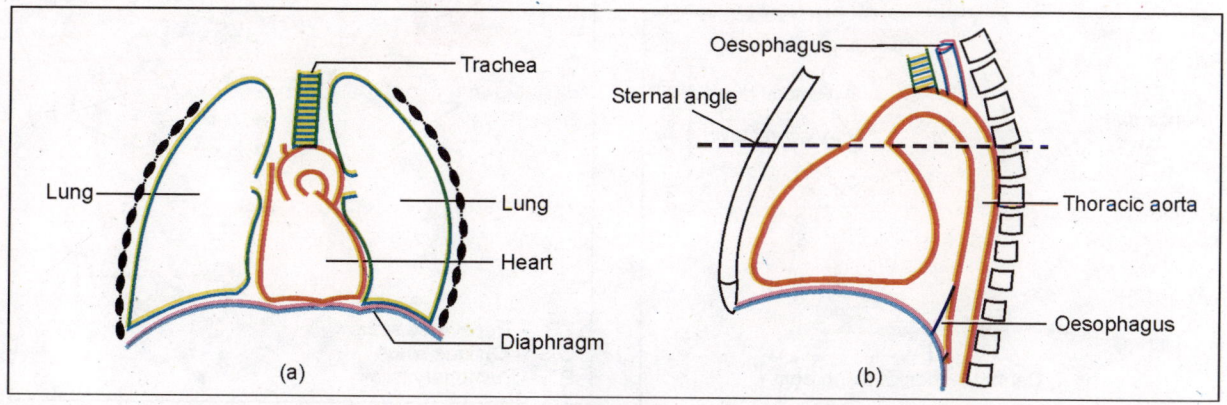

Fig. 5.1

Pericardium (Fig. 5.2)

Pericardium covers the heart. It has two layers – an outer fibrous pericardium and an inner serous pericardium.

Fibrous pericardium

Formed of strong fibrous tissue. Below it blends with the central tendon of diaphragm.

Serous pericardium

Seen inside the fibrous pericardium. It is a thin closed serous sac into which heart is invaginated from behind. Thus it has two layers – inner visceral layer in contact with the surface of heart and outer parietal layer that lines the inner surface of fibrous pericardium. The narrow cavity of serous pericardium contains minimum amount of pericardial fluid that facilitates movement of heart during contraction and relaxation.

Pericardial sinuses (Fig. 5.3)

On the posterior surface, the line of reflection of the serous pericardium from the great veins forms a recess – oblique sinus. Between the lines of reflection on aorta and pulmonary trunk above and pulmonary veins below, a transverse sinus is seen.

HEART

Heart is a hollow muscular organ formed of cardiac muscle – myocardium. Placed in the middle mediastinum, covered by pericardium, it is roughly conical in shape. It has four chambers – two atria and two ventricles.

The right atrium receives impure blood from all parts of the body through superior and inferior vena cavae. This flows into the right ventricle which pumps the blood to the lungs through pulmonary trunk for oxygenation. Oxygenated blood returns to the left atrium through four pulmonary veins and flows into the left ventricle. Left ventricle pumps this pure blood to all parts of body through aorta and its branches. (Fig. 5.3)

Surface features of heart (Fig. 5.4)

Heart is placed obliquely in the thorax behind the sternum.

On the surface of heart a groove separates atria and ventricles – atrioventricular sulcus or coronary sulcus.

Heart has three surfaces.

1. Anterior or sternocostal surface, formed by right atrium, right ventricle and partly by left ventricle. Anterior interventricular sulcus on the anterior surface corresponds to the line of interventricular septum.

2. Inferior or diaphragmatic surface is formed by right and left ventricles. Posterior interventricular sulcus marks the line of

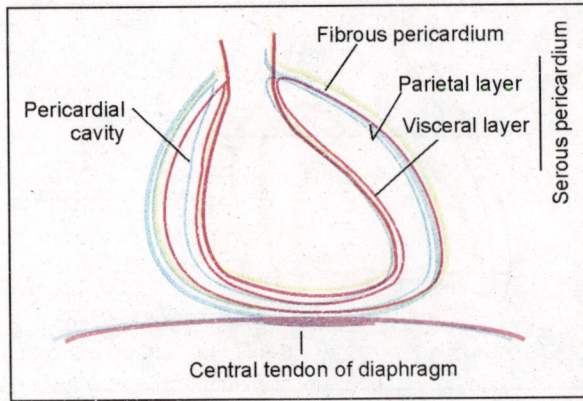

Fig. 5.2

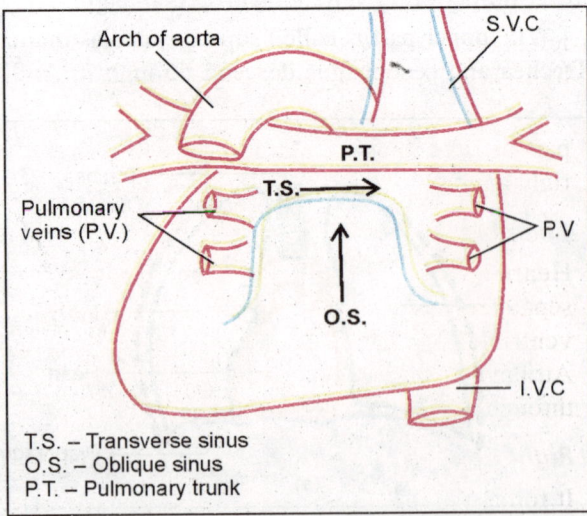

T.S. – Transverse sinus
O.S. – Oblique sinus
P.T. – Pulmonary trunk

Fig. 5.3: Posterior View - Heart

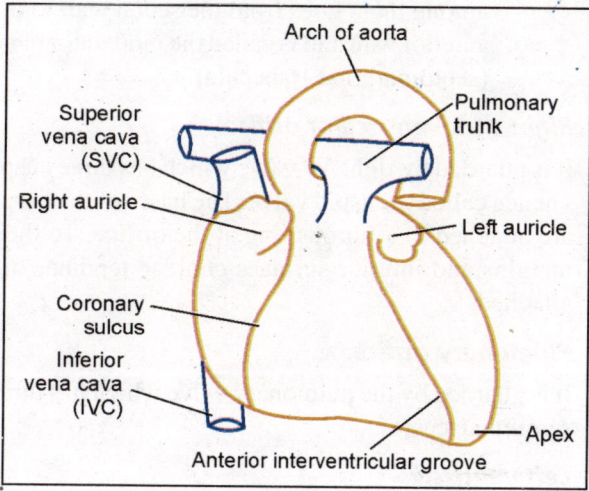

Fig. 5.4: Anterior View - Heart

interventricular septum on the diaphragmatic surface.

3. Posterior surface or base is formed mainly of left atrium and parts of right atrium and left ventricle.

Apex of heart is directed to the left and is formed by left ventricle. It is situated in the left 5th intercostal space about 10 cm form the midline. Here the apex beat of the heart can be seen and palpated in the living.

Right border of heart is formed by right atrium, left border by left ventricle and lower border, mainly by right ventricle.

A small appendage is seen on the upper anterior part of right atrium and left atrium. These are the right and left auricles.

Chambers of heart

Heart has four chambers. Right and left atria separated by interatrial septum and right and left ventricles separated by interventricular septum. Atrium communicates with corresponding ventricle through atrioventricular orifice.

Right atrium

It forms right border of heart. It has a main cavity and a small outpouching, the right auricle.

The interior of right atrium has a smooth posterior wall and rough anterior wall separated by a ridge - crista terminalis which is marked on the surface as sulcus terminalis. (Fig. 5.5) Rough part of the interior is formed by raised bundles of cardiac muscle fibres called musculae pectinati which are present in the auricle also. The smooth walled part of the cavity receives openings of 3 veins – superior vena cava, inferior vena cava and coronary sinus. Opening of inferior vena cava is guarded by a valve – Eustachian valve and that of coronary sinus guarded by Thebesian valve.

On the interatrial septum there is an oval depression, fossa ovalis limited by a sharp edge, limbus fossa ovalis. This represents an opening – foramen ovale that was present during foetal life, permitting blood flow from right atrium to left atrium.

Right atrioventricular orifice is guarded by the tricuspid valve that permits blood to flow from right atrium to right ventricle.

Left atrium

It forms most part of base of heart (posterior surface). The four pulmonary veins open into it. Its interior is smooth and musculae pectinati are present only in the auricle. Left atrioventricular orifice is guarded by a bicuspid valve – mitral valve.

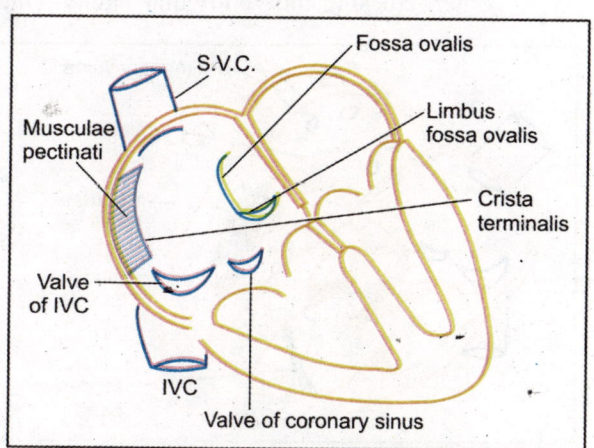

Fig. 5.5: Interior of Right Atrium

Right ventricle

Its anterior surface forms major part of the sternocostal surface of heart, and its inferior surface rests on the diaphragm.

Blood coming to it from the right atrium is pumped into pulmonary trunk through the pulmonary orifice. Near the pulmonary orifice its wall is smooth and funnel shaped and hence this part is called infundibulum. The wall of right ventricle is much thicker than that of right atrium. Its inner surface has a trabeculated appearance due to the thick projecting muscular ridges, collectively called trabeculae carneae.

The ridges are of three types (Fig. 5.6).

1. Prominent muscular bundles forming mere ridges.

2. Longer projections called papillary muscles, which are attached at their bases to the wall of the ventricle. Their apices are connected to the cusps of the atrio ventricular (AV) valve by fine fibrous cords – chordae tendinae. When ventricle contracts papillary muscles also contract and chordae tendinae prevent the cusps of AV valve from being forced into the right atrium. Three major papillary muscles are - anterior, posterior and septal.

3. The third type extends from one wall to the other, crossing the ventricular cavity. One among them goes from the septal wall to the anterior wall and is called the moderator band (septomarginal trabecula).

Right atrioventricular orifice:

It is guarded by right AV valve which has three cusps - hence called tricuspid valve. The bases of the cusps are attached to a fibrous ring at the orifice. To their margins and inferior surfaces chordae tendinae are attached.

Pulmonary orifice:

It is guarded by the pulmonary valve which has three semilunar cusps.

Left ventricle

It forms the major part of the left border and apex of the heart. It has the thickest wall than all other chambers, three times thicker than that of right ventricle. (Fig. 5.7) On cross section the left ventricle is circular and the right ventricle crescentic because the interventricular septum bulges into the right ventricle.

The interventricular septum is thick and muscular in its major lower part and membranous and thin in its upper part.

Left ventricle receives blood from left atrium through left atrio ventricular orifice and pumps it into aorta through aortic orifice. The part of left ventricle near the orifice is smooth – aortic vestibule.

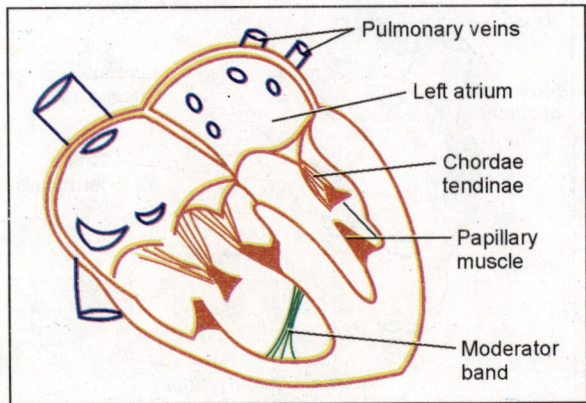

Fig. 5.6

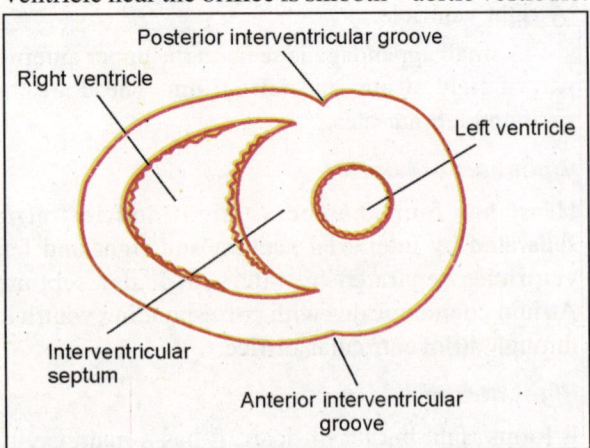

Fig. 5.7: C.S. of Heart at Level of Ventricles

Elsewhere it presents trabaculae carneae and two papillary muscles with chordae tendinae.

Left AV orifice is guarded by the bicuspid mitral valve. The aortic opening leads into ascending aorta and is guarded by the aortic valve, which is tricuspid.

Structure of heart

Wall of the heart is formed of thick layers of cardiac muscle, myocardium. Covered externally by epicardium and internally by endocardium. The spaces between bundles of myocardium are permeated by connective tissue. The collagen is condensed to form a framework around the AV orifices and aortic valve. This is the fibrous skeleton of heart.

Conducting system of heart

Human heart beats about 70 times in a minute. The chambers contract and relax in a sequential manner. The rhythmic contractile process is initiated spontaneously at the pacemaker of the heart – Sinu Atrial node (SA node). From here the impulse travels to other regions of heart through a system of specialized myocardial cells. This forms the conducting system of heart (Fig. 5.8). It consists of SA node, AV node, AV bundle, its right and left bundle branches and subendocardial plexus of Purkinje fibres.

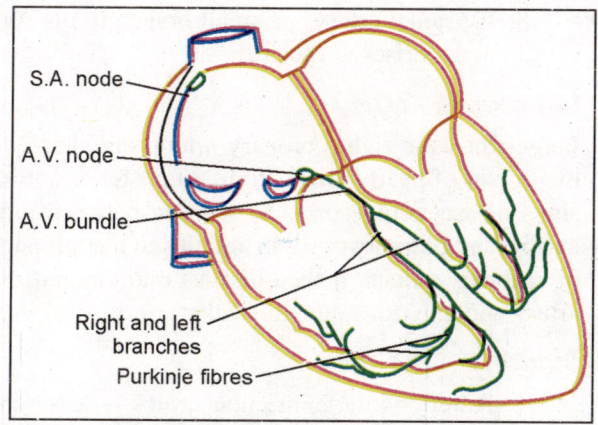

Fig. 5.8: Conducting System of Heart

SA node

Situated in the right atrium, just to the right of superior vena caval opening, at the upper end of crista terminalis. From the SA node, impulses spread through atrial myocardium to reach AV node.

AV node

Located in the lower part of interatrial septum, to the left of the opening of the coronary sinus.

AV bundle

It arises from AV node and descends to the membranous part of interventricular septum. Then it divides into right and left bundle branches. The right branch descends to the apex of heart subendocardially and enters the moderator band to reach the anterior papillary muscle. Here it divides into numerous fine Purkinje fibres which spread into all parts of right ventricular wall.

The left branch descends in the left side of the interventricular septum subendocardially to the bases of papillary muscles. There it breaks into Purkinje fibres in the wall of left ventricle.

The contractile impulse initiated at SA node spreads to atrial musculature and causes atria to contract. The impulses reach the AV node, pass through AV bundle to the Purkinje fibres and thus transmitted to the ventricles to make them contract. Thus contraction of atria is followed by contraction of ventricles.

The contractile cardiac cycle which is initiated at SA node is influenced and harmonized by the autonomic nerves that supply the heart.

Nerve supply of heart

Heart is innervated by sympathetic and parasympathetic parts of autonomic nervous system. The parasympathetic nerves slow the rate of contraction and sympathetic nerves accelerate it.

Sympathetic nerve fibres arise from the neurons of intermediolateral horn of upper 4 to 6 thoracic segments of spinal cord. Parasympathetic fibres are cardiac branches of right and left vagus nerves.

Acute myocardial ischemia (lack of blood supply) due to block of coronary arteries results in oxygen deficiency and accumulation of metabolites in the myocardium. This stimulates sensory nerves of heart and sensation passes through the sympathetic nerves to reach the spinal cord through posterior roots of upper four thoracic spinal nerves. Pain will be refered to areas of skin supplied by the corresponding spinal nerves. So cardiac pain due to myocardial infarction is felt over the left upper thoracic wall, left arm and lower part of neck.

Blood supply of heart

Arterial supply (Fig. 5.9)

The right and left coronary arteries provide arterial supply to the heart. They lie in the coronary (atrioventricular) sulcus.

Right coronary artery

Arises from the right anterior aortic sinus of ascending aorta, comes out between pulmonary trunk

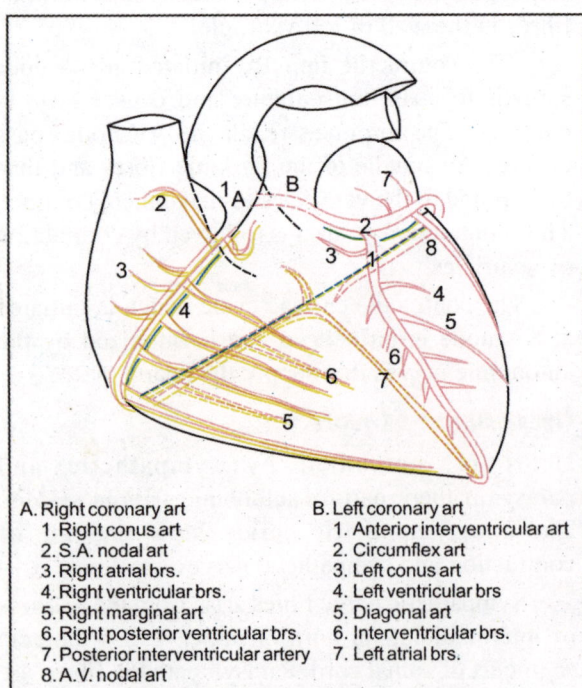

A. Right coronary art	B. Left coronary art
1. Right conus art	1. Anterior interventricular art
2. S.A. nodal art	2. Circumflex art
3. Right atrial brs.	3. Left conus art
4. Right ventricular brs.	4. Left ventricular brs
5. Right marginal art	5. Diagonal art
6. Right posterior ventricular brs.	6. Interventricular brs.
7. Posterior interventricular artery	7. Left atrial brs.
8. A.V. nodal art	

Fig. 5.9: Arterial Supply of Heart

and right auricle. Descends in the right part of atrioventricular (AV) sulcus to the lower end of right border of heart. There it curves to lie in the posterior part of AV sulcus and reaches the crux (junction of the interatrial and interventricular grooves with the posterior part of AV sulcus). Here the artery ends by anastamosing with left coronary artery.

Branches:

1. Right conus artery – supplies upper part of right ventricle.
2. SA nodal artery – supplies SA node and anterior wall of right atrium.
3. Anterior atrial branches – to the anterior wall of right atrium.
4. Anterior ventricular branches – to the anterior wall of right ventricle.
5. Right marginal artery – runs along the lower margin of anterior surface of heart upto the apex – supplies the right ventricle.
6. Right posterior ventricular branches – to the diaphragmatic surface of right ventricle.
7. Posterior interventricular artery – considered as the terminal branch of right coronary artery and descends in the posterior interventricular sulcus. Sometimes it arises as a branch of left coronary artery. Supplies the ventricles and posterior 1/3rd of interventricular septum.
8. AV nodal artery – a small branch to the AV node, arises at the crux.

Left coronary artery

Larger than the right coronary artery and supplies major part of heart. Arises from left posterior aortic sinus of ascending aorta. Appears in between left auricle and pulmonary trunk and lies in the left part of coronary sulcus. It then divides into circumflex artery and anterior interventricular artery.

Branches

1. Anterior interventricular artery – descends in the anterior interventricular (IV) groove,

curves from the apex and enter the lower end of posterior IV groove where it anastamoses with posterior IV artery.

2. Left conus artery – arises from the beginning of anterior IV artery.

3. Left anterior ventricular branches – arise from anterior IV artery and supply the left ventricle. One among them is larger and is known as Diagonal artery.

4. Septal branches – arise from the anterior IV artery and supply anterior 2/3rd of IV septum.

5. Circumflex artery – one of the two terminal branches of left coronary artery, continues in the left part of coronary sulcus, curves round the left border of heart to lie in the posterior part of coronary sulcus. Usually ends at the crux, but sometimes continues as the posterior interventricular artery.

6. Atrial branches to left atrium.

7. Left marginal artery – a branch of circumflex artery, descends along the left border of heart to supply left ventricle.

As mentioned earlier, major part of myocardium is supplied by left coronary artery. In 'right dominance' of blood supply of heart posterior IV artery is branch of right coronary artery. In 'left dominance' it is a branch of left coronary artery. In 'balanced pattern' branches from right and left coronary arteries run in the posterior IV groove. 'Right dominance' is more common.

Applied anatomy

Anastamosis exists between terminal branches of the coronary arteries to establish a collateral circulation. But they are not large enough to provide adequate blood supply if a major branch gets blocked. So the coronary arteries function as end arteries. If any major branch of these arteries gets occluded, the myocardium undergoes necrosis – myocardial infarction.

In angina pectoris, patient experiences pain on exertion and not at rest. The reason is, coronary arteries are narrowed due to atherosclerosis to cause myocardial ischemia on exertion, but not at rest.

Venous drainage (Fig. 5.10)

Most of the venous blood from myocardium is drained through the coronary sinus into the right atrium. Also there are anterior cardiac veins emptying directly into right atrium, and venae cordis minimae (Thebesius' veins) draining into right atrium and other chambers.

Coronary sinus

Lies in the posterior part of coronary sulcus, about 3 cms long. It commences as continuation of great cardiac vein, one of its tributaries. It opens into right atrium to the left of opening of inferior vena cava and the opening is guarded by a valve.

Tributaries

1. Great cardiac vein – lies in the anterior IV sulcus together with the anterior IV artery. Ascends and lies in the left part of coronary sulcus to continue as coronary sinus.

2. Left marginal vein.

3. Posterior vein of left ventricle – lies on the diaphragmatic surface of heart.

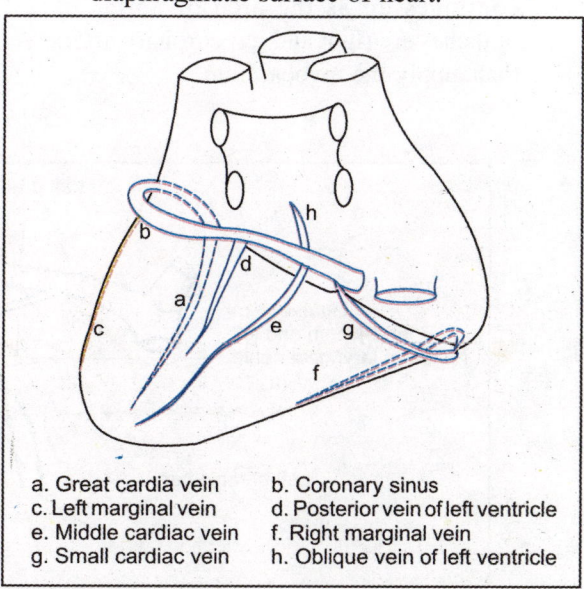

a. Great cardia vein   b. Coronary sinus
c. Left marginal vein   d. Posterior vein of left ventricle
e. Middle cardiac vein   f. Right marginal vein
g. Small cardiac vein   h. Oblique vein of left ventricle

Fig. 5.10: Venous Drainage of Heart

4. Middle cardiac vein – lies in the posterior IV groove.

5. Small cardiac vein – opens into the coronary sinus near its termination.

6. Right marginal vein – opens into small cardiac vein.

7. Oblique vein of left atrium – lies on the posterior surface of left atrium.

Arterial System

MAJOR ARTERIES OF THE BODY

Aorta

Aorta is the main outflow tract of the oxygenated blood from the left ventricle of heart. It is described in different parts-

Ascending aorta, Arch of aorta, Descending thoracic aorta and Abdominal aorta.

1. Ascending aorta:

Begins from the base of left ventricle, ascends behind left half of sternum for about 4-5 cms. Behind the sternal angle, it continues up as the arch of aorta. Its 2 branches are right and left coronary arteries, that supply the myocardium.

2. Arch of aorta. (Fig:5.11)

It is continuous with the ascending aorta at the level of sternal angle. The arch is directed upwards, backwards to the left and then downwards on to the left side of vertebral column. There at the level of sternal angle, it continues as descending thoracic aorta. It lies in the superior mediastinum behind the lower ½ of manubrium sterni. About 2.5 cms is diameter.

Relations of arch of aorta: (Fig. 5.11 & 5.12)

Anteriorly and to the left

1. Mediastinal surface of left lung.
2. Left vagus nerve.
3. Left phrenic nerve.
4. Left superior intercostal vein.
5. Cardiac branches of vagus and sympathetic nerves.

Posteriorly and to the right

1. Trachea
2. Oesophagus
3. Recurrent branch of left vagus
4. Thoracic duct
5. Deep cardiac plexus

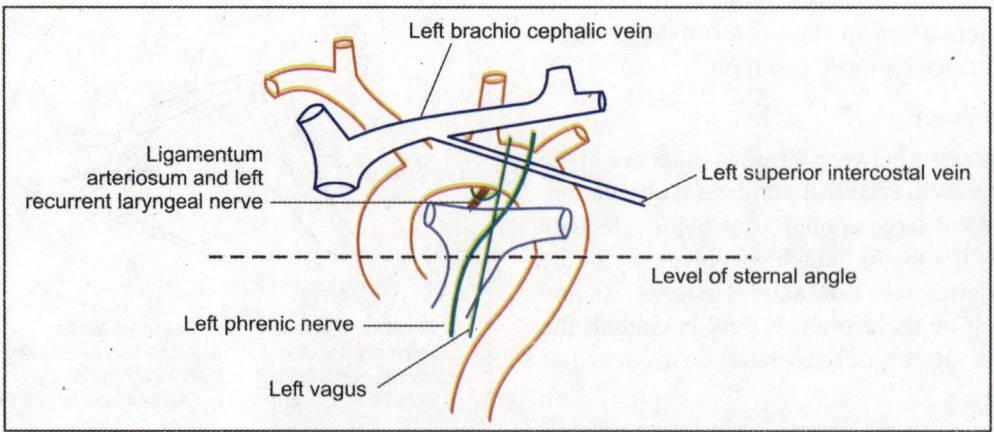

Fig. 5.11: Relations of Arch of Aorta

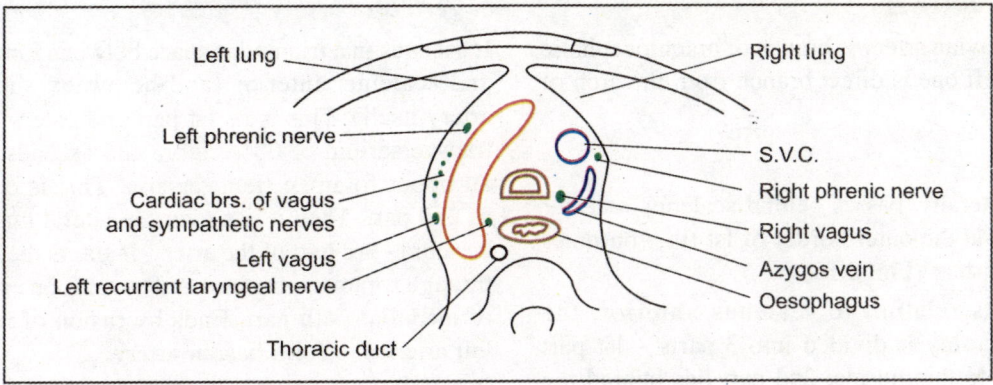

Fig. 5.12: C.S. at Level of T4 Vertebra - Relations of Arch of Aorta

Below:

1. Bifurcation of pulmonary trunk.
2. Ligamentum arteriosum.
3. Left recurrent laryngeal nerve.
4. Superficial cardiac plexus.

Above:

1. Origin of its 3 branches.
2. Left brachiocephalic vein.

Branches of arch of aorta (Fig. 5.13)

1. Brachiocephalic artery.
2. Left common carotid artery.
3. Left subclavian artery.

Through them, blood is distributed to the head and neck and upper limbs

Brachiocephalic artery

It is the largest branch of arch of aorta. About 4 to 5 cm in length, terminates behind right sterno-clavicular joint by dividing into right subclavian and right common carotid arteries. Other than the terminal branches, an inconstant branch, arteria thyroidea ima may arise from it.

Right and left subclavian arteries are stem arteries of upper limb. From origin, upto the outer border of Ist rib, it is called subclavian, thence to the lower border of teres major muscle, it continues as axillary artery and extends along the upper arm as brachial artery to divide into 2 terminal branches radial and ulnar arteries below the elbow.

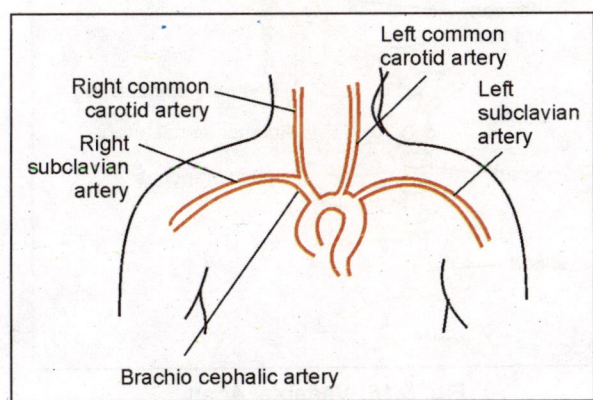

Fig. 5.13: Branches of Arch of Arota

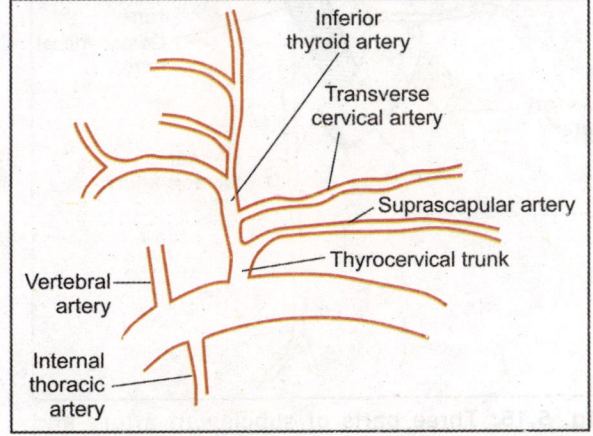

Fig. 5.14: Brs. From 1st Part of Subclavian Artery

Subclavian arteries

Right subclavian artery is branch of brachiocephalic trunk and left one is direct branch from the arch of aorta.

Course

It curves laterally, passes behind scalenus anterior muscle and at the outer border of Ist rib, continues as axillary artery (Fig. 5.15).

With its relation to scalenus anterior, the subclavian artery is divided into 3 parts – Ist part lies medial to the muscle, 2nd part lies behind the muscle and 3rd part lies lateral to the muscle, over the Ist rib.

Branches from Ist part: (Fig. 5.14 and 5.15)

1. Vertebral artery
2. Internal thoracic artery
3. Thyrocervical trunk

Branches from 2nd part: Costocervical trunk

Branches from 3rd part: Dorsal scapular artery

1. Vertebral artery (Fig. 5.16)

It ascends in a triangular space between longus colli and scalenus anterior (and below by subclavian artery itself). This is its Ist part and enters foramen transversarium of C_6 vertebra and ascends through all upper foramen transversaria. This is described as 2nd part. Then it lies over the lateral mass of C_1 vertebra - 3rd part of the artery. It enters the cranium through foramen magnum and ascends on either side of medulla – 4th part. Ends by fusion of right and left arteries to form basilar artery.

Branches

- Muscular branches
- Spinal branches – from its 2nd part.
- Anterior and posterior spinal arteries from its 4th part.
- Posterior inferior cerebellar artery from its 4th part.

2. Internal thoracic artery

Descends in the thorax, behind the costal cartilages, about 1cm lateral to the sternal margin. At the level of 6th intercostal space, ends by dividing into musculophrenic and superior epigastric arteries.

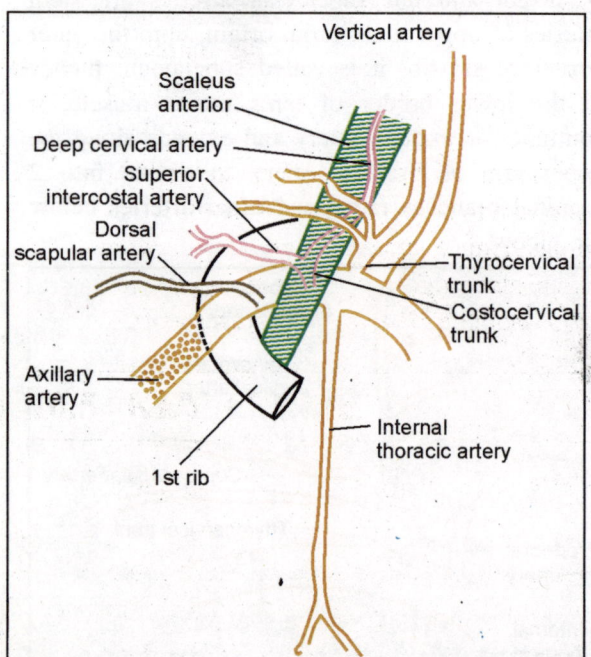

Fig. 5.15: Three parts of subclavian artery and branches

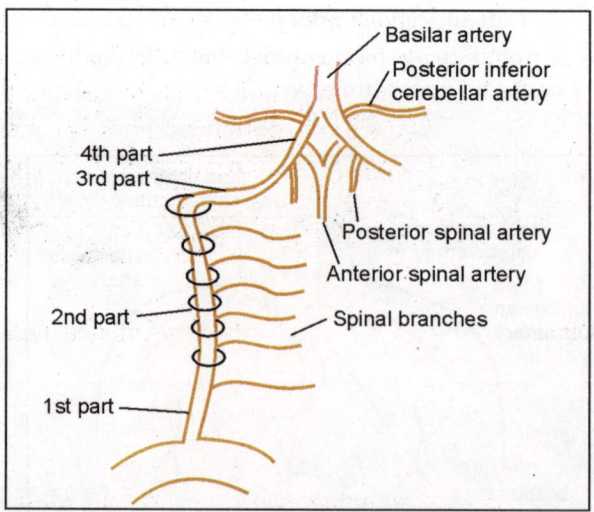

Fig. 5.16: Vertebral Artery

Other branches are:

- Anterior intercostal branches
- Mediastinal arteries
- Pericardiophrenic artery
- Sternal branches
- Pericardial branches
- Perforating branches

3. Thyrocervical trunk

After a very short course from its origin, it divides into

- Inferior thyroid artery
- Suprascapular artery &
- Superficial cervical (transverse cervical) artery

Inferior thyroid artery: Has branches to thyroid gland and also small cervical branches, pharyngeal branches and inferior laryngeal artery.

Suprascapular artery: Crosses the posterior triangle, goes to the scapular region and takes part in scapular anastamosis. (Fig. 5.17)

Transverse cervical artery: Also crosses the floor of posterior triangle and enters the trapezius.

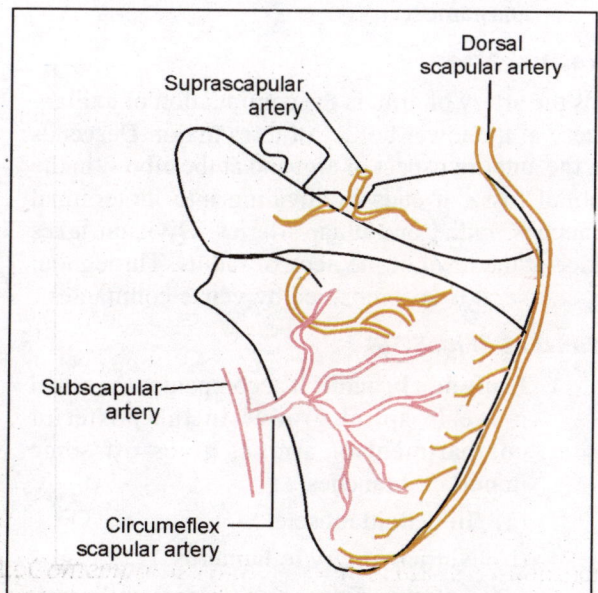

Fig. 5.17: Arterial Anastamosis Around Scapula

Branch from 2nd part of subclavian

Costo cervical trunk

Usually on the left side, it is a branch from 1st part and on right side, from the 2nd part.

It passes posteriorly over the cervical pleura to reach the neck of Ist rib where it divides into

- Superior intercostal artery and
- Deep cervical artery

Superior intercostal artery: descends and divides into posterior intercostal arteries of the Ist and 2nd intercostal spaces.

Deep cervical artery: goes back and ascends among the posterior muscles of neck, supplying them

Branch from the third part of subclavian-

Dorsal scapular artery: (Fig. 5.17)

Passes laterally and posteriorly in a deeper plane to reach the superior angle of scapula. There it descends along the medial margin of the bone deep to rhomboideus. Supplies the muscles there and ends by taking part in scapular anastamosis.

Arteries of upper limb

Axillary artery (Fig. 5.18)

A main content of the axilla, the artery begins as the continuation of subclavian artery at the outer border of Ist rib and ends by continuing as brachial artery at the lower border of teres major. Throughout its course, it is surrounded by the cords and branches of brachial plexus. Axillary vein passes close to it, medially.

Pectoralis minor crosses the artery anteriorly to reach its insertion. Thus conveniently the artery is divided into 3 parts.

Ist part – proximal to pectoralis minor

2nd part – deep to pectoralis minor

3rd part - distal to pectoralis minor

Branches

I. From Ist part, one branch - Superior thoracic artery.

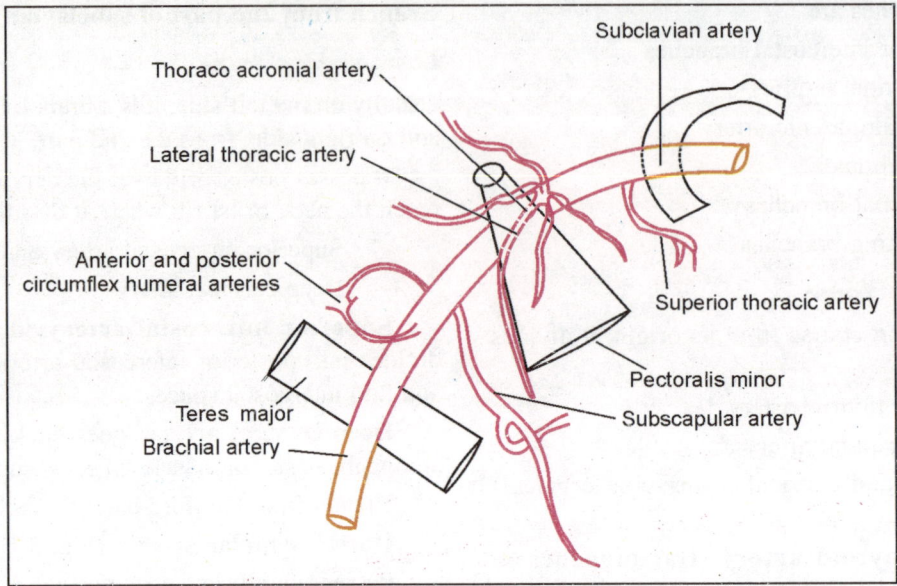

Fig. 5.18: Axillary Artery

II. From 2nd part, two branches
 1. Thoraco-acromial artery
 2. Lateral thoracic artery

III. From 3rd part, three branches
 1. Subscapular artery
 2. Anterior circumflex humeral artery
 3. Posterior circumflex humeral artery

1. **Superior thoracic artery:** A small branch. Distributed to the upper part of thoracic wall.

2. **Thoraco-acromial artery:** It divides into acromial, clavicular, deltoid and pectoral branches which are distributed to the corresponding areas.

3. **Lateral thoracic artery:** Descends along the lateral border of pectoralis minor and distributed in the lateral part of thoracic wall. In female, important due to its supply to mammary gland.

4. **Subscapular artery:** Largest branch. Runs along the lower border of subscapularis muscle till lower angle of scapula. It supplies the muscles around lateral thoracic wall.

Circumflex scapular artery is a major branch from subscapular artery.

5. & 6. - **Anterior circumflex humeral & Posterior circumflex humeral arteries:** Encircle the surgical neck of humerus and anastamose.

Brachial artery

It is the artery of arm, is the continuation of axillary artery at the lower border of teres major. Descends on the anterior aspect of arm and at the elbow, in the cubital fossa, it ends by dividing into its terminal branches, radial and ulnar arteries. Division takes place at the level of the neck of radius. Throughout its course, it is accompanied by venae comitantes.

Branches: (Fig. 5.19)

1. **Profunda brachii:** It accompanies the radial nerve in spiral groove in the posterior compartment of arm. It gives off some important branches:
 (a) To deltoid muscle
 (b) Nutrient artery to humerus.
 (c) Anterior descending (radial collateral) artery.

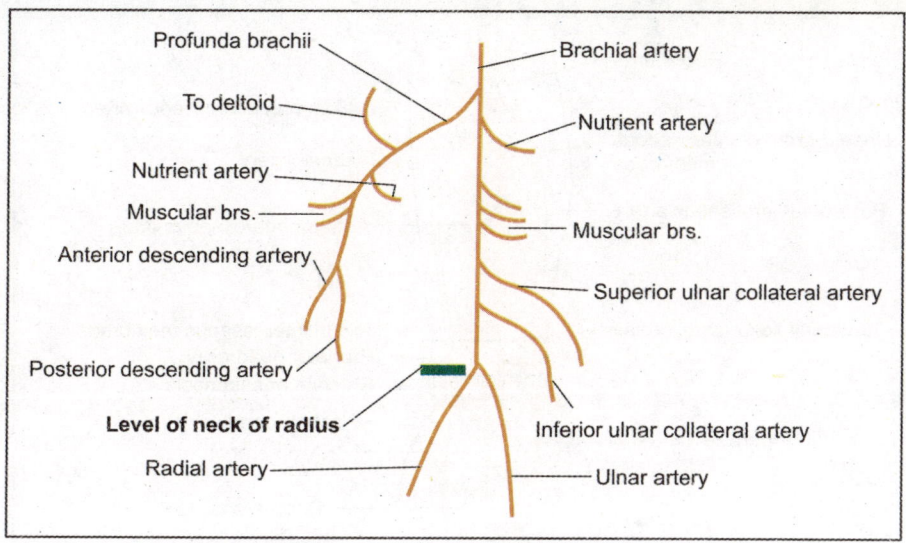

Profunda brachii
To deltoid
Nutrient artery
Muscular brs.
Anterior descending artery
Posterior descending artery
Level of neck of radius
Radial artery

Brachial artery
Nutrient artery
Muscular brs.
Superior ulnar collateral artery
Inferior ulnar collateral artery
Ulnar artery

Fig. 5.19: Brachial Artery and Branches

(d) Posterior descending artery

c and d, are terminal branches and they take part in arterial anastamosis around elbow.

2. **Nutrient artery to humerus**

3. Muscular branches

4. Superior ulnar collateral artery.

5. Inferior ulnar collateral artery

6. Radial artery

7. Ulnar artery

4 & 5 take part in anastamosis around elbow.

Radial Artery (Fig. 5.20,21)

It is the smaller of the 2 terminal branches of brachial artery, but is the direct continuation of brachial artery. It commences about 1cm below the bent of elbow, at the level of neck of radius. It descends deep to brachioradialis and at the lower part of forearm it lies over the lower end of radius, lateral to the tendon of flexor carpii radialis, covered only by skin and fascia. Here radial arterial pulsation is palpated. Then the artery winds round the lateral border of wrist to reach the dorsum of hand, deep to tendons of abductor pollicis longus, extensor pollicis brevis and extensor pollicis longus. Here it lies in the proximal end of Ist intermetacarpal space, in the anatomical snuff box.

Then from the dorsum, it reaches the palm by passing between the 2 heads of Ist dorsal interosseous muscle. In the palm, it curves medially and ends by joining the deep branch of ulnar artery, thus forming the deep palmar arch.

Branches

1. Radial recurrent artery – anastemoses with anterior descending branch of profunda brachii.

2. Muscular branches.

3. Palmar carpal branch – in front of wrist, it passes medially to anastamose with similar branch of ulnar artery to form a palmar carpal arch.

4. Superficial palmar branch – goes to complete superficial palmar arch with the ulnar artery.

5. Dorsal carpal branch – arises on the dorsum of wrist and anastamoses with similar branch of ulnar artery, to form a dorsal carpal arch from which 2nd, 3rd and 4th dorsal metacarpal arteries proceed distally to the dorsum of hand.

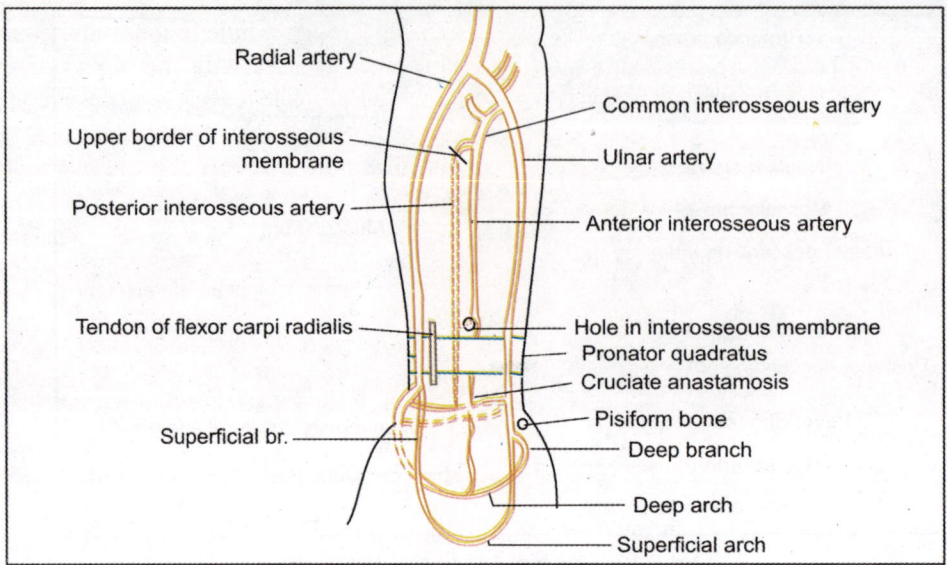

Fig. 5.20: Ulnar and Radial Arteries

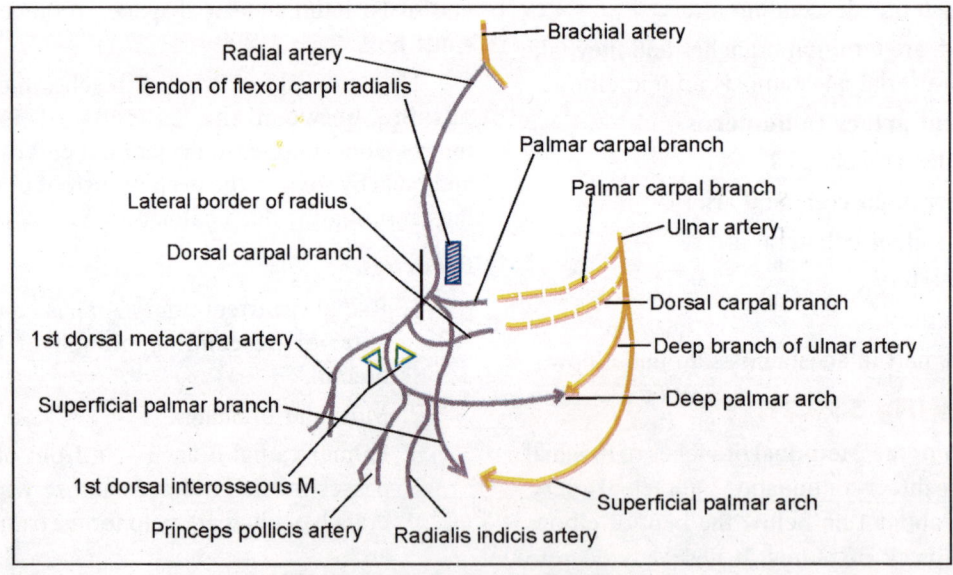

Fig. 5.21: Branches of Radial Artery

6. Ist dorsal metacarpal artery which divides immediately into 2 branches on the adjacent sides of thumb and index finger.

7. Princeps pollicis artery, arises as the radial artery reaches the palm. It divides into 2 branches on the palmar aspect of thumb.

8. Radialis indicis. Last branch from the radial before it forms the deep arch. This descends on the lateral side of index finger.

Ulnar Artery: (Fig. 5.22)

Larger of the 2 terminal branches of brachial artery,

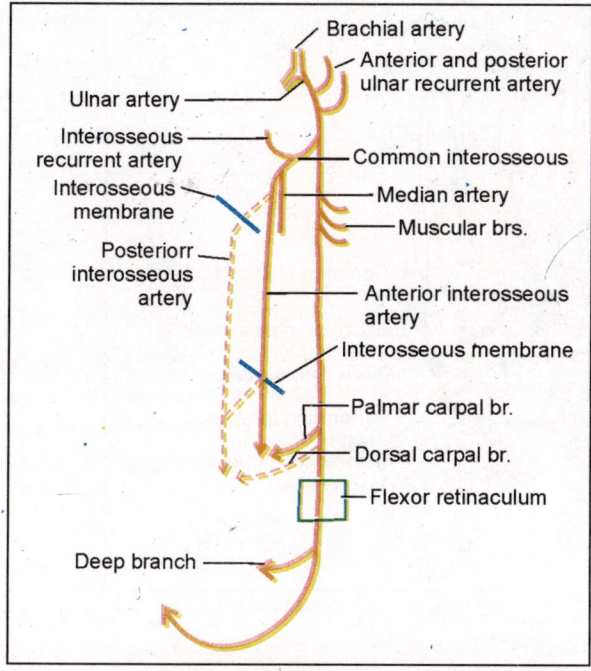

Fig. 5.22: Ulnar Artery

begins at the level of neck of radius. Descends under cover of the flexor muscles on the medial aspect of front of forearm. At the wrist, passes superficial to flexor retinaculum accompanied by ulnar nerve just lateral to pisiform bone and medial to hook of hamate. In the palm ends by forming superficial palmar arch by uniting with superficial branch of radial artery.

Branches

1. Muscular branches to muscles of forearm and hand.
2. Anterior and posterior ulnar recurrent arteries that take part in anastamosis around elbow.
3. Common interosseous artery.

A short trunk, gives an interosseous recurrent branch for anastamosis around elbow and then divides into anterior and posterior interosseous arteries.

Anterior interosseous artery: Descends on the interosseous membrane accompanied by the nerve. Above the pronator quadratus, it passes to the dorsal

aspect through a hole in the introsseous membrane and anastamoses with the posterior interosseous artery. Before it leaves the flexor compartment it gives a branch that descends deep to the pronator quadratus and meets the palmar carpal arch of arteries.

Median artery: is a slender branch of anterior interosseous artery and descends accompanying the median nerve.

Posterior interosseous artery: It passes to the extensor compartment of forearm above the interosseous membrane and descends between deep and superficial extensors accompanying the posterior interosseous nerve. Below it joins with the anterior interosseous artery and takes part in the dorsal carpal arterial arch.

4. Palmar carpal branch.
5. Dorsal carpal branch.
6. Deep palmar branch, in the palm, it joins the radial artery to form the deep palmar arch.

Palmar arterial arches

1. Superficial palmar arch: (Fig. 5.23)

It is an arterial anastamosis formed by the continuation of ulnar artery in the palm joining with the superficial palmar branch of radial artery. The anastamosis froms a curve (arch) directed distally. Lies superficial to flexor tendons.

Branches:

1. Proper palmar digital branch to the medial side of little finger.
2. Three common palmar digital branches which divide into proper digital arteries at the interdigital clefts and go to adjacent sides of the fingers.

2. Deep palmar arch

This arterial arch is formed deep in the palm by the continuation of radial artery joining with the deep branch of ulnar artery. It lies deep to the flexor tendons, proximal to superficial arch, in the concavity of deep branch of ulnar nerve.

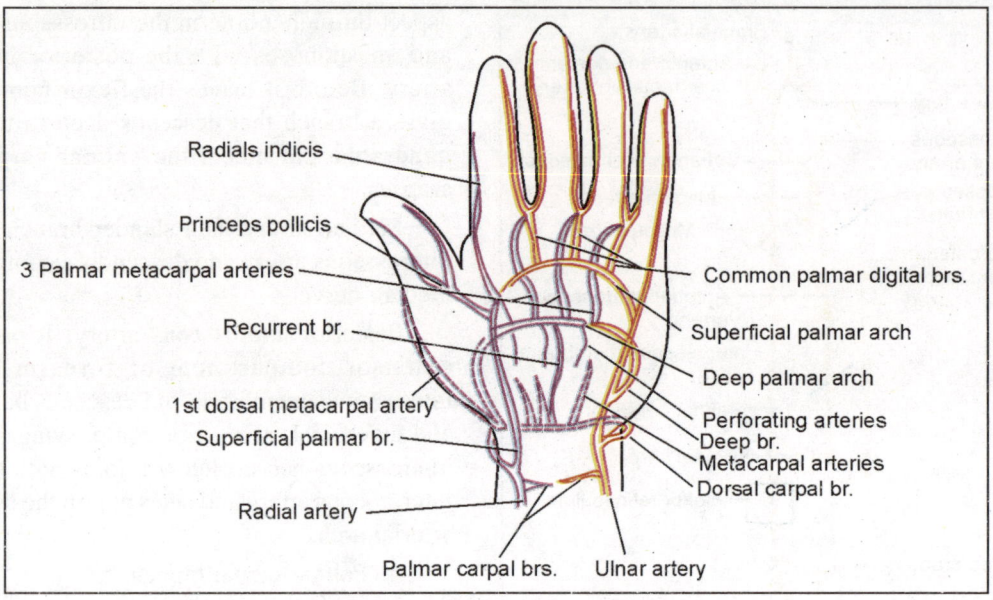

Fig. 5.23: Palmar Arterial Arches

Branches

1. Three palmar metacarpal arteries. They join the 3 common palmar digital branches of superficial arch.
2. Three perforating arteries - go distally to anastamose with dorsal metacarpal arteries which are branches from dorsal carpal arch.
3. Recurrent branch ascends back to join the palmar and carpal arch.

Anastamosis around elbow (Fig: 5.24)

An arterial anastamosis is formed at elbow among the branches of brachial radial and ulnar arteries, as shown in (Fig. 5.24)

Arteries of the Head and Neck

Common carotid arteries

Right common carotid artery is a branch of brachiocephalic trunk and left one, direct branch from the arch of aorta. Both reach the neck behind the sternoclavicular joint. From this level, each artery ascends in the neck to the level of upper border of thyroid cartilage where it terminates by dividing into internal and external carotid arteries. Common carotid artery is enclosed in carotid sheath together with internal juglar vein and vagus nerve.

At the point of division, the common carotid artery shows a localised dilatation, the carotid sinus. It may extend to the beginning of internal carotid artery also. Here the tunica media of the artery is thin and adventitia thick having nerve endings from glossopharyngeal nerve. Carotid sinus is a baroreceptor acting reflexly to changes in blood pressure.

Behind the common carotid bifurcation, 2 small reddish brown structures of about 5-7 mm size are seen. They are carotid bodies, remain connected to or embedded in the adventitia of the vessel. They are chemoreceptors responding to excess CO_2 and low O_2 tension in blood. Supplied by glosso-pharyngeal nerve. Normally common carotid artery has no branches in the neck.

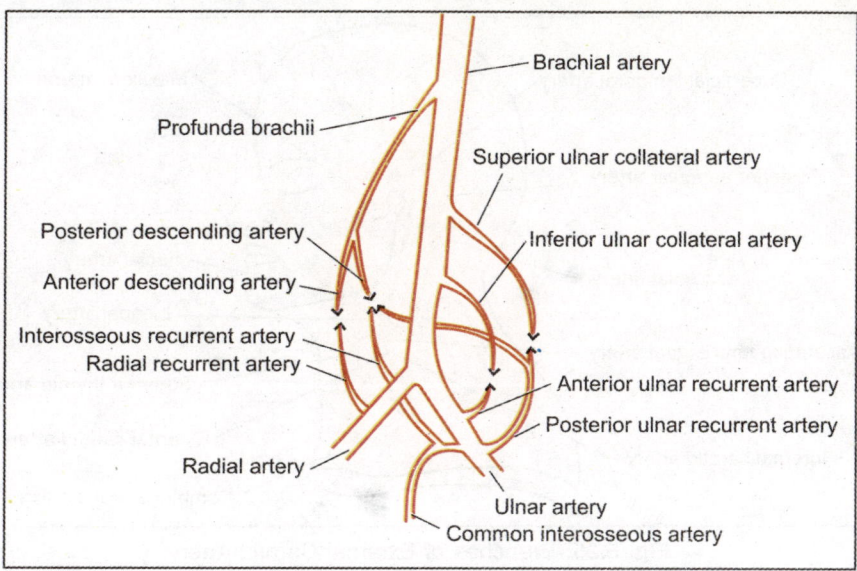

Fig. 5.24: Arterial anastamosis around elbow

External carotid artery

One of the 2 terminal branches of common carotid artery, arises at the level of upper border of thyroid cartilage (upper border of C_4 vertebra) It gives branches to the neck, head, face and outer aspect of cranial cavity.

It ascends in the carotid triangle of neck medial to the internal carotid artery. In the upper part of neck, deep to posterior belly of digastric, it lies lateral to internal carotid artery and enters the posteromedial surface of parotid gland. Within the gland, it divides into the terminal branches - Maxillary and Superficial temporal arteries.

Branches (Fig. 5.25)

1. Ascending pharyngeal artery: smallest and Ist branch of external carotid, ascends in a deeper plane to the Pharynx.

2. Suprior thyroid artery: One of the 2 arteries of the thyroid gland. It also gives a sternomastoid branch, superior laryngeal artery and infrahyoid artery.

3. Lingual artery: It arises from the external carotid artery at the level of tip of greater horn of hyoid borne. It makes a loop and then passes deep to hyoglossus muscle to reach the tongue, to supply it. Its major branches are suprahyoid artery, dorsal lingual artery and sublingual artery.

4. Facial artery (Fig. 5.26): Arises just above the lingual artery. It goes upwards, grooves the posterior surface of submandibular salivary gland and passes between the gland and body of mandible. Reaches the face crossing the lower border of mandible at the anteroinferior angle of masseter. It ascends on the face medially among the muscles of facial expression related to angle of mouth, about 1cm lateral to it, and to the ala of nose. It ends at the medial angle of eye. It has a tortuous course on the face to accommodate for the movements of the muscles of the face. Its branches are, ascending palatine, tonsillar, glandular and submental - in the neck; inferior labial superior labial, and lateral nasal - on the face.

5. Occipital artery: Arises near the facial artery, runs back to the back of scalp to supply that

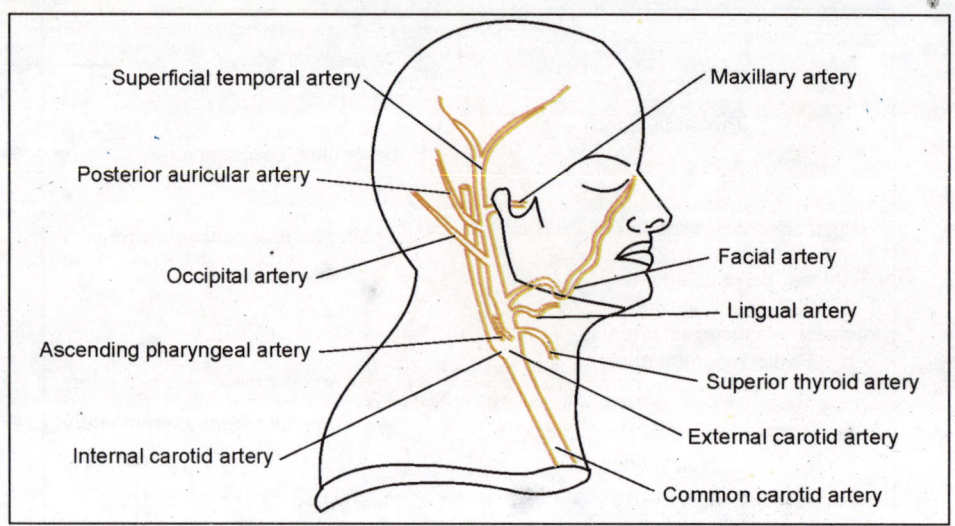

Fig. 5.25: Branches of External Carotid Artery

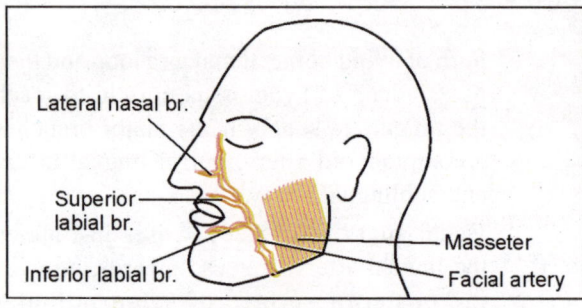

Fig. 5.26: Facial Artery on Face

region. Its branches are stylomastoid artery, mastoid artery and auricular branch.

6. Posterior auricular artery: From its origin, it runs posteriorly above the posterior belly of digastric to the region behind the auricle. Its branches are stylomastoid, auricular and occipital branches.

7. Superficial temporal artery: It is the smaller of the 2 terminal branches of external carotid artery, arises within the parotid gland. Ascends in front of the auricle and divides into anterior and posterior branches which supply the corresponding parts of the temporal region.

8. Maxillary artery: (Fig. 5.27) It is the larger of the 2 terminal branches. Arises in the parotid gland behind the neck of mandible. Runs medially in the infratemporal fossa in relation to lateral pterygoid muscle. Leaves the fossa by passing through the pterygomaxillary fissure and reaches pterygopalatine fossa where it ends.

Branches of maxillary artery are described in 3 parts.

Ist part of the artery in relation to neck of mandible – **mandibular part.**

2nd part in relation to lateral pterygoid muscle – **pterygoid part.**

3rd part in the pterygopalatine fossa - **pterygopalatine part.**

Branches from the Ist part:

1. Deep auricular artery – goes to external acoustic meatus.

2. Anterior tympanic artery – goes to middle ear cavity.

3. Middle meningeal artery – goes to the cranial cavity through foramen ovale. Inside the cranium, its anterior branch lies over the precentral gyrus – the mortor area of brain.

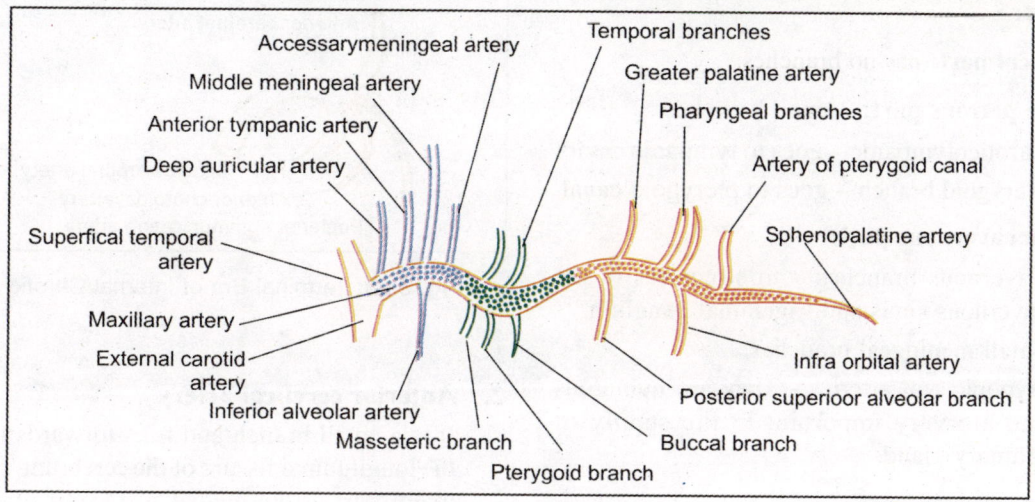

Fig. 5.27: Maxillary Artery

So haemorrhage from this artery will affect motor activity of the opposite side of body.

4. Accessary meningeal artery – goes to cranial cavity through foraman spinosum.

5. Inferior alveolar artery - passes through the mandibular canal.

Branches from 2nd part

1. Masseteric branches
2. Temporal branches
3. Pterygoid branches
4. Buccal branches

Branches from the 3rd part

1. Posterior superior alveolar artery.
2. Infra orbital artery.
3. Greater palatine artery.
4. Pharyngeal branches.
5. Artery of pterygoid canal.
6. Sphenopalatine artery – the terminal branch, ends in the nasal cavity.

Internal carotid artery (Fig. 5.28)

One of the 2 terminal branches of the common carotid artery, begins in the neck at the level of upper

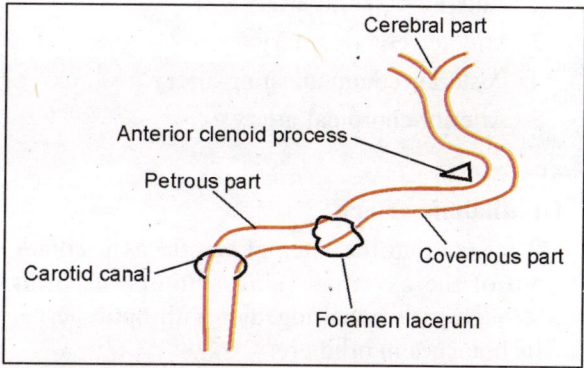

Fig. 5.28: Course of Internal Carotid Artery

border of thyroid cartilage. It supplies most part of the brain, eye, forehead and part of nose.

It ascends in the neck covered in the carotid sheath and gives no branches in the neck.

At the base of skull, it passes anteriorly through the carotid canal, in the petrous part of temporal bone. Enters the cranium through the foramen lacerum, and runs anteriorly through cavernous sinus. Then turns up medial to anterior clenoid process and runs backwards and upwards to reach the anterior perforated substance of brain where it divides into the 2 terminal branches – anterior and middle cerebral arteries.

Branches

Cervical part: has no branches.

In the petrous part: 2 small branches

1. Caroticotympanic – goes to tympanic cavity
2. Pterygoid branch – goes to pterygoid canal

In the cavernous part:

1. Cavernous branches – to structures in the cavernous sinus and trigeminal ganglion.
2. Small meningeal branches.
3. Hypophyseal arteries - They are numerous and are very important in the supply of pituitary gland.

In the cerebral part:

1. Ophthalmic artery
2. Anterior cerebral artery
3. Middle cerebral artery
4. Posterior communicating artery
5. Arterior choroidal artery

Major branches:

1. Ophthalmic artery

It arises from the internal carotid as it comes out of the cavernous sinus. Enters the orbit through optic canal together with optic nerve. Its branches in orbit are:

(a) Central artery of retina.
(b) Muscular branches
(c) Ciliary arteries
(d) Lacrimal artery
(e) Supratrochlear and supra orbital arteries which come to the forehead region.

After giving off the ophthalmic branch, the internal carotid artery bends upwards to reach the region below anterior perforated substance of brain. Here it terminates by dividing into anterior cerebral and middle cerebral arteries. At the terminal division, it gives off 2 smaller branches – posterior communicating artery and anterior choroidal artery. (Fig. 5.29)

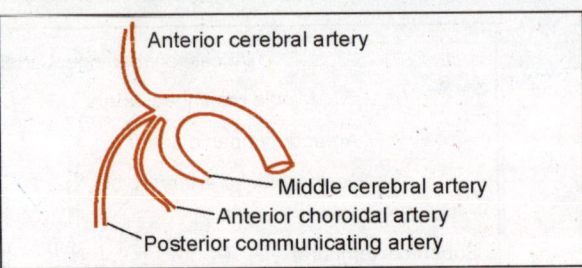

Fig. 5.29: Terminal Brs of Internal Carotid Art.

2. Anterior cerebral artery

It is a small branch and runs forwards to enter the longitudinal fissure of the cerebrum, supplies major part of the medial surface of brain. The anterior cerebral arteries of both sides are connected by a short anterior communicating artery at the base of brain.

3. Middle cerebral artery

It is the largest branch of internal carotid artery. It runs laterally to enter the lateral sulcus of cerebrum. Supplies major parts of the lateral surface of brain.

4. Posterior communicating artery

It is a short vessel, helps to complete an arterial circle at the base of brain, by joining the posterior cerebral artery.

5. Anterior choroidal artery

It is a small branch, enters the inferior horn of lateral ventricle through the choroid fissure and ends in choroid plexus. It gives branches to the neighbouring regions of brain before ending in the choroid plexus.

Circle of Willis (Fig. 5.30)

The terminal branches of internal carotid arteries are involved in the formation of an arterial circle of anastamosis, the circle of Willis or **Circulus arteriosus** at the base of brain. The circle is completed by two posterior cerebral arteries which are branches of basilar artery, formed by the union of 2 vertebral arteries.

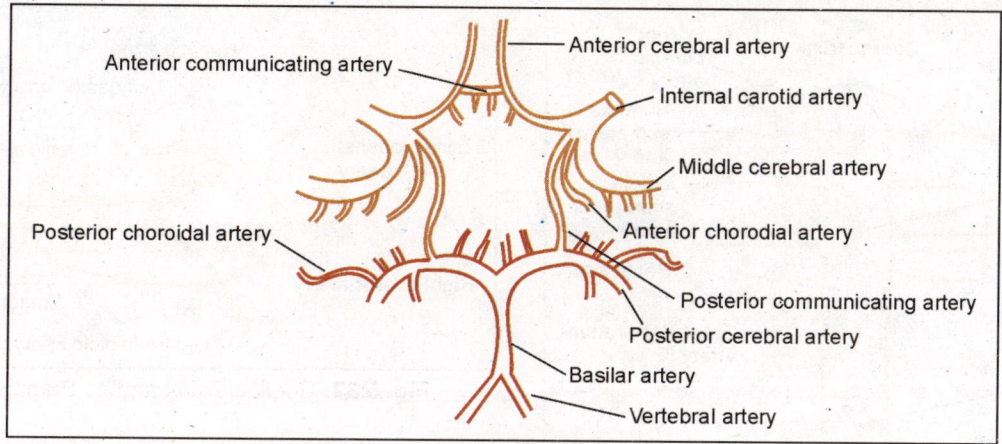

Fig. 5.30: Circle of Willis

The circle is formed by:

The 2 anterior cerebral arteries connected by the anterior communicating artery, and the posterior communicating arteries connected to the posterior cerebral arteries, as shown in the diagram.

The anterior and middle cerebral arteries of the internal carotid artery, the posterior cerebral arteries of basilar artery and the other branches of Circle of Willis supply various parts of brain. Details will be described in the blood supply of brain.

THORACIC AORTA

It is the continuation of the arch of aorta at T_4 level. Descends in front of vertebral column, in the posterior mediastinum of thorax. At the level of lower border of T_{12}, it passes through the aortic opening in diaphragm and becomes abdominal aorta.

In its course, it is closely related to the oesophagus which is to the right of the aorta above and in front of it below.

Branches:

1. Pericardial branches.
2. Posterior intercostal arteries.
3. Subcostal artery, the last of the intercostals.
4. Bronchial arteries- They vary in Number- usually one on right side and 2 on left side.

5. Oesophageal arteries
6. Mediastinal branches
7. Phrenic branches – to upper surface of diaphragm.

ABDOMINAL AORTA

It is the continuation of the thoracic aorta at the level of T_{12} behind the median arcuate ligament of diaphragm. Descends in front of lumbar vertebrae and at level of L_4 vertebra, terminates by dividing into right and left common iliac arteries, accompanied by the inferior vena cava on its right side.

Branches (Fig. 5.31)

I. **Ventral branches (unpaired)**
    (a) Coeliac trunk
    (b) Superior mesenteric artery
    (c) Inferior mesenteric artery

II. **Lateral branches (paired)**
    (a) Inferior phrenic
    (b) Middle suprarenal
    (c) Renal
    (d) Testicular / ovarian
    (e) Terminal branches – Right and Left common iliac.

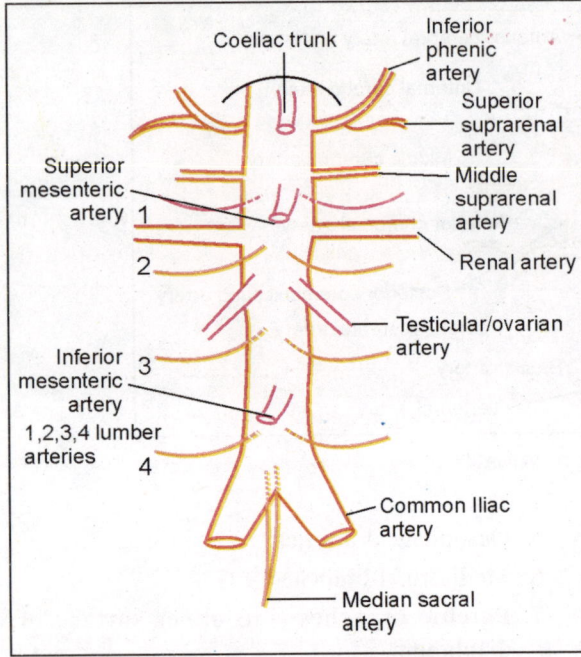

Fig. 5.31: Branches of Abdominal aorta

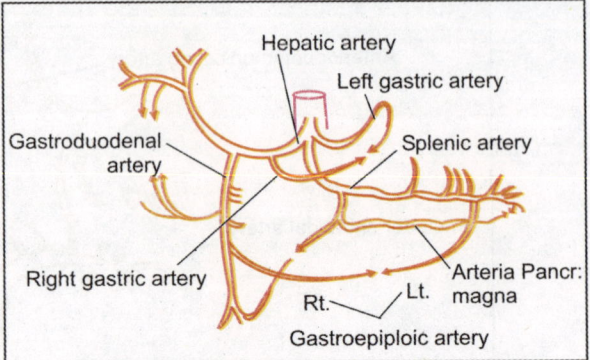

Fig. 5.32: Coeliac Trunk and its Branches

III. Dorsal branches

(a) Four lumbar arteries (paired)

(b) Median sacral artery (unpaired)

Ventral Branches

I. Coeliac trunk (Fig. 5.32)

Ist ventral branch, arises from the aorta immediately below the aortic opening of diaphragm. It is about 1.25 cms long and immediately divides into 3 branches – Left gastric, common hepatic and splenic arteries.

(a) **Left gastric artery:** From its origin, first it runs upwards and to the right. Then near the cardiac end of stomach, it turns forwards to lie in the lesser curvature of stomach between the 2 layers of lesser omentum. Supplies branches to lower oesophagus and both surfaces of stomach. Ends by anastamosing with the right gastric artery.

(b) **Hepatic artery:** It ascends in the free margin of lesser omentum accompanied by portal vein and bile duct. At the porta hepatis, ends by dividing into right and left branches.

Branches of the hepatic artery are:

(i) Right gastric artery: runs along the lesser curvature to anastamose with left gastric artery. Supplies branches to both gastric surfaces.

(ii) Gastroduodenal artery: Arises from hepatic artery above the duodenum, descends behind the duodenum, between it and neck of pancreas, and at the lower border of Ist part of duodenum, divides into right gastroepiploic and superior pancreaticoduodenal arteries.

Right gastroepiploic artery runs along the greater curvature of stomach to the left and anastamoses with left gastroepiploic artery. It gives branches to both surfaces of stomach and to greater omentum.

Superior pancreaticoduodenal artery divides into anterior and posterior branches which anastamose with corresponding branches of inferior pancreatico duodenal artery of superior mesenteric artery.

(iii) Cystic artery: May arise from the hepatic artery or from its right branch.

(c) **Splenic artery:** It is the longest branch of coeliac truck. It has a course to the left along the upper border of pancreas behind the stomach and lesser sac. Passing through the lienorenal ligament, it reaches the hilum of spleen, where it divides into terminal branches.

Branches of splenic artery

(i) Pancreatic branches – numerous: Of these, a dorsal branch descends behind the pancreas and divides into right and left branches. Right one anastamoses with an ascending branch from the anterior division of superior pancreatico duodenal artery to make a prepancreatic arterial arch. The left branch runs to left, to the tail of pancreas and anastamoses with a branch from splenic artery at the hilum of spleen – arteria pancreatica magna.

(ii) Short gastric arteries.

(iii) Posterior gastric artery.

(iv) Left gastro epiploic artery: Arises near the termination of splenic artery. Runs along the greater curvature of stomach to the right, anastamoses with the right one and supplies branches to both surfaces of stomach and greater omentum.

(v) Terminal branches in the spleen.

II. Superior mesenteric artery (Fig. 5.33 a,b)

It is the artery of midgut, supplying the region of alimentary tract from the middle of 2nd part of duodenum to the junction of right 2/3rd & left 1/3 rd of transverse colon.

Arises 1cm below the coeliac trunk, at level of L_1 or L_2 vertebra, descends behind the pancreas, then anterior to its uncinate process and 3rd part of duodenum. Enters the root of mesentery. As it descends in the mesentery with a curve to the right, crosses the inferior vena cava, right ureter and psoas major. Ends in the right iliac fossa by dividing into branches which anastamose with branches of ileocolic artery.

Branches

1. Inferior pancreaticoduodenal artery.
2. Jejunal and ileal branches.
3. Ileocolic artery.
4. Right colic artery.
5. Middle colic artery: Its supplies branches upto the right 2/3rd of transverse colon.

III. Inferior mesenteric artery (Fig. 5.34)

Arises 3 to 4 cm above aortic bifurcation behind the horizontal part of duodenum. Enters sigmoid mesocolon. Continues in it to lesser pelvis as superior rectal artery. Supplies left 1/3 rd of transverse colon, descending colon and most part of rectum.

Latleral branches (Fig. 5.35)

1. **Inferior phrenic arteries:** Supply diaphragm. They give superior suprarenal arteries also.

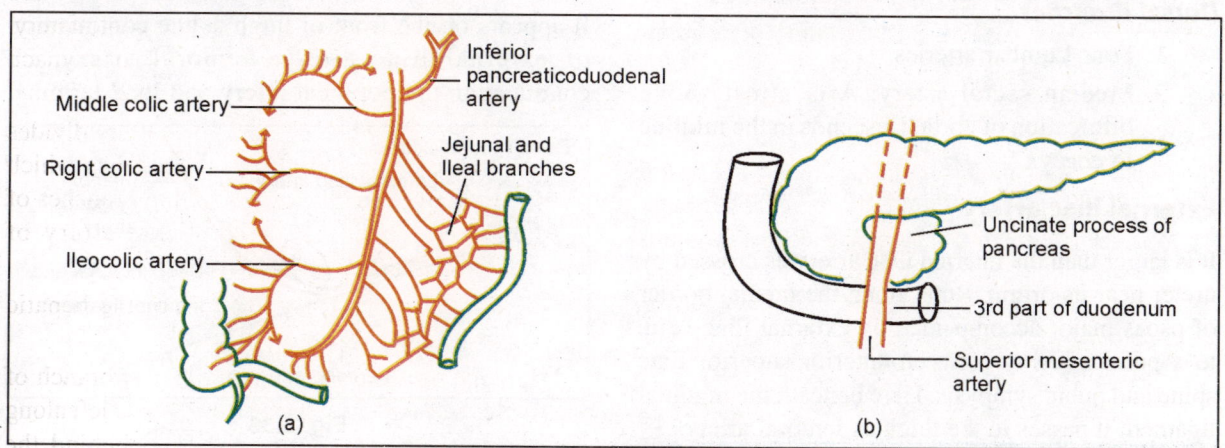

Fig. 5.33: Superior Mesenteric Artery

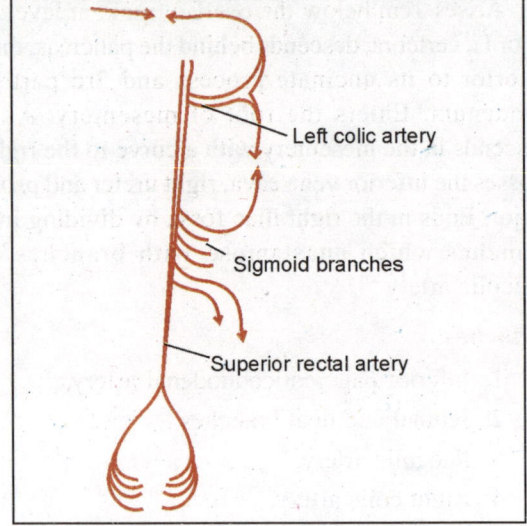

Fig. 5.34: Inferior Mesenteric Artery

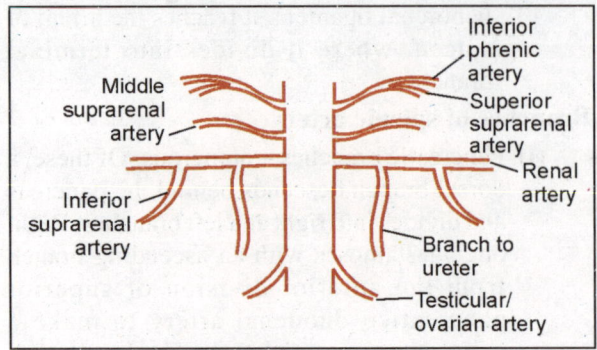

Fig. 5.35: Lateral Brs. of Aorta

2. **Middle suprarenal artery**
3. **Renal arteries:** They give inferior suprarenal artery and branches to ureter.
4. **Testicular artery:** Descends on psoas major, crosses ureter and external ileac artery, passes to deep inguinal ring to enter spermatic cord.

Ovarian artery: Descends to the lesser pelvis, crosses external iliac artery and enters true pelvis. Turns medially into broad ligament. Gives branches to tube, ovary ureter and uterus.

Dorsal Branches

1. Four Lumbar arteries.
2. Median sacral artery: Arises just above bifurcation of aorta. Descends in the midline to coccyx.

External iliac artery

It is larger than the internal iliac artery, is crossed by ureter near its origin. Runs along the medial border of psoas major accompanied by external iliac vein, to a point midway between anterior superior iliac spine and pubic sympysis. Here beneath the inguinal ligament it passes to the thigh as femoral artery.

Branches (Fig. 5.36)

Two branches arise near its termination.

1. Inferior epigastric artery. Ascends obliquely along the medial border of deep inguinal ring on the deep surface of anterior abdominal wall. Lies in the rectus sheath deep to rectus muscle. Ends by anatamosing with superior epigastric artery. Cremasteric artery is one of its branches.

2. Deep circumflex iliac artery. Runs laterally deep to inguinal ligament towards anterior superior iliac spine and iliac crest.

Arteries of the lower limb

Femoral artery (Fig. 5.37 a,b)

It appears on the front of thigh as the continuation of external iliac artery. Femoral artery, its continuation the popliteal artery and its 2 terminal

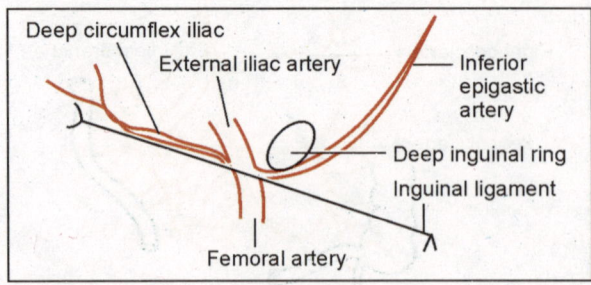

Fig. 5.36

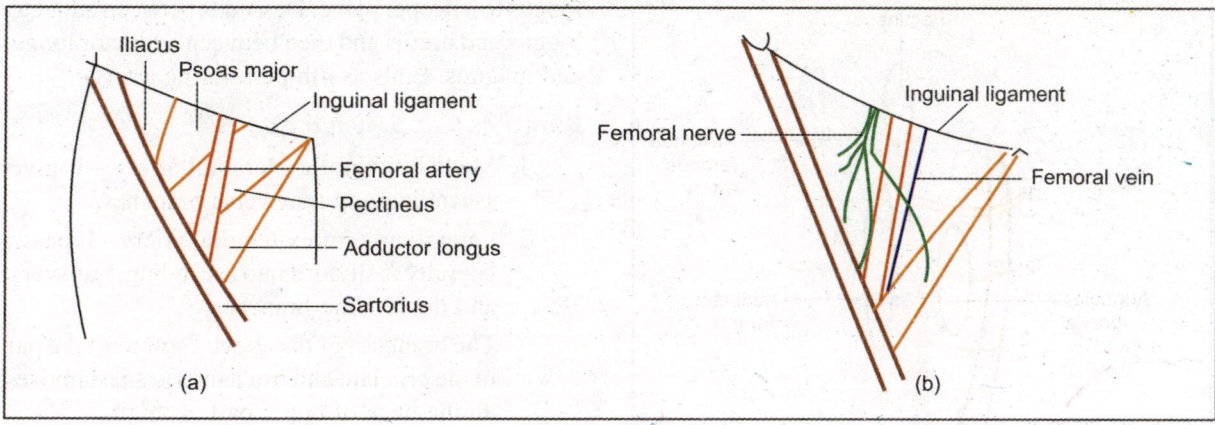

Fig. 5.37

branches – anterior and posterior tibial arteries provide the major arterial supply to the lower limb.

Femoral artery enters the thigh behind inguinal ligament midway between anterior superior iliac spine and pubic symphysis. In the front of thigh, it lies in the femoral triangle. Down, it lies in the adductor canal and leaves the space by passing through adductor hiatus to the popliteal region as popliteal artery.

Important relations (Fig. 5.37 a, b)

In the femoral triangle, it lies over psoas major, pectineus and adductor longus. Femoral vein is medial to it and femoral nerve, lateral. In the upper 3 cms of the triangle, the 2 vessels are covered by femoral sheath.

In the adductor canal it lies over adductor longus and then over adductor magnus accompanied by saphenous nerve. Sartorius overlies it.

Branches (Fig. 5.38, 5.41)

1. Superficial circumflex iliac artery - directed towards anterior superior iliac spine.
2. Superficial epigastric artery - directed towards umbilicus.
3. Superficial external pudental artery - goes to the skin of scrotum or labium majus.
4. Deep external pudental artery - to the skin of scrotum.

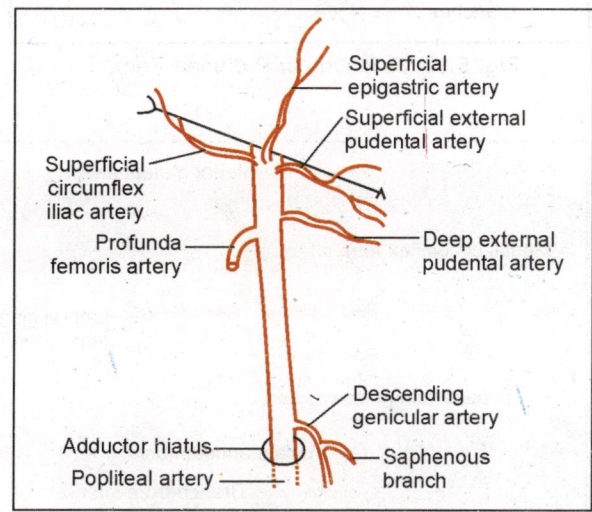

Fig. 5.38: Branches of Femoral Artery

5. Profunda femoris artery.
6. Descending genicular artery - arises near its lower end. A branch of it, saphenous artery accompanies saphenous nerve.
7. Muscular branches

Profunda femoris artery (Fig. 5.39)

Largest branch of femoral artery, is the main artery to the muscles of thigh.

Arises about 4 cms below the inguinal ligament and descends behind the femoral artery. Leaves the triangle by passing between pectineus and adductor

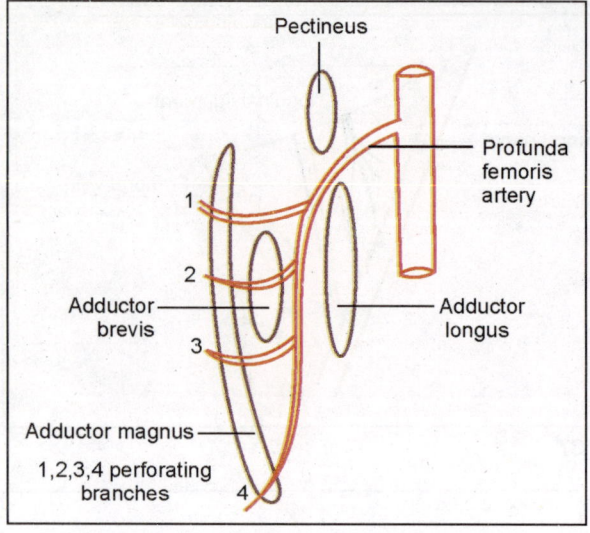

Fig. 5.39: Relations of Profunda Femoris

longus to a deeper plane. Descends between adductor longus and brevis and then between adductor longus and magnus. Ends as 4th perforating artery.

Branches (Fig. 5.40 a,b,c,d,)

1. Medial circumflex femoral artery - It gives ascending and transverse branches.
2. Lateral circumflex femoral artery - It passes laterally & divides into ascending, transverse and descending branches.

   The branches of the above 2 arteries take part in the cruciate and trochanteric anastamoses, on the back of upper part of thigh.

3. Perforating branches - 4 in number - They give numerous branches to the muscles of back of thigh. All these pierce the adductor magnus near its attachment along linea

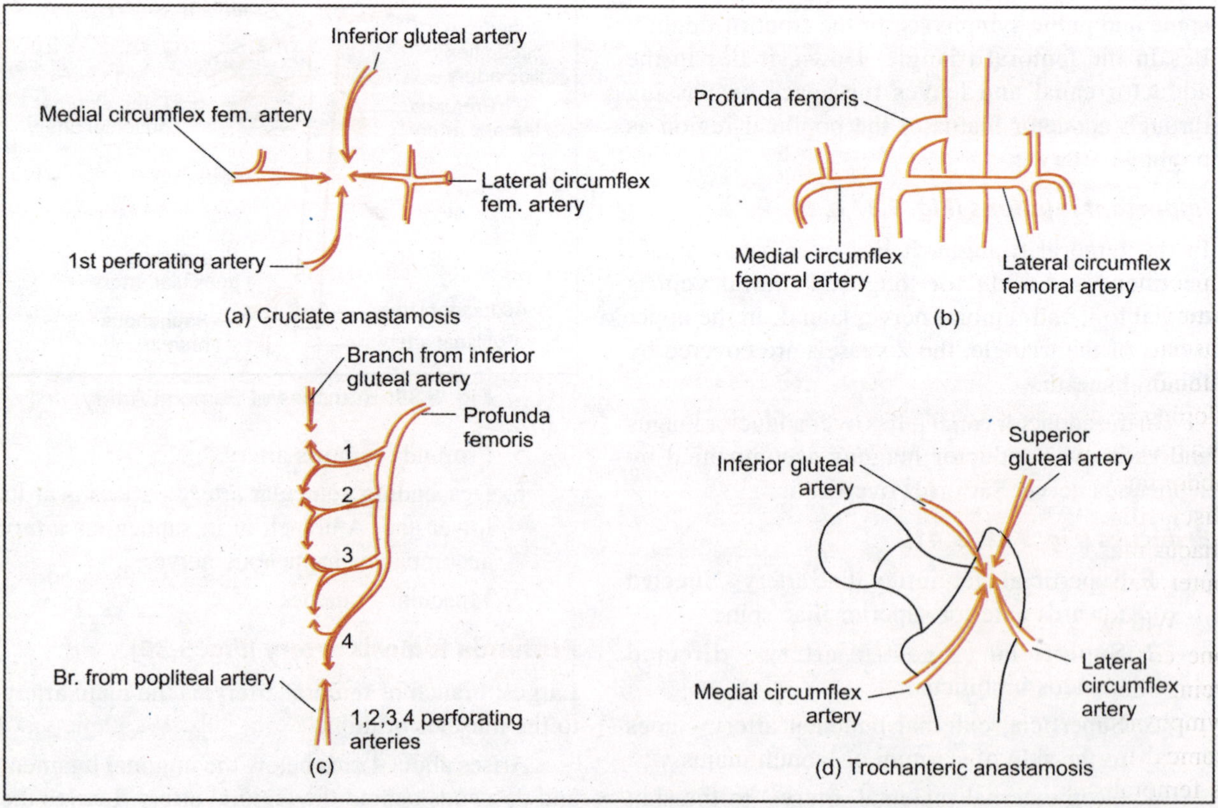

(a) Cruciate anastamosis

(b)

(c)

(d) Trochanteric anastamosis

Fig. 5.40: Branches of Profunda Femoris and their Anastomoses

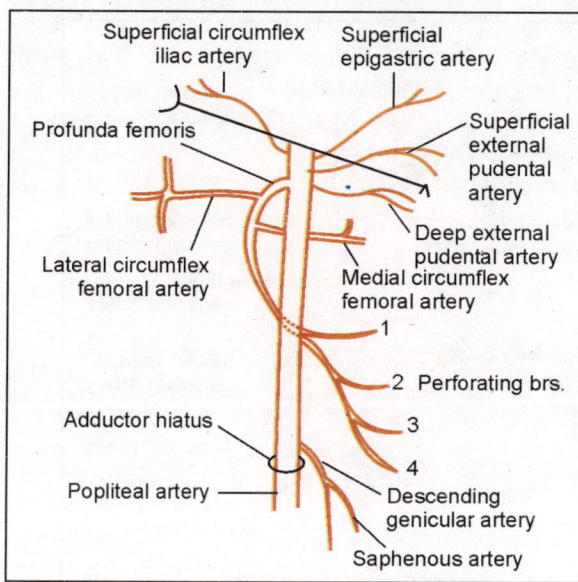

Fig. 5.41: Femoral Artery - Branches

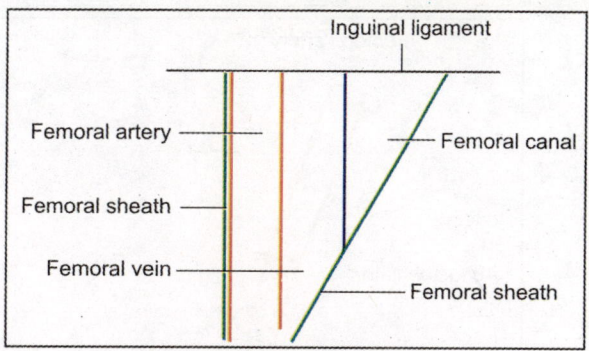

Fig. 5.42: Femoral Sheath

aspera and go posteriorly where they are connected by vertical anastamotic channels. 4th perfortaing artery is the terminal part of profunda femoris. It anastamoses whith the upper muscular branch of popliteal artery.

Femoral Sheath (Fig. 5.42 a)

In the femoral triangle, upper part of the femoral artery and vein, for about 3-4 cms are covered by a fascial sheath, the femoral sheath. It is somewhat funnel shaped having a vertical lateral wall and sloping medial wall. The anterior layer of the sheath is a prolongation of fascia transversalis from anterior abdominal wall. Posterior layer is prolongation from fascia iliaca from abdomen, where it covers the iliacus muscle. Lower end of the sheath, fuses with outer wall of the vessels.

Within it, there are 3 compartments. Lateral one contains femoral artery. Middle one, femoral vein. Medial one contains areolar tissue and a lymph node and is called femoral canal which is conical in shape. Above its opening into abdomen is femoral ring and is closed by condensed areolar tissue, femoral septum. Femoral ring is bounded medially by lacunar ligament, laterally by femoral vein anteriorly by inguinal ligament and posteriorly by pectineus.

Femoral hernia

Contents of abdominal cavity can herniate through femoral ring into femoral canal. It will protrude anteriorly through the saphenous opening. More common in female where femoral ring is larger.

Popliteal artery (Fig. 5.43 a,b)

It is the continuation of femoral artery from the level of adductor hiatus. Descends through popliteal fossa and at the lower border of popliteus muscle, ends by dividing into anterior and posterior tibial arteries.

In its course, it lies on the popliteal surface of femur, capsule of knee joint and popliteal fascia over the muscle. Overlapped by popliteal vein and tibial nerve.

Branches (Fig. 5.43 b)

1. Cutaneous branches to the skin of popliteal region.
2. Superior muscular branches to the lower part of thigh.
3. Several branches – to muscles of back of leg.
4. Genicular branches
   (a) Medial and lateral superior genicular arteries.
   (b) Medial and lateral inferior genicular arteries.

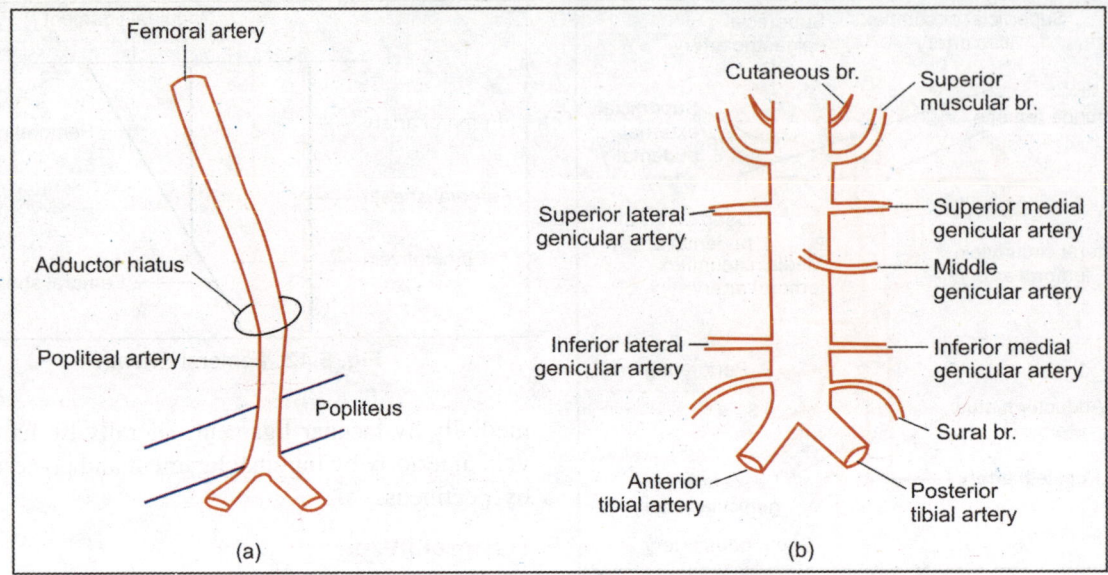

Fig. 5.43: Popliteal artery

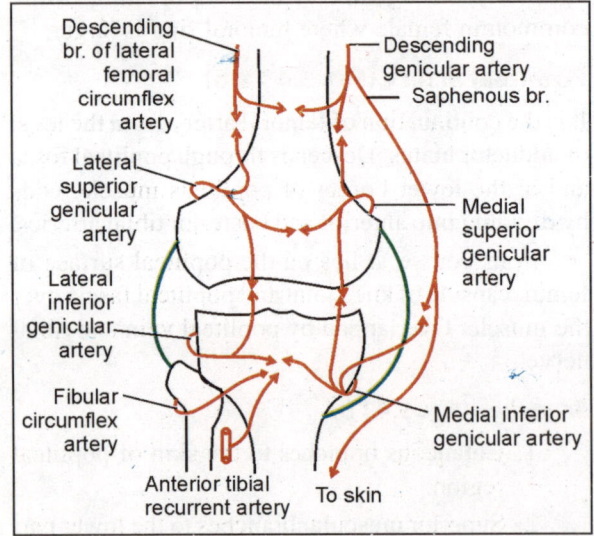

Fig. 5.44: Arterial anastamosis around knee

(c) Middle genicular artery. Middle genicular artery pierces capsule of knee joint. Other genicular arteries take part in the anastomosis around knee (Fig. 5.44)

5. Terminal branches: anterior and posterior tibial arteries.

Anterior tibial artery (Fig. 5.45)

One of the 2 terminal branches of popliteal artery, begins at the lower border of popliteus. From the posterior compartment of leg, it passes through an opening in the upper part of interosseous membrane to reach the anterior compartment. Descends on the interosseous membrane and lower down, it lies on tibia. Passes deep to the extensor retinacula. Midway between the medial & lateral malleoli, beyond the ankle joint, it continues as the dorsalis pedis artery on the dorsum of foot. In its course in the leg, it is accompanied by the deep peroneal nerve.

Branches

1. Posterior tibial recurrent artery.
2. Anterior tibial recurrent artery.
3. Muscular branches to the muscles of anterior compartment of leg.
4. Anterior medial malleolar artery.
5. Anterior lateral malleolar artery.

Dorsalis pedis artery (Fig. 5.45)

Continuation of anterior tibial artery distal to the ankle. It reaches the proximal part of 1st

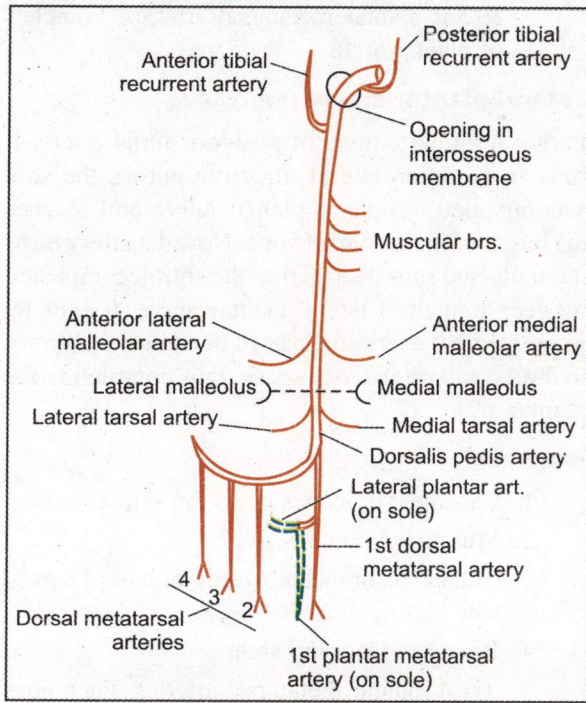

Fig. 5.45: Anterior tibial artery

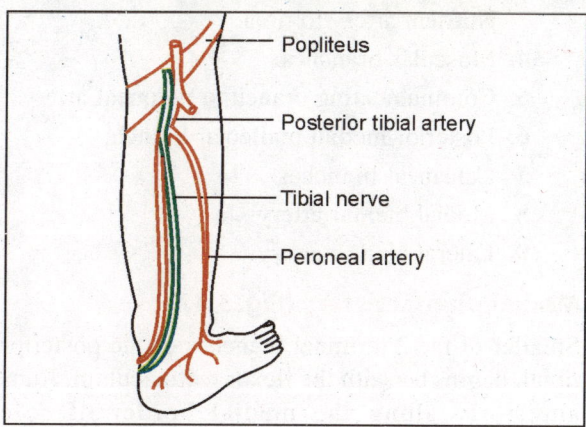

Fig. 5.46: Posterior tibial artery

Posterior tibial artery (Fig. 5.46)

One of the 2 terminal branches of popliteal artery, begins at the upper part of back of leg, at the lower border of popliteus muscle. Descends between the superficial and deep groups of flexor muscles, accompanied by tibial nerve and 2 veins. Lower part of the medial side of back of leg, it is superficial, covered by skin & fasciae only. Under the flexor rectinaculum, deep to the abductor hallucis, it terminates by dividing into medial and lateral plantar arteries.

Branches

1. Circumflex fibular artery.
2. Peroneal artery: A large branch, arises about 2.5 cms below the origin of posterior tibial. Descends in relation to fibula, covered by flexor hallucis longus. At the lower tibiofibular joint, it terminates by dividing into numerous calcaneal branches which ramify on the lateral & posterior surfaces of calcaneus. Other branches of peroneal artery are:

(a) Muscular branches.

(b) Nutrient artery to fibula.

(c) Perforating artery: Its branches make anastamoses with anterior lateral malleolar artery & lateral tarsal artery.

(d) Communicating branch to posterior tibial artery.

intermetatarsal space. Turns to the sole between the heads of 1st dorsal interosseous muscle and in the sole, joins with the lateral plantar artery to complete the plantar arterial arch.

Often palpated for aterial pulsation.

Branches

1. Lateral tarsal artery. Passes deep to extensor digitorum brevis.

2. Medial tarsal artery

3. Arcuate artery – Passes laterally deep to extensor tendons over the bases of metatarsal bones, ends by anastamosing with lateral tarsal, lateral anterior malleolar & lateral plantar arteries. It gives off 2nd, 3rd, 4th dorsal metatarsal arteries.

4. 1st dorsal metatarsal artery

1st plantar metatarsal arises from the junction of dorsalis pedis & lateral plantar arteries.

3. Nutrient artery to tibia.
4. Muscular branches.
5. Communicating branch to peroneal artery.
6. Posterior medial malleolar branch.
7. Calcaneal branches
8. Medial plantar artery
9. Lateral plantar artery

Medial plantar artery (Fig. 5.47)

Smaller of the 2 terminal branches of the posterior tibial, begins beneath the flexor rectinaculum. Runs anteriorly along the medial border of sole accompanied by medial plantar nerve and between abductor hallucis and flexor digitorum brevis. It ends by supplying the medial side of big toe.

Branches

1. Muscular branches.
2. Three digital branches which join the 1st, 2nd

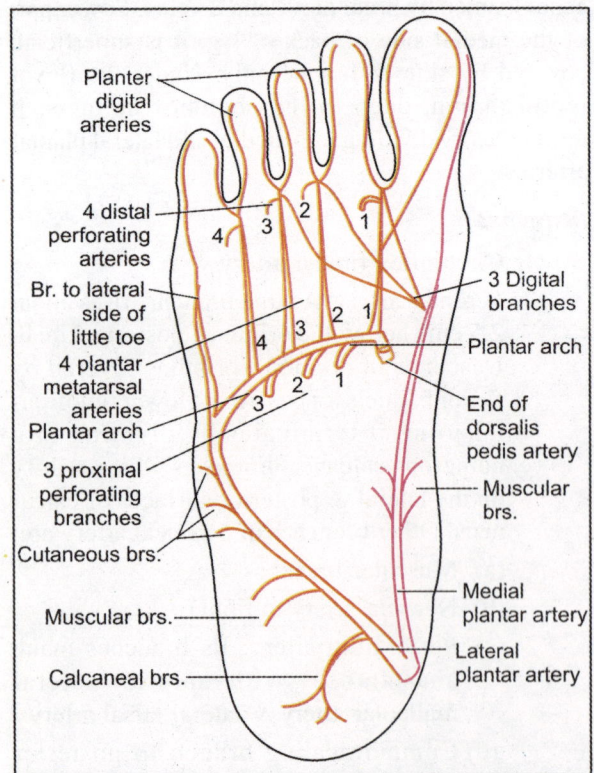

Fig. 5.47: Medial and Lateral Plantar Arteries

& 3rd plantar metatarsal arteries, branches of plantar arch.

Lateral plantar artery (Fig. 5.47)

Larger terminal branch of posterior tibial artery. It runs in an anterolateral direction across the sole accompanied by lateral plantar nerve and reaches the base of 5th metatarsal bone. Now the artery turns medially and runs deep across the sole accompanied by deep branch of lateral plantar nerve. It ends by joining with the terminal part of dorsalis pedis artery in the 1st intermetatarsal space, thus completing the plantar arch.

Branches

1. Calcaneal branches go to the skin of heel.
2. Muscular branches.
3. Cutaneous branches to skin of lateral part of sole.
4. Branches from the arch.
   (i) 4 Plantar metatarsal arteries. Each goes to the interdigital cleft and divides into plantar digital arteries to the adjacent sides of the toes.
   (ii) 3 proximal perforating arteries which go through the 2nd, 3rd and 4th intermetatarsal spaces to join the proximal parts of corresponding dorsal metatarsal arteries.
5. A branch to the lateral side of little toe arises from the lateral plantar, before it arches.

INTERNAL ILIAC ARTERY

Internal iliac artery is one of the 2 terminal branches of common iliac artery, begins in front of the sacroiliac joint. It descends to the upper margin of greater sciatic foramen where it divides into an anterior trunk and a posterior trunk.

Branches (Fig. 5.48)

From anterior trunk-

1. **Superior vesical artery:** Supplies the upper part of urinary bladder. Artery to the vas is a branch from it, usually.

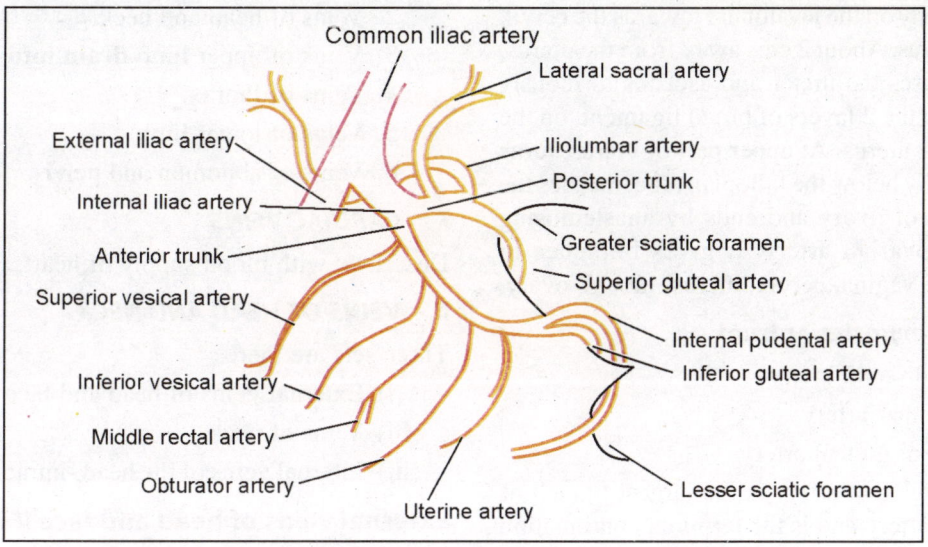

Fig. 5.48: Branches of internal iliac artery

2. **Inferior vesical artery:** Supplies the lower part of the urinary bladder, seminal vesicle, prostate, lower ureter. Artery to vas may arise from this.

In female, replaced by vaginal artery.

3. **Middle rectal artery:** It supplies lower part of rectum and anastamoses with superior and middle rectal arteries. Branches are given to prostate and seminal vesicle also.

4. **Internal pudendal artery:** In leaves the pelvis through greater sciatic foramen to enter the gluteal region. Crosses the ischial spine and through the lesser sciatic foramen it enters the perineum and lies in the lateral wall of ischiorectal fossa, in a fascial canal - pudendal canal.

Branches:

(a) Muscular branches

(b) Inferior rectal artery

(c) Perineal branch

Inferior rectal artery & perineal artery are its major branches.

(d) Artery to bulb of penis.

(e) Urethral artery

(f) Deep artery of penis

(g) Dorsal artery of penis

(f) and (g) are two terminal branches of the internal pudendal artery.

5. **Inferior gluteal artery:** Largest branch of internal iliac. Arises within the pelvis. Passes to gluteal region through greater sciatic foramen, below piriformis. Descends in the gluteal region deep to gluteus maximus and extends to upper part of thigh.

6. **Obturator artery:** From origin, it runs on the obturator fascia downwards and forwards accompanied by obturator nerve. Leaves pelvis through obturator canal. Outside the pelvis divides into anterior and posterior terminal branches.

Branches:

(a) Iliac branches to iliac fossa.

(b) Vesical branch to urinary bladder.

(c) Pubic branch.

(d) Anterior & posterior terminal branches-encircle the margin of obturator foramen.

7. **Uterine artery (in the female):** It runs

medially on the levator ani towards the cervix of uterus. About 2 cms away from the uterus, it crosses the ureter and ascends tortuously within the 2 layers of broad ligament, on the side of uterus. At upper part of uterus, turns laterally below the fallopian tube, reaches the hilum of ovary and ends by anastemosing with ovarian artery. It gives branches to ureter, vagina, cervix, uterus, tube & ovary.

Branches from posterior trunk

1. Lateral sacral artery
2. Iliolumbar artery
3. Superior gluteal artery

Superior gluteal artery is the largest branch of internal iliac artery and is the terminal continuation of the posterior trunk. It leaves the pelvis through greater sciatic foramen above piriformis. In the gluteal region, it divides into superficial and deep branches, deep to gluteus maximus.

VENOUS SYSTEM

Three main groups of veins are present.

I. **Pulmonary veins** – bring oxygenated blood from lungs to the heart.

II. **Systemic veins** – bring venous blood from most part of body except from abdominal organs, to the heart.

III. **Portal vein** – Collects venous blood from the abdominal organs passes through liver and empties into the systemic vein.

1. Pulmonary veins

They begin as tiny capillaries in the walls of alveoli of lungs. They emerge as 2 pulmonary veins from each lung. The 4 pulmonary veins open into the posterosuperior part of left atrium.

2. Systemic veins

There are six sets-

1. Cardiac veins – drain the myocardium and open into the heart itself.

2. Veins of head and neck.
3. Veins of upper limb **drain into S.V.C**.
4. Veins of thorax.
5. Veins of lower limb.
6. Veins of abdomen and pelvis.

I.   CARDIAC VEINS

Described with blood supply of heart.

II.   VEINS OF HEAD AND NECK

Three sets are there.

(i) External veins of head and face
(ii) Veins of neck
(iii) Internal veins of the head -intracranial veins.

External veins of head and face (Fig. 5.49)

1. **Supratrochlear vein**: Starts on the forehead and converges towards medial angle of eye. Drains the neighbouring area.

2. **Supraorbital vein**: Seen lateral to supratrochlear vein, joins with it to form facial vein.

3. **Facial Vein**: Formed by union of supratrochlear and supraorbital veins at the medial angle of eye. Here it is known as angular vein and has connection with ophthalmic veins. Descends posterolaterally, crosses the lower border of mandible and joins with anterior division of retromandibular vein to form common facial vein, below the angle of mandible. Finally it ends in the internal jugular vein.

It is connected to the cavernous sinus by 2 routes -Ist, through ophthalmic veins which drain into cavernous sinus and 2nd, through deep facial vein which connects facial vein to pterygoid venous plexus which in turn is connected to cavernous sinus.

A rectangular area including lower part of nose and upper lip is regarded as dangerous area of face, as infection from this part can easily be conveyed to the cavernous sinus.

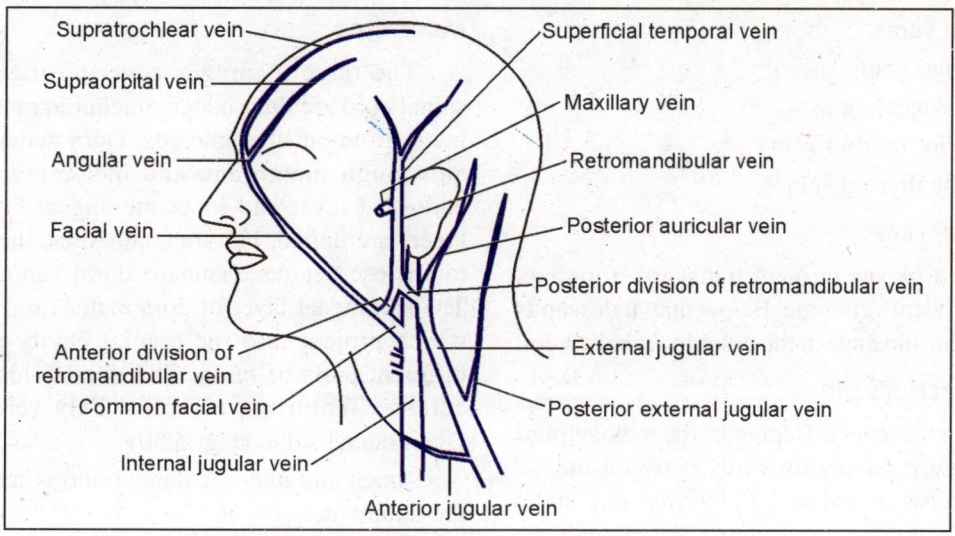

Fig. 5.49: External Veins of Head and Neck

4. **Superficial temporal vein:** Drains the side of the scalp.

5. **Maxillary vein:** Drains the infratemporal region and joins with the superficial temporal vein to form retromandibular vein.

6. **Retromandibular vein:** Is formed inside the parotid gland. Descends in it and divides into anterior and posterior divisions. Anterior division joins with facial vein to form common facial vein which empties into internal jugular vein. Posterior division joins with the posterior auricular vein to form the external jugular vein.

7. **Occipital veins:** Drain the posterior part of scalp and join the deep cervical and vertebral veins.

Veins of the neck

1. External jugular vein

Formation: Joining the posterior division of retromandibular vein and posterior auricular vein below and behind the angle of mandible.

Descends obliquely over sternomastoid and behind the middle of clavicle, ends by joining the subclavian vein.

Tributaries:

1. Posterior external jugular vein from posterior part of neck.

2. Transverse cervical vein.

3. Suprascapular vein

4. Anterior jugular vein: Formed near the hyoid bone in front of neck. Descends on either side of midline of neck. Turns laterally deep to sternomastoid and ends in the external jugular vein. In the lower part of neck, veins of both sides are joined by a short jugular venous arch.

2. Internal Jugular vein

This large vein drains venous blood from the skull, brain, superficial parts of face and neck.

Begins as continuation of sigmoid venous sinus as it comes out of skull through jugular foramen. Descends in the neck together with internal carotid and common carotid arteries, covered in the carotid sheath. Behind the sternal end of clavicle, ends by joining with the subclavian vein to form the brachiocephalic vein.

Tributaries:

1. Inferior petrosal sinus.

2. Facial vein
3. Linguial vein
4. Pharryngeal veins
5. Superior thyroid vein
6. Middle thyroid vein

3. Vertebral vein

Descends as a plexus through transverse foramina of upper 6 cervical vertebrae. Below that, it descends as a single vein and ends in the brachiocephalic vein.

4. Deep cervical vein

Accompanies the artery. Begins in the suboccipital region. Below it passes forwards between the C_7 transverse processes and neck of Ist rib to end in the vertebral vein.

INTRACRANIAL VEINS

Different venous channels present inside the cranium are:

1. Diploic veins: present within the thickness of skull bones. They drain into dural venous sinuses.
2. Meningeal veins: Lie on the dura mater and drain into dural venous sinuses.
3. Emissary veins: not restricted to cranial cavity. They connect intracranial venous sinuses to extracranial veins. They are special in that their walls are very thin and do not have valves.
4. Cerebral and cerebellar veins: drain different parts of brain into venous sinuses.

Meninges

The three meninges covering the brain and spinal cord are dura mater, arachnoid mater and pia mater from outside, inwards. Dura mater is a thick and tough membrane and has 2 layers. Outer endosteal layer and inner meningeal layer. The 2 layers are united, but at certain sites, they separate to enclose venous channels, dural venous sinuses. The meningeal layer of dura mater form four folds which project into the cranial cavity separating different parts of brain. The dural folds are, Falx cerebri, Tentorium cerebilli, Falx cerebelli and Diaphragma sella. (Fig. 5.50)

Arachnoid mater is thinner and is seen inner to the dura mater.

Pia mater is the thinnest layer and closely invests the brain and spinal cord. Between the arachnoid mater and pia mater, is the subarachnoid space in which the cerebrospinal fluid circulates.

Dural Venous sinuses (Fig. 5.51)

They are venous channels between the 2 layers of dura mater. They drain venous blood from the brain, orbit and skull bones. Blood from these sinuses finally reach the internal jugular vein.

Dural venous sinuses are classified into 2 groups – **paired and unpaired**

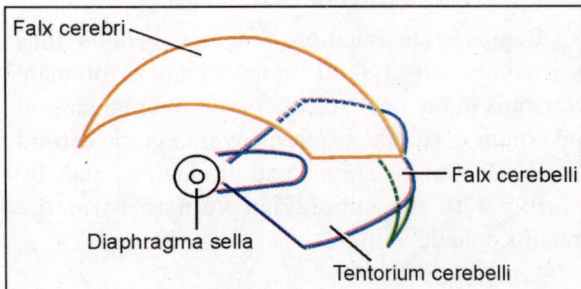

Fig. 5.50: Dural Folds

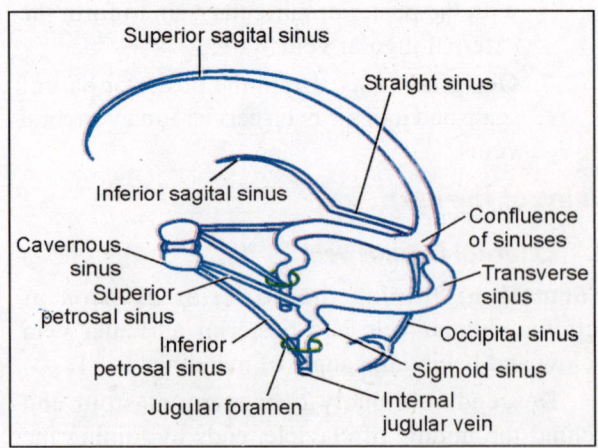

Fig. 5.51: Dural Venous Sinuses

Paired:

1. Cavernous sinus
2. Transverse sinus
3. Sigmoid sinus
4. Superior petrosal sinus
5. Inferior petrosal sinus
6. Sphenoparietal sinus

Unpaired:

1. Superior sagital sinus
2. Inferior sagital sinus
3. Straight sinus
4. Occipital sinus
5. Basilar plexus

Cavernous sinus: Seen on either side of body of sphenoid bone, lateral to the pituitary gland, about 2 cms long and 1 cm wide. Both sinuses are connected by 2 intercavernous sinuses.

Tributaries and connections of the cavernous sinus are shown in Fig:5.52.

Internal carotid artery and abducent nerve, 3rd, 4th, ophthalmic and maxillary nerves pass through the cavernous sinus separated from the blood by endothelium.

Fracture of the base of skull can involve the cavernous sinus and may result in an arteriovenous communication.

The cavity of cavernous sinus contains many fine fibrous trabeculae making it similar to a cavernous tissue. So blood flow is not smooth as in any other vein and hence chances of venous thrombosis are more.

Carvernous sinus is connected to veins outside the cranial cavity through emissary veins and through them any infection outside the skull can spread to cavernous sinus.

Transverse sinus: Seen along the transverse sulcus in the posterior cranial fossa, along the attached margin of tentorium cerebelli.

Sigmoid sinus: is the continuation of transverse sinus, lies in sigmoid sulcus and goes out of cranial cavity through jugular foramen, and becomes the internal jugular vein.

Superior petrosal sinus: is seen on the sharp upper border of petrous part of temporal bone, along

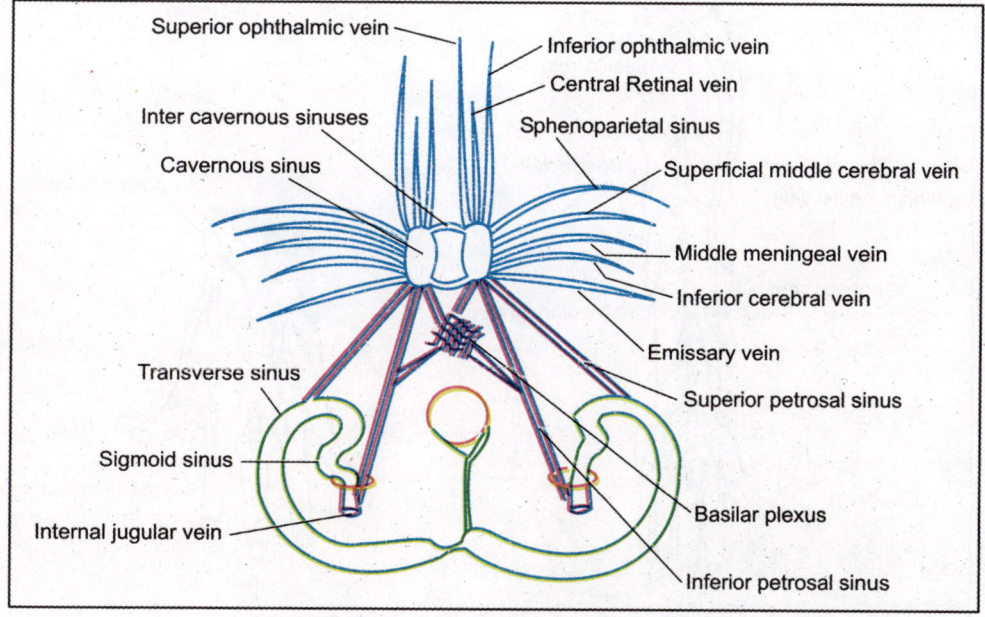

Fig. 5.52: Connections of Cavernous Sinus

the attached margin of tentorium cerebelli. It drains the cavernous sinus to transverse sinus.

Inferior petrosal sinus: is seen between the petrous part of temporal bone and occipital bone. Drains the cavernous sinus to internal jugular vein.

Sphenoparietal sinus: Seen along the posterior border of lesser wing of sphenoid.

Superior sagital sinus: Seen along the upper attached convex margin of falx cerebri and posteriorly continues as the transverse sinus of right side usually, or of left side.

Inferior sagital sinus: Seen along the free concave margin of falx cerebri, along its posterior 2/3rd.

Straight sinus: seen along the junction between posterior broad end of falx cerebri and upper surface of tentorium cerebelli. Formed by union of inferior sagital sinus and great cerebral vein. Posteriorly ends in the confluence of sinuses which is the dilated posterior end of superior sagital sinus, where transverse sinus also begins.

Occipital sinus: Seen along the attached margin of falx cerebelli, drains into confluence of sinuses.

Basilar plexus: Seen over basilar part of occipital bone; drains cavernous sinus to inferior petrosal sinus.

Blood from all these venous sinuses finally reach internal jugular vein.

VEINS OF UPPER LIMB

They are superficial and deep veins, both sets interconnected at certain regions. They have valves, permitting blood flow in the cephalic direction only.

Superficial veins (Fig. 5.53)

On the dorsum of hand, a dorsal venous plexus is seen which drains the digital veins from fingers and dorsal metacarpal veins from dorsum of hand.

Cephalic vein: From the radial end of the dorsal plexus, continues proximally crossing anatomical snuff box. It curves round the radial border of distal

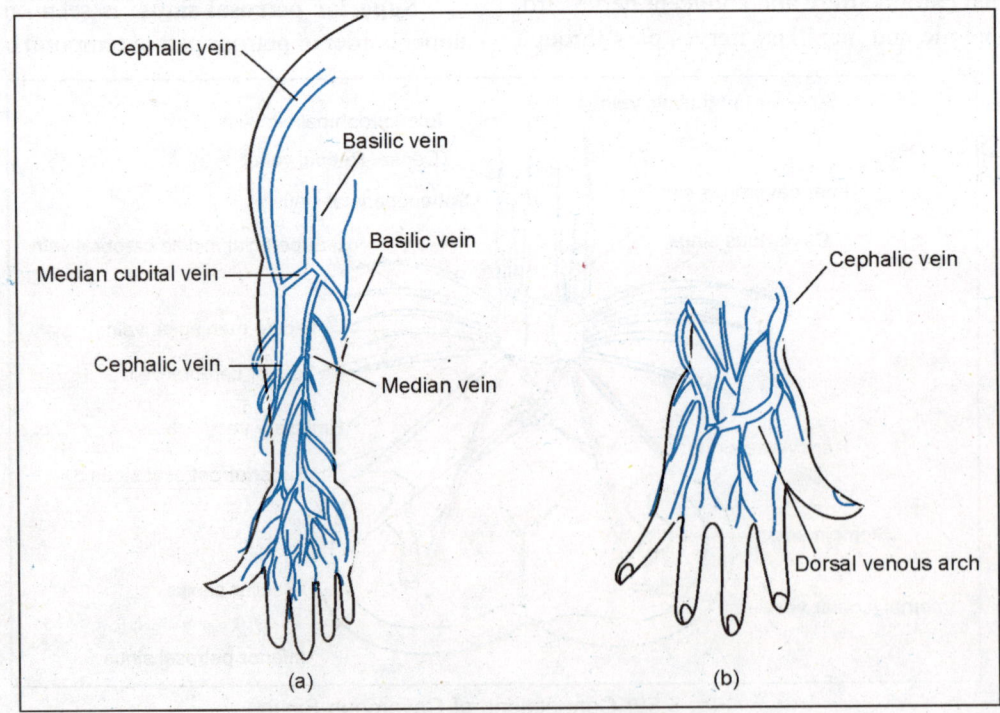

(a)   (b)

Fig. 5.53: Superficial Veins of Upper Limb

part of forearm and continues on the ventral surface, receiving neighbouring veins.

Basilic Vein: Continues from the medial end of dorsal plexus proximally. Nearing the elbow, it turns to ventral surface.

Just distal to the elbow, a median cubital vein connects cephalic vein to the basilic vein.

Cephalic vein ascends in front of elbow, through the lateral part of upper arm and above, it lies in the delto-pectoral groove. Basilic vein ascends in front of medial part of elbow and about the middle of upper arm, it pierces deep fascia and ascends in a deeper plane, to the lower border of teres major muscle. Here onwards, it continues as **axillary vein**, a deep vein of upper limb.

Cephalic vein continuing in the delto-pectoral groove, pierces the clavipectoral fascia below the clavicle and joins the axillary vein.

Median vein of forearm drains the superficial palmar veins and continues up in front of forearm to end in basilic vein or median cubital vein.

Applied Aspects

Median cubital vein or commencement of cephalic vein over anatomical snuff box are usually chosen for intravenous injections, transfusion or catheterisation.

Deep Veins

Deep veins form venae comitantes that accompany the arteries in pairs which are connected by short links.

From the hand, veins accompanying superficial and deep palmar arterial arches – Venus arches - join the veins accompanying radial and ulnar arteries.

They ascend in the forearm and above the elbow, ascend as paired brachial veins, with the brachial artery. At the wrist and elbow they are connected to the superficial veins.

Brachial veins ascend on either side of brachial artery and end in the axillary vein, at the lower border of subscapularis muscle.

Axillary vein

It is the continuation of basilic vein from the level of lower border of teres major. It continues medially and at the outer border of Ist rib, it continues as subclavian vein. Cephalic vein, brachial veins and veins corresponding to branches of axially artery, are its tributaries.

Subclavian vein

It is the continuation of axillary vein from the outer border of Ist rib and ends at the medial border of scalenus anterior muscle, behind medial end of clavicle, by joining with internal jugular vein to form the brachio cephalic vein. (Fig. 5.54)

VEINS OF THORAX

1. Brachiocephalic veins (Fig. 5.55)

Formed by the union of subclavian and internal jugular veins behind the sternal end of clavicle.

The right vein is shorter (2.5cms) runs almost vertically downwards to behind the sternal end of Ist right costal cartilage.

Left vein is longer (6 cms), runs obliquely downwards and to the right just behind upper 1/2 of manubrium sterni. Behind the sternal end of Ist right costal cartilage, joins with the right vein to form superior vena cava.

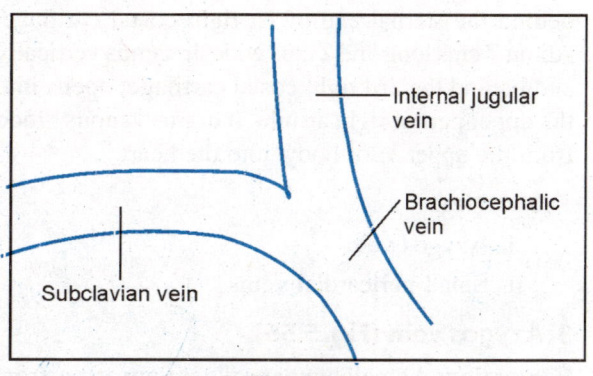

Fig. 5.54

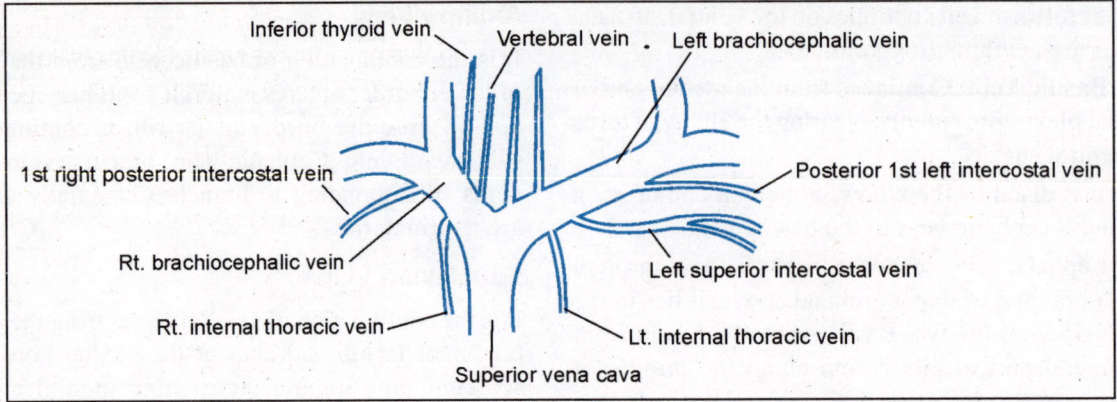

Fig. 5.55

Tributaries

Right brachiocephalic:

- Inferior thyroid vein
- Vertebral vein
- Internal thoracic vein
- Ist right posterior intercostal vein.

Left brachiocephalic:

- Inferior thyroid vein
- Vertebral vein
- Internal thoracic vein
- Ist left posterior intercostal vein
- Left superior intercostal vein.

2. Superior Vena Cava (SVC)

Formed by the union of the 2 brachiocephalic veins, behind the sternal end of Ist right costal cartilage. About 7 cms long and 2 cms wide descends vertically and behind the 3rd right costal cartilage, opens into the upper part of right atrium. It drains venous blood from the upper ½ of body, into the heart.

Tributaries:

- i. Axygos vein
- ii. Small pericardial veins

3. Azygos vein (Fig. 5.56)

Formation: A small lumbar azygos vein arises from the posterior aspect of inferior vena cava and ascends

behind it, in front of the upper lumbar vertebrae. Another vein is formed at the upper lumbar levels by the union of subcostal vein and ascending lumbar vein. Lumbar azygos vein is joined by this vein in front of T_{12} vertebra to form the azygos vein.

Course: It ascends to the thorax through the aortic opening of diaphragm. In close contact with the descending thoracic aorta and thoracic duct, it ascends in front of the lower 8 thoracic vertebrae in the posterior mediastinum.

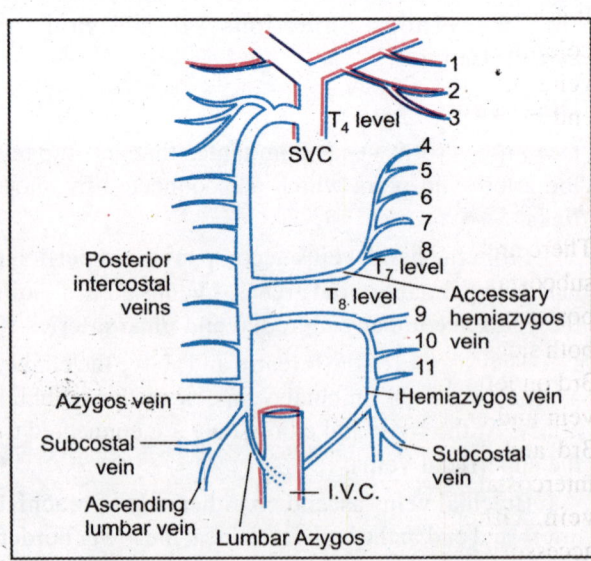

Fig. 5.56: Azygos Venous System

Termination: At the level of T_4 vertebra, it arches forwards above the hilum of right lung and opens into the superior vena cava.

Tributaries

1. Posterior right intercostal veins except, Ist
2. Hemiazygos vein
3. Accessary hemiazygos vein
4. Oesophageal veins
5. Mediastinal veins
6. Pericardial veins
7. Right bronchial veins

4. Hemiazygos Vein

Origin: On the left side, like the origin of azygos.

Course: Ascends to T_8 vertebral level, where it crosses to the right side, behind aorta, oesophages and thoracic duct and ends in azygos vein.

Tributaries:

1. Left lower 3 posterior intercostal veins.
2. A vein formed by union of left ascending lumbar and subcostal veins.

5. Accessory Hemiazygos vein

It is a vein that descends on the left side of vertebral column receiving 4th to 8th left posterior intercostal veins. Crosses the T_7 vertebra to the right side to end in azygos vein.

Left bronchial veins end in it.

6. Posterior intercostal veins

There are 11 pairs of intercostal veins and 1 pair of subcostal vein draining the venous blood from the posterior parts of intercostal spaces. The Ist ones on both sides empty into brachiocephalic veins. 2nd and 3rd on left side join to form left superior intercostal vein and ends in the left brachiocephalic vein. 2nd 3rd and 4th on right side form a right posterior intercostal vein and opens into the arch of azygose vein. Others join the azygos, hemiazygos and accessory hemiazygos as shown in the figure.

Anterior intercostal veins draining the anterior parts of intercostal spaces end in the internal thoracic vein.

7. Veins of vertebral column (Fig. 5.57)

They are:

(a) External vertebral venous plexuses:
- Anterior plexuses seen anterior to vertebral bodies.
- Posterior plexuses seen on posterior surfaces of vertebrae.

(b) Internal vertebral venous plexuses:
- Anterior and posterior plexuses, seen anteriorly and posteriorly in vertebral canal in the extra dural space.

(c) Basivertebral veins: Short, but wide channels, seen to emerge from the posterior surface of vertebral bodies and end in internal vertebral venous plexuses.

(d) Intervertebral veins: Seen to emerge through intervertebral foramina. They receive internal and external venous plexuses and end in vertebral, posterior intercostal, lumbar and lateral sacral veins.

Vertebral venous plexuses anastamose freely and they do not have valves.

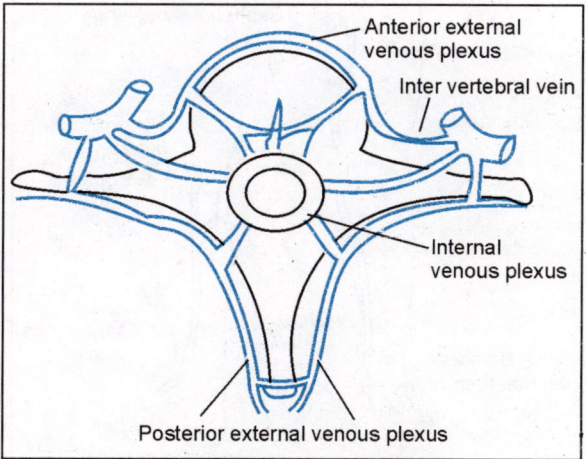

Fig. 5.57: Veins of Vertebra

VEINS OF LOWER LIMB

1. Superficial veins present in the superficial fascia.
2. Deep veins seen deep to deep fascia, accompanying major arteries.

All have valves.

Superficial veins (Fig. 5.58 a & b)

They are:

1. **Great Saphenous vein**
2. **Short (small) Saphenous vein**

On the dorsum of foot, there is a dorsal venous arch formed, receiving the digital and metatarsal veins. On the medial and lateral borders of the foot, medial and lateral marginal veins, draining the veins of sole, join the dorsal venous arch, at its medial and lateral ends.

1. Great Saphenous Vein

It begins as upward continuation of dorsal venous arch, in front of medial malleolus.

It ascends accompanied by saphenous nerve, on the medial aspect of leg. It passes behind the medial

side of knee and then recurves to the front of medial side of thigh and ascends in the thigh. It passes through the saphenous opening in the deep fascia of thigh and ends in the femoral vein. This point is about 3 cms inferolateral to the pubic tubercle. Behind the knee, it is connected to small saphenous vein.

It has about 10-20 valves in it, and is connected to deep veins by means of perforating veins, plenty in the leg.

Along its course it receives tributaries from the front of leg and from the thigh. The main named tributaries are superficial external pudental, superficial epigastric, superficial circumflex ileac and deep external pudental veins.

2. Small (Short) Saphenous vein

Begins as a continuation of lateral marginal vein, joined with the lateral end of dorsal venous arch. Ascends behind the lateral malleolus, accompanied by sural nerve. It runs up in the middle of back of leg and about 5 cm above the knee joint, ends in the popliteal vein. It also has numerous valves.

It gets tributaries from the back of leg and communicating veins to great saphenous veins and deep veins.

Deep Veins of lower limb

1. **Anterior tibial veins:** Accompany anterior tibial artery.
2. **Posterior tibial veins:** Accompany posterior tibial artery.
3. **Popliteal vein:** Formed by the union of anterior tibial and posterior tibial veins. Ascends behind the knee and passes through the opening in the adductor magnus to become femoral vein.
4. **Femoral Vein:**

Begins as continuation of popliteal vein through adductor hiatus and ascends in the adductor canal accompanied by femoral artery. Passes in the upper part of front of thigh, inside the femoral sheath and behind the inguinal ligament, continues as the

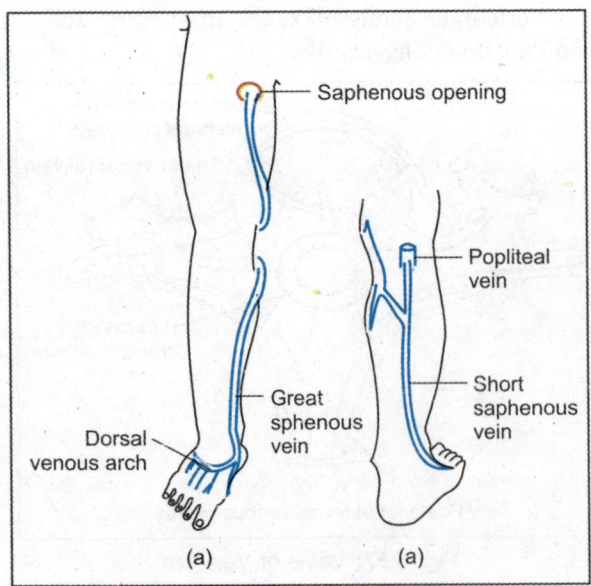

Fig. 5.58: Superficial Veins of lower Limb

external iliac vein. Profunda femoris vein and great saphenous vein are its large tributaries.

Applied anatomy (Fig. 5.59)

There are perforating veins connecting the superficial and deep veins in the leg, and they have valves preventing blood flow from deep to superficial veins.

Venous return from the lower limb depends mostly on the contraction of the calf muscles – 'Calf pump'. During the contraction of calf muscles, blood is pumped towards heart, through deep veins, but does not flow to the superficial veins due to the valves in perforating veins. When muscles relax, blood from superficial veins is partially drained into the deep veins through perforating veins. If the valves of perforating veins become incompetent, blood from deep veins flow to superficial veins which become dilated – varicose veins.

VEINS OF ABDOMEN AND PELVIS

IN THE PELVIS

1. External iliac vein

It is the upward continuation of femoral vein from behind the inguinal ligament. Ascends along the pelvic brim and in front of sacroiliac joint, joins with internal iliac vein to form the common iliac vein. Its major tributaries are inferior epigastric vein and deep circumflex iliac vein.

2. Internal iliac vein

It is formed by joining of all the veins that correspond to the branches of internal iliac artery.

3. Common iliac vein

Formed by the union of external and internal iliac veins in front of the sacroiliac joint. Iliolumbar vein, and lateral sacral veins empty into it. Both common iliac veins join to form inferior vena cava in front of L_5, vertebra, slightly to the right side.

IN THE ABDOMEN

1. Inferior Vena Cava (I.V.C)

Formed by the union of the 2 common iliac veins in front of the L_5 vertebra. Ascends in front of vertebral column, on the right side of Aorta. Pierces the central tendon of diaphragm at level with T_8 vertebra and opens into the posteroinferior part of right atrium, where it is guarded by valve of I.V.C. It conveys major part of the venous blood from structures below diaphragm to the right atrium. Along its course, it has no valves.

Tributaries (Fig. 5.60)

1. *Lumbar veins:* 4 pairs. They are interconnected among them.

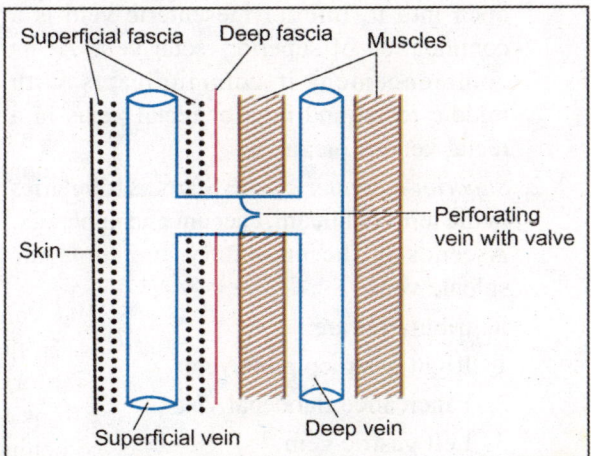

Fig. 5.59

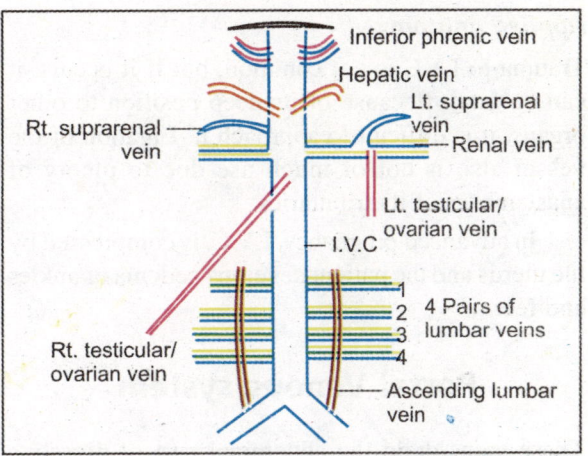

Fig. 5.60

2. *Ascending lumbar vein:* Below it is connected to the common iliac and internal iliac veins. Ascends interconnecting the lumbar veins. It is joined by the subcostal vein. The vein thus formed, joins the small lumbar azygos vein in front of T_{12} vertebra to form the azygos vein on the right and hemiazygos vein on the left side.

3. *Testicular veins (in male):* Begin in the testis and epididymis as pampiniform plexus and pass through the spermatic cord and reach the abdomen through deep inguinal ring. The right testicular vein directly opens into the inferior vena cava and the left one, into the left renal vein.

4. *Ovarian veins (in female):* Begin as a plexus near ovary and tube in the broad ligament and end as the testicular veins do.

5. *Renal veins:* Left renal vein, about 7.5cms long and right one, about 2.5 cms long.

6. *Suprarenal veins:* Right one ends directly in superior vena cava and left one, in left renal vein.

7. *Inferior phrenic veins:* From inferior surface of diaphragm

8. *Hepatic veins:* They empty into inferior vena cava as it passes grooving the posterior surface of liver.

Applied anatomy

Trauma to I.V.C is not common, but if it occurs, it can be fatal. Because of its deep position to other organs, it is difficult to approach it. Ligation of the vessel also is not of much use due to plenty of anastamoses of its tributaries.

In advanced pregnancy, I.V.C. is compressed by the uterus and the patient develops oedema of ankles and feet.

Portal Venous system

These veins drain the abdominal part of digestive tract except lower end of anal canal, and also the spleen, pancreas and gall bladder. Portal vein and tributaries do not have valves.

Portal Vein (Fig. 5.61)

It is formed by the union of splenic and superior mesenteric veins, behind the neck of pancreas, in front of I.V.C. at level with L_2 vertebra; about 8 cms long. It ascends to the right, behind the Ist part of duodenum and enters the lesser omentum to lie in the anterior border of epiploeic foramen. Here it is accompanied by bile duct and hepatic artery. Reaches the right end of porta hepatis and divides into right and left divisions.

Portal venous tributaries begin as capillaries like an artery, and join to form larger vein. In the liver, again it branches and ramify as the capillaries of an artery, which end in sinusoids. From the sinusoids, hepatic veins are formed which end in I.V.C.

Hence portal circulation begins as capillaries and ends as capillaries.

Tributaries

1. *Splenic vein:* Comes from the hilum of spleen, passes through leinorenal ligament with the splenic artery. Joins with superior mesenteric vein to form portal vein. Short gastric veins, left gastroepiploeic vein, inferior mesenteric vein and pancreatic veins open into it. Inferior mesenteric vein is a continuation of superior rectal vein. At its commencement it communicates with middle rectal and inferior rectal veins in a rectal venous plexus.

2. *Superior mesenteric vein:* Starts as tributaries in the terminal ileum, caecum and appendix. Ascends in the mesentery and joins the splenic vein.

    Its tributaries are:

    1. Right gastroepiploic vein
    2. Pancreatico duodenal veins
    3. Left gastric vein
    4. Right gastric vein

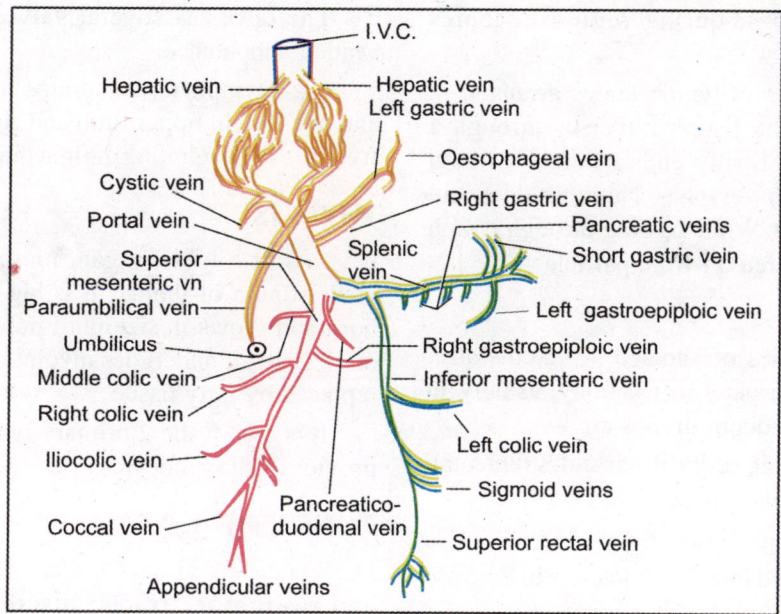

Fig. 5.61: Portal Venous System

5. Para umbilical veins - Start from the anterior abdominal wall and run in the falciform ligament. Largest of them ends in the left branch of portal vein.

6. Cystic veins – from gall bladder.

Applied anatomy

Certain conditions like cirrhosis of liver, tumours of liver, carcinoma of the head of pancreas or enlarged lymph nodes in the lesser omentum – can compress the portal vein. Obstruction to portal vein can cause ascites.

In portal obstruction, regions where there are anastamoses between portal and systemic veins, establish a collateral circulation (porto systemic anastamosis). The small venous channels enlarge and become varicose, at sites of portosystemic anastamosis.

Such sites are:

1. Lower end of Oesophagus.
2. Wall of rectum and anal canal.
3. Para umbilical veins.

LYMPHATIC SYSTEM

It is associated with cardio vascular system. It consists of lymphoid tissues or organs and lymphatic vessels.

Lymphoid tissue has large collections of lymphocytes and are thymus, lymph node, spleen, tonsil, and Peyer's patches of small intestine. Lymph nodes are associated with lymph vessels which carry tissue fluid (lymph) from tissue spaces.

Lymphocytes are involved in the defensive mechanism of body by producing antibodies against antigens. Precursors of lymphocytes are present in bone marrow and reach the thymus where they mature into lymphocytes and pass into other sites.

Lymph in the lymphatics is a clear fluid. Lymphatics remove unwanted materials as cell debris, foreign particles etc. from tissue spaces. They begin as blind ended thin walled capillaries. They are permiable to larger particles as micro organisms. They join to form larger vessels and traverse through groups of lymph nodes. If the lymphatics get obstructed, the neighbouring region becomes oedematous.

There are groups of lymph nodes arranged in different regions. The lymph traverses through a series of nodes and finally ends in venous blood through large lymph vessels - Thoracic duct and Right lymphatic duct. While passing through lymph nodes, lymph is filtered off from particles.

Lymph nodes

They are small bodies of about 0.1 – 2.cms size, arranged in different parts of the body, usually in groups. Some of the major groups are –

1. Submandibular, cervical, parotid, submental, supraclavicular – in head and neck.
2. Axillary groups – in axilla.
3. Intercostal and internal thoracic – in thoracic wall.
4. Mediastinal, tracheobronchial - in thorax.
5. Para aortic, hepatic, coeliac, mesenteric, gastric, internal and external iliac – in abdomen and pelvis.
6. Superficial and deep inguinal – in the inguinal region.

Lymphatics are absent in CNS, eye ball, internal ear, cartilage, bone and epidermis.

THORACIC DUCT

It begins as the continuation of an elongated and dilated lymph sac, the cisterna chyli, that lies in front of L_1 and L_2 vertebrae. It ascends to the thorax passing through the aotic opening of diaphragm, on the right side of aorta. In the posterior mediastinum of thorax, it turns to left side at level with T_4 vertebra. Again it ascends and reaches root of neck. At level with transverse process of C_7 vertebra, it turns downwards to end in the beginning of left brachiocephalic vein – at junction of left subclavian and left internal jugular veins.

It drains lymph from the lower limbs, abdomen and pelvis, left side of thorax, left upper limb and left side of head and neck.

The duct has several valves which give it a beaded appearance.

Right lymphatic duct drains the right side of head and neck, right upper limb and right side of thorax. It ends in the beginning of right brachiocephalic vein.

THYMUS

It is a soft bilobed organ, present in the anterior mediastinum of thorax. It is big in infant and new born and grows in size until puberty. After the age of 15 years, it undergoes involution and is gradually replaced by fatty tissue.

It is one of the 2 primary lymphoid organs and provides T lymphocytes.

TONSILS (Fig. 5.62)

In the mucosa around the openings into digestive and respiratory tracts, discrete collections of lymphoid tissue are seen, somewhat in a ring like arrangement – (Waldeyer's ring). They include lingual tonsil, palatine tonsil, tubal tonsil and pharyngeal tonsil. Lymphocytes from these tissues are involved in local mucosal defence and immune activities.

Lingual tonsil: Small lymphoid nodules in the mucosa of posterior 1/3 rd of tongue.

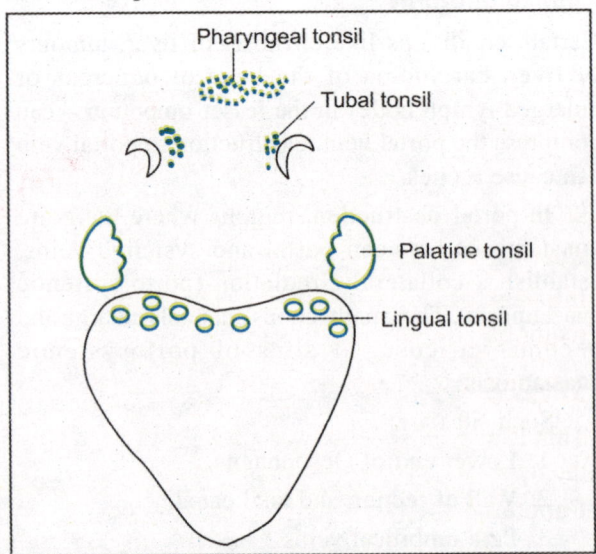

Fig. 5.62: Waldeyer's Ring of Tonsils.

Tubal tonsil: in the lateral wall of nasopharynx, behind the opening of auditory tube, as a small collection of lymphoid tissue.

Pharyngeal tonsil: In the roof of nasopharynx.

Palatine tonsil

It is the largest of the members of Waldeyer's ring.

It is an almond shaped mass of lymphoid tissue on either side of the lateral wall of oropharynx. Situated in a depression called tonsillar sinus, bounded by palatopharyngeal fold behind and palatoglossal fold in front. It has maximum size in children and later diminishes in size.

Covered on its medial surface by mucosa having stratified squamous epithelium. This surface presents deep grooves – tonsillar crypts.

Its lateral surface is covered by a fibrous capsule deep to which the para tonsillar vein descends.

Above, it reaches soft palate and below, posterior part of tongue.

Palatine tonsil contains collections of lymphoid tissue that produce lymphocytes.

Blood Supply

Main artery is tonsillar artery. It also gets branches from lingual, ascending palatine, ascending pharyngeal and greater palatine arteries. Venous drainage is through paratonsillar vein which ends in facial vein.

Lymphatic drainage

Into jugulo digastric nodes of upper deep cervical group of lymph nodes.

Applied anatomy

Inflamation leads to tonsilitis. Recurrent episodes require tonsillectomy.

SPLEEN (Fig. 5.63)

This is a lymphoid and vascular organ, situated in the upper left part of abdomen posteriorly.

Functions:

1. Phagocytosis
2. Immune responses and defensive activities.

3. In human foetus, a site of haemopoeisis.

Its shape varies with its relation to neighbouring organs – roughly a curved wedge. About 12 cms long, 7cms broad and 3-4 cms thick. Lies against 9th, 10th and 11th ribs and its long axis is along 10th rib.

Spleen has a diaphragmatic surface, related to diaphragm, visceral surface related to various organs. On the visceral surface, a linear groove is seen – hilum. It has an upper border and lower border and posterior and anterior ends. Posterior end is about 4 cms. lateral to the posterior midline of the body at level with T_{10} vertebral spine. Anterior end is broader, directed anteriorly and downwards.

Spleen is completely covered with peritoneum and two major peritoneal folds connect it with kidney and stomach – lienorenal ligemant and gastrosplenic ligament.

Blood supply

Spleen is supplied by splenic artery, a branch of coeliac trunk. Splenic vien ends in portal vein.

Applied Anatomy

1. Enlargement of spleen – splenomegaly – occurs in certain diseases as malaria and other haemolitic diseases. Then spleen becomes palpable per abdomen.
2. Splenectomy is done in certain conditions. Spleen is not essential for survival, but immune responses of the individual reduces after that.

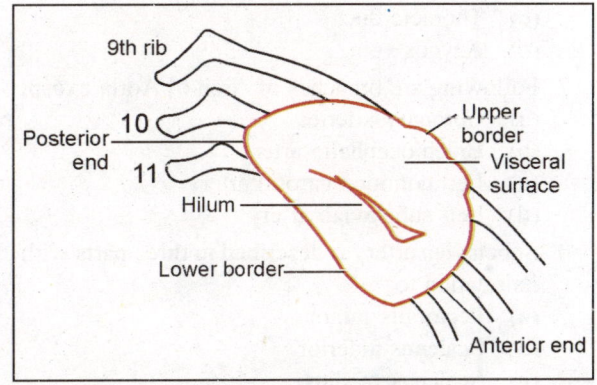

Fig. 5.63: Spleen

Single Best Response M.C.Qs

1. Heart is situated in the
   (a) Superior mediastinum
   (b) Anterior mediastinum
   (c) Middle mediastinum
   (d) Posterior mediastinum

2. Following Anatomical events occur at lower border of T_4 vertebra except.
   (a) Separation between superior and inferior mediastina
   (b) Sternal angle
   (c) Bronchi enter the lungs
   (d) Arch of aorta begins and ends

3. In the heart, mitral valve guards
   (a) Right atrioventricular orifice
   (b) Left atrioventricular orifice
   (c) Aortic orifice
   (d) Pulmonary orifice

4. Musculae pectinati is found in
   (a) Right atrium
   (b) Left atrium
   (c) Right ventricle
   (d) Left Ventricle

5. Following are correct about coronary sinus except
   (a) It lies in posterior part of coronary sulcus.
   (b) It is a continuation of great cardiac vein.
   (c) Anterior cardiac veins open into it.
   (d) It opens into right atrium

6. Structure that is not related to Arch of Aorta is
   (a) Left superior intercostal vein
   (b) Left phrenic nerve
   (c) Thoracic duct
   (d) Azygos vein

7. Following are branches of Arch of Aorta except
   (a) Coronary arteries
   (b) Brachiocephalic artery
   (c) Left common carotid artery
   (d) Left subclavian artery

8. Subclavian artery is described in three parts with its relation to
   (a) Pectoralis minor
   (b) Scalenus anterior
   (c) Scalenus medius
   (d) Scalenus posterior

9. Following are correct about vertebral artery except.
   (a) It arises from Ist part of subclavian artery.
   (b) It ascends through foramen transversaria of all cervical vertebrae
   (c) It lies over posterior arch of atlas.
   (d) Inside cranium, it joins with the artery of opposite side to form basilar artery.

10. Following are correct about radial artery except.
    (a) It begins from brachial artery at the level of neck of radius.
    (b) It is direct continuation of brachial artery.
    (c) At lower end of forearm it is lateral to tendon of flexor carpi radialis.
    (d) In the palm, it ends by forming superficial palmar arch.

11. Following are branches of facial artery except.
    (a) Ascending pharyngeal
    (b) Glandular
    (c) Tonsillar
    (d) Submental

12. Middle meningeal artery is a branch of
    (a) External carotid artery
    (b) Internal carotid artery
    (c) Maxillary artery
    (d) Superficial temporal artery

13. Following are branches of internal carotid artery except.
    (a) Anterior cerebral artery
    (b) Middle cerebral artery
    (c) Posterior communicating artery
    (d) Anterior communicating artery

14. Artery that is not a direct branch of coeliac trunk is
    (a) Left gastric
    (b) Right gastric
    (c) Common hepatic
    (d) Splenic

15. Following statements are correct about femoral sheath except.
    (a) Its anterior layer is formed by fascia iliaca

(b) Its posterior layer is formed by fascia transversalis.

(c) It covers femoral artery, vein and nerve.

(d) Its medial compartment is femoral canal.

16. Dorsalis pedis artery is the continuation of
    (a) Anterior tibial artery
    (b) Posterior tibial artery
    (c) Peroneal artery
    (d) Saphenous artery.

17. Venous sinus that is not related to Falx cerebri is.
    (a) Superior sagital sinus
    (b) Inferior sagital sinus
    (c) Transverse sinus
    (d) Straight sinus.

18. Inferior petrosal sinus drains cavernous sinus into
    (a) Transverse sinus
    (b) Sigmoid sinus
    (c) Occipital sinus
    (d) Internal jugular vein.

19. Axillary vein is the continuation of
    (a) Cephalic vein
    (b) Basilic vein
    (c) Median cubital vein
    (d) Median vein of forearm.

20. Azygos vein empties into
    (a) Superior vena cava
    (b) Inferior vena cava
    (c) Right brachiocephalic vein
    (d) Hemiazygos vein.

M.C.Qs - Answers

1. (c), 2. (c), 3. (b), 4. (a), 5. (c), 6. (d), 7. (a), 8. (b), 9. (b), 10. (d), 11. (a), 12. (c), 13. (d), 14. (b), 15. (c), 16. (a), 17. (c), 18. (d), 19. (b), 20. (a)

Essays

I. Describe external features of heart and the right atrium of heart.

II. Describe the ventricles of heart

III. Describe the blood supply of heart. Discuss its clinical importance

IV. Describe the extent, relations and branches of arch of aorta.

V. Describe the axillary artery and branches.

VI. Describe the external carotid artery and its branches.

VII. Describe the femoral artery and its branches.

VIII. Classify dural venous sinuses and describe cavernous sinus in detail.

IX. Describe the Azygos vein and its tributaries.

X. Describe the portal vein.

Short notes

1. Coronary sinus
2. Conducting system of heart
3. Pericardium
4. Vertebral artery
5. Palmar arterial arches.
6. Facial artery
7. Facial vein
8. Great saphenous vein
9. Venous drainage of lower limb
10. Dorsalis pedis artery
11. Profunda femoris artery
12. Femoral sheath
13. Portosystemic anastamosis
14. Thoracic duct
15. Spleen.

6 Respiratory System

PARTS

1. External nose
2. Nasal Cavity and Paranasal air sinuses
3. Larynx
4. Trachea
5. Bronchi
6. Lungs

EXTERNAL NOSE

The framework of external nose is formed of the nasal bones, frontal processes of maxillae, nasal part of frontal bone, nasal cartilages and septal cartilage.

The external opening of nose is nostril or anterior nares, bounded laterally by ala of nose.

NASAL CAVITY (Fig. 6.1)

A single cavity of nose is divided into right and left nasal cavities by a median nasal septum. Each cavity is about 5 cms in height, 5 to 7 cms deep and 1.5 cms transversely below and 2 mm transversely above. Anteriorly each cavity opens to exterior by anterior nares and posteriorly by posterior nares into nasopharynx.

Skeleton of nasal cavity

Lateral wall (Fig. 62.a,b)

Lateral wall of each cavity is formed of mainly by medial surface of maxilla, labyrinth of ethmoid above and perpendicular plate of palatine bone behind.(Fg: 6.2 b.) From the ethmoid, 2 curved shelves project into to the cavity - superior and middle conchae. A separate bone, inferior concha articulates with part of maxilla.

Septum (medial wall): (Fig. 6.3)

It is formed by vomer, perpendicular plate of ethmoid and septal cartilage. Also along their edges, there are contributions from nasal, frontal, maxilla, palatine bone and sphenoid.

Floor

Formed by hard palate - Anterior 3/4th by palatine processes of maxillae and posterior 1/4th byhorizontal plates of palatine bones.

Roof (Fig. 6.4)

It is very narrow. Anteroposteriorly formed by nasal bone and frontal bone form the anterior sloping

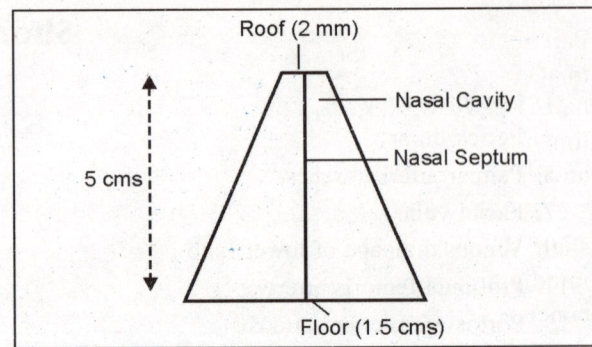

Fig. 6.1: Nasal Cavity - Dimensions

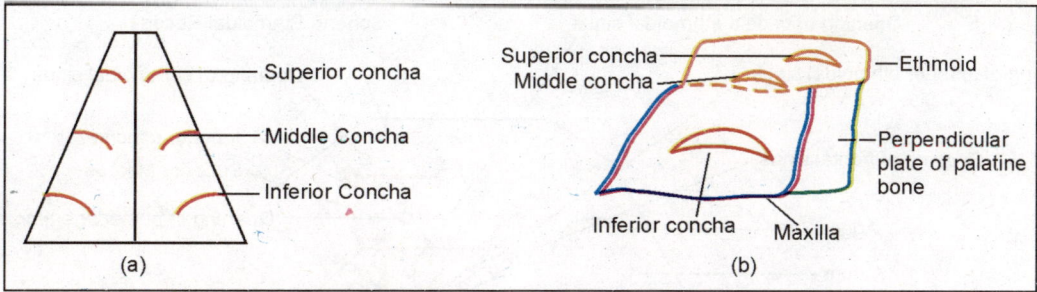

Fig. 6.2: (a) Nasal Cavities (b) Lateral Wall-Bony Framework

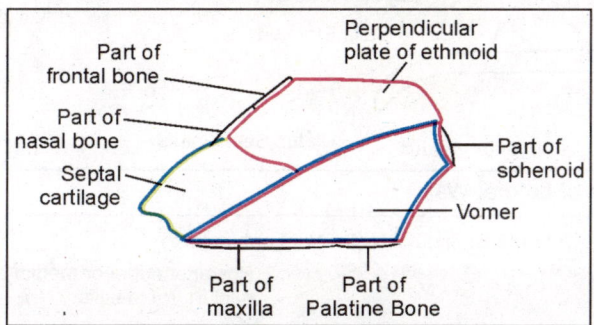

Fig. 6.3: Septum-Constituent Parts

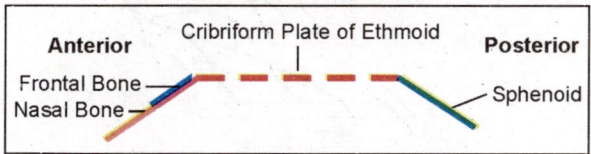

Fig. 6.4: Roof-Constituent Parts

part. Middle horizontal part formed by cribriform plate of ethmoid and posterior sloping part by body of sphenoid.

Features of lateral wall of nasal cavity (Fig. 6.5)

Part of lateral wall just above the anterior nares, deep to ala of nose is called vestibule, lined by skin with hair. Vestibule is limited above by a curved line, limen nasi. Above the vestibule, a more depressed area is seen - atrium, limited above by agger nasi.

Behind these, the lateral wall shows 3 curved shelf like projections into the cavity - superior, middle and inferior conchae. Spaces below these conchae are superior, middle and inferior meatuses. A small space above and behind superior concha is sphenoethmoidal recess.

Structures opening into nasal cavity through the lateral wall:

Into sphenoethmoidal recess, sphenoidal air sinus opens. Into superior meatus, posterior ethmoidal sinus opens. Middle meatus shows a rounded elevation, bulla ethmoidalis produced by middle ethmoidal sinus, which opens into the surface of bulla. Below the bulla, there is a curved groove, hiatus semilunaris. Into it opens the maxillary air sinus, anterior ethmoidal sinus and frontal sinus. Anterior part of inferior meatus receives the opening of nasolacrimal duct.

Nerve supply and blood supply

See diagrams (Fig. 6.6 a,b and 6.7 a,b)

Venous drainage of nasal cavity is into maxillary vein, ophthalmic vein and facial vein.

PARANASAL AIR SINUSES

They are air filled spaces present in the bones surrounding nasal cavity and are lined by mucous membrane, continuous with that of nasal cavity. All of them open through lateral wall into nasal cavity by small openings. Their function is to give resonance to voice and to lighten the bones. They are absent at birth and grow during childhood upto puberty.

The sinuses are

Frontal - Right and left

Ethmoidal - Anterior, middle and posterior group on either side.

Sphenoidal - Right and left

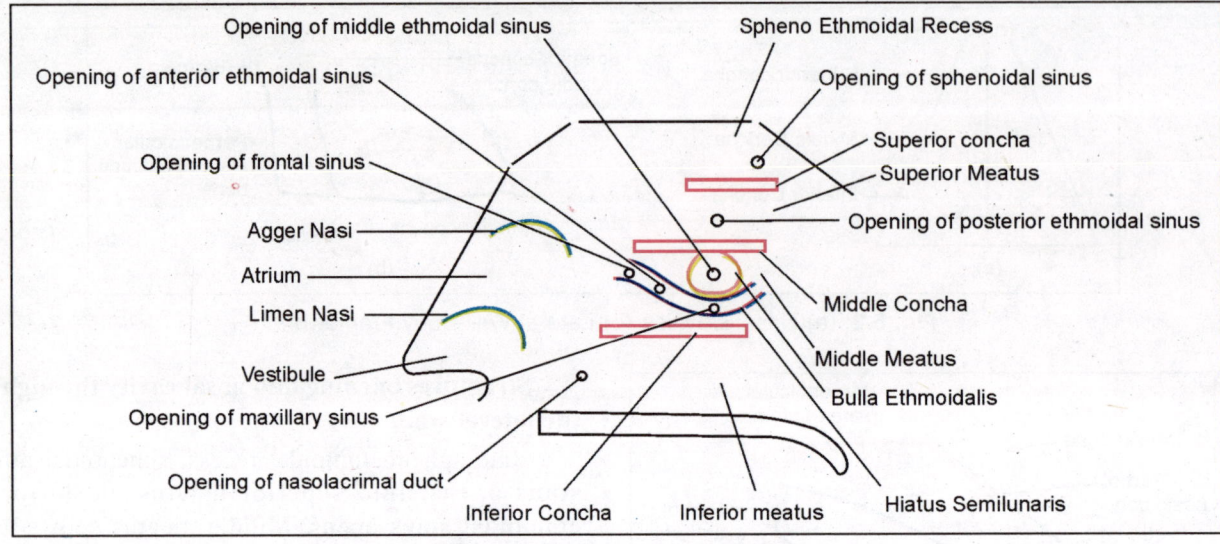

Fig. 6.5: Features of Lateral Wall

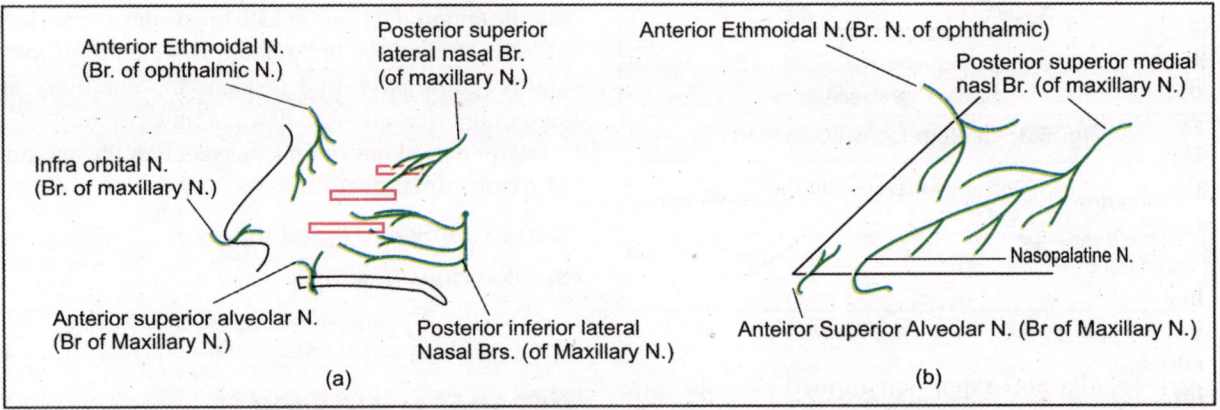

Fig. 6.6: (a) Sensory Nerve Supply-Lateral Wall (b) Sensory Nerve Supply-Medial Wall

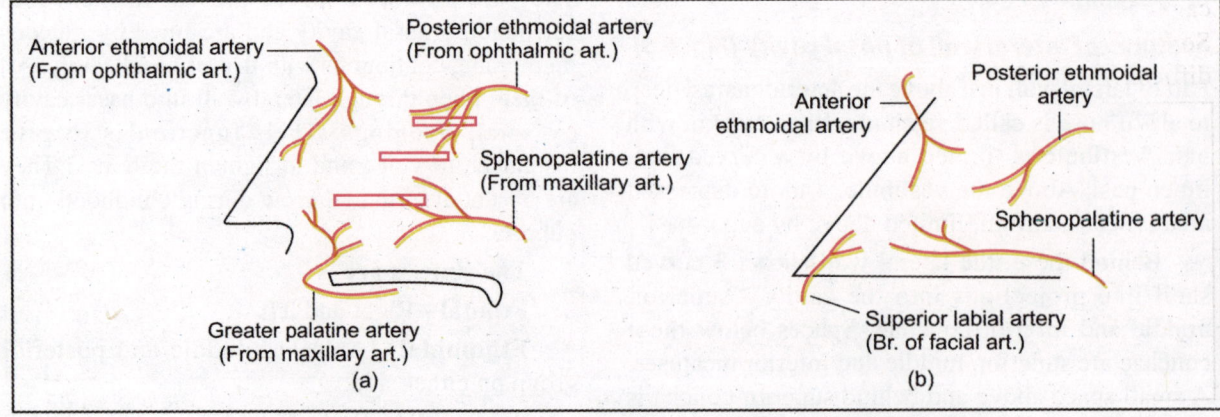

Fig. 6.7: (a) Arteries of Lateral Wall (b) Arteries of Medial Wall

Maxillary - Right and left

Frontal Sinus

In the anteroinferior parts of frontal bone. They open into upper end of hiatus semilunaris.

Ethmodial Sinus

Present in the labyrinth of ethmoid, 3 large and about 18 small ones, on each side, between the upper part of nasal cavity and orbit. Open into superior and middle meatuses.

Sphenoidal Sinus

In the body of sphenoid. Opens into sphenoethmodial recess.

Maxillary sinus

Largest of the sinuses, present in the body of maxilla, it opens into the hiatus semilunaris of middle meatus. It has pyramidal shape with base at the lateral wall of nasal cavity. Apex directed laterally-into the zygomatic process of maxilla and roof is orbital floor. Its floor is maxilla's alveolar processes. Roots of first 2 molars and sometimes of premolars project into the floor.

The opening of maxillary sinus: Maxillary hiatus is very large in size but in articulated skeleton, in life, it is reduced in size by- uncinate process of ethomoid bone, perpendicular plate of palatine bone, inferior nasal concha and descending process of lacrimal bone. The opening of this hiatus into nasal cavity is at a higher level than the floor of the sinus. So natural drainage of any accumulated fluid is difficult. Infection into sinuses (Sinusitis) is usually by spread from nasal cavity. But maxillary sinusitis can be by spread from infected roots of teeth also.

Chronic infection of maxillry sinus requires aspiration through inferior meatus.

Nerves and vessels of the sinuses extend from nasal cavities.

LARYNX (Fig. 6.19)

Larynx is not only an organ of respiration but also of phonation.

Formation

Frame work of larynx is made of cartilages connected together by ligaments and membranes. A number of muscles are attached to the cartilages. Interior of larynx is lined by mucous membrane.

Cartilages

3 Unpaired - Thyroid, Cricoid and Epiglottic.

3 Paired - Arytenoid, Corniculate and Cuneiform.

Thyroid Cartilage (Fig. 6.8)

It is the largest of all. Formed of hyaline cartilage, has two laminae which meet at the anterior angle which is 90° in males and 120° in females (Fig. 6.8). This angulation makes the laryngeal prominence. From its free posterior border superior cornu projects upwards and inferior cornu projects downwards. Oblique line on the lamina gives attachment to many muscles.

Cricoid Cartilage (Fig. 6.9)

Also of hyaline type, is ring shaped, posterior part of which is a broad lamina. The two arytenoid

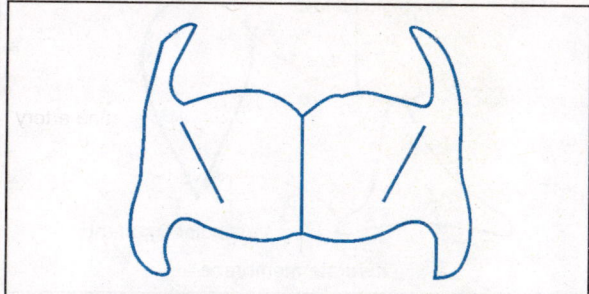

Fig. 6.8: Thyroid Cartilage

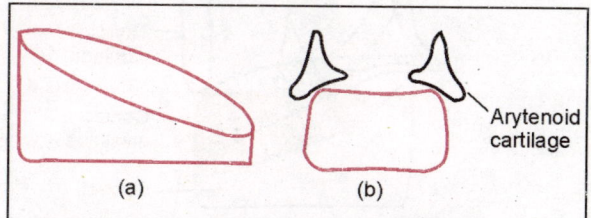

Fig. 6.9: (a) Cricoid Cartilage–Lateral View (b) Cricoid Cartilage–Posterior View

cartilages articulate with the upper border of posterior lamina of cricoid cartilage.

Epiglottic Cartilage (Fig 6.10)

A leaf shaped elastic cartilage, attached to the inner aspect of angle of thyroid cartilage. Situated behind the root of tongue.

Arytenoid Cartilages (Fig. 6.11)

Roughly pyramidal in shape, articulated at the upper broder of cricoid lamina. At its apex, corniculate cartilage is placed. from the base, a vocal process projects anteriorly and muscular process projects laterally.

Corniculate Cartilage (Fig. 6.11)

A small conical cartilage at the apex of arytenoid cartilage. A fold of mucous membrane, aryepiglottic fold passes from arytenoid cartilage to side of epiglottic cartilage. Corniculate is seen in the posterior end of the fold.

Cuneiform Cartilage (Fig : 6.11)

A small rod shaped cartilage, in the aryepiglottic fold, near the cuneiform.

Ligaments and Membranes

Extrinsic ligaments

1. Thyrohyoid membrane - from upper border of thyroid cartilage to upper border of hyoid bone.
2. Cricotracheal ligament - from lower border of cricoid cartilage to 1st tracheal ring.
3. Hyoepiglottic ligament - from anierior suface of epiglottis to hyoid bone.

Intrinsic ligaments

1. **Cricothyroid membrane** (Cricovocal membrane) (Fig. 6.12). Below, attached to the upper margin of ring of cricoid cartilage. Above, its anterior end only is attached to the inner surface of the lower part of angle of thyroid cartilage. Behind that it forms a thick free border, the vocal ligament, the posterior end of which is attached to the vocal process of arytenoid cartilage. Its thickend median part is conus elasticus.

2. **Quadrate membrane** (Fig : 6.13): A thin membrane that stretches from the margin of arytenoid cartilage to the margin of epiglottic

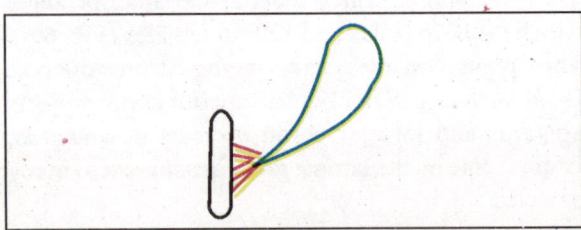

Fig. 6.10: Epiglottic Cartilage

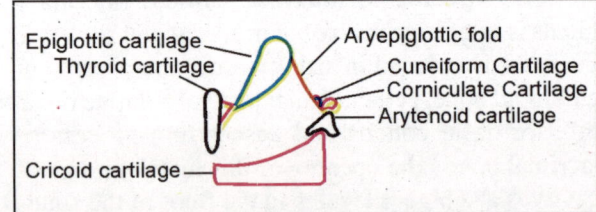

Fig. 6.11: Laryngeal Cartilages-Articulated

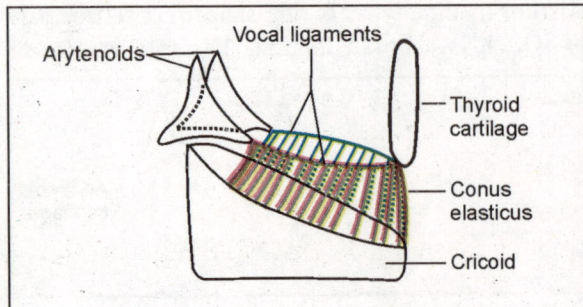

Fig. 6.12: Cricothyroid Membrane

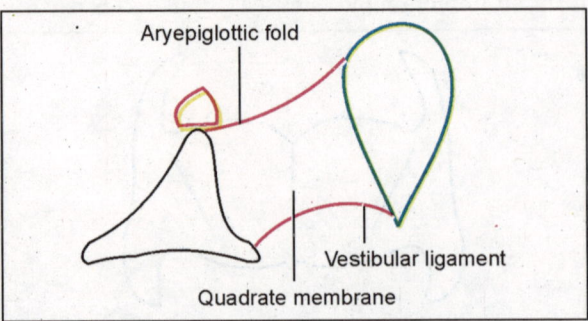

Fig. 6.13: Quadrate Membrane

cartilage. Its lower free border forms the vestibular ligament and upper border, aryepiglottic fold.

3. **Thyroepiglottic ligament** (Fig. 6.14)

Connects lower end of epiglottis to inner surface of thyroid angle.

Interior of larynx

Larynx opens above into laryngopharynx through the inlet.

Inlet (Fig. 6.15)

Bounded by upper margin of epliglottis, two aryepiglottic folds and posteriorly interarytenoid fold.

The cavity of larynx extends from the inlet, down to the lower border of cricoid cartilage, where it becomes continuous with trachea. (Fig. 6.16)

Two pairs of mucosal folds pfoject into the cavity from the lateral walls. Upper is the vestibular folds that overlie vestibular ligaments and lower is vocal folds that overlie vocal ligaments.

The cavity of larynx is thus divisible into-

1. Vestibule-Part above vestibular folds.
2. Sinus (Ventricle)-small part between vestibular and vocal folds.
3. Space between the 2 vestibular folds is called rima vestibuli.
4. Space between the 2 vocal folds is rima glottidis or glottis.
5. Infraglottic Part - Below the vocal folds.

A pouch Extends up from the side of sinus, deep to thyroid lamina-the saccule. It contains mucous glands whose secretion lubricates the vocal folds.

Vocal Folds (Vocal Cords) (Fig. 6.17)

Extend from the inner surface of angle of thyroid

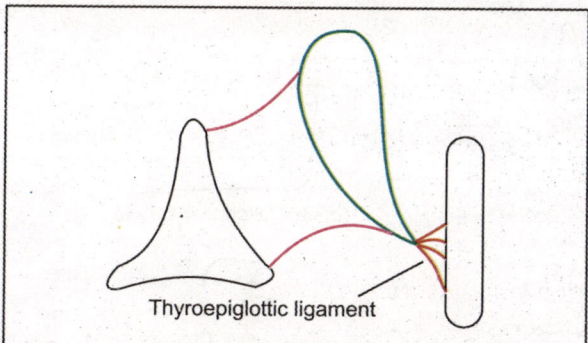

Fig. 6.14

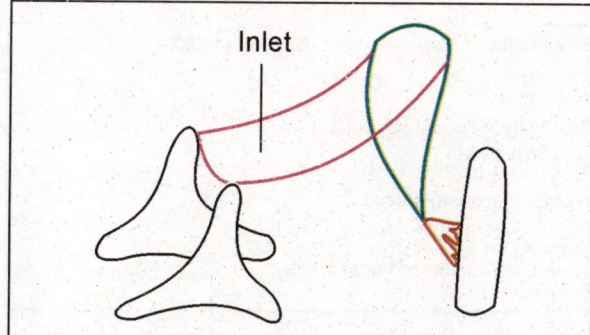

Fig. 6.15: Inlet of Larynx

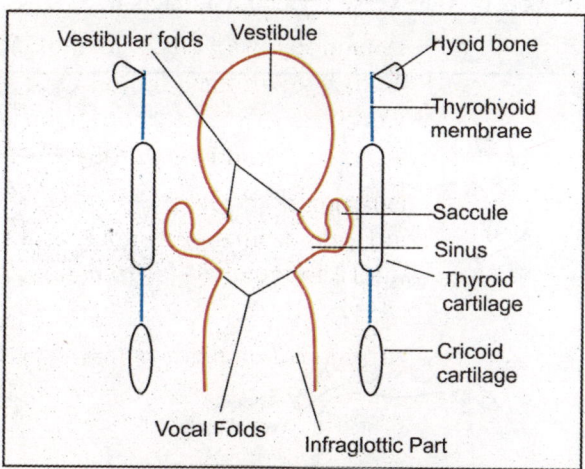

Fig. 6.16: Interior of Larynx

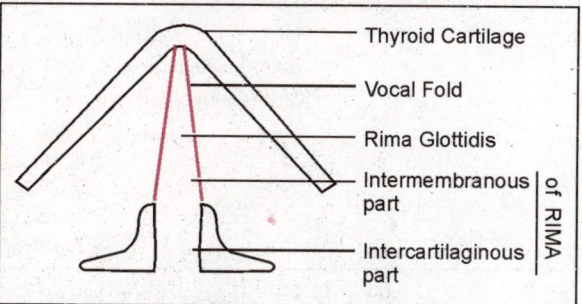

Fig. 6.17: Vocal Folds

cartilage to the vocal processes of arytenoid cartilages. They are formed of the vocal ligament and some muscle fibres - vocalis, both coverd by mucous membrane. Vocal folds appear white in colour.

Rima glottidis is the region of cavity of larynx between the two vocal folds and it is the narrowest part of larynx. Anterior 3/5 of rima is intermembranous and posterior 2/5th is intercartilaginous.

Length of vocal fold is 17 mm in female and 23mm in male. Vocal folds are acted upon by muscles of larynx to alter their tension and shape of rima glottidis. When vocal folds are tensed, pitch of voice is increased. While whispering, the 2 folds come close. Cricothyroid muscle tenses vocal fold. Thyroarytenoid relaxes it. Posterior cricoarytenoid abducts it. Transverse arytenoid adducts it.

Muscles of Larynx

Extrinsic muscles

Connect larynx to neighbouring structures:-

1. Thyrohyoid
2. Sternothyroid
3. Inferior constrictor of pharynx

Intrinsic muscles (Fig. 6.18 A to G)

1. Cricothyroid
2. Posterior Cricoarytenoid
3. Lateral Cricoarytenoid
4. Transverse Arytenoid
5. Oblique Arytenoid
6. Aryepiglotticus
7. Thyroarytenoid
8. Vocalis
9. Thyroepiglotticus **(Details in the diagrams)**

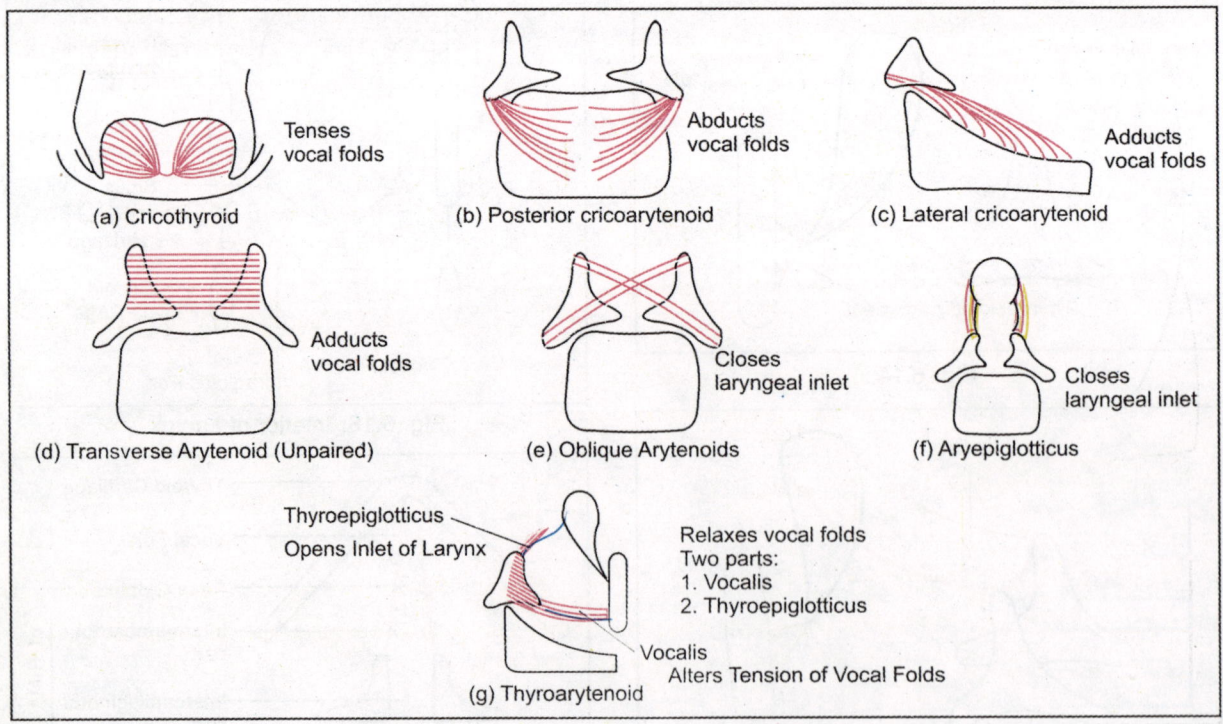

Fig. 6.18: Intrinsic muscles and their actions

Nerve Supply of Larynx

Sensory

Above the level of vocal folds, mucosa is supplied by the internal laryngeal nerve. Below, by recurrent laryngeal nerve.

Motor

Recurrent laryngeal nerve supplies all muscles except cricothyroid which is supplied by external laryngeal nerve.

Blood Supply

Branches of superior and inferior throyid arteries supply larynx.

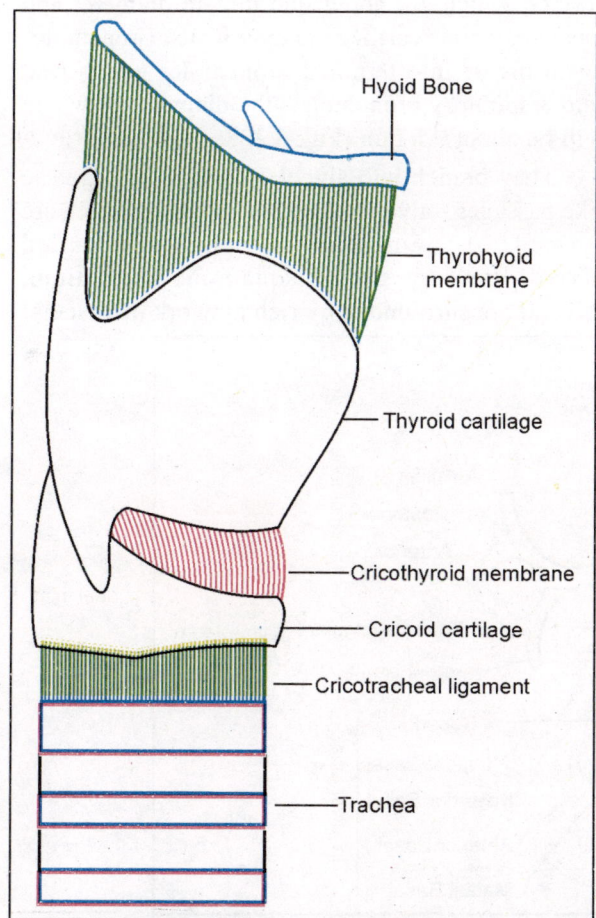

Fig. 6.19: Larynx - External Aspect

TRACHEA (Fig. 6.20)

A fibrocartilagenous-tube of about 13 cms long and 2.5 cms diameter. Continuous above wth the lower end of larynx at level of C_6 vertebra, below cricoid cartilage. Ends below at level of sternal angle (T_4 vertebra) by dividing into 2 Bronchi. Its frame work is formed of about 15-20 C shaped hyaline cartilagenous rings, connected by fibroelastic tissue. Posteriorly the fibroelastic tissue connecting the free ends of the C shaped cartilages contain a smooth muscle called - Trachealis. Internally the mucosa is lined by pseudostratified ciliated columnar epithelium.

In the neck it descends along the midline, in front of oesophagus. Isthmus of thyroid gland crosses it anteriorly against 2nd and 3rd rings. Below that, the inferior thyroid vein, thyroidea ima artery and jugular venous arch are important relations in the neck.

In the thorax also, it descends in front of oesophagus, in the superior mediastinum. Here it is crossed anteriorly by the arch of aorta, brachiocephalic trunk and left common carotid artery.

Applied anatomy

Tracheostomy is done in patients with severe laryngeal damage causing airway obstruction. The

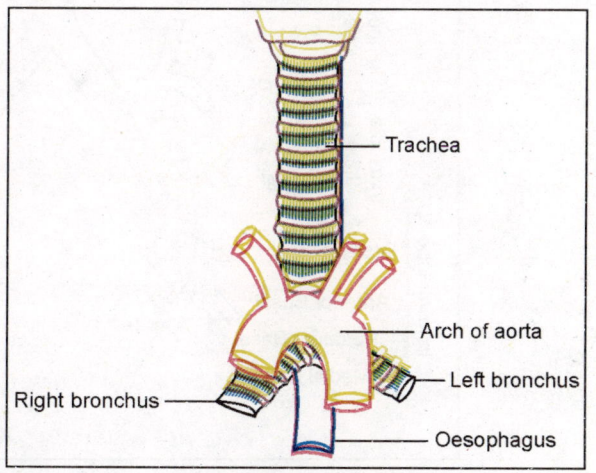

Fig. 6.20: Trachea

site usually chosen is at second tracheal ring, by retracting isthmus of thyroid gland downwards.

Blood Supply

Arteries - Inferior thyroid arteries.

Veins - To left brachiocephalic vein.

Nerve Supply - Branches of vagus and sympathetic nerves.

BRONCHI

Lower end of trachea divides in the thorax at level of lower border of T_4 vertebra into right and left principal bronchi. Right bronchus is shorter, wider and more vertical, about 2.5cm long. It enters the right lung at the hilum and inside the lung, divides into three lobar (Secondary) bronchi, to the three lobes of right lung. Left bronchus, about 5 cms long, in the left lung divides into two lobar(secondary) bronchi to the 2 lobes of the left lung.

In each lobe of both lungs the lobar/secondary bronchi divide into segmental or tertiary bronchi and into bronchioles. The bronchioles ramify into a functionally independant unit of lung, broncho-pulmonary segment.

Bronchopulmonary Segment (Fig. 6.21)

It is the independant unit of lung that is aerated by the division of a tertiary/segmental bronchus. It is supplied by a tertiary division of pulmonary artery.

Applied anatomy

Knowledge of bronchopulmonary segments is essential during bronchoscopy and to interpret bronchograms. In diseases limited to a segment, ressection of that particular segment can be performed instead of lobectomy or pneumonectomy.

Bronchioles

In bronchopulmonary segments, the segmental bronchus divides repeatedly and bronchioles are formed which are about one mm in diameter and have no hyaline cartilage in their walls. Bronchioles again divide into terminal bronchioles which lead into respiratory bronchioles, the diameter of which will be about 0.5 mm (Fig. 6.22).

They branch into alveolar ducts which are sac like passages - alveolar sacs, the walls of which are formed of numerous outpouchings called alveoli, lined by simple squamous epithelium. Alveoli are surrounded by rich network of vascular

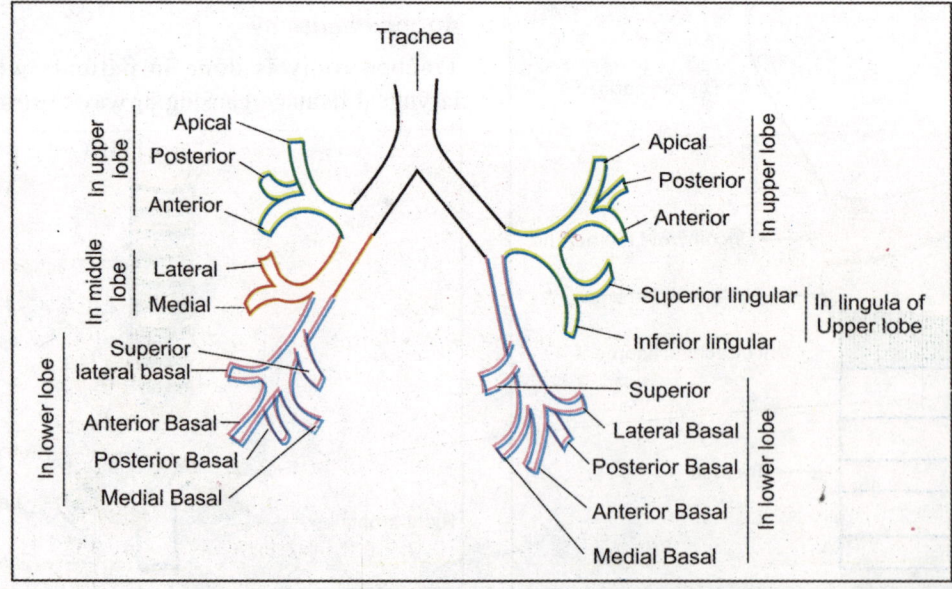

Fig. 6.21: Bronchopulmonary Segments of the 2 Lungs

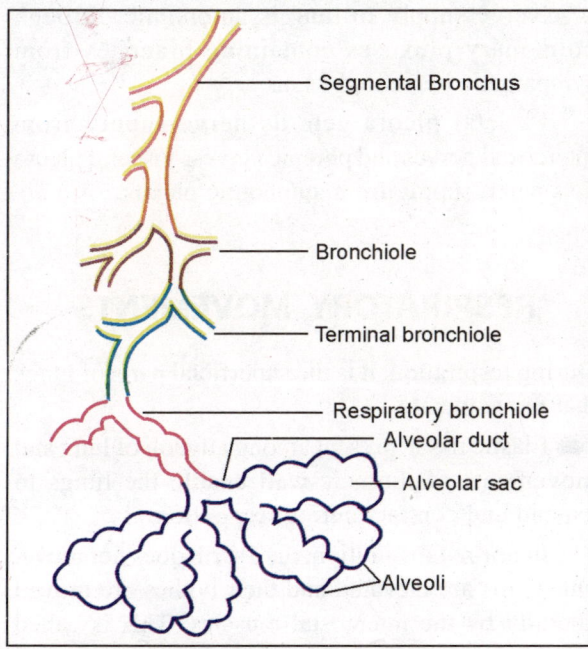

Fig. 6.22: Respiratory Tree

Each lung is conical in shape with an apex reaching root of neck, base, that rests on diaphragm, a costal surface, related to the thoracic wall and a mediastinal surface facing medially. About the middle of this surface, a depressed area is seen, hilum, through which bronchi, blood vessels, nerves and lymphatics enter and leave the lung. These structures constitute the root of lung and are covered by pleura.

Lung has two borders - posterior blunt border, near the vertebral column and anterior sharp border.

The right lung has two fissures - oblique and horizontal, thus dividing the lung into upper, middle and lower lobes (Fig. 6.23).

Left lung has a single oblique fissure dividing it into upper and lower lobes (Fig. 6.24) Its anterior border-shows a cardiac notch where it overhangs the heart. Lower end of cardiac notch shows a small process - lingula.

Structure: Lung tissue contains ramifications of bronchial tree with alveoli, separated by rich capillary plexus, connective tissue fibres and cells.

capillaries. Exchange of gases takes place between air in lungs and blood in capillaries.

LUNGS

The right and left lungs are spongy and elastic organs, present in the thoracic cavity on each side of the mediastinum. It is invaginated into the pleural cavity and hence covered by the 2 layers of pleura - visceral pleura, closely investing the lung and parietal pleura, which lines the thoracic wall.

Pleura

It is a serous membrane formed as a closed sac, into which the lung is invaginated. Thus it has an outer parietal layer and an inner visceral layer, continuous with each other at the hilum, covering the structures forming the root of lung. Between the two layers, a potential space is seen - the pleural cavity where a thin film of serous fluid lubricates the surfaces.

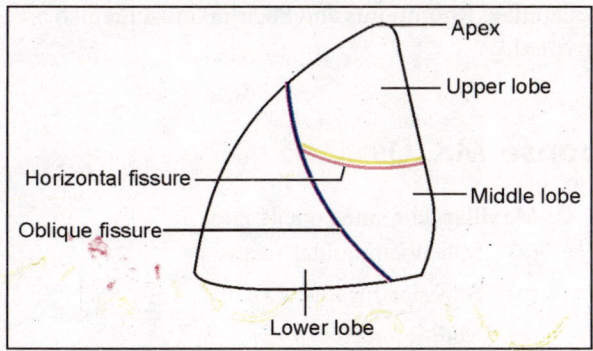

Fig. 6.23: Right Lung - Fissures and Lobes

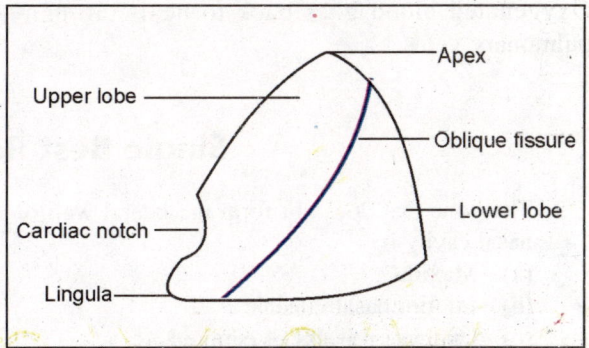

Fig. 6.24: Left Lung - Fissures and Lobes

Corresponding to the different parts of lung, pleura is also customoraly described as costal pleura, mediastinal pleura, cervical pleura and diaphragmatic pleura. From the root of lung, the mediastinal pleura extends down a short distance as a fold forming pulmonary ligament to allow movements of structures at the root.

Pleural recesses

1. Costodiaphragmatic recess.

   In normal respiration, the lower margin of the lung does not extend down to the line of pleural reflection of costodiaphragmatic surface. This slit like space is called costodiaphragamatic recess. In conditions of fluid or pus collection in pleural cavity it tracts down to this recess.

2. Costomediastinal recess.

   Similar small space is present in the anterior border of lung, between lung and pleura.

Applied Anatomy

Inflamation of pleura causes friction between visceral and parietal layers and leads to severe pain.

Fluid collection - plerual effusion.

Air in plerual cavity -Pneumothorax.

Nerve supply of lung and pleura

Parenchyma of lung and pleura get blood supply from bronchial arteries and its venous drainage is to azygos vein. Deoxygenated blood reaches around alveoli through branches of pulmonary arteries and Oxygenated blood goes back to heart through-pulmonary veins.

Nerve supply to lung is autonomic, through pulmonary plexuses containing branches from sympathetic nerve and vagus.

Parietal pleura gets its nerve supply from intercostal nerves and phrenic nerves. Visceral pleura gets nerve supply from autonomic plexus.

RESPIRATORY MOVEMENTS

During respiration, it is the superficial parts of lungs that move mostly.

Elastic tissue present among allveoli of lung and movements of thoracic wall enable the lungs to expand and contract during respiration.

In normal inspiration, the 1st rib does not move. Other ribs are elevated and their bodies are moved laterally by the intercostal muscles. This is called "bucket handle" movement of ribs. Also the sternum moves up and forwards. Thus transverse and anteroposterior diameters of thorax increase. Diaphragm descends causing increase in vertical diameter of thorax.

In expiration, there is elastic recoil of thoracic wall, depression of ribs and sternum moves back. This is "pump handle" movement. Diaphragm also rises. Air is expelled out.

In deep inspiration, scalene muscles and sternomastoid muscles also act.

In forced respiration, Trapezius, Lavator secapulae, Rhomboids and Pectoral muscles also are involed.

Single Best Response M.C.Qs

1. The bone that does not form the lateral wall of nasal cavity is
   (a) Maxilla
   (b) Inferior nasal concha
   (c) Uncinate process of ethmoid
   (d) Perpendicular plate of palatine bone.

2. Maxillary air sinus opens into
   (a) Sphenoethmoidal recess
   (b) Superior meatus
   (c) Middle meatus
   (d) Inferior meatus

3. Superior meatus receives the opening of
   - (a) Sphenoidal sinus
   - (b) Anterior ethmoidal sinus
   - (c) Middle ethmoidal sinus
   - (d) Posterior ethmoidal sinus
4. Muscle that tenses vocal cord is
   - (a) Cricothyroid
   - (b) Thyroarytenoid
   - (c) Transverse arytenoid
   - (d) Posterior cricoarytenoid.
5. Following are correct about trachea except.
   - (a) It begins at level of C_6 vertebra
   - (b) Its framework has C shaped fibrocartilages.
   - (c) It descends in front of oesophagus
   - (d) It divides into bronchi at the level of sternal angle.
6. Following are correct about Lungs except.
   - (a) Right lung has 3 lobes and left lung has 2 lobes
   - (b) Apex of lungs reach the root of neck.
   - (c) They are lined by parietal pleura
   - (d) Lingula is present in the left lung.

7. Maxillary hiatus is reduced in size in living by the following except.
   - (a) Uncinate process of ethmoid bone.
   - (b) Perpendicular plate of palatine bone.
   - (c) Descending process of lacrimal bone
   - (d) Middle nasal concha.
8. Of the following cartilages of larynx, paired one is
   - (a) Thyroid
   - (b) Cricoid
   - (c) Arytenoid
   - (d) Epiglottic
9. Air sinus that opens into sphenoethmoidal recessis
   - (a) Sphenoidal sinus
   - (b) Anterior ethmoidal sinus
   - (c) Posterior ethmoidal sinus
   - (d) Frontal sinus
10. Muscle that abducts the vocal folds is
   - (a) Cricothyroid
   - (b) Posterior cricoarytenoid
   - (c) Lateral cricoarytenoid
   - (d) Oblique arytenoids

M.C.Qs - Answers

1. (c), 2. (c), 3. (d), 4. (a), 5. (b), 6. (c), 7. (d), 8. (c), 9. (a), 10. (b)

Essays

I. Name the paranasal air sinuses and describe the maxillary sinus

II. Describe the lateral wall of nasal cavity

III. Describe the muscles and ligaments of larynx. Give the nerve supply of larynx.

IV. Describe the right / Left lung.

Short Notes

1. Nasal septum
2. Middle meatus
3. Vocal folds
4. Interior of larynx
5. Rima glottides
6. Cricothyroid muscle
7. Bronchopulmonary segments
8. Pleura
9. Trachea
10. Bronchi

7   Alimentary System

DIGESTIVE SYSTEM – GASTROINTESTINAL TRACT

The alimentary tract is an epithelium lined muscular tube extending from the mouth, to the anal canal. The ingested food is broken down by teeth, propelled down the tract and is exposed to digestive enzymes which convert it into small molecules. They pass through the epithelial lining of the tract, enter the blood capillaries to be used up in the whole body. Undigested parts of the food is expelled out as faecal matter. Glands along the epithelial lining provide enzymes and other materials required for digestion and absorption. Larger glands associated with the function of digestion are located out side the tubular tract. They are:

1. 3 pairs of salivary glands that pour their secretion – saliva into the mouth.
2. Liver - that secretes bile.
3. Pancreas - that secretes pancreatic juice.

PARTS OF ALIMENTARY TRACT (DIGESTIVE TRACT)

From cranial to caudal end, the parts are

1. Oral cavity (mouth)
2. Pharynx
3. Oesophagus
4. Stomach
5. Small intestine
6. Large intestine
7. Rectum and anal canal

Oral Cavity

The 2 lips surround the oral opening anteriorly. Mouth has a major part, the oral cavity proper and a narrow part – vestibule – between the teeth and cheek.

The 2 incisors, one canine, 2 premolars and 3 molar teeth in each quadrant of the upper and lower jaw separate the major oral cavity from vestibule.

Roof of mouth is bounded by hard and soft palates. Floor has the tongue in the major part and also the mucous membrane overlying the muscle – mylohyoid.

Posteriorly mouth is continuous with the oropharynx at the oropharyngeal isthmus bounded laterally by the palatoglossal arch.

Tongue

A muscular organ for speech, taste and deglutition.

In the mouth, it is attached to the mandible, hyoid bone, styloid process, soft palate and pharyngeal wall by muscles.

It has a root, apex, dorsal and ventral surfaces and 2 margins. Root is attached to the floor of the mouth posteriorly.

Covered by mucous membrane having stratified squamous epithelium.

Dorsum is rough due to projections of mucous membrane called papillae. Dorsum is divided into anterior 2/3 rd and posterior 1/3 rd by a ∧ shaped sulcus – sulcus terminalis, the point at the apex of which is foramen caecum (Fig. 7.1). Posterior 1/3 rd does not show papillae but only scattered projections of lingual tonsil.

Papillae are

1. Circumvallate papillae seen in front of sulcus terminalis, parallel to it (10-12- in No.)
2. Fungiform - more on the margins and also scattered on dorsum.
3. Filiform – scattered on dorsum.
4. Foliate papillae - 4 or 5 vertical folds on the posterior part of the margins.

Taste buds are seen in relation to the epithelium of papillae. From the specialised taste cells of taste buds, the gustatory nerves carry the sensation to brain.

Ventral surface (Fig. 7.2) of tongue is smooth and mucosa is reflected to floor of mouth. Along its midline, a mucosal fold is seen – frenulum. Lateral to it the deep lingual veins are seen through mucosa. Lateralmost, a **fimbriated** fold is seen, plicae fimbriata.

Muscles of the tongue

I. Intrinsic muscles

1. Superior longitudinal
2. Inferior longitudinal
3. Transverse
4. Vertical

II. Extrinsic muscles: (Fig. 7.3)

1. Styloglossus – From styloid process, to the side of tongue, pulls tongue upwards and backwards.
2. Palatoglossus – From soft palate, to side of tongue. Elevates the back of tongue. It produces palatoglossel fold which is the boundary between mouth and pharynx.
3. Hyoglossus – From hyoid bone, to side of tongue. It depresses the tongue.
4. Genioglossus – From the superior genial tubercle on the back of symphysis menti. The fibers fan out to the whole extent of tongue, intermingle with all muscles. It protrudes the tongue.

Nerve supply of tongue:

Motor – All muscles except palatoglossus, by hypoglossal nerve. Paltoglossus, by cranial accessary.

Sensory – anterior 2/3 rd - lingual nerve (of mandibular) posterior 1/3 rd – Glossopharyngeal.

Taste – anterior 2/3 rd - chorda tympani (of facial nerve) posterior 1/3 rd – Glossopharyngeal nerve.

Posteriormost part – Vagus

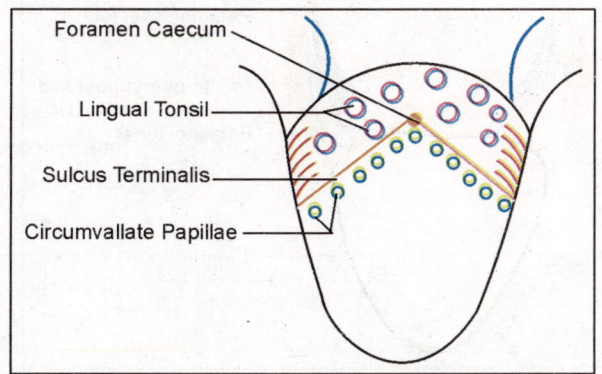

Fig. 7.1: Tongue - Dorsum

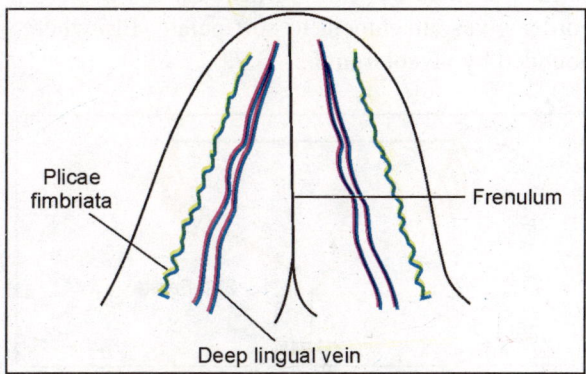

Fig. 7.2: Tongue Ventral Surface

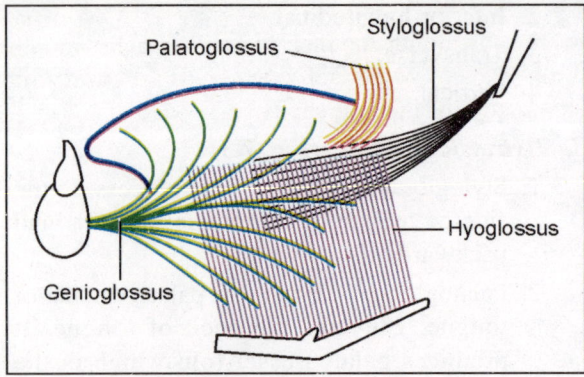

Fig. 7.3: Tongue - Extrinsic Muscles

Blood supply of tongue

Lingual artery – branch of external carotid artery. It also gets branches from ascending palatine, ascending pharyngeal and tonsillar arteries.

Venous drainage is through lingual veins into internal jugular vein.

Lymphatic drainage – to the submental, submandibular, jugulodigastric and juguloomohyoid nodes.

Palate (Fig. 7.4)

Palate forms the roof of mouth. It has an anterior part, hard palate and posterior part, soft palate.

Hard palate

Formed of palatine processes of the 2 maxillae and horizontal plates of 2 palatine bones. Its under surface is lined by mucoperiosteum. Its posterior border gives attachment to soft palate. Elsewhere, bounded by alveolar arch.

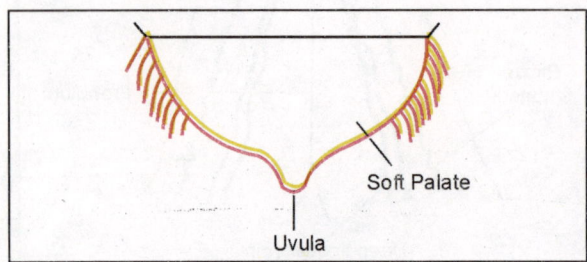

Fig. 7.5: Soft Palate

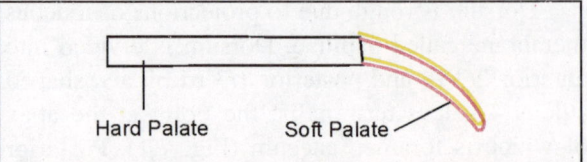

Fig. 7.4

Soft palate (Fig. 7.5)

It is a curved fibromuscular flap attached to the posterior border of hard palate.

Its sides blend with the pharyngeal wall. Posterior free border presents a small conical projection, uvula.

Formed of an aponeurosis, the palatine aponeurosis, palatine muscles, lymphoid tissue and mucous glands; all covered by mucous membrane.

From the sides of the soft palate, two mucosal folds curve downwards; the anterior one to the tongue, palatoglossal fold, formed by palatoglossus muscle; posterior one to the pharynx, palatopharyngeal fold, formed by palatopharyngeus muscle (Fig. 7.6) between these two folds, palatine tonsil is located.

Muscles of soft palate

1. Tensor palati: Its tendon is flattened to form palatine aponeurosis, attached to posterior border of hard palate and forms the fibrous skeleton of soft palate.

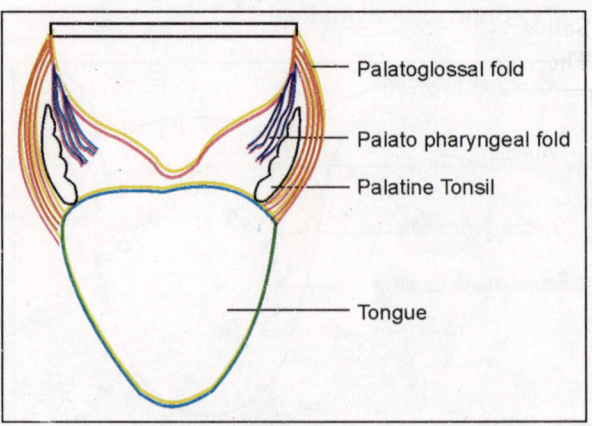

Fig. 7.6

2. Levator palati
3. Palatopharyngeus
4. Palatoglossus
5. Musculus uvulae.

Nerve supply

Motor – All muscles except tensor palati are supplied by pharyngeal plexus - fibres of cranial accessory, through branches of vagus. Tensor palati is supplied by branch of mandibular nerve.

Sensory – Branches of maxillary nerve and glossopharyngeal nerve.

Blood supply

Arteries – Ascending palatine artery
Ascending pharyngeal artery
Greater palatine artery.
Veins – Veins drain into tonsillar veins and pterygoid venous plexus.
Lymphatic drainage to deep cervical nodes.

Congenital anomalies

Palate develops from 2 palatine processes and an anterior premaxilla. The three parts fuse normally. Failure of fusion or defective fusion of the parts, leads to cleft palate of varying degrees. Some are associated with cleft lip.

SALIVARY GLANDS

Salivary glands secrete saliva into the oral cavity. There are paired major salivary glands situated outside the mouth and their secretion reaches mouth through ducts. Minor salivary glands are located in the mucosa of the oral cavity.

The major glands are

1. Parotid glands
2. Submandibular glands
3. Sublingual glands

Parotid gland (Fig. 7.7)

Largest of the 3 salivary glands, purely serous in nature.

Position: Below the external acoustic meatus, in the hollow between ramus of mandible and sternocleidomastoid muscle.

Shape (Fig. 7.8): Roughly pyramidal in shape, with three sides, apex and base. Base is directed upwards, around the external acoustic meatus. Apex directed downwards. Surfaces are superficial, anteromedial and posteromedial. Anteromedial and posteromedial surfaces meet at the medial border.

The gland has 4 processes or extensions.

1. Glenoid process from base, extends up behind temporomandibular joint.
2. Facial process – from anterior border, extends over masseter muscle.
3. Accessory part – a detached part of the facial process, seen above the duct.
4. Pterygoid process – from anteromedial

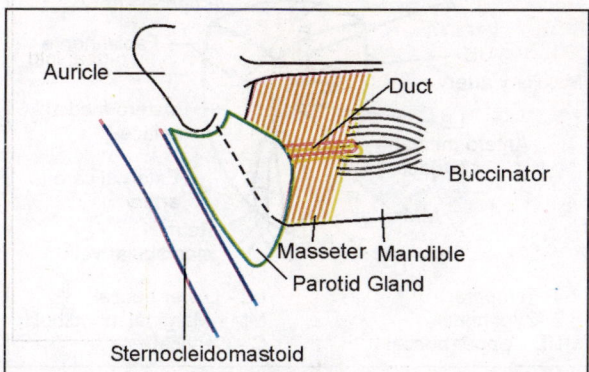

Fig. 7.7

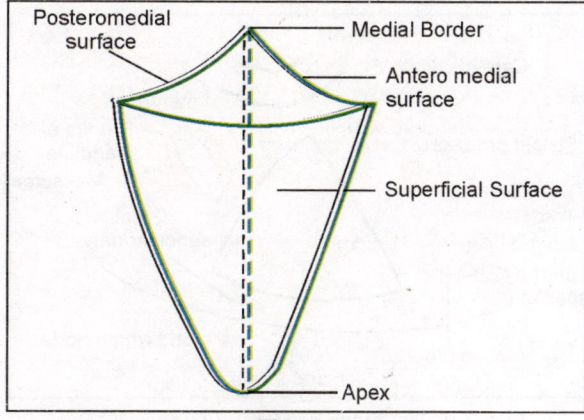

Fig. 7.8

surface, to between ramus of mandible and medial pterygoid muscle.

Coverings: It has a fibrous capsule of its own. Outside that, a dense parotid fascia is seen, an extension from the general investing layer of deep cervical fascia.

Relations (Fig. 7.9)

1. **Structures related to its outer aspect:**

   Superficial surface: Covered by skin and fascia, has branches of greater auricular nerve and parotid lymph nodes.

   Anteromedial surface: Related to posterior border of ramus of mandible with medial pterygoid and masseter on its 2 surfaces.

   Posteromedial surface: Mastoid process with posterior belly of digastric and sternomastoid.

   Deeper to that, styloid process and attached structures. Deepest, carotid sheath with contents.

   Base: Related to external acoustic meatus, temporomandibular joint and auriculo-temporal nerve.

   Medial Border: Reaches the side of pharynx.

   Apex: Reaches carotid triangle in neck.

2. **Structures passing through the gland** (Fig. 7.10)

   (a) External carotid artery enters the gland through its posteromedial surface, divides into superficial temporal and maxillary branches inside the gland which emerge through the upper part of anteromedial surface.

   (b) Retromandibular vein is formed by union of superficial temporal vein and maxillary vein. Descends in the gland and divides into 2 divisions.

   (c) Facial nerve. Enters the gland through the upper part of posteromedial surface, divides into its terminal branches which emerge along the anterior border of gland into the face.

Parotid Duct

Emerges from the anterior border of gland, about 5 cms long. Crosses masseter, turns inwards, pierces buccal pad of fat, buccopharyngeal fascia buccinator and buccal mucous membrane to open into vestibule of mouth at the level of upper 2nd molar tooth.

Nerve Supply: Secretomotor (Fig. 7.11)

Preganglionic fibres arise from inferior salivatory nucleus in the brain stem, pass through IX cranial nerve. Then through its tympanic branch to tympanic plexus. From there, come through lesser petrosal nerve to the otic ganglion. Fibres relay there, postganglionic fibres reach the gland through auriculotemporal nerve.

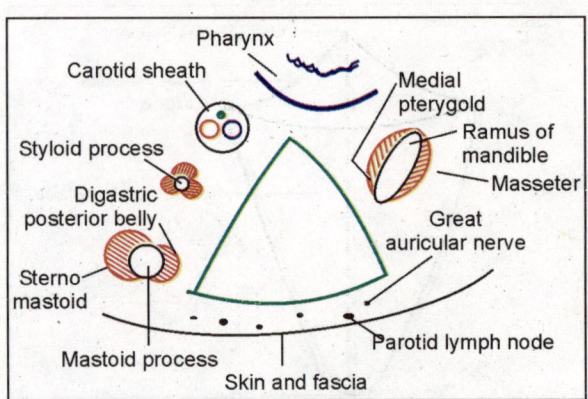

Fig. 7.9: Relations of Parotid Gland - C.S.

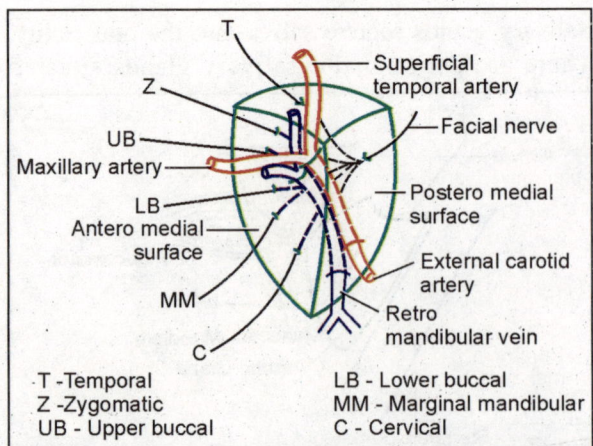

Fig. 7.10: Structures Passing Through Parotid Gland

Histology

Contains serous acini

Submandibular gland

It is a mixed salivary gland located partly under cover of mandible, near its angle, in the digastric triangle.

It has a large superficial part and smaller deep part, both continuous around the posterior border of mylohyoid muscle. (Fig. 7.12)

Superficial part (Fig. 7.13)

Has inferior, medial and lateral surfaces. Inferior and medial surfaces are covered by an extension from general investing layer of deep cervical facia.

Relations

Inferior surface: Covered by skin, platysma, deep fascia; crossed by facial vein and cervical branch of facial nerve. Submandibular lymphnode is related.

Lateral surface: In contact with medial pterygoid on the medial surface of ramus of mandible. Facial artery grooves the posterior end of the gland and comes in between the lateral surface and ramus of mandible to emerge on to the face.

Medial surface (Fig. 7.14): Related to mylohyoid, hyoglossus, hypoglossal nerve, lingual nerve and submandibular ganglion.

Anterioly it is related to anterior belly of digastric and posteriorly to the posterior belly of digastric and stylohyoid.

Deep part of the gland

Continuous with the superficial part around the posterior border of mylohyoid. Lies between the mylohyoid and hyoglossus.

Lingual nerve, submandibular ganglion and hypoglossal nerve are related to it on the hyoglossus. (Fig. 7.14)

Blood Supply

Arteries: Branches from facial and lingual arteries.
Veins: Correspond to arteries.

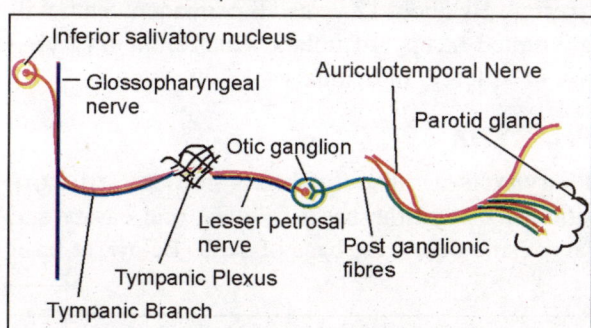

Fig. 7.11: Secretomotor Nerve Supply to Parotid Gland

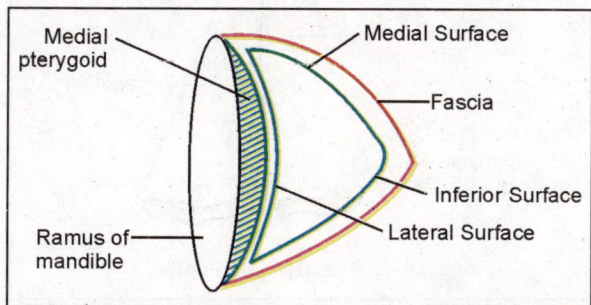

Fig. 7.13: Superficial Part of Submandibular Gland - Vertical Section

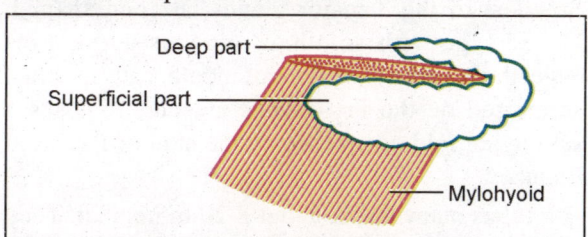

Fig. 7.12: Submandibular Gland

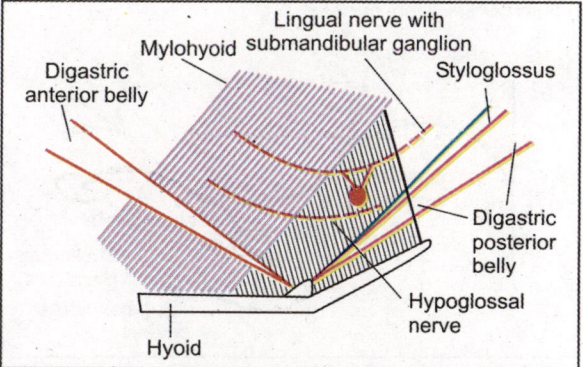

Fig. 7.14: Deep Relations of Submandibular Gland

Nerve Supply (Fig. 7.15)

Secretomotor, preganglionic fibres originate from superior salivatory nucleus in brain stem. Pass through the VII cranial nerve, its chorda tympani branch and reach lingual nerve, branch of mandibular nerve. Relay in the sub mandibular ganglion & post ganglionic fibres reach the gland.

Lymphatic drainage: To submandibular & deep cervical nodes.

Histology

Contains mucous and serous acini

Duct

Emerges from the anterior end of deep part of the gland. Passes anteriorly beneath the mucosa of floor of mouth, crossed by lingual nerve. Opens into the mouth at the summit of sublingual papilla on the side of frenulum of tongue.

Sublingual gland (Fig. 7.16)

Smallest of the 3 major glands, almond shaped. Mixed type with serous & mucous acini. Lies beneath the mucosa of floor of mouth, near midline, supported on the mylohyoid muscle. It raises a sublingual fold of mucosa on the side of frenulum linguae.

It has many ducts, about 8-20 in number. They open on the summit of sublingual fold, separately.

A major duct may open with submandibular duct, through the sublingual papilla.

Teeth

There are 20 deciduous teeth, replaced by 32 permanent teeth, in both jaws.

Deciduous teeth: - in each ½ of a jaw,

two incisors – one central and one lateral,

one canine and

two molars

Permanent teeth:– In each ½ of a jaw,

Two incisors,

One canine,

Two premolars and

Three molars.

The deciduous teeth Ist to erupt are lower central incisors. They start eruption by 6-12 months and all teeth will be erupted by 2 – 2 ½ years. They start shedding by 6th year when permanent teeth begin to erupt. By about 12 years all permanent teeth will be erupted except 3rd molars, which erupt in varying age in different individuals – 17-30 years.

PHARYNX

Pharynx is a musculofibrous conical structure situated behind the nasal cavities, oral cavity and larynx and below the base of skull. Below, at level

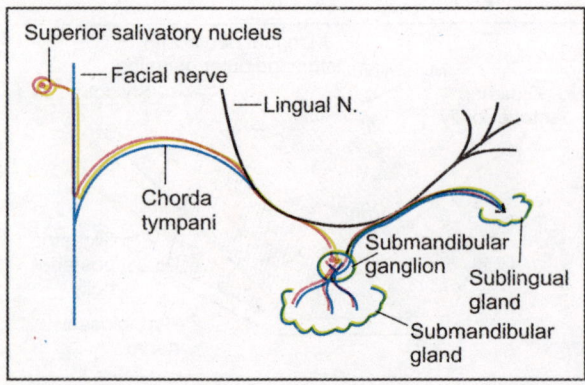

Fig. 7.15: Secretomotor Nerve Suppy to Submandibular Gland

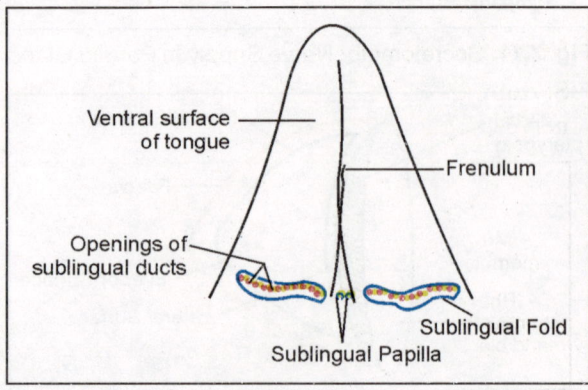

Fig. 7.16

with C$_6$ vertebra, it becomes continuous with oesophagus, which is the narrowest part of alimentary tract- pharyngo oesophageal junction.

Its anterior wall is incomplete (Fig. 7.17) as it opens into the nasal cavity, mouth and larynx. So it has three parts -Nasopharynx, Oropharynx and Laryngopharynx.

Structure

Internally lined by mucous membrane.

Thickness of its wall is formed of muscles, inner aspect of which is lined by a membrane pharyngobasilar fascia and outer aspect by buccopharyngeal fascia.

Muscles of pharynx

1. **Three constrictors:** Superior, middle and inferior.

   They are circularly arranged in an overlapping manner (Fig. 7.18). They arise from the base of skull, mandible, hyoid bone, thyroid and cricoid cartilages. From origin, they cover the lateral surface of pharynx and get inserted into a common median posterior raphe. They act to propel food down to pharynx.

2. **Three Longitudinal muscles:**

   Stylophraryngeus, palatopharyngeus and salpingopharyngeus, descending and merging into the wall of pharynx. They elevate the pharynx during deglutition.

Nerve Supply

Stylopharyngeus supplied by glossopharyngeal nerve and others by pharyngeal plexus.

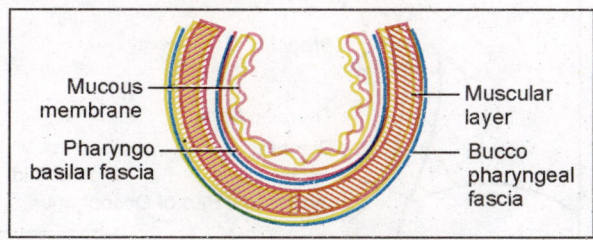

Fig. 7.17: C.S of Wall of Pharynx

- Mucous membrane
- Pharyngo basilar fascia
- Muscular layer
- Bucco pharyngeal fascia

Parts of pharynx (Fig.7.19)

1. **Nasopharynx:** part behind the nasal cavities.

   Its lateral wall has opening of auditory tube, bounded by tubal elevation, due to projecting cartilagenous end of the tube. From the tubal elevation a mucosal fold descends, salpingopharyngeal fold, caused by salpingopharyngeus muscle.

   Behind it, there is collection of tubal tonsil and posterior to which, there is a depression, pharyngeal recess or forsa of Rossenmuller. Upper part of the posterior wall, near its roof, nasopharynx has pharyngeal tonsil.

2. **Oropharynx:** Part behind the mouth. Oropharynx commuinicates above with nasopharynx through isthumus of pharynx. During swallowing, oropharynx is shut off from nasopharynx by elevation of soft palate. In the lateral wall of oropharynx, there is the palatine tonsil, between palatoglossal and palatopharyngeal arches.

3. **Laryngopharynx:** Lies behind the larynx. Anteriorly, above it communicates with larynx through laryngeal inlet. Below at level of cricoid cartilage or C$_6$ vertebral level, it becomes continuous with oesophagus.

Sensory nerve supply of pharynx: - Branches of glossopharyngeal nerve and maxillary nerve.

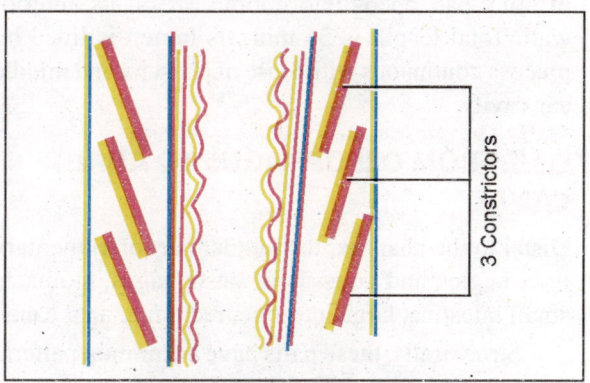

3 Constrictors

Fig. 7.18: L.S of Pharynx

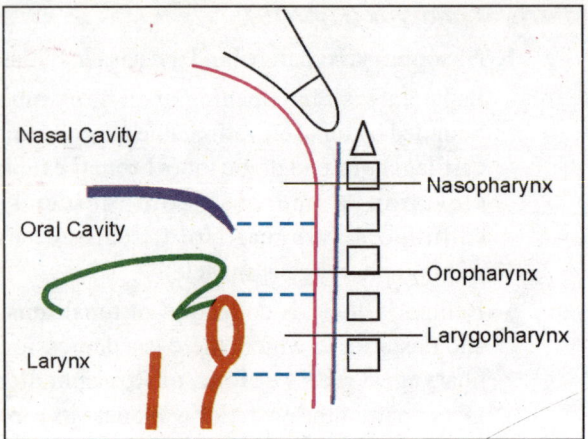

Fig. 7.19: Parts of Pharynx

Blood Supply

Arteries: Branches of ascending pharyngeal artery, facial artery, lingual artery and maxillary artery.

Veins: Drain to pharyngeal plexus.

Lymphatics: to deep cervical and retropharyngeal nodes.

Auditory tube

(Pharygotympanic tube, Eustacian tube)

Connects the nasopharynx with middle ear. Function is to equalise pressure in middle ear with atmospheric pressure.

It has a medial cartilagenous part formed of elastic cartilage and lateral bony part. End of cartilagenous part opens into nasopharynx and end of bony part opens into middle ear on its anterior wall. Total length is 36 mm. Its lumen is lined by mucosa continuous with those of pharynx and middle ear cavity.

G.I.T. FROM OESOPHAGUS TO ANAL CANAL

Distal to the pharynx, the tubular part of alimentary tract begins and consists of oesophagus, stomach, small intestine, large intestine, rectum & anal canal.

Structurally, these parts have a common pattern, arranged in layers. Inner to outer, they are:

1. Mucosa – has a lining epithelium, lamina propria of loose connective tissue & muscularis mucosa – of smooth muscle.
2. Submucosa formed of connective tissue.
3. Muscularis externa of smooth muscle layers.
4. Serosa – thin layer of connective tissue.

In oesophagus, mucosa is folded. In stomach, mucosa shows short narrow canals called gastric pits. In small intestine, it shows narrow projections-villi. In large intestine, mucosa shows folds.

Mucosa of stomach has gastric glands & that of small intestine has intestinal glands – crypts of Lieberkuhn. In duodenum, submucosa has Brunner's glands.

OESOPHAGUS

Oesophagus is a muscular tube, about 25 cms long, continuous above with the pharynx at level of C_6 vertebra. It passes through the superior and posterior mediastinum of thorax, pierces diaphragm at level with T_{10} vertebra and opens into stomach at level with T_{11} vertebra. Thus it has a cervical part, thoracic part and very short abdominal part.

In the neck, it is in front of vertebral column, behind the trachea and the lobes of thyroid gland lie lateral to it.

In the thorax, it lies behind the trachea, left bronchus and left atrium. It is in front of the thoracic part of vertebral column, azygos vein, thoracic duct and descending thoracic aorta. (Fig. 7.20)

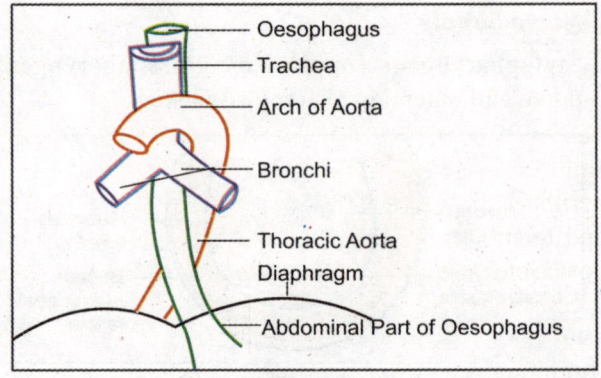

Fig. 7.20

When it goes through the opening in the diaphragm to the abdomen, it is accompanied by the right and left vagus nerves.

Blood Supply

Arteries: Branches from thyroid arteries, thoracic aorta and left gastric artery.

Veins: from upper part, to inferior thyroid veins, from middle part, to azygos vein and from lower end, to portal vein through left gastric vein.

Sites of constriction of oesophagus

1. At its commencement – 15 cm from incisor teeth.
2. Where it is crossed by arch of aorta - 22.5 cm from incisors.
3. Where it is crossed by left bronchus – 27.5 cm from incisor teeth.
4. Where it pierces the diaphragm – 40 cm from incisor teeth.

Abdomen

To learn the relative positions of the abdominal organs, anterior abdominal wall is divided into different regions by certain planes. (Fig. 7.21)

Peritoneum

It is a thin serous membrane lining the inner surface of abdominal and pelvic cavities and reflected on to the viscera to cover them. Its surface has a thin film of serous fluid for smooth inter movements of viscera.

Peritoneal folds extend from the abdominal wall to organs or between organs connecting them or retaining their relative positions. The folds carry vessels and nerves to organs. Also they form ligaments. Omentum (lesser and greater) are peritoneal folds that extend from stomach to liver and to transverse colon. Mesentery extends from posterior abdominal wall to small intestine, to cover it. Similarly mesocolon, to large intestine. Peritoneal folds extend between kidney and spleen as lienorenal ligament; between stomach and spleen as gastrosplenic ligament. Peritoneal folds form most

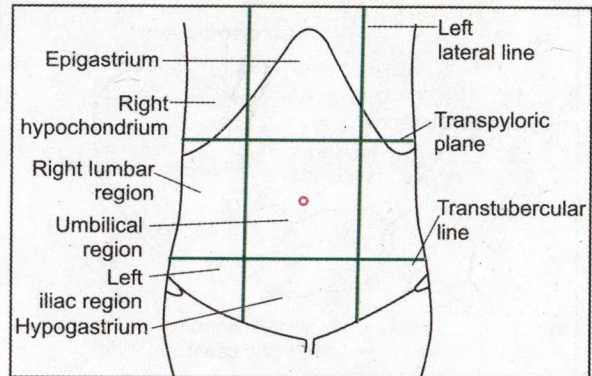

Fig. 7.21: Regions of Abdomen

of the ligaments of liver. Greater omentum has a major role in storing fat and limiting spread of infection.

Short peritoneal folds form recesses in relation to organs – e.g., duodenal recesses and ileocaecal recesses. These form sites where internal herniation of a segment of intestine can occur. If it is not released, leads to strangulation of the hernia.

Peritoneum can be considered as a blown up balloon on which organs are invaginated. Thus the layer of peritoneum covering organs is visceral peritoneum and the layer lining the abdominal wall is parietal peritoneum. Cavity of peritoneum is peritoneal cavity, the greater sac. From the major peritoneal cavity a sac like extension goes behind the stomach - the lesser sac.

STOMACH (Fig. 7.22)

Most dilated part of alimentary tract. Situated in the epigastric, umbilical and left hypochondriac regions. Shape and position are modified by changes within itself and by the surrounding viscera.

Mean capacity is 1500 ml in adults. Has 2 orifices, 2 borders (curvatures) and 2 surfaces.

Orifices

Above, oesophagus opens into stomach at the cardiac orifice.

Below, it opens into duodenum at pyloric orifice. This is marked on the surface of the organ by pyloric

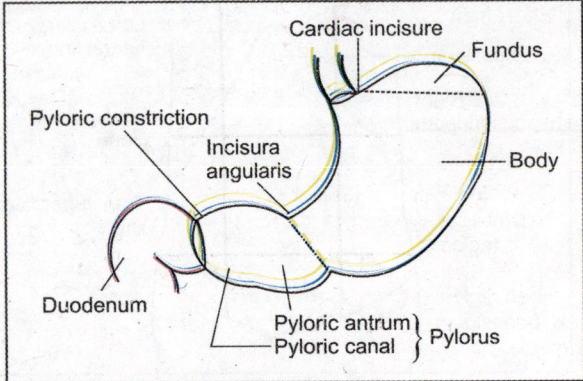

Fig. 7.22

constriction indicating pyloric sphincter. Prepyloric vein crosses vertically on its anterior surface. This orifice lies about 1.25 cms to the right of midline at level with lower border of L_1 vertebra and the plane is known as transpyloric plane.

Borders (Curvatures)

Lesser curvature – descends from the right side of oesophageal end to the pylorus. At the most dependent part of this border, there is a notch – incisura angularis. Lesser omentum is attached along this border and right and left gastric arteries lie on it.

Greater curvature: Longer, starts from the left side of oesophageal opening, ascends up and then descends to the right, to reach pyloric end. At its beginning where it ascends, there is a depression, cardiac incisure. Before it ends at pyloric end, there is a bulge along the curvature, it corresponds to pylorus of stomach.

Parts of stomach

  Fundus

  Body

  Pylorus – Antrum and Canal

Peritoneal folds attached along the greater curvature are gastropherinic ligament above, then gastrosplenic ligament and along the major part, greater omentum. Right and left gastroepiploeic vessels lie here.

Major relations

Anterior

Anterior abdominal wall, liver, diaphragm, spleen (near the fundus)

Posterior (Fig.7.23)

Posterior surface of stomach is separated from structures of posterior abdominal wall by lesser sac. These structures collectively form the stomach bed. They are - Diaphragm, Left kidney, Left suprarenal, Pancreas, Spleen, Left colic flexure, Splenic artery and Transverse mesocolon.

  Blood Supply: (Fig. 7.24)

  Arteries: Branches of coeliac trunk.

  Veins: drain to portal vein.

Lymphatic drainage: (Fig. 7.25)

Different parts of stomach drain to specific groups of lymph nodes, as shown.

Nerve supply

Sympathetic - from coeliac plexus. Parasympathetic – Vagus

Interior

Mucosa is thrown into folds – rugae that stretch when the organ is distended. Mucosa has tubular glands.

SMALL INTESTINE

Longest part of the alimentary tract, about 6-7 metres long. Extends from pyloric orifice of stomach, to the ileocaecal junction where it opens into large intestine.

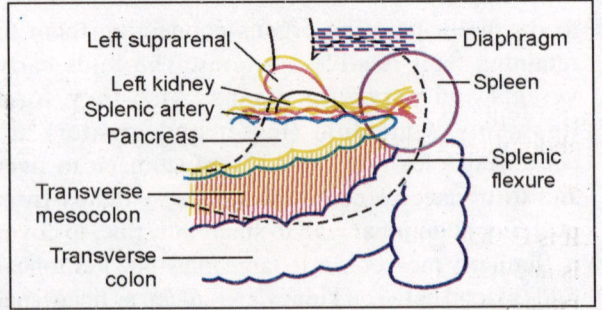

Fig. 7.23: Posterior Relations of Stomach (Stomach Bed)

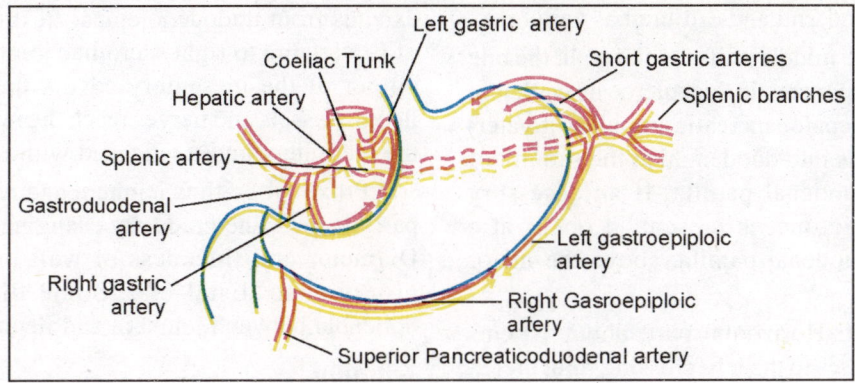

Fig. 7.24: Arterial Suppy of Stomach

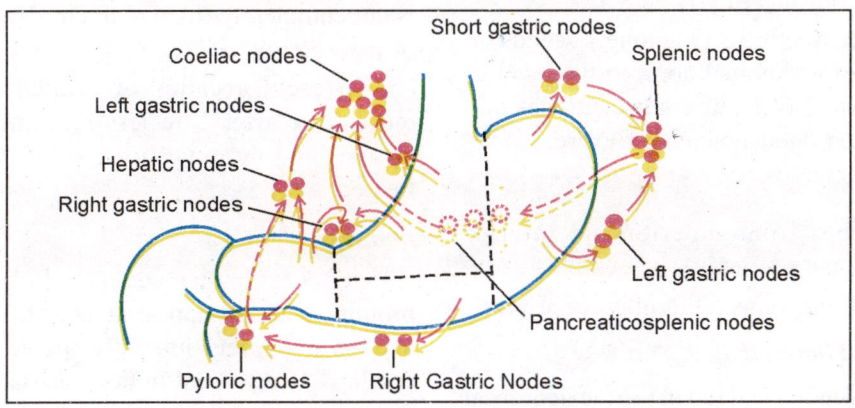

Fig. 7.25: Lymphatic Drainage of Stomach

Parts

1. Short curved sessile part, Duodenum.
2. Jejunum – proximal 2/5 th of the remaining mobile and coiled part.
3. Ileum: Distal 3/5th of the remaining mobile and coiled part.

Jejunum and ileum are attached to posterior abdominal wall by a peritoneal fold, mesentery.

1. Duodenum (Fig. 7.26)

It is C shaped - Curves around head of pancreas and is about 25 cms long.

Divisible into 4 part.

(a) **Ist part** – ascends from the pylorus, on the right side of L_1 vertebra. About 5 cm long, and partially covered by peritoneum.

(b) **2nd part**: descending part. About 7.5 cms long, descends in front of hilum of right

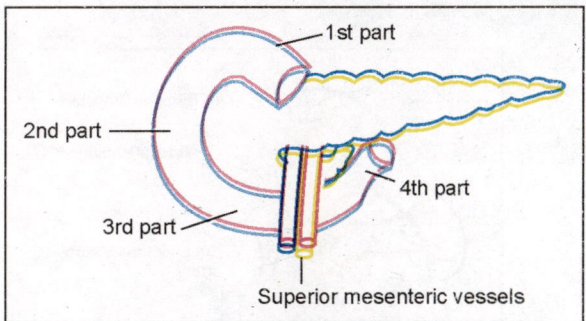

Fig. 7.26: Duodenum

kidney and 2nd and 3rd lumbar vertebrae.

About the middle of its medial wall, the bile duct and pancreatic duct pierce its wall, join to form hepatopancreatic ampulla (of Vater) that opens into duodenum at the summit of major duodenal papilla. If an accessory pancreatic duct is present, it opens at a minor duodenal papilla, above the major one.

(c) **3rd part**: Horizontal part, about 10 cms long. Passes to the left, crossing right ureter, inferior vena cava and abdominal aorta, Anteriorly it is crossed by root of mesentery and superior mesenteric vessels.

(d) **4th part:** About 2.5 cms long, ascends on the left of abdominal aorta to the level of upper border of L_2 where it continues into jujunum at duodenojejunal flexure.

Blood supply

Arteries: Branches from superior and inferior pancreaticoduodenal arteries.

Veins: Corresponding veins drain into portal vein.

2. Jejunum and ileum (Fig. 7.27 a & b)

Extend from duodenojejunal flexure to the ileocaecal junction, about 6 ms long, form coils and are freely mobile. Attached to the posterior abdominal wall by a double layer of fan shaped peritoneal fold – Mesentery. Root of mesentery attached to posterior abdominal wall is about 15 cms long and its intestinal border is about 6 metres long. Attachment of root extends from dudodenojejunal flexure – on the left of L_2 vertebra to right sacroiliac joint. The long free border of the mesentery covers the jejunum and ileum. Vessels and nerves reach the intestine through the mesentery and it is loaded with fat.

Proximal 2/5th is jejunum and remaining distal part, ileum – one gradually changing into the other. Diameter and thickness of wall decreases from proximal to distal end. Some differences are noticable between jejunum and ileum:

Jejunum

Diameter – about 4 cms. Mucosa shows prominent foldings - plicae circulares and long villi. Mesentery is not completely filled with fat – only near the root of mesentery.

Artereal arcades of branches of superior mesenteric artery are less in number – one or 2 arcades and terminal branches of the vessels are longer.

Ileum

About 3.5 cm in diameter. Plicae circulares are less prominent and disappear at its end. Villi are smaller and fewer. Aggregations of lymphoid tissue – Peyer's patches -- are present in the mucosa.

Arterial arcades in the mesentery are more in number, 3 to 6 and terminal vessels are shorter.

Blood supply:

Arteries: To jejunum and ileum, from branches of superior mesenteric artery.

Veins: - Drain to superior mesenteric vein.

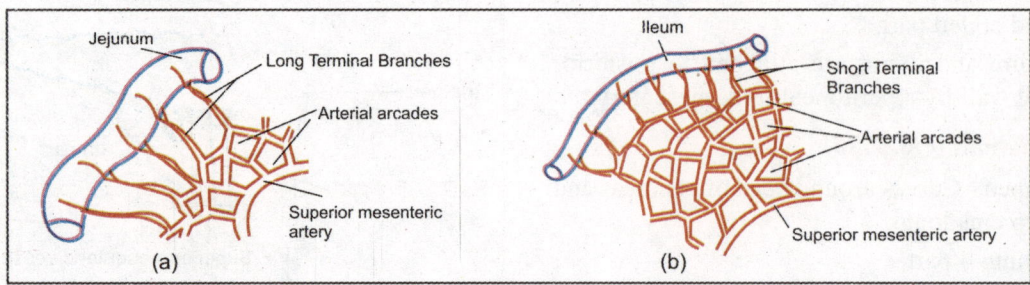

Fig. 7.27

LARGE INTESTINE (Fig. 7.28)

Function is to absorb fluid and solutes. About 1.5 metres long, starts in the right iliac region as a dilated part, caecum, in to which the ileum of small intestine opens. Next to caecum, it continues as ascending colon upto lever. There, at right colic flexure, continues to left as transverse colon, to the region of spleen. Here, at left colic flexure, continues down as descending colon. In the lesser pelvis, it continues as a S shaped sigmoid colon which continues down in the posterior wall of pelvis as rectum and anal canal.

Differences from small intestine

1. Larger in calibre.
2. Its longitudinal muscles in the wall concentrate into 3 longitudinal taeniae coli.
3. Due to taeniae coli, wall of colon shows sacculations.
4. Small fat projections - appendices epiploicae are present on the outer surface of colon except at caecum and rectum.
5. Vermiform appendix emerges from caecum, below ileocaecal junction.

Most part is fixed to the posterior abdominal wall, but transverse colon and sigmoid colon have folds of peritoneum –transverse mesocolon and sigmoid mesocolon.

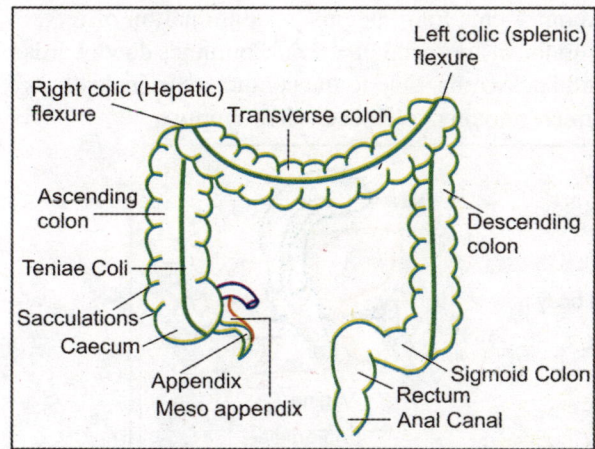

Fig. 7.28: Large Intestine

Caecum and appendix

Caecum is the most dilated part, receives ileoceacal opening, guarded by an ileocaecal valve.

Vermiform appendix is a narrow worm like diverticulum from posteromedial wall of caecum, below ileal end. The most common position of appendix, is retrocaecal. Others are pelvic, subcaecal (below ileum), pre ileal and post ileal.

Appendix vary in length - 2-20 cms, average being 9 cms. It has a short triangular peritoneal fold, connecting to the ileum, mesoappendix. In it, the appendicular vessels run. Its lumen is continuous with that of caecum. It is considered as a specialized, vestigeal structure.

Arterial supply: Appendicular arteries, branches of ileocolic artery.

Surface marking: Base of appendix is marked at McBurney's point – junction between lateral 1/3rd and middle 1/3 rd of a line joining umbilicus and anterior superior iliac spine.

Ascending colon

15 cms long. Covered by peritoneum on three sides. Reaches upto hepatic flexure.

Transverse colon

50 cms long. Covered by peritoneum and transverse mesocolon connects it to the pancreas on the posterior abdominal wall.

Descending colon

25 cms long. Extends upto pelvic brim covered by peritoneum, but no mesocolon.

Sigmoid colon

About 40 cms long. Continues from descending colon through pelvic inlet (brim) into lesser pelvis. Below it becomes continuous with rectum at level with S3 vertebra. It is covered by peritoneum and a fold of peritoneum sigmoid mesocolon attaches it to posterior pelvic wall.

Arterial supply: Ascending colon, and proximal 2/3rd of transverse colon are supplied by branches of superior mesenteric artery. Distal 1/3 rd of transverse colon, descending colon and sigmoid colon are supplied by branches of inferior mesenteric artery.

Veins: Follow arteries and end in superior and inferior mesenteric veins.

RECTUM (Fig. 7.29 a & b)

Continuous with sigmoid colon in front of S_3 vertebra. It descends corresponding to the curvature of sacrum showing a sacral flexure and ends to continue as anal canal after piercing the pelvic diaphragm about 2-3 cms in front of and just below the tip of coccyx at level of apex of prostate in male. It is about 13 cms long. Lower end is slightly dilated-ampulla, and from here, canal bends backwards and downwards – this bent is called perineal flexure of rectum. Rectum also shows 3 lateral flexures.

Rectum is covered by peritoneum on its anterior and lateral surfaces in upper 1/3 rd, only on anterior surface in middle 1/3 rd, and lower 1/3 rd is not covered by peritoneum. Sacculations are absent in rectum and the taeniae coli get spread to form anterior and posterior longitudinal muscular bands.

The mucosa on the interior of rectum shows 3 horizontal semilunar folds which become more marked in rectal distension, in contrast to numerous longitudinal folds which get effaced in distension.

Major relation

Anteriorly upper 2/3 rd is related to sigmoid colon and coils of ileum in the rectovesical pouch in male and rectouterine pouch in female. Lower 1/3rd is related to bladder, seminal vesicle and prostate in male and to vagina in female.

Arteries

1. Superior rectal artery – continuation of inferior mesenteric artery.
2. Middle rectal artery – branch from internal iliac artery.
3. Inferior rectal artery – branch of internal pudental artery.

Veins

1. Superior rectal vain drains into portal vein.
2. Middle rectal vain drains into internal iliac vein.
3. Inferior rectal vein drains into internal pudential vein.

2 and 3 are tributaries of systemic veins. So this is an important site of portocaval anastamosis.

Nerves

Nerve Supply of upper part is autonomic. That of lower part, somatic-inferior rectal nerve.

Lymphatic drainage

Lymphatics from upper part, to para rectal and inferior mesenteric nodes. From lower part, to superficial inguinal nodes.

ANAL CANAL (Fig. 7.29 a & b)

About 4 cms long, begins as continuation of rectal ampulla at anorectal junction. Continues downwards and backwards. Due to the sphincters in its wall, its lumen remains collapsed when empty.

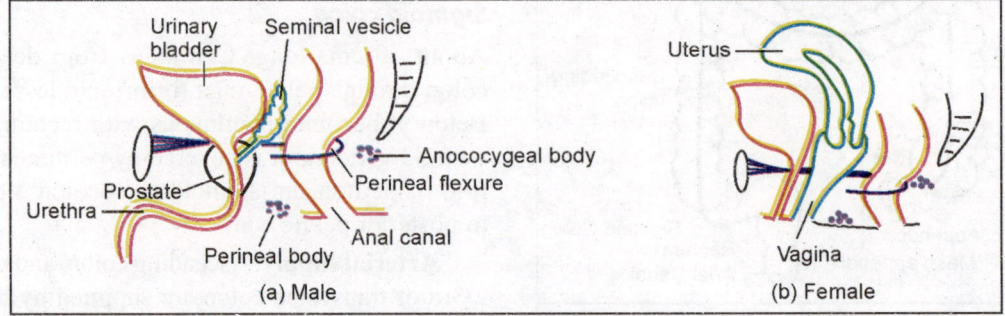

Fig. 7.29

Relations

Male: Anteriorly, perineal body, membraneous urethra and bulb of penis.

Posteriorly, anococcygeal body.

Laterally ischiorectal fossa.

Female: Anteriorly, perineal body and lower part of vagina and urethra.

Posteriorly, anococcygeal body.

Laterally ischiorectal fossa.

Interior of anal canal

The upper 1/3 rd of the mucosa of anal canal is reddish in colour, lined by columnar epithelium, presents about 8-10 vertical columns – anal columns. Deep to anal columns, lie the terminal radicles of superior rectal artery and vein – enlargement of which leads to internal haemorrhoids. Lower ends of anal columns are joined by anal valves, along a line – pecctinate line. (Fig.7.30). Small spaces above anal valves are anal sinuses.

Applied anatomy: Anal glands open into these spaces. If they get infected, leads to abscess formation and fistula. Also a hard faecal matter can tear off an anal valve and cause a long ulcer and anal fissure.

Middle 1/3 rd called pecten, lined by stratified squamous epithelium, is bluish in colour, the lower end of which is marked by White line of Hilton.

Lower 1/3rd is whitish in colour and lined by skin.

Anal musculature (Fig.7.30)

Anal wall has got an inernal anal sphincter and external anal sphincter.

Internal anal sphincter is continuous with the smooth muscle layer of the rectal wall and reaches upto the level of White line.

External anal sphincter is of skeletal muscle, surrounds the hole length of anal canal in 3 parts – subcutaneous, superficial and deep parts.

Tone of the muscle keeps anal canal closed.

The external sphincter is supplied by pudental nerve $(S_2 S_3)$ and S_4 nerves.

Between the external and internal sphincters, there is vertical fibroelastic layer, lower ends of the fibres, being attached to perianal skin. This attachment causes corrugation of the skin there.

Blood supply of Rectum and Anal Canal

Arteries:

1. Superior rectal artery – continuation of inferior mesenteric artery.
2. Middle rectal artery – branch from intrrnal iliae artery.
3. Inferior rectal artery – branch from internal pudental artery.

Veins: (Fig. 7.31)

3 veins and 2 venous plexuses

Superior rectal vein

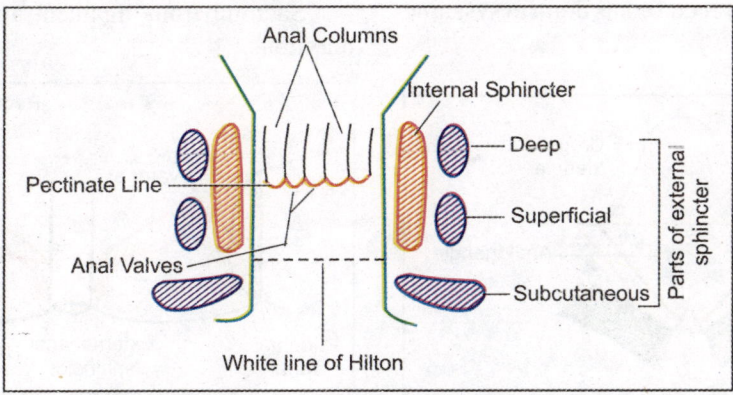

Fig. 7.30: Interior of Anal Canal and Musculature

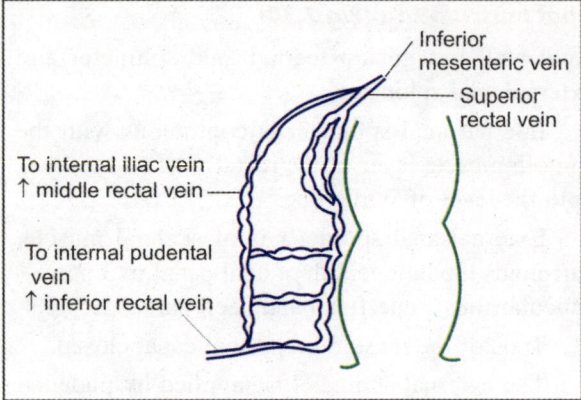

Fig. 7.31

Middle rectal vein

Inferior rectal vein and

Internal and external venous plexuses.

Internal plexus is deep to the mucosa and external being outside the musculature. Both plexuses are interconnected.

Superior rectal vein begins from the upper end of internal venous plexus and continues up as inferior mesenteric vein, thus to portal vein. It also drains upper pat of external venous plexus.

Middle rectal vein drains into internal iliac vein – from internal and external plexuses.

Inferior rectal vein begins from the lower part of external plexus and drains into internal pudental vein.

Middle and inferior rectal veins drain to systemic veins.

This shows, there is communication between portal and systemic venous system in the wall of rectum and anal canal, a site of portocaval (portosystemic) anastamosis.

Applied anatomy: Haemorrhoids (Piles) due to engorgement of venous plexus.

Nerve supply: Upper part has autonomic nerves and lower part, somatic nerve – inferior rectal nerve.

Lymphatic drainage: To internal iliac and superficial inguinal nodes.

Ischiorectal fossa (Fig. 7.33)

Perineum is divisible into 2 triangles by a transverse line that passes just anterior to the ischial tuberosities and anal opening. Anterior one is urogential triangle and posterior one is anal triangle.(Fig.7.32)

In the anal triangle there is a weldge shaped space on either side of rectum and anal canal – seen between ischium and rectum, hence ischiorectal fossa. It is a fascia lined fat filled space, about 5 cm high, 5 cm deep and 2.5 cm wide.

Its base is directed towards the perineum and the apex is along the line of meeting of obturator internus and levator ani.

Boundaries (Fig. 7.33)

Laterally - Ischium and obturator internus.

Medially - rectum and anal canal to which levator ani and sphincter ani externus are applied.

Posteiorly -

Sacrotuberous ligament and overlying gluteus maximus.

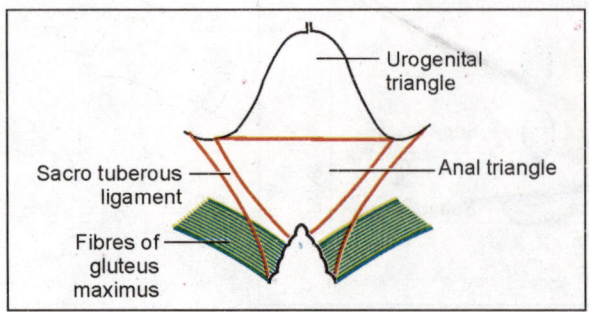

Fig. 7.32

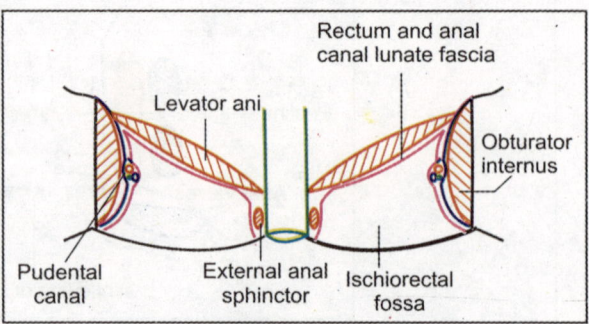

Fig. 7.33: Ischiorectal Fossa

Anteriorly – Posteior border of urogenital diaphragm.

Floor is formed by skin of perineum.

In the formation of the fossa, large pad of fat fills the space deep to the skin and lifts up the deep fascia, towards the fascia covering obturator internus and levator ani muscles and merges with those fasciae. This is the lunate fascia.

Contents

Apart from fat,

1. Internal pudental vessels
2. Pudental nerve

They pass through a fascial canal called pudental canal or Alcock's canal on the lateral wall of the fossa. The canal runs forwards and is formed by obturator fascia and lunate fascia.

Applied anatomy

Abscess in the fossa is rare, but if occurs, it may rupture externally to produce an external sinus. It may also repture into anal canal leading into a fistula.

Pancreas and Liver

They are accessory organs associated with gastrointestinal tract.

PANCREAS (Fig. 7.34, 7.35 a & b)

It is a soft lobulated gland, about 15 cms long, lies almost horizontally across the posterior abdominal

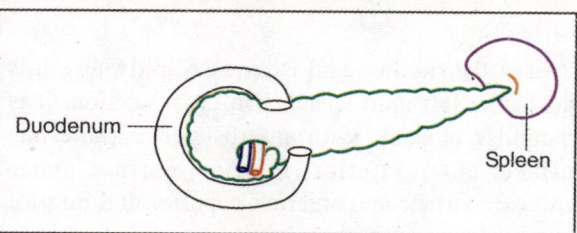

Fig. 7.34

wall, from the duodenum, to the spleen, in the epigastrium and left hypochondrium.

It has both endocrine and exocrine parts. Endocrine part – islets of Langerhans, produces insulin and glucagon. Exocrine part – acini, produces pancreatic juice, conveyed to duodenum through pancreatic duct.

The gland is retroperitoneal and has a Head, Neck, Body and Tail.

Head

Flattened anteroposteriorly, lies in the concavity of duodenum. From its lower part, a hook like part projects to the left, behind the superior mesenteric vessels – the uncinate process. Superior and inferior pancreatico duodenal arteries run and anastamose between head of pancreas and duodenum.

Neck

It is the constriction between head and body. Anterior to it lies the gastro-duodenal artery and posterior to it, the portal vein is formed by union of superior mesenteric and splenic veins.

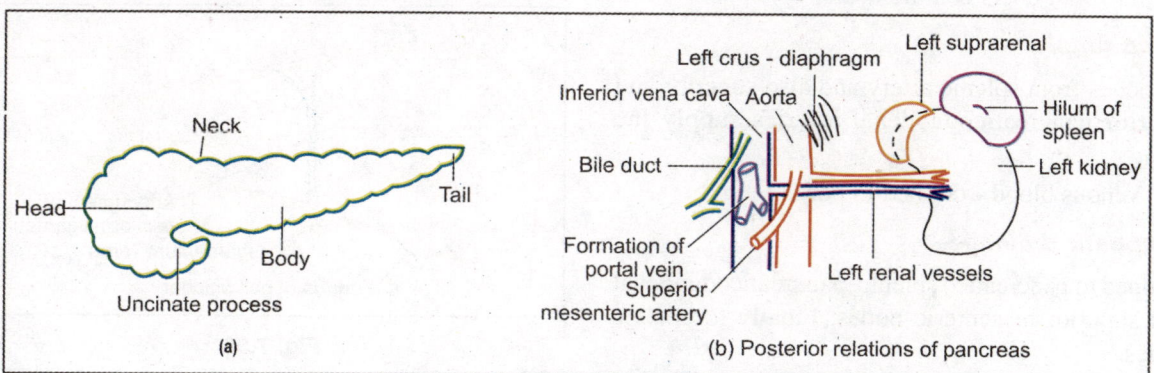

Fig. 7.35

Body

Crosses the midline and extends slightly upwards and to the left upto spleen. On cross section, it is triangular is shape with anterosuperior (anterior) surface, anteroinferior (inferior) surface and a posterior surface and anterior, superior and inferior borders.

Tail

Reaches the hilum of spleen, contained in the lienorenal ligament together with splenic vessels.

Major relations

Anteriorly: From right to left, Ist part of duodenum, transverse colon, attachment of transverse mesocolon and stomach.

Posteriorly: From right to left, bile duct, formation of portal vein, inferior vena cava, aorta with origin of superior mesenteric artery, left crus of diaphragm, left renal vessels, left suprarenal gland, left kidney and hilum of spleen.

Ducts

Main duct of pancreas (of Wirsung), begins in the tail and runs to the right, by receiving numerous small ducts on its way. It joins with the bile duct and opens into the 2nd part of duodenum on the summit of the major duodenal papilla.

Accessory duct (of Santorini) when present, drains the upper part of head and opens a little above the opening of main duct, at the minor duodenal papilla. Both ducts communicate.

Blood supply

Branches from splenic artery and also superior and inferior pancreaticoduodenal arteries supply the gland.

Venous blood - drained to portal vein.

Lymphatic drainage

Drained to pancreatico splenic, pancreaticoduodenal and superior mesenteric nodes. Finally to coeliac nodes.

Applied aspects

1. Pancreatitis – inflammation of pancreas.
2. Carcinoma of head of pancreas.
3. Annular pancreas – due to failure of proper fusion of ventral pancreatic bud with dorsal bud during development.

LIVER

Liver is the largest gland in the body,. Weighs about 1.5 kg. It secretes bile and is involved in carbohydrate, protein and fat metabolisms.

It is soft and friable, reddish brown in colour and highly vascular.

Location

Situated in the upper right part of the abdomen, below the diaphragm, occupying the right hypochrondrium, extending through the epigastrium, into leflt hypochondrium. Most part of it lies under cover of lower ribs and costal cartilages. But at the epigastrium, for about one hand's breadth, it is in contact with anterior abdominal wall.

General features (Fig. 7. 36)

It has superior, arterior, right lateral, posterior and inferior (visceral) surfaces.

A sharp inferior border separates the visceral surface from anterior and right lateral surfaces. This border is notched by ligamentum teres just on the left of midline. About 5 cms to the right of midline,

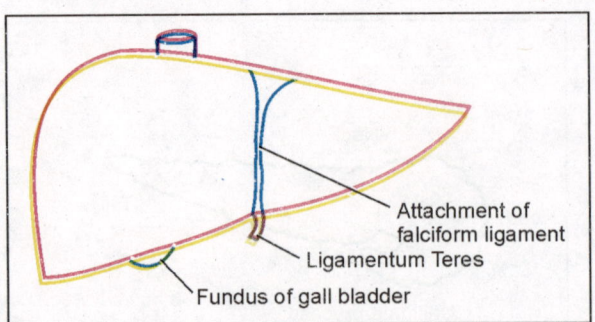

Attachment of falciform ligament
Ligamentum Teres
Fundus of gall bladder

Fig. 7.36

fundus of gall bladder projects below this border. Liver is traditionally divided into right and left lobes along the line of attachment of ligamentum teres.

The organ is almost completely covered by peritoneum except at a small triangular area posteriorly – the bare area. A number of peritoneal folds connect liver to neighbouring organs, as ligaments.

Surfaces and relations

Visceral surface (Fig. 7.37)

Covered by peritoneum except at porta hepatis and fossa for gall bladder.

Porta is a deep transverse fissure and here the portal vein and hepatic artery enter liver and hepatic ducts emerge.

At the left end of porota hepatis, fissure for ligamentum teres meets fissure for ligamentum venosum. In front of the porta hepatis, the quadrate lobe of liver is seen and behind the porta, the caudate lobe and its process, a small extension of caudate lobe, into right lobe of liver.

On the visceral surface of the left lobe, is a large gastric impression, related to stomach. To its right side, an elevated area of liver is tuber omentale; behind which is a shallow groove for oesophagus.

On the right border of quadrate lobe, fossa for gall bladder is seen, where gall bladder is situated.

To its right side, are the duodenal, renal and colic impressions.

Posterior surface

Generally convex, bare area is seen on this surface, as a triangular area of liver, devoid of peritoneum. A deep groove for inferior vena cava is present along the base of the bare area, next to the caudate lobe. Lowr part of bare area shows impression of right suprarenal gland.

Ligaments of liver

1. **Falciform ligament:** A cresentic fold of pepritoneum connects liver to the diaphragm and anterior abdominal wall. From its attachment to the anterior and superior surfaces of liver the two layers of the fold stretch on to the right and left lobes. The free concave border of falciform ligament contains the ligamentum teres.

2. **Coronary ligament:** Connects the posterior and superior surfaces of liver to diaphragm. It has 2 layers upper and lower, both layers enclose the bare area of liver.

3. **Right triangular ligament:** Upper and lower layers of coronary ligament extend to the right and meet to form the right triangular ligament which also connects liver to diaphragm.

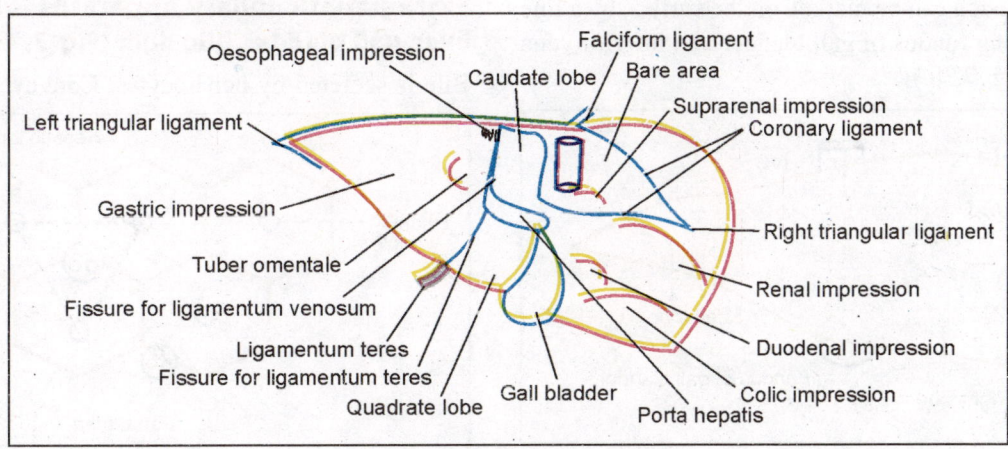

Fig. 7.37: Visceral Surface of Liver

4. **Left triangular ligament:** Extends from the left end of left lobe to the diaphragm. Its two layers – anterior and posterior – are continuous with the peritoneum on superior surface and visceral surface.

5. **Lesser omentum:** Extends from the lesser curvature of stomach and proximal part of duodenum to the porta hepatis and fissure for ligamentum venosum. Between its two layers bile duct, hepatic artery and portal vein are present.

6. **Ligamentum teres:** It is not a peritoneal fold, but a thick ligament present in the free concave margin of falciform ligament. Extends from umbilicus to liver. It is the remnant of obliterated left umbilical vein during development.

Lobes of Liver

Liver is customarily divided into a large right and a smaller left lobe based on certain surface features.

With recent development of imaging methods, it is rational to divide liver into right and left lobes, based on the vascular and biliary duct patterns.

Liver is drained off bile by right and left hepatic ducts which join to form common hepatic duct. The territory drained by right duct is now considered as right lobe and that drained by left duct, left lobe. This division can be marked on the surface by a line connecting fundus of gall bladder and inferior vena cava (Fig. 7.38.)

Segmentation

Each lobe is divisible into a number of segments based on the pattern of hepatic ducts inside liver. 9 (nine) such segments are described.

Lobulation (Fig. 7. 39)

Microscopic structure of liver shows, liver cells (hepatocytes) arranged in radial plates from a central hepatic venule. This hexagonal unit is hepatic lobule of 1 mm diameter. At its corners portal triad can be seen. (branches of hepatic artery, portal vein and bile duct).

A portal lobule is also described, with the portal triad at the centre and portions of 3 adjacent hepatic lobules, around.

Blood Supply of Liver

Artery: Hepatic artery, branch of coeliac trunk enters as 2 branches through porta.

Veins: Portal vein enters through porta as 2 divisions, conveys venous blood from gastrointestinal tract, rich in products of digestion.

Venous blood from liver drains through central veins, to hepatic veins (right and left) which open into inferior vena cava.

Lymphatics: Lymphatics drain to nodes at prota, coeliac nodes and from bare area, to posterior mediastinal nodes.

Extra hepatic billary apparatus – Ducts of liver, gall bladder, bile duct (Fig. 7. 40)

Bile is secreted by hepatocytes. Conveyed through

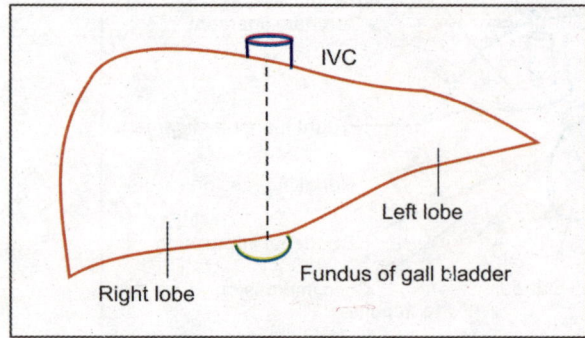

Fig. 7.38

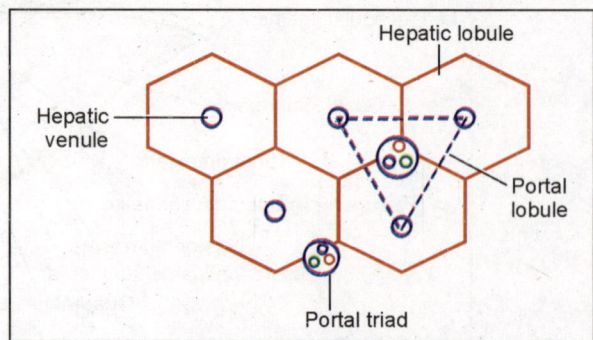

Fig. 7.39: Lobulation of Liver

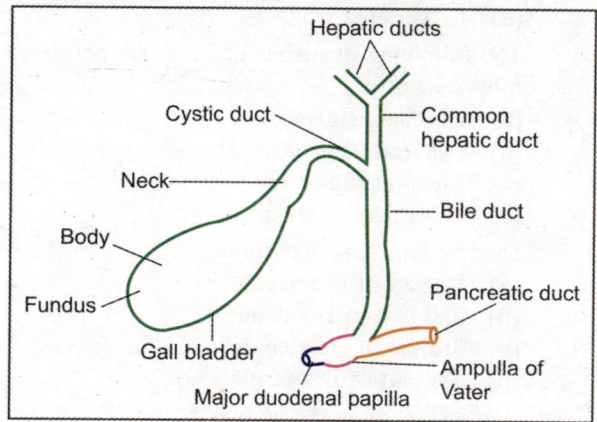

Fig. 7.40

Bile duct is about 8 cms long and descends in the lesser omentum and lies behind the head of pancreas. It pierces middle of the 2nd part of duodenum – on its medial wall where it is joined by pancreatic duct, to form a short dilated duct-hepatopancreatic ampulla (of Vater). The distal narrow end of the ampulla opens into the lumen of 2nd part of duodeum at the summit of major duodenal papilla. The terminal narrow part of the duct (ampulla) is surrounded by a sphincteric muscle (Sphincter of Oddi).

When digestion of fatty food is required, as it enters the duodenum, duodenal mucosa releases the hormone, cholecystokinin. It causes gall bladder to contract and bile is released through cystic and bile ducts, to reach duodenum.

Gall Bladder

This sac, having capacity of about 30 – 50 ml is located on the under surface of liver, in its fossa. It has a fundus, body and neck.

Fundus is rounded, projects below the lower border of liver at level with tip of 9th costal cartilage.

Body lies in contact with under surface of liver, covered by peritoneum.

Neck is continuous with body.

Neck narrows into cystic duct which joins common hepatic duct to form bile duct.

hepatic ducts, to gall ladder, where it is concentrated. Thence conducted to 2nd part of duodenum through bile duct. This system consists of:

- Right and left Hepatic ducts
- Common Hepatic duct
- Cystic duct
- Gal bladder and
- Bile duct

Right and Left hepatic ducts emerge from the two lobes through porta and join to form common hepatic duct.

Common hepatic duct is a about 4 cms long and descends in the free border of lesser omendum. It is joined by cystic duct from gall bladder to from the bile duct.

Single Best Response M.C.Qs

1. Average length of oesophagus is
   (a) 10 cms
   (b) 15 cms
   (c) 20 cms
   (d) 25 cms
2. The main motor nerve of Tongue is
   (a) Facial
   (b) Glossopharyngeal
   (c) Hypoglossal
   (d) Accessary
3. Structure that does not pass through parotid gland is
   (a) Facial artery
   (b) Facial nerve
   (c) Retromandibular vein
   (d) External carotid artery
4. Vertebral level at which oesophagus pierces diaphragm is
   (a) T_6
   (b) T_8

(c) T_{10}
(d) T_{12}

5. Structures along the lesser curvature of stomach are the following except.
   (a) Short gastric arteries
   (b) Right gastric artery
   (c) Left gastric artery
   (d) Lesser omentum

6. Longest part of alimentary tract is
   (a) Oesophagus
   (b) Small intestine
   (c) Large intestine
   (d) Rectum and anal canal

7. Transpyloric plane is at level with
   (a) T_{10} vertebra
   (b) T_{12} Vertebra
   (c) L_1 Vertebra

(d) L_2 Vertebra

8. The following ligaments of Liver are peritoneal folds except
   (a) Coronary ligament
   (b) Falciform ligament
   (c) Ligamentum teres
   (d) Triangular ligament

9. Duct of Pancreas opens into
   (a) Ist part of Duodenum
   (b) 2nd part of Duodenum
   (c) 3rd pat of Duodenum
   (d) 4th part of Duodenum

10. Largest gland in the body is
    (a) Liver
    (b) Pancreas
    (c) Pituitary
    (d) Thyroid

M.C.Qs - Answers

1. (d), 2. (c), 3. (a), 4. (c), 5. (a), 6. (b), 7. (c), 8. (c) , 9. (b), 10. (a)

Essays

I. Name the different parts of digestive tract and describe the stomach.
II. Name the salivary glands and describe the parotid gland.
III. Name the parts of digestive tract and describe the liver.

Short notes

1. Tongue
2. Pharynx
3. Oesophagus
4. Pancreas
5. Liver
6. Gall bladder
7. Duodenum
8. Vermiform appendix
9. Rectum an anal canal
10. Extrahepatic biliary apparatus
11. Lesser omentum
12. Blood supply of stomach

8 Genitourinary Systems

URINARY SYSTEM (EXCRETORY SYSTEM)

Consists of two kidneys, 2 ureters, urinary bladder and urethra. (Fig. 8.1)

Kidneys control the water and electrolyte balance, maintain the acid base balance in the body and excretes the waste products of metabolism as urine. Urine formed in the kidneys is conveyed through the ureters to the urinary bladder which stores it temporarily and is expelled out through urethra.

KIDNEYS (Fig. 8.2)

Bean shaped organs, situated retroperitonially on each side of vertebral column, at level from T_{11} to L_3 vertebrae. It has an upper pole, lower pole, convex lateral margin and concave medial margin, called hilum. Hilum is a vertical slit which leads into a cavity in the kidney, renal sinus. It is through the hilum, the renal vessels enter and leave the kidney and the upper expanded end of ureter, the renal pelvis reaches kidney. (Fig. 8.3) Hilum is at level with transpyloric plane (L_1). Kidneys are obliquely placed, upper pole being 2.5 cms lateral to midline, hilum 5 cms from midline and lower pole, 7.5 cms from midline. Right kidney is slightly at lower level due to the presence of liver. Each is about 11 cms long, 6 cms broad, 3 cms thick and 130–150 gms in weight.

On the dorsal body surface, the position of kidney can be shown to contain in a parallelogram – Morrison's parallelogram as shown in Fig. 8.4. Upper and lower lines, at levels with T_{11} and L_3

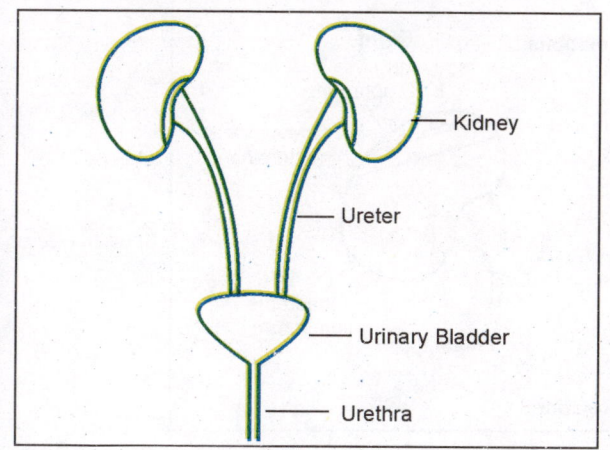

Fig. 8.1

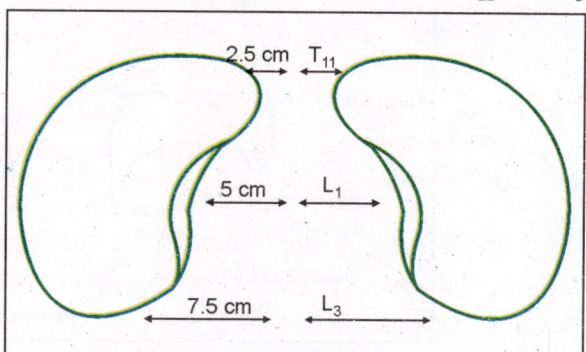

Fig. 8.2

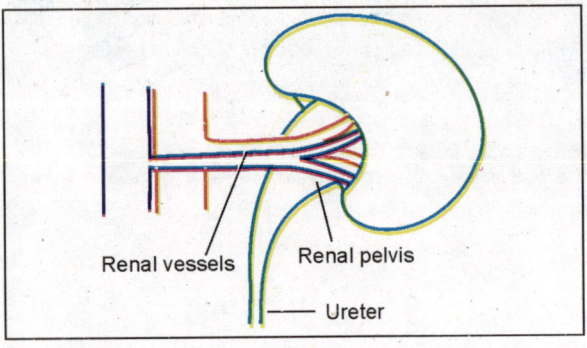

Fig. 8.3

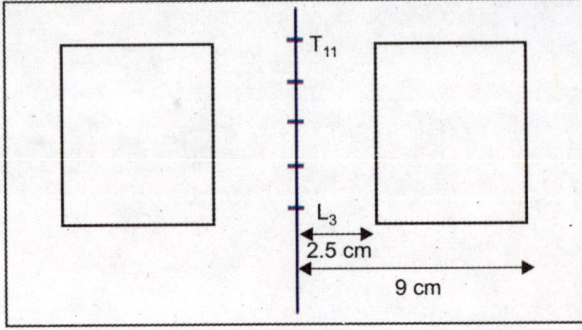

Fig. 8.4

vertebrae. Vertical lines, 2.5 cms and 9 cms from midline.

Coverings of kidney

It has a fibrous capsule of its own. Outside that, a fatty covering, perirenal fat. Next covering is a fascia, renal fascia. Outermost is again an amount of fatty layer – Para renal fat.

Relations of the kidneys are shown in the Fig. 8.5.

General structure of kidney

In a sagital section, kidney has an outer cortex and an inner medulla. Medial border has the renal hilum, through which the upper expanded end of ureter, renal pelvis enters the kidney and divides into 2 or 3

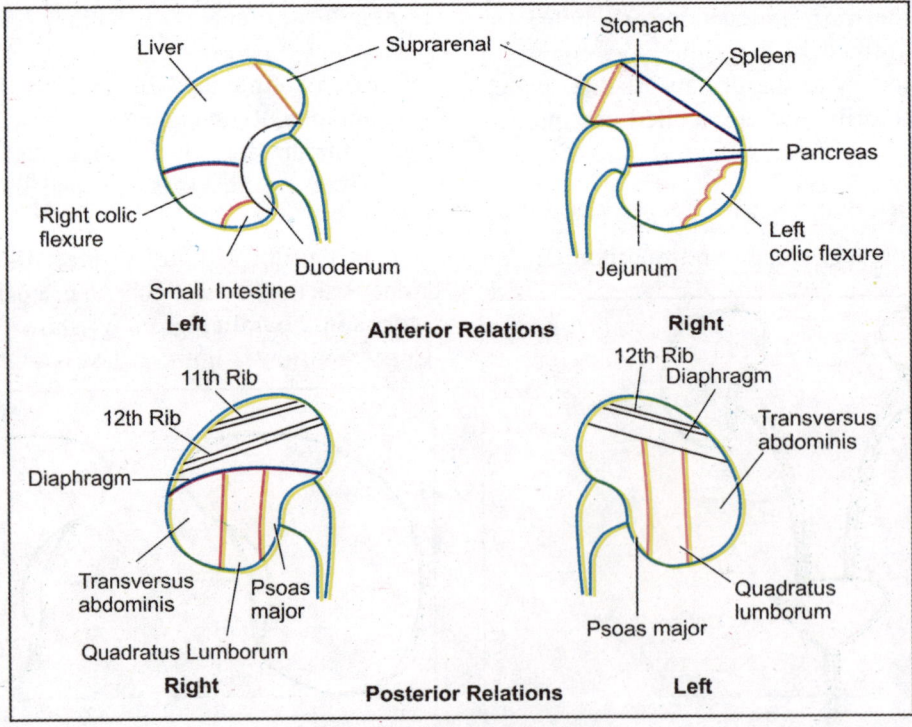

Fig. 8.5: Relations of Kidneys

major calyces and 7 – 14 minor calyces in the sinus of the kidney (Fig. 8.6).

Medulla has conical structures, the renal pyramids, bases of which are directed peripherally and apices are papillae, which project into minor calyces. Outer part is the cortex. A pyramid, capped by the cortex is a **renal lobe.**

Microstructure (Fig. 8.7)

Kidney has many uriniferous tubules. Tubule has a functional unit, the nephron that produces urine and a collecting tubule.

Nephron consists of a renal corpuscle (malpighian), concerned with filtration from plasma and a renal tubule concerned with reabsorption of the filtrate from urine.

Renal corpuscle has a central collection of convoluted capillaries, the glomerulus, surrounded by a Bowman's capsule lined by thin squamous epithelium. From the blood in the capillaries of glumerulus, filtration of excess water and metabolic waste products pass in to the urinary space in Bowman's capsule. From here, filtrate passes through the renal tubule which has proximal convoluted tubule, loop of Henle, distal convoluted tubule which finally leads into the collecting duct. The tubules are concerned with selective reabsorption of the glomerular filtrate to form urine. The ducts open at the apices of pyramids (papillae).

The corpuscles and convoluted tubules occupy the renal cortex and the other tubules and ducts, in the pyramids, in the medulla of kidney.

Blood supply

Kidneys are supplied by renal arteries, branches of abdominal aorta and drained by renal veins into IVC.

At the hilum of kidney, renal artery divides into anterior and posterior divisions and further into segmental arteries. Pattern of branching of the renal artery and their areas of distribution form the basis of renal vascular segmentation. 5 segments are described.

Lymphatic drainage – Into para aortic lymph nodes.

Development

Secretory part – From metanephric blastema

Collecting part – From ureteric bud

Failure of establishment of continuity between these two parts leads to congenital polycystic kidney.

Other anomalies – Pelvic kidney, Horse shoe

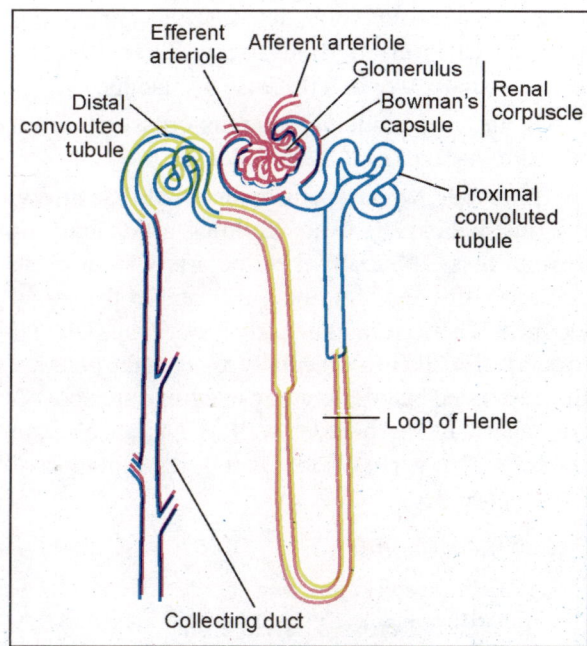

Fig. 8.7: Nephron

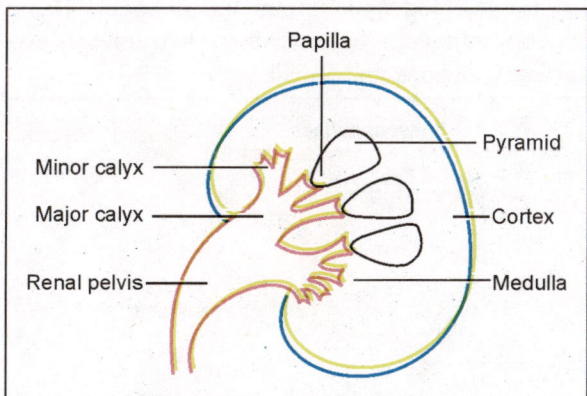

Fig. 8.6: Internal Structure - Kidney

kidney, Pancake kidney, Hilum directed laterally and both kidneys on the same side.

Clinical aspects

1. Infection – Nephritis, pylonephritis
2. Tumours – Mostly cancerous – Hypernephoma, Nephoblastoma
3. Renal failure – Requires renal transplantation
4. Calculi (stone) formation is very common in urinary tract.

URETER (Fig. 8.1)

A narrow muscular tube that conveys urine from kidney to the urinary bladder. Each is about 3 mm in diameter, 25 cms long and half its length is in the abdomen and half in the pelvis.

Continuous above with the renal pelvis. Descends behind the peritoneum, on the psoas major muscle, just lateral to the tips of lumbar transverse processes. In its descent, it crosses genitofemoral nerve and is crossed by gonadal vessels. Each reaches the pelvic brim and enters the lesser pelvis. It turns posterolaterally in front of sacroiliac joint, greater sciatic notch and reaches ischial spine, lying anterior to internal iliac artery. Then it turns anteromedially to reach the base of bladder.

In the male, ductus deferens crosses it from lateral to medial, near the bladder.

In female, where it crosses internal iliac artery, it is just behind the ovary, forming a boundary of ovarian fossa. Medially, Uterine artery is in close contact with ureter for about 2.5 cms in the broad ligament. Then it turns anteriorly about 2 cms lateral to cervix. Finally turns medially to reach the bladder. In a distended bladder ureteric openings are about 5 cms apart. In the bladder wall, it has an oblique course so that when bladder is full, regurgitation of urine is avoided.

Sites of constriction

1. Pelvi ureteric junction.
2. Where it crosses pelvic brim.
3. Where it pierces bladder wall – narrowest.

Structure

Its inner wall mucosa is lined by transitional epithelium. Outer to that, a thick smooth muscle coat and outermost is a fibrous adventitia.

Blood vessels: Along its course, it gets arterial supply from branches of different arteries – renal, abdominal aorta, gonodal, common iliac, internal iliac and vesical arteries.

Lymphatics: Drained to para aortic, common iliac and internal iliac nodes.

Nerves: Autonomic plexus – T_{11} to L_2 segments.

Development – From ureteric bud.

Clinical aspects

Ureteric calculus is common. When it passes through ureter, causes severe spasmodic pain to the surface of the body, in the area supplied by $T_{11} – L_2$ nerves, ie. from loin to groin.

Anomalies

1. Bifid or completely duplicated ureter.
2. Ureter may open into rectum, prostatic urethra, vagina etc.

URINARY BLADDER (Fig. 8.8)

A reservoir of urine, situated in the pelvis, in the adult. But when distended with urine, expands into abdominal cavity. Its average capacity is 120–320 ml. Micturition occurs usually at about 300 ml. Maximum capacity is 500 ml when it gets distended.

Empty bladder is tetrahedral in shape. Has a superior surface, a base (fundus), two inferolateral surfaces, an apex and a neck.

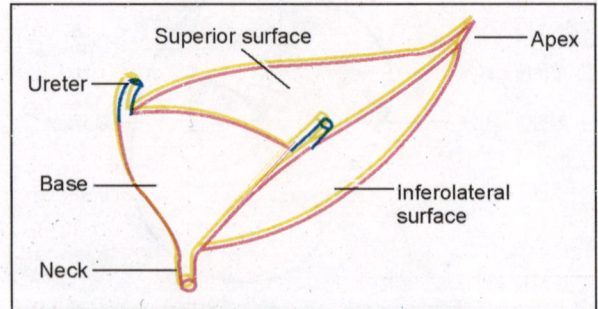

Fig. 8.8: Urinary Bladder

Shape, surfaces and relations (Fig. 8.9)

Base

Its posterior surface, often referred to as fundus or base, is triangular. At its upper two corners, the ureters enter the bladder. Its narrow lower end is the neck, about 3 – 4 cms behind the lower part of pubic symphysis. It is the most fixed part. In male the neck rests on prostate. Urethra emerges from the neck. In male lower part of the base is related to ductus deferens and seminal vesicle. In female, base is in contact with anterior wall of vagina.

Superior surface

It is also triangular having 2 lateral borders, apex directed anteriorly and posterior border, which is the upper border of base. It is completely covered by peritoneum in male and forms rectovesical pouch, behind. From the apex, a median umbilical ligament and fold extends to umbilicus. In female, in its posterior part, the peritoneum gets reflected on to the uterus forming vesicouterine pouch.

Inferolateral surfaces: not covered by peritoneum

When distended, bladder becomes ovoid and its upper part comes in contact with anterior abdominal wall, devoid of peritoneum. There the bladder can be approached through anterior abdominal wall, above pubic symphysis.

Ligaments

1. Pubovesical ligament on each side.
2. Pubourethral in female and Puboprostatic ligament in male.
3. Median umbilical ligament – remnant of urachus.

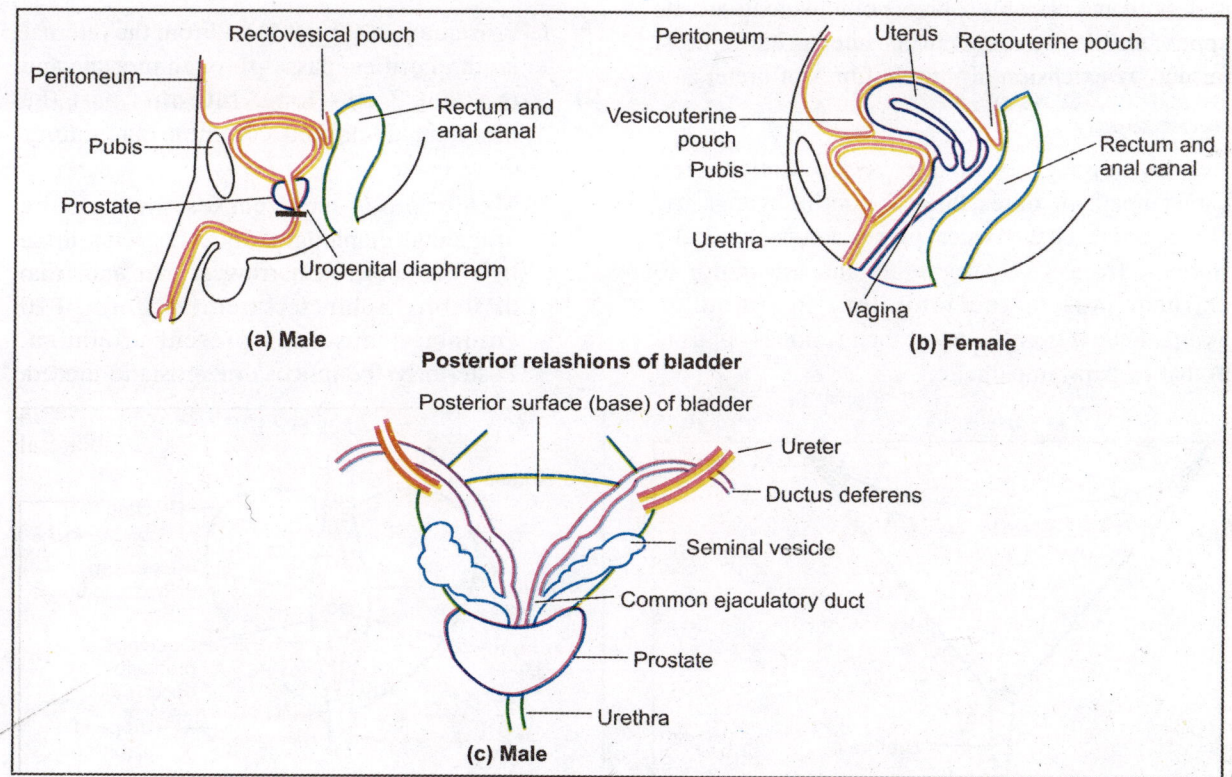

Fig. 8.9: Relations of urinary bladder

4. False ligaments – They are peritoneal folds. Median unbilical fold over the median ligament and 2 medial umbilical folds over obliterated umbilical areteries.

Structure

It has an inner mucosa, lined by transitional epithelium. Mucosa is loosely attached to the deeper lying muscularis except at trigone, to allow distention.

Muscular layer, called detrusor muscle arranged in complex interlacing network is formed of smooth muscle. 3 layers of network are seen generally. This acts as a single unit. Outer surface has a serosal lining.

Trigone (Fig. 8.10)

The triangular space inside the bladder, between the openings of 2 ureters and urethra is devoid of folds, is smooth and has only 2 layers of muscle tissue. Its upper border is prominent as inter ureteric crest formed by extension of muscle fibres of ureter.

Nerve supply

Nerve supply is from sympathetic and parasympathetic fibres, through inferior hypogastric plexus and reach the vesical plexus. Parasympathetic fibres – from S_2–S_4 segments and are motor to detrusor muscle and inhibitory to sphincter. Sympathetic is from T_{11} to L_2; their action is opposite to that of parasympathetic.

Arteries: Superior and inferior vesical arteries form internal iliac.

Veins: Drain to internal iliac vein.

Lymphatic drainage: To external iliac nodes.

Clinical aspects

1. Ectopia vesica-due to malformation of anterior wall of bladder and anterior abdominal wall.
2. Hourglass bladder – constriction at middle.

URETHRA

Male urethra

Extends from the neck of urinary bladder at the internal urethral orifice, to the external meatus at the end of the penis. About 20 cms long and 6 mm in diameter.

Male urethra is described in 3 parts

1. Prostatic part (Fig. 8.11) – From the internal urethral orifice, passes through prostate and is about 3 cms long. Into this part the prostatic ducts and common ejaculatory ducts open.
2. Membranous part, passes through the urogenital diaphragm, about 1.5 cms long. It is the shortest, narrowest part and least dilatable. Sphincter urethrae, formed of voluntary muscle is present around it. Posteriorly the mucosa of prostatic urethra

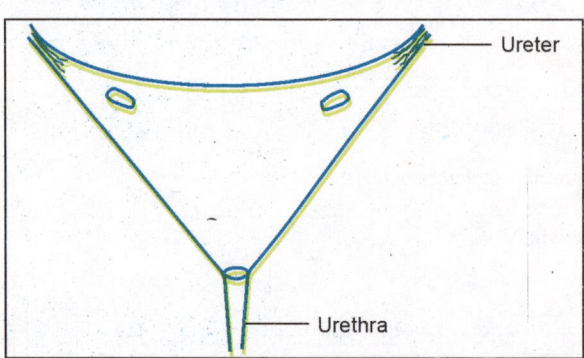

Fig. 8.10: Trigone of Bladder

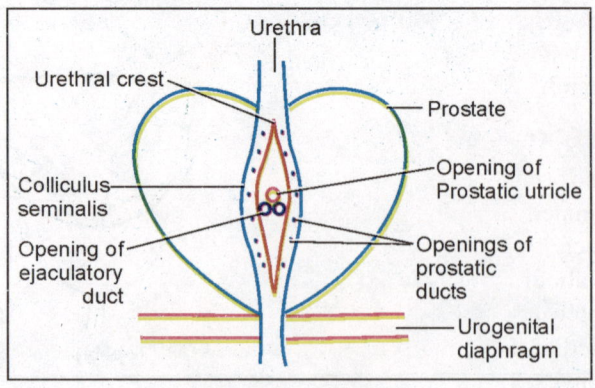

Fig. 8.11: Prostate

has a median crest – urethral crest having a dilation on its middle, colliculus seminalis.

3. Penile part, about 15 cms long. Bulbourethral glands and other small glands open into this part.

Sphincters

1. Internal sphincter – at the neck of uinary bladder, formed of smooth muscle.
2. External sphincter – Sphincter urethra, surrounds membranous urethra. Formed of striated voluntary muscle.

Female Urethra

About 4 cms long and 6 mm in diameter. It is closely related to the anterior wall of vagina.

Epithelium of urethra

Upto membranous part, mucosa in male is lined by transitional epithelium. Beyond that, epithelium is pseudostratified and stratified columnar epithelium. Distal end has stratified squamous epithelium. Mucosa of female urethra is lined by stratified squamous epithelium.

GENITAL SYSTEM – REPRODUCTIVE SYSTEM

MALE REPRODUCTIVE SYSTEM

The male genital organs are the Testes, Epididymis, Vas deferens, Ejaculatory duct and Penis. Associated with these structures are accessory glands – seminal vesicle, prostate and bulbourethral glands.

Testis

The primary reproductive organ or gonad in the male, situated in the scrotal sac, the right and left testis. Each is ellipsoidal in shape, compressed laterally. It is about 4 – 5 cms long, 2.5 cms broad and 3 cms anteroposteriorly. About 10 – 15 gms in weight. Medial and lateral surfaces and anterior border are convex. Posterior border is almost straight.

Situated in the scrotum, having an outer skin and closely lined on inside by a layer of smooth muscle-dartos. Inner to dartos there are the external spermatic fascia, cremasteric fascia and internal spermatic fascia surrounding the testis and its coverings in the scrotal sac.

Coverings of testis are:

1. Outermost layer – Tunica vaginalis, having a visceral layer and parietal layer of serous membrane.
2. Tunica albugenia, a fibrous layer.
3. Tunica vasculosa – formed of a plexus of blood vessels.

Structure (Fig. 8.12):

Inside the testis, it contains numerous convoluted seminiferous tubules inside which spermatogenesis takes place. Among the seminiferous tubules, there are interstitial cells of Leydig which are endocrine in function and produce testosterone.

Seminiferous tubules of testis lead posteriorly as straight tubules, then as a network of small tubules, rete testes in the thick posterior part of tunica albugenia (mediastinum testes). From the rete, the tubules proceed as efferent ductules at the upper pole of testes.

Blood supply of testis

Testicular artery, a branch of abdominal aorta. It descends and reaches the testis by passing through the inguinal canal, in the spermatic cord.

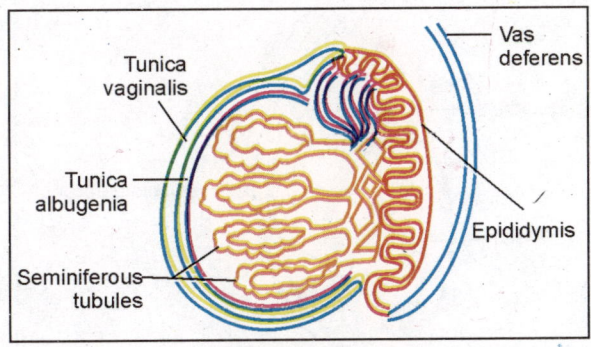

Fig. 8.12: Testis

Testicular vein starts as a venous plexus – Pampiniform plexus, passes back through the spermatic cord and at the deep inguinal ring, forms the testicular vein. Right vien empties into inferior vena cava and left one into left renal vein.

Lymphatic drainage

Lymphatics reach the lateral aortic nodes.

Nerves

Sympathetic – from T_{10} and T_{11} segments of spinal cord.

Development

Develops from the intermediate mesoderm of the embryo, in relation to the posterior abdominal wall and then descends to reach the scrotum. Descent is facilitated by a peritoneal pouch, the processus vaginalis, which gets attached to the developing testis: It descends and passes through the lower end of anterior abdominal wall through a passage which forms the inguinal canal and reaches the scrotum. Here the testis is seen to be invaginated into the distal end of processus vaginalis, where it is known as tunica vaginalis. Remaining part of tunica vaginalis gets obliituated.

Anomalies

1. Anomalous decent of testis. One or both testis may fail to reach the scrotal sac. It may remain in the lumbar region or iliac fossa or inguinal canal. Condition is called cryptorchidism.
2. Persistance of processus vaginalis leads to inguinal hernia.
3. Persistance of processus vaginalis in the testis can lead to accumulation of fluid with in it – hydrococle.
4. Testis may not develop.

Epididymis (Fig. 8.13)

The efferent ductules from the testis go to form the epididymis. The tubules become highly convoluted to form the head of epididymis behind the upper end of testis. The lesser convolution below form the body and tail of epididymis. At the tail, the duct of epididymis forms the ductus deferens. Thus epididymis is applied to the posterior border of testis.

Ductus deferens (Fig. 8.14) (Vas deferens)

Continues from the tail of epididymis. Ascends along the posterior aspect of testis and enters the spermatic cord attached to the upper end of testis. Inside the spermatic cord, it traverses the inguinal canal and enters the abdomen through deep inguinal ring. It hooks round the inferior epigastric artery and descends to the lesser pelvis to reach the posterior surface of urinary bladder, crossing the ureter. Here each duct joins with the duct of seminal vesicle of

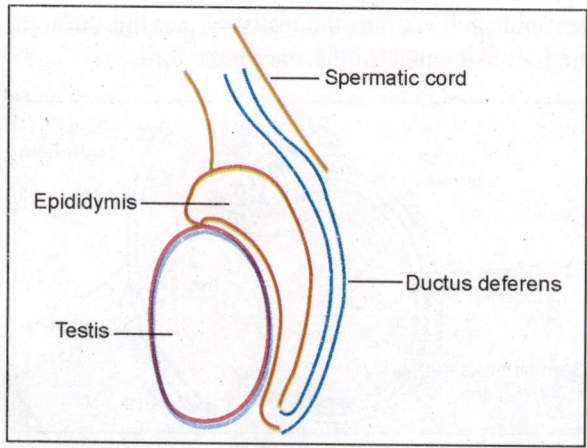

Fig. 8.13

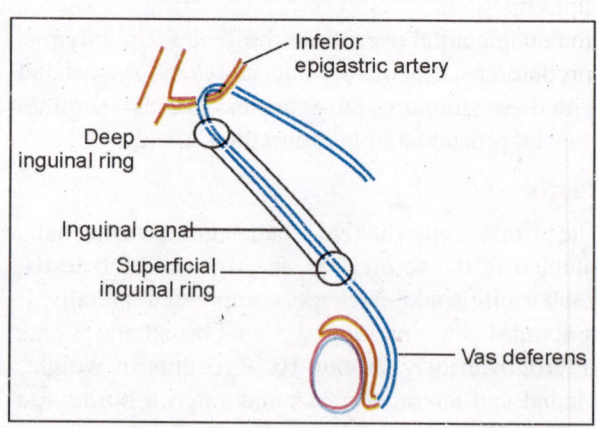

Fig. 8.14

that side and forms the ejaculatory duct. They pass through the prostate and open in the prostatic urethra on the colliculus seminalis on either side of opening of prostatic utricle.

Vas deferens has a narrow lumen and is thick walled by smooth muscle tissue. So it is palpable as a cord. Throughout, it is a straight tube except at the posterior surface of bladder near its termination, where it is dilated and slightly tortuous. Its lumen is lined by simple columnar epithelium. Artery that supplies it is a branch from superior vesical artery.

Penis

It has a fixed part, root fixed to the perineum and a free part or body. The distal end of penis is slightly enlarged, the glans penis.

The substance of penis is formed of three masses of spongy erectile tissue, covered by a fibrous sheath, superficial fascia and skin. (Fig. 8.15 a b) The two dorsal masses are corpora cavernosa and the ventral mass is corpus spongiosum, which is traversed by the penile part of urethra.

At the root of penis, the 2 corpora cavernosa separate and are called crura, which are attached to the right and left borders of the bony pubic arch. At the root, the corpus spongiosum is enlarged (bulb of penis) and is attached to inferior surface of perineal membrane.

The skin covering the penis is loosely attached upto the glans, where it is firmly attached. Anterior to that, glans is covered by a loose fold of skin called prepuse, upto the tip.

Blood supply

Arteries – Deep and dorsal arteries of penis, branches of internal pudendal artery.

Veins – Superficial and deep dorsal veins which are unpaired. Superficial vein ends in external pudendal vein and deep vein ends in internal iliac vein.

Lymphatics – Drained into superficial inguinal nodes. From the glans penis, into deep inguinal nodes.

Nerve – Dorsal nerve of penis, branch of pudendal nerve.

Seminal vesicles (Fig. 8.9 c)

They are two sacculated structures, each about 5 cms long, present between the bladder and rectum. Its upper broader part is seen laterally and narrow lower tubular part joins with vas deferens to form the ejaculatory duct. In structure, it is a highly coiled tube with many diverticula, the inner lining epithelium has goblet cells. Secretion of seminal vesicle adds about 70 % of the seminl fluid and also it modifies the sperms activity.

Prostate (Fig. 8.16 a b)

Prostate is a fibromuscular and glandular organ seen below the bladder, surrounding the initial part of male urethra. It has a base in contact with the neck of the bladder, an apex directed downwards, is behind the lower border of symphysis pubis and pubic arch. It has also a posterior, anterior and 2 inferolateral surfaces. It is about 4 cms transversely,

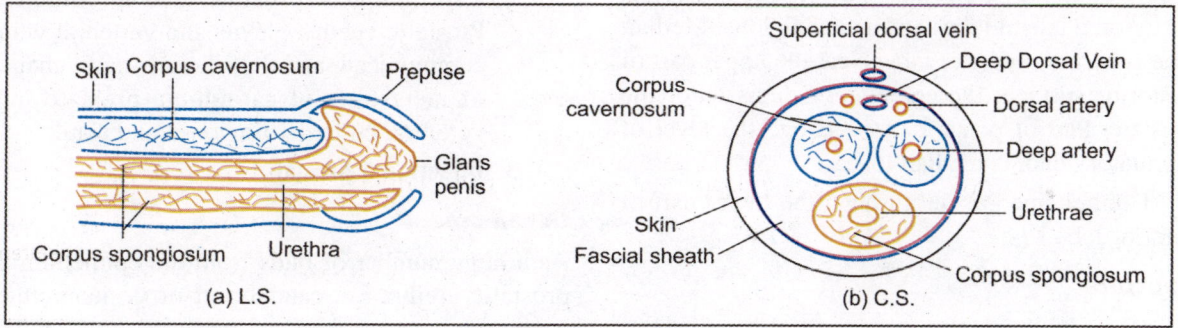

Fig. 8.15: Penis

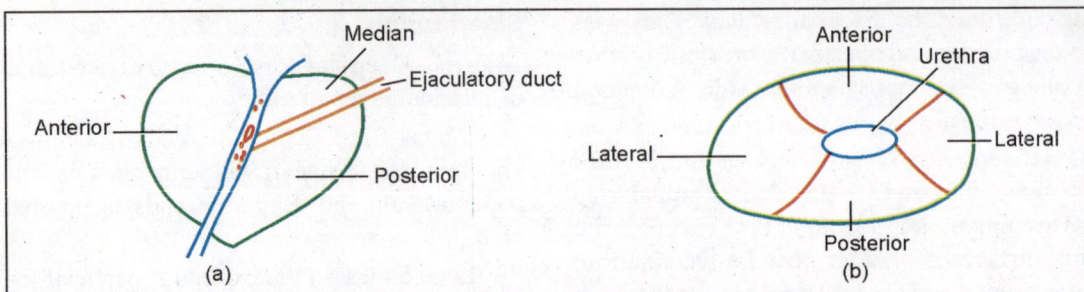

Fig. 8.16: Prostate - Lobes

3 cms vertically, 2 cms anteroposteriorly and 8 gms in weight. The urethra, ejaculatory duct and prostatic utricle are seen to pass through prostate. Prostate is a remnant of lower end of paramesonephric duct.

Relations

Anteriorly connected to the pubic bones by right and left puboprostatic ligaments. Posterior surface is in contact with the ampulla of rectum through which prostate can be palpated. The posterior surface is seperated from the rectum by a fascial septum which is formed by fusion of 2 layers of rectovesical peritoneal pouch. The septum is called Denonvillier's fascia. Inferolateral surfaces are in contact with levator ani muscles.

It has a fibrous capsule of its own and outside that, a fibrous sheath formed by condensation of pelvic fascia. Between the two, there is a venous plexus.

Lobes of prostate

Traditionally 5 lobes are described. Anterior, posterior, 2 lateral lobes and a median lobe. Median lobe is part of posterior lobe. Near the upper part of posterior surface, the ejaculatory ducts enter the prostate. Part of posterior lobe above the level of ejaculatory duct is median lobe.

Urethra emerges out through the lower part of anterior lobe.

Structure

Has glandular tissue separated by fibrous-muscular bundles – muscle being smooth muscle. Glandular tissue is formed of follicles and papillae, lining cells being columnar. About 14–20 prostatic ducts open into the sinus of prostatic urethra. Prostatic and seminal vesicle's secretions form the bulk of seminal fluid.

Blood supply

Arteries – Branches from inferior vesical, middle rectal and internal pudendal arteries.

Veins – Prostatic venous plexus drains into internal iliac vein.

Nerves – Autonomic nerves from inferior hypogastric plexus.

Lymphatics – To internal and external iliac nodes.

Applied aspects

1. Benign enlargement in old age – adenoma. Mostly seen in median lobe. It can cause obstruction to flow of urine.

2. Carcinoma of prostate also is common. Prostatic venous plexus and vertebral veins communicate and thus there is more chance of metastasis of carcinoma prostate into vertebral column, hip bones and skull.

3. Infection – prostatitis.

Development

As a large number of buds from the epithelium of prostatic urethra i.e. caudal part of vesicourethral canal.

Bulbourethral glands

The two glands right and left arc seen on either side of membranous urethra, in the sphincter urethra. Their ducts open into penile part of urethra and secretion adds to seminal fluid.

FEMALE REPRODUCTIVE SYSTEM

The female reproductive organs include the ovaries, fallopian tubes, uterus and vagina (all situated in the pelvis) and the external genital organs.

OVARIES (Fig. 8.17)

Ovaries are the female gonads that produce the female gametes, ova. Each is almond shaped and in nulliparous woman, about 3.5 cms long, 1.5 cms broad and 1 cm thick. Lies in relation to the lateral pelvic wall, in the ovarian fossa, behind the broad ligament of uterus. Broad ligament is a double fold of peritoneum that stretches from the sides of uterus to lateral pelvic wall and floor of pelvis. From the posterior surface of the broad ligament, a fold – mesovarium extends to get attached to the ovary and covers it. Part of broad ligament from the ovary to lateral pelvic wall is called suspensory ligament of ovary. From the lower pole of ovary, the ligament of ovary passes between the 2 layers of broad ligament to get attached to the uterus, near the tubal opening. The medial surface of ovary is overhung by the fimbriated end of uterine tube.

Structure of ovary

On section, it has an outer cortex which is the seat for oogenesis (production of ova). Inner medulla is a fibrovascular area. In the cortex, varying stages of follicles grow, which contain developing ova. During reproductive life of a female, every month, one follicle will grow into Graafian follicle in which mature ovum will be formed. Tissue surrounding the Graafian follicle is called thecal gland and liberates oestrogen. One ovum will be discharged from one ovary every month. The remaining part of follicle changes into corpus luteum that liberates progesterone.

Blood supply

Branches from uterine artery and ovarian artery.

Ovarian veins start as a plexus and join to form the right and left ovarian veins. Right one empties into inferior vena cava and left one ends in left renal vein.

Lymphatics :– go to para-aortic nodes.

Nerves :– Autonomic nerves.

Uterine tube (fallopian tube) (Fig. 8.17)

Each tube, about 10 cms long lies in the upper free margin of broad ligament. Its medial end opens into the corresponding side of the uterus, below the fundus. This is the narrowest part of the tube and is called intra-mural part. Next part is thick walled and narrow and is the isthmus. Next about 5 cms is the

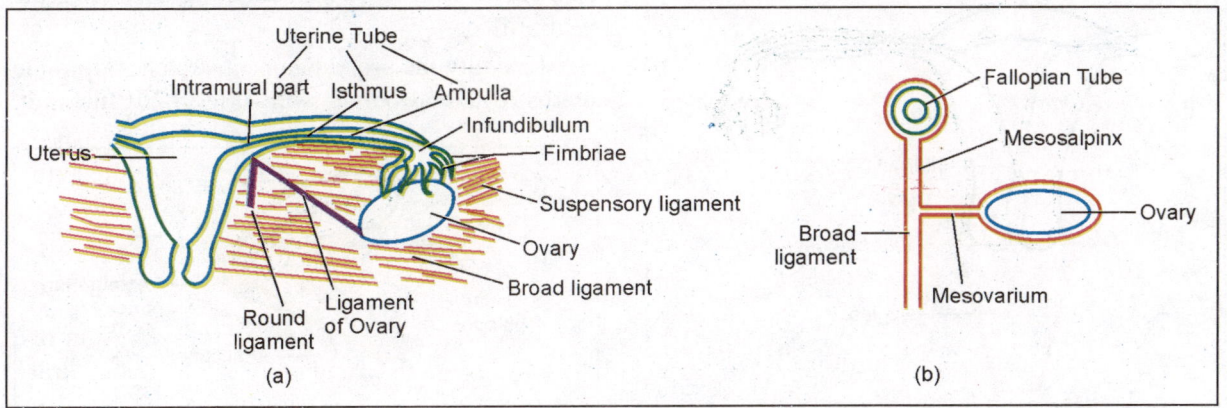

Fig. 8.17

thin walled widest part, ampulla. Usually fertilisation of gametes takes place in the ampulla. Lateral end of the tube is infundibulum. From the infundibulum, finger like processes – fimbriae hang over the ovary. This sucks in the ovum liberated from the ovary. The lumen of fallopian tube has mucosa, lined by ciliated columnar epithelium which helps in the transportation of fertilized egg. Part of broad ligament that extends up to cover the fallopian tube is mesosalpinx.

Blood supply

Branches from the uterine and ovarian arteries. Veins accompany the arteries. **Lymphatics** drain into para aortic nodes.

Nerve supply

Autonomic nerves. Sympathetic, from T_{10}–L_2 spinal segments Parasympathetic, from Vagus and pelvic splanchnic nerves.

UTERUS (Fig. 8.18)

Uterus is a hollow muscular organ situated in the lesser pelvis between rectum and bladder. After conception, as the embryo and foetus grows inside the uterus, it grows into the abdomen.

Nulliparous uterus is 7.5 cms long, 5 cms wide (at its broadest part) and 2.5 cms thick. The fallopian tubes open into the uterus at the upper part of its sides.

Parts

Part above the level of opening of fallopian tubes is fundus.

Main part below that is the body. The narrower lowest part is cervix. The uterine cavity narrows at internal os where it becomes continuous with the cervical canal. Cervix opens distally into the anterior aspect of the upper part of vagina at the external os.

Position of uterus (Fig. 8.21)

The long axis of the body of uterus is bent at an angle of about 170 degrees with the long axis of cervix. This is the position of anteflexion.

Long axis of uterus as a whole is bent at an angle of 90 degrees with the long axis of vagina. This is the position of anteversion. When the uterus is bent back, it is retroverted and retroflexed.

Relations (Fig. 8.19)

Anterior surface is bent on the superior surface of urinary bladder. Peritoneal reflection from the uterus to the upper surface of bladder forms the uterovesical fold and the space is vesicouterine pouch. Posteriorly related to the rectum, the peritoneum from the posterior surface of uterus, cervix and upper vagina, being reflected to the front of rectum, forming the rectouterine pouch of Douglas. The base of pouch of Douglas is at level with about 5.5 cms from the anal orifice.

Laterally the broad ligament stretches from the uterus to lateral pelvic wall. (Fig. 8.20) Inside it,

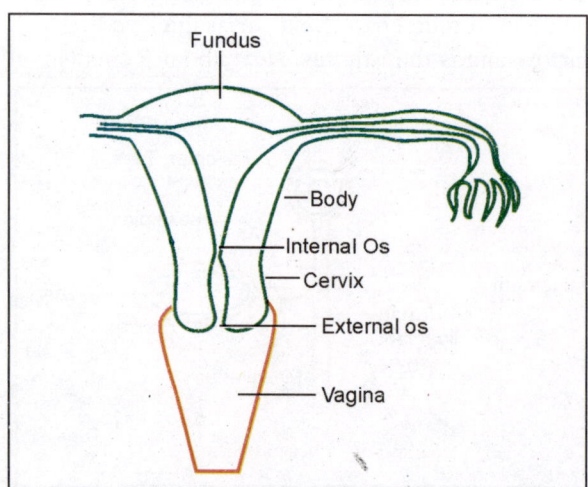

Fig. 8.18

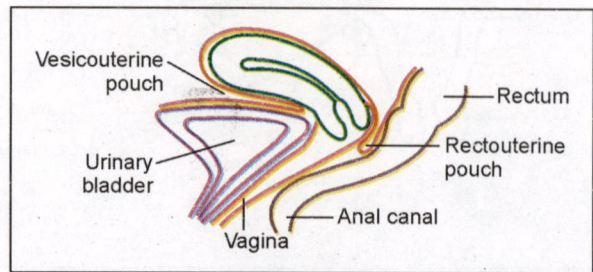

Fig. 8.19

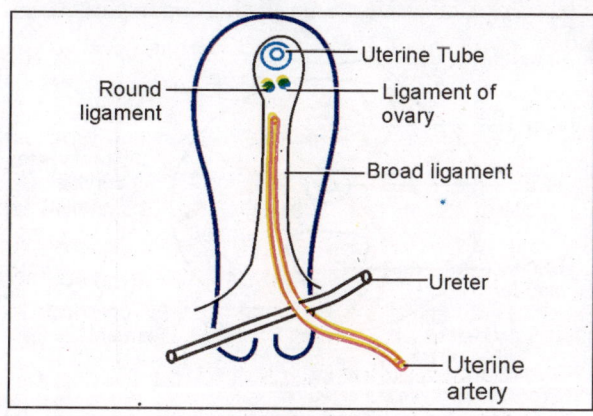

Round ligament

Uterine Tube

Ligament of ovary

Broad ligament

Ureter

Uterine artery

Fig. 8.20

structures, closely related to uterus are from below upwards, uterine vessels, ureter, round ligament of uterus, ligament of ovary and uterine end of fallopian tube.

Blood supply

Uterine artery and branches from ovarian artery supply the uterus.

Veins drain into internal iliac vein.

Nerve supply

Sympatheic and parasympathetic – from inferior hypogastric plexus.

Lymphatic drainage (Fig. 8.22)

From the cervix, drained to external iliac, internal iliac, rectal and sacral nodes.

From the lower part of body, to external iliac nodes, together with cervical lymphatics.

From the upper part of body, fundus, fallopian tubes and ovaries, lymphatics go to the pre- and lateral aortic nodes.

From the region of tubal attachment, lymphatics accompany the round ligament and reach the superficial inguinal lymph nodes.

Supports of uterus

Muscular and ligamentous factors support the uterus.

Muscular

Levator ani and perineal body form the musculofascial support. Levator ani that forms major part of pelvic diaphragm is broad and gives effective support to the uterus. Perineal body also has an equal role in giving support to uterus. If it is torn during child birth, prolapse of uterus can develop later.

Ligamentous (Fig. 8.23)

They are condensations of connective tissue of pelvic floor and give strong support to uterus.

1. Transverse cervical or Meckendrot's ligament or cardinal ligament. This is the most important and strongest ligament, stretches from the sides of cervix and upper vagina to the lateral wall of pelvis.

2. Pubocervical ligament. From the posterior surface of pubic bones to the anterior surface

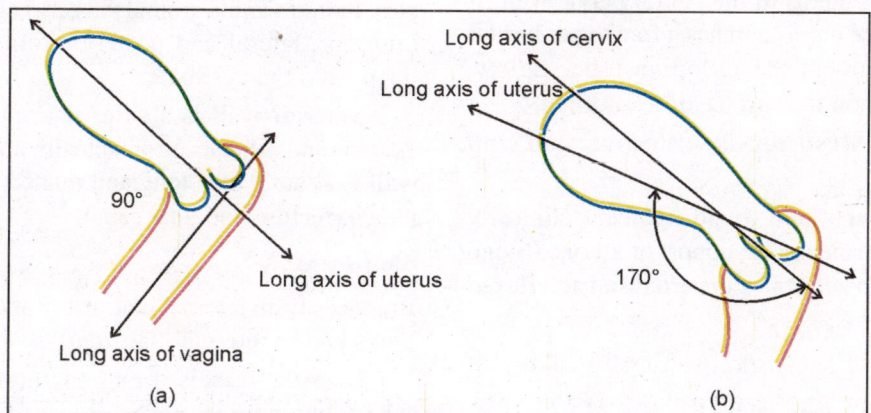

Long axis of cervix

Long axis of uterus

90°

Long axis of uterus

Long axis of vagina

(a)

170°

(b)

Fig. 8.21

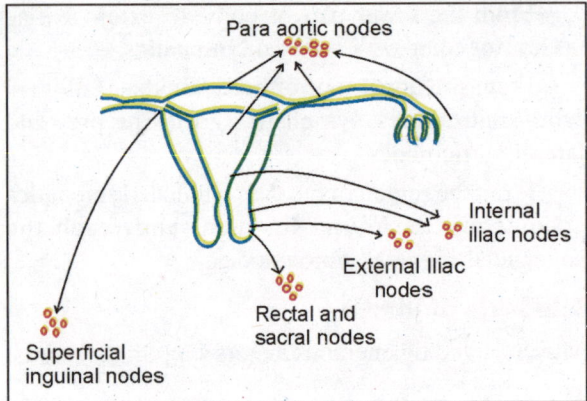

Fig. 8.22: Lymphatic Drainage

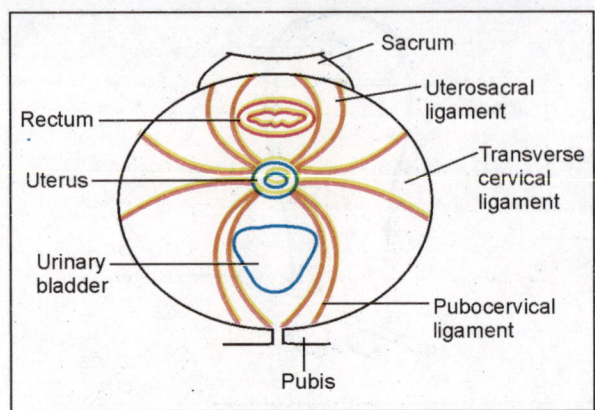

Fig. 8.23

of uterus and upper vagina, around the urethra.

3. Uterosacral ligament. From the back of cervix and lower uterus, to the sacrum around the rectum.

4. Round ligament is a narrow flat band that stretches from near the tubal attachment of uterus, passes through the inguinal canal and finally splits into strands in the connective tissue of labia majora. Round ligament and ligament of ovary are continuous and are remnants of the same embryological tissue.

5. Broad ligament – It is a broad double layered peritoneal fold, extending from the lateral aspect of uterus to the lateral pelvic wall. It covers the uterus and has a free upper border which covers the fallopian tube. Below, diverges on the surface of levator ani.

Parts are Mesosalpinx, mesovarium and mesometrium.

Broad ligament and round ligament clinically play very minor role in the support of uterus. Round ligament helps to keep the anteverted and anteflexed positions of uterus.

Structure

Uterus has three layers.

Innermost is the endometrium lined by simple columnar epithelium. Endometrium has the uterine glands and blood vessels in the endometrial stroma.

Outer to that is the thick muscle wall formed of smooth muscles, myometrium. Outermost is a serosal covering, perimetrium.

Development

From the fused lower ends of Mullarian (paramesonephric) ducts.

VAGINA

It is a muscular tube with anterior and posterior walls.

Cervix opens into the anterior aspect of its upper part. Part of vagina around the cervix is called fornix. (anterior, lateral and posterior fornices) Below it opens into the vestibule.

Anterior wall is shorter than posterior wall – 7.5 cms and is in close contact with urethra. Posterior wall is about 9 cms long and related to rectouterine pouch, rectum and anal canal.

Blood supply

Branches from internal iliac artery and uterine artery. Veins end in internal iliac vein.

Lymph vessels - end in internal iliac and superficial inguinal nodes.

External genital organs

1. Mons pubis – It is the raised hair bearing area of skin in front of pubis.
2. Labia majora – They are two prominent longitudinal hear bearing folds extending back from the mons to the perineal body.
3. Labia minora – They are 2 smaller hairless folds of soft skin, seen medial to the labia majora. Around the vaginal orifice, they go posteriorly and meet to form a sharp fold. Their anterior ends split to enclose the clitoris.
4. Vestibule – It is the space between the labia minora and contains the external orifices of urethra, vagina and greater vestibular glands (of Bartholin) similar to bulbourethral glands in male.
5. Clitoris – Situated at the upper end of vestibule, formed of erectile tissue, homologus with the penis.
6. Vaginal orifice and Hymen – Vaginal orifice is seen below the urethral orifice. Hymen is a thin fold of mucous membrane with a central hole, protecting the vaginal orifice. Seen in virgins.

Single Best Response M.C.Qs

1. Following are correct about kidneys except.
   (a) They are retroperitoneal
   (b) They extend from T_{11} to L_3 vertebral levels vertically.
   (c) Left kidney is slightly at lower level.
   (d) Medial concave margin is hilum.
2. Vertebral level of hilum of kidney is
   (a) T_{12}
   (b) L_1
   (c) L_2
   (d) L_3
3. Renal pyramids are present in
   (a) Cortex
   (b) Medulla
   (c) Sinus
   (d) Pelvis
4. Bowman's capsule is lined by
   (a) Simple squamous epithelium
   (b) Simple cuboidal epithelium
   (c) Simple columnar epithelium
   (d) Transitional epithelium
5. Length of the ureter is about
   (a) 15 cms
   (b) 20 cms
   (c) 25 cms
   (d) 30 cms
6. Sites of constriction of ureter are the following except.
   (a) Pelviureteric junction.
   (b) Where it crosses pelvic brim
   (c) Where it is crossed by uterine artery in female and vas deferens in male.
   (d) Where it pierces bladder wall.
7. Maximum capacity of urinary bladder is
   (a) 200 ml
   (b) 300 ml
   (c) 400 ml
   (d) 500 ml
8. Length of male urethra is about
   (a) 25 cms   (b) 20 cms
   (c) 15 cms   (d) 10 cms
9. Ejaculatory ducts open into
   (a) Urinary bladder
   (b) Prostatic urethra
   (c) Membranous urethra
   (d) Penile urethra
10. Part of peritoneal fold that extends from ovary to lateral pelvic wall is
    (a) Suspensory ligament
    (b) Ligament of ovary
    (c) Mesovarium
    (d) Round ligament.

M.C.Qs - Answers

1. (c), 2. (b), 3. (b), 4. (a), 5. (c), 6. (c), 7. (d), 8. (b), 9. (b), 10. (a)

Essays

  I. Name the parts of urinary system and describe the urinary bladder.
 II. Describe the kidneys
III. Describe the position, parts, relations, blood supply, lymphatic drainage and supports of uterus.

Short notes

1. Ureter
2. male urethra
3. Testis
4. Vas deferens
5. Prostate
6. Ovary
7. Fallopian tube
8. Supports of uterus
9. Nephron
10. Trigone of bladder.

9 Endocrine System

It includes glands of internal secretion i.e., they are ductless glands and their secretion – hormones pass directly into blood. Endocrine glands are highly vascular not only for their own metabolic needs, but also for transport of secretion to different parts of body.

They are: Pituitary gland (hypophysis cerebri)

Thyroid gland

Parathyroid glands

Adrenal (suprarenal) glands

Also epithelial cells present scattered or in groups in certain organs have endocrine function.

PITUITARY GLAND

The hormones secreted by the pituitary gland influence the activities of other endocrine glands. So it is known as **master endocrine gland.**

Located in the middle cranial fossa, over the surface of body of sphenoid, in the sella tursica (pituitary fossa). It is continuous with the hypothalamic region of brain through a hollow stalk – infundibulum. Sella tursica and pituitary gland are roofed by a fold of dura mater, diaphragma sella. Infundibulum passes through a hole in the diaphragma.

Pituitary gland is roughly ovoid in shape, 12 mm broad, 8mm anteroposteriorly and 7mm vertically.

Important relations

Below – sphenoidal air sinus

Anterosuperiorly - optic chiasma

Laterally – on either side, the carvernous sinus with III, IV, V_1 and V_2, VI cranial nerves and internal carotid artery, inside it.

A tumour in pituitary can cause pressure effects on all the important neighbouring structures.

Parts (Fig. 9.1)

Pars anterior

Pars intermedia

Pars posterior - neurohypophysis

(pars nervosa)

Pars anterior and pars intermedia developmentally have same origin from Rathke's pouch of stomatodeum.

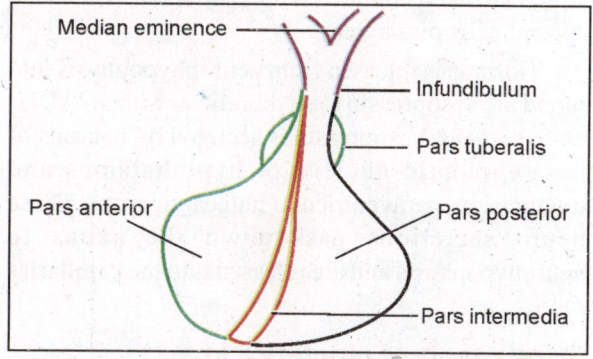

Fig. 9.1: Pitutary Gland (Hypophysis Cerebri)

There is a cleft between them which usually obliterates in childhood. Adenohypophysis has a small extension upwards around the infundibulum – called pars tuberalis.

Pars posterior is continuous with infundibular stem and median eminence part of hypothalamus. It is known as neurohypophysis and develops as a down growth from the floor of III ventricle of brain.

Structure and secretions

Adenohypophysis - Pars anterior contains secretory cells arranged in groups or chords, separated by sinusoids. They are chromophil cells and chromophobe cells with various subtypes.

Secretions from pars anterior are –

Growth hormone (GH)

Lactogenic hormone (LTH)

Adreno cortico tropic hormone (ACTH),

Thyroid stimulating hormone (TSH)

Gonado tropic hormones (FSH and LH in female) and

Interstital cells stimulating hormone (ICSH in male)

Pars intermedia of adenohyphophysis is not well developed in human. Some cells secrete melanocyte stimulating hormone (MSH) and some, ACTH .

Secretion from anterior pituitary is controlled by the hypothalamus.

Pars nervosa – contains neumerous nerve fibres which are axons of nuclei of hypothalamus and also special cells pituicytes.

Hormones released from neurophypophysis into blood are vasopressin (anti diuretic hormone- ADH) and oxytocin. Vasopressin is secreted by neurons of the supraoptic nucleus of hypothalamus and oxytocin, by paraventricular nuclear neurons. These neuro secretions pass down the axons to neurohypophysis and are released into the capillaries there.

Blood supply of pituitary (Fig. 9.2)

It is a highly vascular organ. Arteries are several.

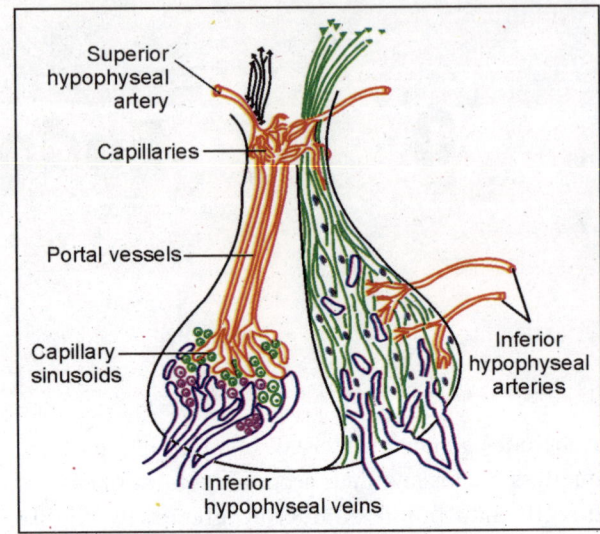

Fig. 9.2: Blood Supply of Hypophysis

Superior hypophysial arteries and a single inferior hypophysial artery from internal carotid arteries of both sides supply it.

The superior hypophysial arteries end in a capillary network in the region of median eminence and infundibulum. From this, straight portal vessels arise and descend to pars anterior. There they divide again into branches that open into sinusoids that lie in close contact with the secretory cells. These portal vessels carry hormone releasing factors or hormone inhibitory factors from the hypothalamic neurons to the secretory cells of adenohypophysis. These cells release their hormones as per the signals thus received, into the venous sinusoids around them.

The arterial supply to anterior pituitary is known as hypothalamohypophysial portal circulation.

The inferior hypophysial arteries supply mainly neurohypophysis which gets branches from superior arteries also.

Venous Drainage

Drained by inferior hypophysial veins into neighbouring dural venous sinuses. The venous blood from pituitary carries the hormones from the gland to their destination.

Pineal body (epiphysis cerebri)

It is a small pear shaped organ situated just above the superior colliculus of midbrain, about 8 mm size. It is connected to the brain by a stalk which divides into 2 laminae. Upper lamina contains habenular commissure and lower contains posterior commissure. Between the stalk, is the pineal recess of 3rd ventricle.

The structure contains prolygonal cells pinealocytes and supporting cells.

Pineal secretes hormones which regulate functions of other endocrine glands.

Thyroid gland

A highly vascular endocrine gland situated in front of the lower part of neck, anterior to larynx and trachea.

It extends from the level of C_5 vertebra to T_1 vertebra. (Fig. 9.3) It has right and left lobes connected by a median narrow istumus. The lobes are conical in shape and their upper ends reach the oblique line of thyroid cartilage. Bases reach down to the level of 4th or 5th tracheal rings. Each lobe is about 5 cm long, 3 cm wide and 2 cm thick.

Isthmus, about 1.25 cm in size connects the lower parts of the 2 lobes lying across the 2nd and 3rd tracheal rings. Gland is about 25 grams in weight.

Gross features (Fig. 9.3, 9.4)

Each lobe has a superficial (lateral) surface, medial surface and posterolateral surface, a thin anterior border and blunt posterior border. The gland has a connective tissue capsule. Outside this, it is surrounded by a false capsule, derived from the pretracheal layer of deep cervical fascia. From the medial surface a thickened band of this fascia connects the gland to the cricoid cartilage – the ligament of Berry. As the pretracheal fascia is attached to hyoid bone and cricoid cartilage, thyroid gland moves up and down during deglutition.

Relations

Lateral surface (superficial): (Fig. 9.5 & 9.6)

It is generally convex and covered by sternothyroid, sternohyoid, inferior belly of omohyoid and anterior margin of sternomatoid.

Medial surface: Structures related to this surface are

1. Larynx
2. Trachea
3. Oesphagus
4. Inferior constrictor
5. cricothyroid
6. Recurrent laryngeal nerve
7. External laryngeal nerve

Posterolateral surface: Related to carotid sheath and contents.

Anterior border: Anterior branch of superior thyroid artery descends along this border.

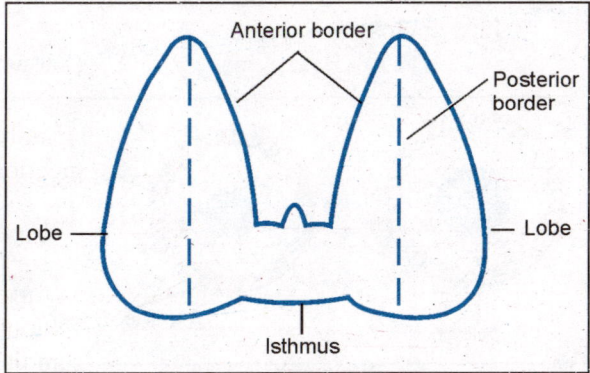

Fig. 9.3: Thyroid Gland

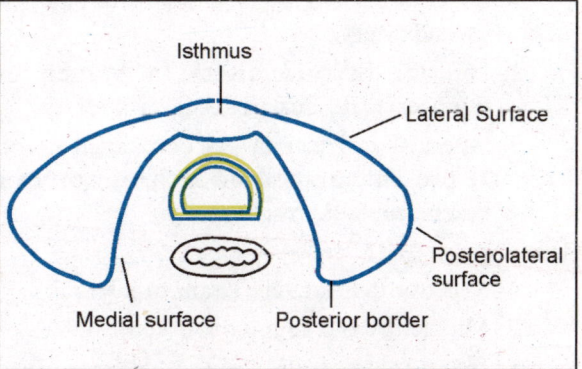

Fig. 9.4: Thyroid - Gross Features

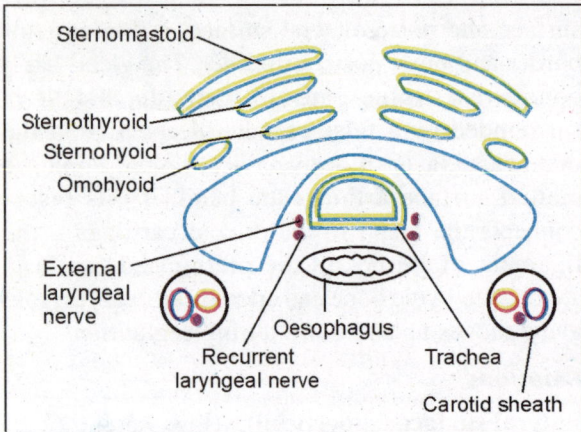

Fig. 9.5: Thyroid - Relations

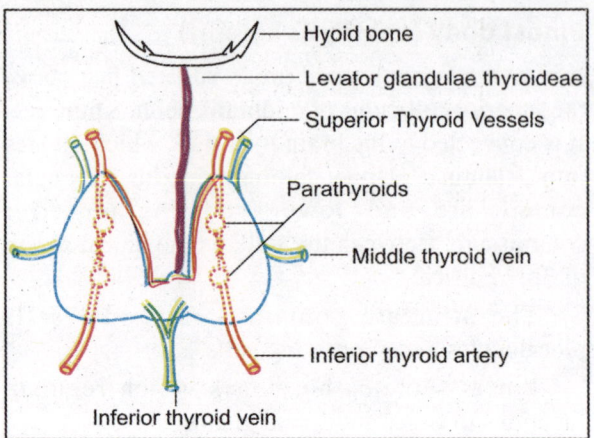

Fig. 9.6

Posterior border: Inferior thyroid artery ascends along the border and anastamoses with posterior branch of superior thyroid artery. Parathyroid glands are embedical along this border.

Isthmus: Branches of superior thyroid arteries anastamose along its upper border and inferior thyroid vein leaves its lower border.

A small pyramidal projection may be present usually from the upper border of isthumus – pyramidal lobe. A fibrous or fibrovascular band connects the pyramidal lobe to the hyoid bone – levator glandulae thyroideae. It is the remnant of thyroglossal duct from which thyroid develops.

Blood supply:

Arteries:

1. Superior thyroid artery, a branch of external carotid artery.
2. Inferior thyroid artery, a branch of thyrocervical trunk of subclavian artery.
3. Arteria thyroidea ima – an occasional artery. If present, branch of arch of aorta or brachiocephalic trunk.

Veins:

1. Superior thyroid vein Drain to internal.
2. Middle thyroid vein jugular vein.
3. Inferior thyroid vein – drains into brachiocephalic vein.

Nerve supply: From cervical sympathetic trunk.

Development: From lower end of thyroglossal duct.

Structure (Fig. 9.7): Thyroid gland has follicles lined by cuboidal or columnar or flat cells. Follicles contain colloid, the secretion of the gland containing T_3 and T_4 which are precursors of thyroid hormone. Thyroid activity is controlled by TSH from anterior pituitary. Apart from follicular cells follicle contains parafollicular cells or C cells that secretes thyrocalcitonin which regulates calcium metabolism.

Applied anatomy

1. As superior thyroid artery descends to the thyroid lobe it is in close contact with external laryngeal nerve, but close to the lobe, the nerve moves away from artery. So in thyroidectomy, superior thyroid artery is ligated close to the lobe.

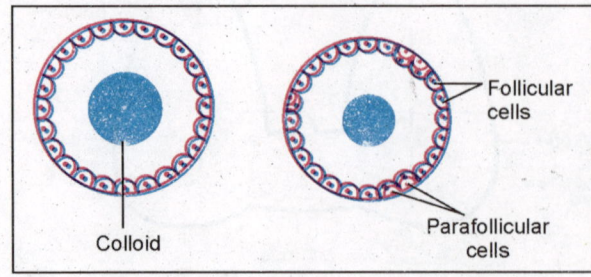

Fig. 9.7: Microscopy – Thyroid gland

But inferior thyroid artery is very close to the recurrent laryngeal nerve, near the lower part of thyroid lobe. So during surgery, the inferior thyroid artery is ligated away from the thyroid lobe. (Fig. 9.8)

2. Enlargement of thyroid gland – Goitre.
   Presses trachea and nerves
3. A benign enlargement of the gland can be due to hypothyroidism - Myxoedema
4. In infants hypothyroidism leads to Cretinism
5. Hyperthyroidism – thyrotoxicosis. This also can cause goitre.
6. Benign or malignant tumours occur with thyroid gland.
7. Inflammation of thyroid gland – thyroiditis

PARATHYROID GLANDS (Fig. 9.6)

There are four parathyroid glands – 2 superior and 2 inferior, situated along the posterior border of thyroid gland. They are small oval bodies about 50 mg in weight, lie inside or outside the capsule of thyroid gland. The cells of the gland produce the hormone-parathormone which helps to maintain calcium level in blood. When blood calcium level decreases, parathormone secretion is increased, it mobilizes calcium from storage sites and brings back the calcium level to normal.

SUPRARENAL GLANDS (Fig. 9.9 & 9.10)

Situated in the abdomen at the upper pole of kidneys, enclosed by the renal fascia. Weighs about 5gms, 5 cm vertically, 3 cm horizontally and 1cm anteroposteriorly. Right one is roughly pyramidal in shape and left one, semilunar in shape.

The right gland is related to the liver, inferior vena cava and diaphragm. Left gland is related to the cardiac end of stomach, pancreas and diaphragm.

Blood supply (highly vascular):

1. Superior suprarenal artery – from inferior phrenic artery.

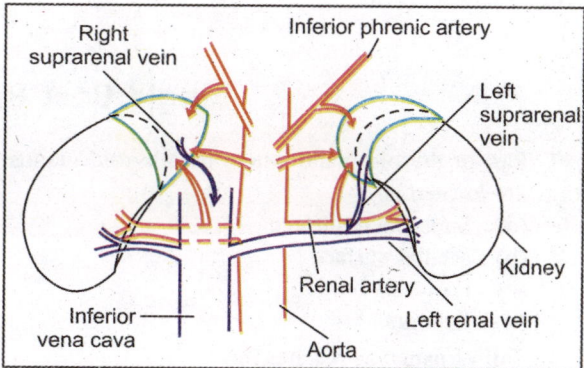

Fig. 9.9

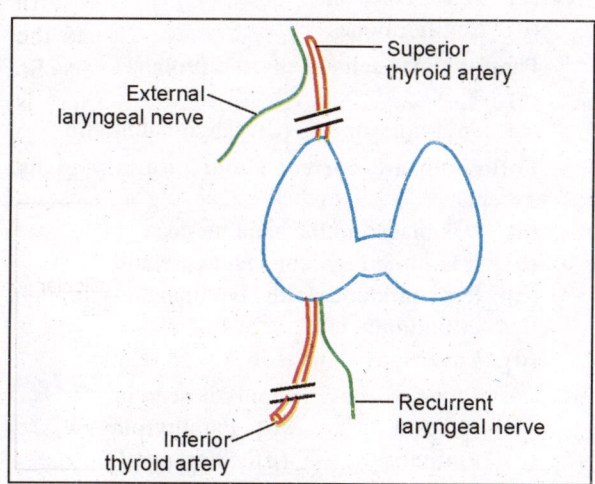

Fig. 9.8

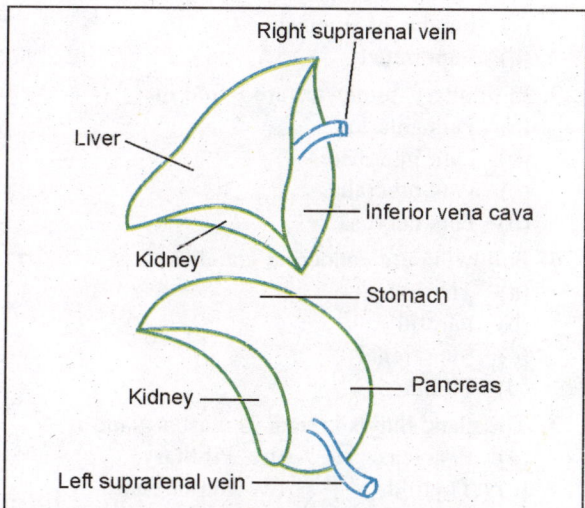

Fig. 9.10: Relations – Suprarenal

2. Middle suprarenal artery – from aorta.

3. Inferior suprarenal artery – from renal artery.

Veins

Right supra renal vein drains into IVC, left one drains into renal vein.

Structure and secretion

It has an outer cortex and inner medulla. Cells of cortex secrete aldosterone, hydrocortisone and sex hormones – oestrogen, progesterone and androgens. Medulla has chromaffin cells and secrete adrenalin and nor adrenalin. ACTH from pituitary controls cortial secretion. Medulla is controlled by sympathetic nerves.

Development

Cortex develops from intermediate mesoderm. Medulla develops from neural crest.

Clinical conditions

Atrophy of cortex leads to Addison's disease. Increased cortical secretion leads to Cushing's syndrome.

Tumour of medulla – Pheochromocytoma

Apart from pituitary, thyroid, parathyroid and suprarenal some other organs also contain endocrine tissue. They are:

1. Islets of Langerhans in pancreas.

2. Interstitial cells of Leydig in testis.

3. Corpus luteum and theca interna in ovary.

Single Best Response M.C.Qs

1. Part of thyroid gland where parathyroid glands are located is
   (a) Superficial surface
   (b) Medial surface
   (c) Posterior border
   (d) Isthmus

2. Tail of pancreas reaches the
   (a) Hilum of spleen
   (b) Hilum of Kidney
   (c) Fundus of stomach
   (d) Suprarenal

3. In pituitary, pituicytes are found in
   (a) Pars anterior
   (b) Pars intermedia
   (c) Pars tuberalis
   (d) Pars nervosa

4. Following are endocrine glands except
   (a) Thyroid
   (b) Parotid
   (c) Suprarenal
   (d) Pituitary

5. The gland that is known as master gland is
   (a) Pancreas   (b) Pituitary
   (c) Thyroid   (d) Suprarenal

6. Isthmus of thyroid gland usually overlies
   (a) 6th tracheal ring
   (b) 4th and 5th tracheal rings
   (c) 3rd and 4th tracheal rings
   (d) 2nd and 3rd tracheal rings.

7. Hormone that is not secreted by adrenal cortex is
   (a) Adrenaline
   (b) Aldosterone
   (c) Hydrocortisone
   (d) Sex hormones

8. Parafollicular cells of thyroid produce
   (a) T_3 (b) T_4
   (c) Parathormone   (d) Thyrocalcitonin

9. Following are correct about pituitary gland except.
   (a) It is placed in the sella tursica
   (b) It is roofed by tentorium cerebelli
   (c) It is continuous with Hypothalamus through infundibulum
   (d) Cavernous sinus is its lateral relation

10. Portal type of arterial supply is seen in
    (a) Thyroid   (b) Parathyroid
    (c) Pituitary   (d) Suprarenal

M.C.Qs - Answers

1. (c), 2. (a), 3. (d), 4. (b), 5. (b), 6. (d), 7. (a), 8. (d), 9. (b), 10. (c)

Essays

  I. Name the endocrine glands and describe the thyroid gland.
 II. Name the endocrine glands and describe the pituitary gland.

Short notes

1. Suprarenal glands
2. Parathyroid glands.
3. Blood supply of pituitary gland.

VISION

The special sensory cells for vision, the photoreceptors are present in the eye balls.

EYE BALL

Eye ball is a spherical structure, formed by parts of 2 spheres. Posterior 5/6th is part of a large sphere, about 2.5 cm in diameter. Anterior 1/6th is part of a smaller sphere, about 1.5 cm in diameter.

Wall of eye ball has three layers (Fig. 10.1) – outermost being **sclera, then choroid and innermost, retina.**

Sclera

This is the outermost fibrous layer. Just medial to the posterior pole of eye ball, optic nerve is attached to the sclera. Extrinsic muscles of eye ball are attached to the outer surface of sclera. Anteriorly the sclera becomes continuous with the transparent

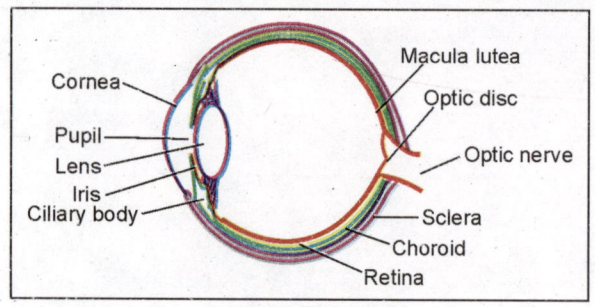

Fig. 10.1: Eye ball

part of this fibrous layer, the **cornea**, at the sclerocorneal junction, marked on surface as a shallow groove – sulcus sclerae.

Cornea has five layers, in its structure. They are from outer to inwards,

Corneal epithelium – Stratified squamous.

Anterior membrane – Bowman's membrane

Substantia propria – Formed of layers of specialized collagen fibres and cells.

Posterior membrane – Descemet's membrane.

Posterior epithelium – of small cuboidal cells.

Injury to cornea leads to corneal opacity and thus blindness. Corneal grafting is done for this.

Changes in curvature of cornea is the clinical condition called astigmatism.

Choroid

It is the vascular layer, formed of a network of blood vessels and connective tissue having plenty of pigmented cells which gives dark colour to the layer and interior of eye ball. Veins from this layer emerge as 5 venae vorticosae through the outer surface of sclera.

Anteriorly choroid continues as the **ciliary body** which continues further as **iris.**

Proximal part of ciliary body shows shallow grooves and is called ciliary ring. Distal part projects as ciliary processes about 70 in number. They are infoldings of the surface of the ciliary body

(Fig. 10.2). To the ciliary processes, the suspensory ligaments of lens are attached, and they secrete the thin fluid aquous humour present in anterior and posterior chambers of eye ball.

Ciliary body contains a smooth muscle, ciliaris, supplied by parasympathetic fibres coming through oculomotor nerve. Its action is to relax the suspensory ligaments and thus to make lens more convex.

Iris is the anterior continuation of ciliary body and presents as a diaphragm in front of the lens. Its central opening is the pupil. Pupil regulates the amount of light entering the eye by contracting and dilating. These are done by 2 smooth muscles, Sphincter pupillae and dilator pupillae. Sphincter is supplied by parasympathetic fibres through oculomotor nerve and dilater pupillae by sympathetic nerve.

Iridocorneal angle (Fig. 10.2) is the angle between peripheral margin of cornea and iris. Laterally there is the sinus venosus sclerae around the angle. Medially there is pectinate ligament, formed of interlacing fibrous filaments with spaces among them. The aquous humor secreted into the posterior chamber by ciliary processes, passes into anterior chamber through the pupil and passes through the spaces of pectinate ligament, into the sinus venosus sclerae and finally drained into the veins. Blockage of the spaces affects drainage of the fluid and leads to glaucoma.

Retina (Fig. 10.3)

The special sensory layer of eye ball. This innermost layer of eyeball has an outer pigmented layer of simple cuboidal cells and inner nervous layer that has the photoreceptors and other nerve cells. Developmentally, these 2 layers are derived from the outer and inner walls of optic cup. The pigmented layer remains attached to the choroid. In certain disease conditions, the nervous layer gets detached from the pigment epithelium – retinal detachment.

The special sensory cells, photoreceptors of nervous layer convert the light stimulus that falls on it, into nerve impulses. The 2 types of photoreceptors are cones and rods. Many millions of them are present. Cones are concerned with bright vision and rods with dim vision. They are arranged intermingled, but at the posterior pole of eye, there is a small area, macula lutea, 2 mm in diameter where cones are more and is the site of maximum vision. Central point of macula lutea is called fovea centralis where only cones are present. Near the posterior pole, there is a circular area at which optic nerve is attached – optic disc (1.5 mm diameter) and here there are no photoreceptors – Blind spot.

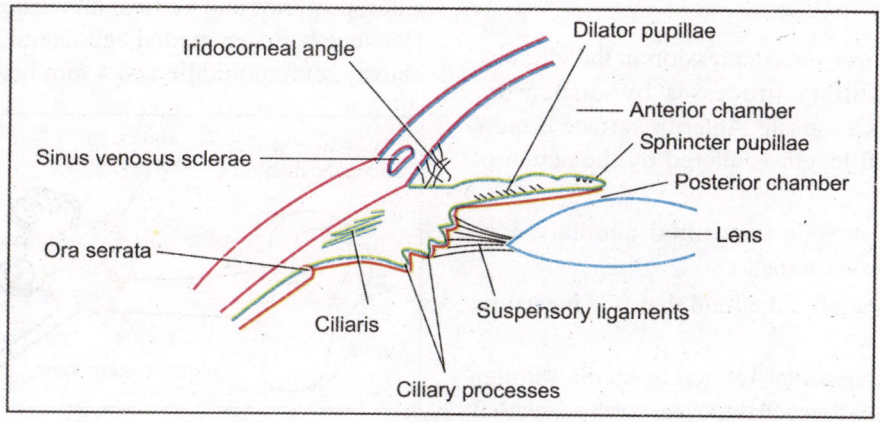

Fig. 10.2

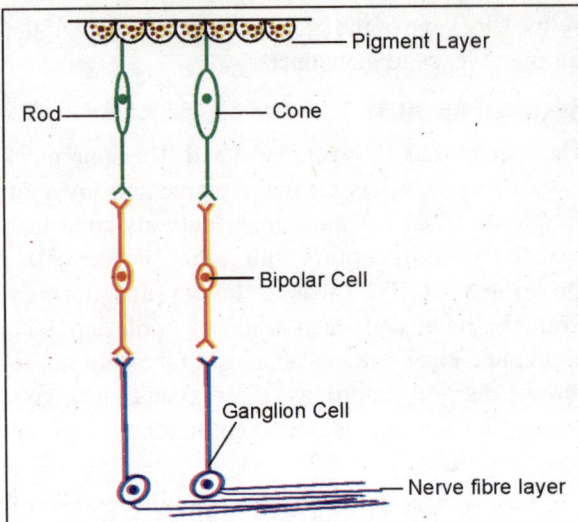

Fig. 10.3: Structure of Retina

Rods, concerned with dim vision, are more numerous near the periphery of retina.

Anterior limit of nervous layer of retina is just behind sclerocorneal junction and is called ora serrata. Nerve impulses produced in the photoreceptors are transmitted through their central processs to bipolar cells; from them, the impulses reach the ganglion cells. Central processes of ganglion cells constitute the nerve fibre layer and emerge as optic nerve which goes to the brain as optic tract, optic radiation, to the visual cortex of occipital lobe of brain.

Lens

Lies behind the iris, on a depression in the vitreous. Connected to ciliary processes by suspensory ligaments. It has a capsule. Anterior surface is more convex. Its focal length is altered by the action of ciliary muscles.

In old age or as a congenital anomaly, lens becomes opaque – cataract.

Vitreous is a jelly like fluid that fills the cavity of eye ball.

Thus the transparent refracting media through which light passes to reach retina are cornea, aqueous humor, lens and vitreous.

AUDITION (HEARING)

EAR

Ear has got three pats – external ear, middle ear and internal ear (Fig. 10.4). Middle and internal ear are situated in the temporal bone. Internal ear contains cochlea in which the special sensory organ for hearing, the spiral organ of Corti is situated.

Internal ear also contains end organs concerned with information of positions and movements of head, in the vestibule and semicircular canals.

External ear

External ear consists of the auricle and a tube leading from auricle internally – the external acoustic meatus. The external acoustic meatus is about 24 mm long, its outer 8 mm is cartilaginous and inner 16 mm is bony. Its medial end is limited by tympanic membrane which forms the lateral wall of middle ear. External acoustic meatus is lined by skin which has numerous ceruminous glands (modified sweat glands) which secrete cerumen, the ear wax. Auricle and external ear conveys the sound waves to impinge on the tympanic membrane.

Middle ear

Middle ear is a small box shaped cavity with 6 walls situated in the petrous part of temporal bone, its lateral wall being the tympanic membrane. Its anteroposterior and vertical dimensions are 15 mm. Distance between medial and lateral walls is 6 mm above, 2mm at middle and 4 mm below. Its medial

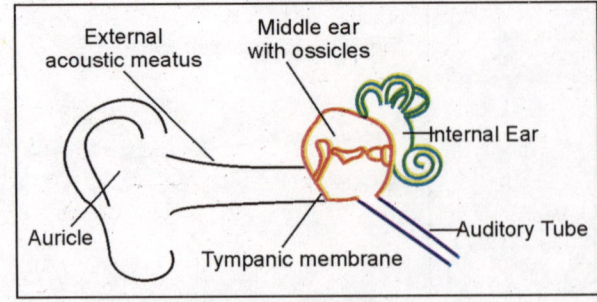

Fig. 10.4: Ear

wall separates it from internal ear. It communicates with nasopharynx through auditary tube (Pharyngotympanic tube / eustacian tube) and thus contains air. Auditary tube opens through the anterior wall. It has two small muscles – stapedius and tensor tympani. Also 3 small bones–ossicles- Malleus, Incus and Stapes arranged in a chain articulating with each other. Handle of malleus is attached to tympanic membrane and base of stapes is fitted over a small opening – fenestra vestibuli in the medial wall of middle ear. Middle ear communicates with a large air space – mastoid antrum, in the petrous part of temporal bone.

Sound waves falling on the tympanic membrane, make vibrations on it, which are transmitted to the internal ear through the chain of ossicles.

Tympanic membrane

It is roughly an oval membrane of about 8 mm diameter, forms the lateral boundary of middle ear. It has three layers structurally – outer cuticular layer, middle fibrous layer and inner mucous layer – each derived embryologically from ectoderm, mesoderm and endoderm. To its inner surface handle of malleus is attached. Chorda tympani nerve is in very close relation with the inner surface of the membrane. A small triangular area in its upper part is loose – pars flaccida and remaining major part is tense – pars tensa.

Applied aspects

Stapedius and tensor tympani contract to reduce the force of sound vibrations reaching the internal ear.

Paralysis of stapedius leads to hyperacousis.

Internal ear

It forms a complex intercommunicating cavities in the petrous part of temporal bone, medial to middle ear. It is called bony labyrinth. Inside the bony labyrinth, there is a corresponding system of membranous labyrinth, which contains endolymph. Space between bony and membranous labyrinth contains perilymph.

Posterior part of the labyrinth has 3 semicircular canals, each placed at right angles to the other (Fig. 10.5). Central part of labyrinth is vestibule. The semicircular canals open into the vestibule. Anterior to the vestibule, there is the cochlea. It has a conical bony central part modiolus around which a bony canal makes 2 ½ turns like a snail shell.(Fig. 10.6)

Inside the bony labyrinth, the membranous labyrinth shows semicircular ducts in the semicircular canals. In the vestibule, there are the saccule and utricle. In the cochlea, there is the cochlear duct. Cochlear duct contains the special sensory hair cells of hearing that form the spiral organ of Corti. It lies over a basilar membrane in the duct (Fig. 10.7). Organ of Corti contains special hair cells. Sound vibrations transmitted to the internal ear through the ossicles of middle ear, reach the perilymph and cause vibration of basilar membrane. The special sensory hair cells over the basilar membrane convert the vibrations into nerve impulses. These impulses are carried along the cochlear part of vestibulecochlear nerve (8th nerve),

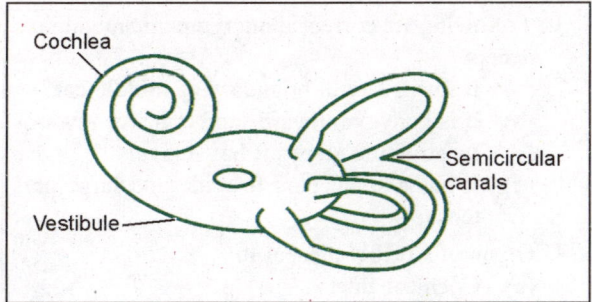

Fig. 10.5: Labyrinth of Internal Ear

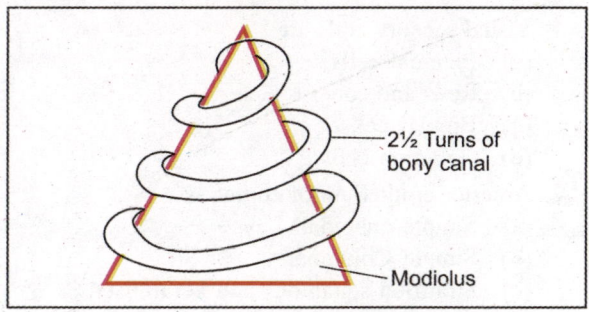

Fig. 10.6: Cochlea

which are formed by central processes of ganglion cells in the cochlea. Through the cochlear nerve, the auditary impulses reach the cochlear nuclei in brain stem.

Similarly vestibular impulses reach the special organs in the semicircular canals and vestibule. They also have specialized sensory cells which covert the mechanical impulses into nerve impulses. They are carried to the vestibular nuclei of brain stem through the vestibular part of 8th nerve, which are fibres of vestibular ganglion situated in the internal acoustic meatus. Vestibular part of the nerve is concerned with regulation of positions and movements of head.

OLFACTION

The special sensory cells of smell or olfaction are the olfactory receptor cells situated in the epithelium of roof of nasal cavity. Their central processes form the olfactory nerve and reach the olfactory bulb in the brain. From these, the olfactory tract leads to the olfactory cortex of brain.

TASTE

The special sensory end organs for taste are taste buds, located in the surface epithelium of tongue. Taste buds are oval bodies formed of taste cells or gustatory cells (lightly staining) and darker sustentacular cells (Fig. 10.8). They are elongated cells. At their apices, taste hairs (long microvilli) project into a tiny space, taste pore.

Taste sensations from the cells of taste buds travel through different nerves – Chorda tympani, Glossopharangeal and vagus – reach the brain stem and end in the nucleus of tractus solitarius.

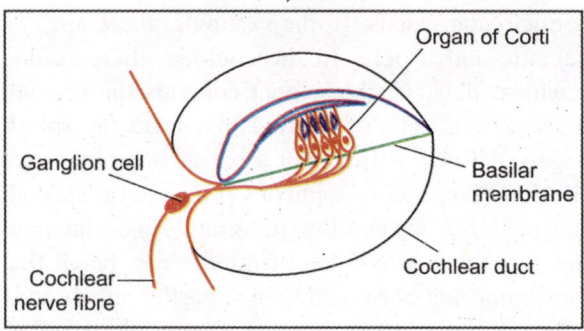

Fig. 10.7: Organ of Corti

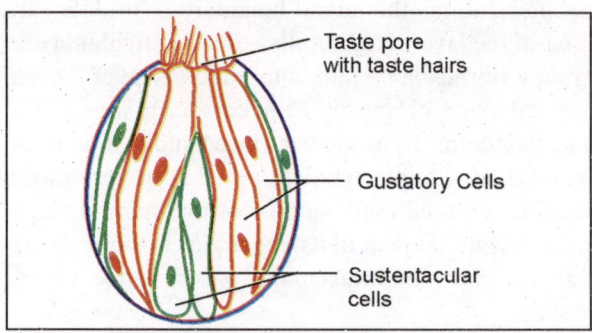

Fig. 10.8: Taste bud

Single Best Response M.C.Qs

1. Visual sensory cells are
   (a) Pigment cells
   (b) Rods and cones
   (c) Bipolar cells
   (d) Ganglion cells
2. Anterior epithelium of cornea is
   (a) Simple cuboidal
   (b) Simple Columnar
   (c) Stratified squamous non keratinised
   (d) Stratified squamous keratinised

3. Following are correct about tympanic membrane except
   (a) It forms lateral boundary of middle ear.
   (b) It is convex outwards and concave inwards
   (c) Its structure shows it has 3 layers.
   (d) It has a small pars flaccida and large pars tensa.
4. Organ of Corti is present in
   (a) Cochlear duct
   (b) Semicircular canals

(c) Vestibule

(d) Endolymphatic duct

5. Dilator pupillae is supplied by
(a) Sympathetic nerve
(b) Parasympathetic nerve
(c) Optic nerve
(d) Ophthalmic nerve

6. Optic nerve is constituted by the central processes of
(a) Rods
b Cones
(c) Bipolar cells
(d) Ganglion cells

7. Aqueous humour is secreted by
(a) Retina
(b) Lens
(c) Ciliary processes
(d) Iris

8. The nerve that does not carry taste sensation from tongue is
(a) Hypoglossal nerve
(b) Glossopharyngeal nerve
(c) Vagus
(d) Chorda tympani

9. Ciliaris muscle of eye is supplied by
(a) Sympathetic nerve
(b) Parasympathetic nerve
(c) Trochlear nerve
(d) Abducent nerve

10. The media through which light passes to reach retina are the following except
(a) Cornea
(b) Iris
(c) Lens
(d) Vitreous

M.C.Qs - Answers

1. (b), 2. (c), 3. (b), 4. (a), 5. (a), 6. (d), 7. (c), 8. (a), 9. (b), 10. (b)

Essays

I. Name the layers of the wall of eye ball and describe the vascular layer.

II. Describe the Middle ear cavity.

Short Notes

1. Cornea

2. Retina

3. Ciliary body

4. Tympanic membrane

5. Cochlea

11 Nervous System

Human nervous system is subdivided into two parts – Central Nervous System and Peripheral Nervous System.

Central Nervous System consists of **Brain and Spinal Cord**.

Peripheral Nervous System includes **Cranial nerves, Spinal nerves, Autonomic nerves and Special Sensory nerves and associated structures.**

SPINAL CORD

It occupies the vertebral canal. About 45 cms long, a cylindrical structure. Average diameter is 1.25 cm.

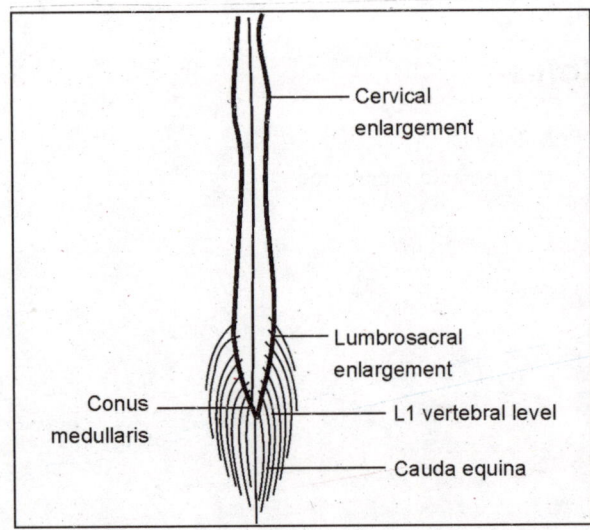

Fig. 11.1

Begins at the upper border of C_1 vertebra as the continuation of Medulla Oblongata of brain. Lower end is conical in shape – Conus Medullaris – reaches up to the lower border of L_1 vertebra in adults. (Fig. 11.1)

Anteriorly along the midline, a deep vertical groove is present, the anterior median fissure. Posteriorly along the midline, a shallow groove, posterior median sulcus is seen.

31 pairs of spinal nerves are attached to the spinal cord, each by a dorsal root and a ventral root. (Fig. 11.2) Each root has a number of rootlets at its attachment to the cord. The stretch of the cord that gives attachment to the rootlets of a spinal nerve is called a spinal segment. (Fig. 11.3)

There are 8 cervical, 12 thoracic, 5 lumbar, 5 sacral and 1 coccygeal spinal nerves.

Diameter of spinal cord is not uniform along its whole length. It has two enlargements – Cervical and Lumbar – where it gives attachment to the nerves that supply upper limb and lower limb. They

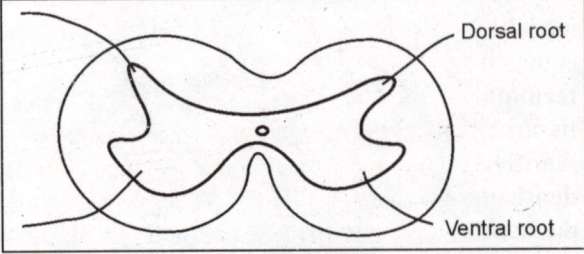

Fig. 11.2

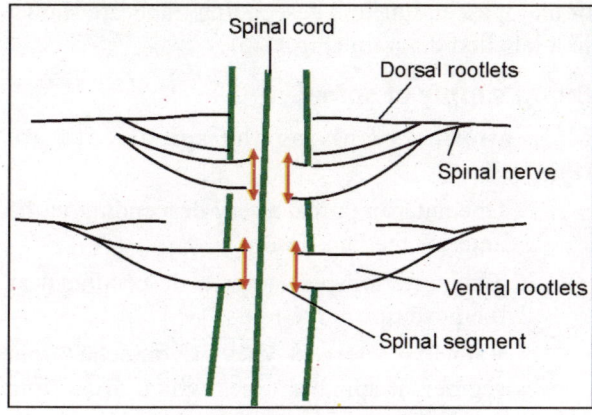

Fig. 11.3: Spinal Segments

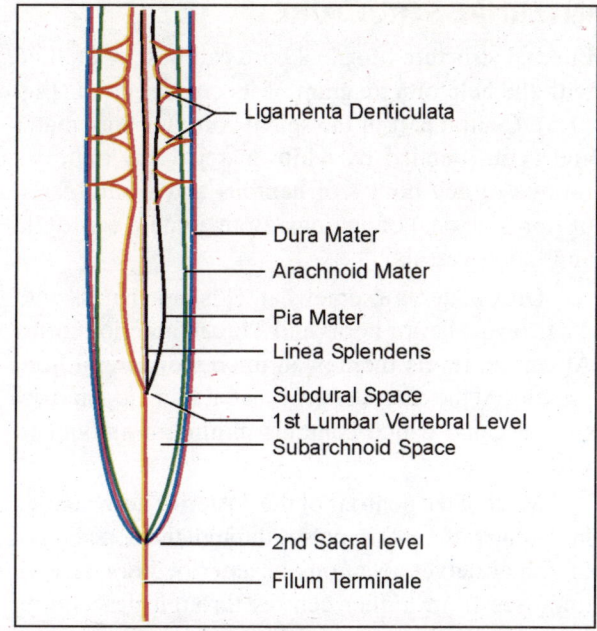

Fig. 11.4: Spinal meninges and spaces

correspond to C_5 to T_1 segments and L_1 to S_3 segments of the cord. (Fig. 11.1)

Spinal nerves generally emerge through the corresponding intervertebral foramina. But the lower ones have an oblique course before they can emerge out of the vertebral canal. They appear as a bundle of nerves below the conus medullaris and is known as cuada equina. (Fig.11.1)

SPINAL MENINGES

The three meninges Dura mater, Arachnoid mater and Pia mater cover the spinal cord from without inwards. They are continuous with cranial meninges that cover the brain. Dura mater is thick and tough membrane. Deep to that arachnoid mater is thin and membranous. The deepest pia mater is very delicate and closely covers the spinal cord. Dura and arachnoid end at the level of S_2 vertebra and pia mater ends at conus medullaris.

Pia mater extends down from the conus medullaris as a thin thread among the nerves of cauda equina to get attached to the coccyx. It is the **filum terminale.** (Fig. 11.4). Along the anterior median fissure, the pia is thickened – the **linea splendens**. Another pial modification is **ligamentum denticulatum**. On each side of spinal cord between the attachments of dorsal and ventral nerve roots, pia mater forms triangular or tooth like processes

which extend laterally through the arachnoid to dura mater. There are about 21 pairs of such ligamenta denticulata. They help to suspend the spinal cord in the normal position.

MENINGEAL SPACES

(Fig. 11.4) Space between dura and vertebral canal is the extra dural or epidural space. It contains loose connective tissue, fat and veins. Space between dura and arachnoid is subdural space, it is only a potential space. Larger space, subarachnoid space is between arachnoid and pia mater and contains cerebro spinal fluid (CSF).

Lumbar puncture

CSF can be withdrawn form the subarachnoid space for investigative purposes, theraputic purpose or to give spinal anaesthesia. For this the needle is safely introduced through the intervertebral space below L_1 into the subarachnoid space, without damaging the spinal cord. Usually selected space for lumbar puncture is between L_3 and L_4 vertebrae.

INTERNAL STRUCTURE

Internal structure of spinal cord can best be studied with the help of a diagram of its cross section (Fig. 11.5). Central part of the spinal cord has grey mater and is surrounded by white mater. Grey mater is formed of cell bodies of neurons and white mater, of fibres (axons) of neurons. Both contain neuroglia and blood vessels.

Grey mater is a somewhat 'H' shaped mass with 2 narrow posterior horns and 2 broad anterior horns. At certain levels there is an intermediolateral horn present. At the centre of grey mater, there is a narrow central canal which contains minimum amount of CSF.

Most of the neurons of the posterior horn receive incoming (afferent) impulses through the dorsal roots of spinal nerves. Neurons of anterior horn receive impulses from higher centres through descending axons which relay in them.

The intermediolateral horn of grey mater contains preganglionic neurons of the sympathetic and parasympathetic (autonomic) nervous system.

Neurons of grey mater are arranged in groups as nuclei and layers.

White mater

Contains myelinated nerve fibres descending form higher centres of brain to various levels of spinal cord and ascending fibres through spinal cord to various centres of brain. They are arranged in discrete bundles and hence called fibre tracts. They occupy specific positions in the spinal cord. The arrangement of major ascending and descending tracts are shown in a labelled diagram (Fig.11.6)

Blood supply of spinal cord

Main arteries supplying the spinal cord are (Fig.11.7):

1. One anterior spinal artery descending in the anterior median fissure.
2. Two posterior spinal arteries descending near the posterior nerve roots.
3. Radicular arteries:- They are branches from segmental spinal arteries which arise from arteries outside vertebral canal (as deep cervical, intercostals and lumbar arteries). Radicular arteries reach the spinal cord along with anterior and posterior nerve roots and reinforce the anterior and posterior spinal arteries up to the lower end of spinal cord.

Venous drainage

Venous blood is drained through internal vertebral venous plexus into intersegmental veins. They communicate with intracranial veins.

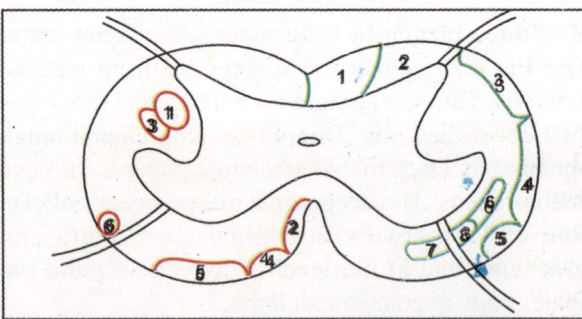

Ascending Tracts
1. Fasciculus Gracilis.
2. Faciculus Cuneatus.
3. Posterior Spinocerebell:Tr.
4. Anterior Spinocerebell:Tr.
5. Spino Olivary Tr.
6. Lateral Spinothalamic Tr.
7. Anterior Spinothalamic Tr.
8. Spino Tectal Tr.

Descending Tracts
1. Lateral Corticospinal Tr.
2. Anterior Cortico-Spinal Tr.
3. Rubrospinal Tr.
4. Tectospinal Tr.
5. Vestibulospinal Tr.
6. Olivospinal Tr.

Fig. 11.6: Fibre Tracts in White Mater

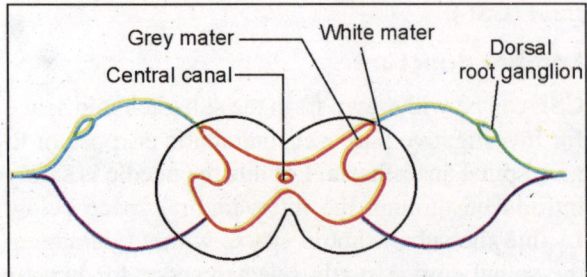

Fig. 11.5: Cross section of Spinal cord

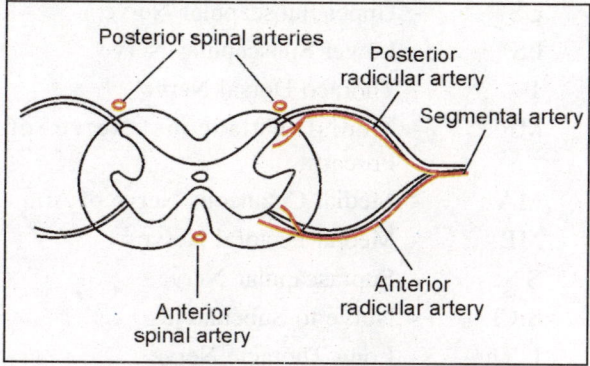

Fig. 11.7: Arteries of Spinal Cord

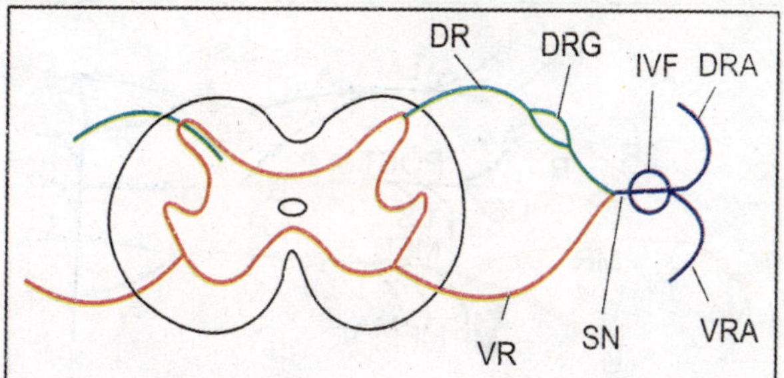

DR - Dorsal Root	VR - Ventral Root
DRG - Dorsal Root Ganglion	SN - Spinal Nerve
IVF - Intervertebral Foramen	DRA - Dorsal Ramus
VRA - Ventral Ramus	

Fig. 11.8: Spinal Nerve

SPINAL NERVES

31 pairs attached to the spinal cord by anterior and posterior roots. Anterior roots contain axons of the neurons of anterior horn of the grey mater of spinal cord. They carry information away form the Central Nervous System (CNS) and are motor fibres. Posterior root is formed by fibres of the neurons of dorsal root ganglion (Fig.11.8). They convey general sensory information form different parts of body to CNS and are sensory fibres. Near the intervertebral foramen, the anterior and posterior roots join to form the spinal nerve which thus contains sensory and motor fibres. Outside the vertebral canal each spinal nerve divides into a dorsal ramus and a ventral ramus. Dorsal ramus and its branches supply skin and muscles of the back. Ventral ramus divides into branches that supply skin and muscles of anterior and lateral body wall and limbs.

Ventral rami of upper 11 thoracic nerves are intercostal nerves and of the 12th one is the subcostal nerve. Intercostal nerves run in the intercostal spaces and supply skin and muscles of the spaces and also parietal pleura.

The thoracic spinal nerves have connecting branches – grey and white rami communicantes to the sympathetic trunk.

NERVE PLEXUSES

At the root of neck and roots of upper and lower limbs the ventral rami of spinal nerves form irregular network - nerve plexuses. Their branches supply the regions of neck, upper limb and lower limb. In the plexuses nerve fibres from different spinal segments intermingle. So branches from the plexuses will contain fibres from more than one spinal segment.

Major nerve plexuses formed of ventral rami of spinal nerves are:

1. Cervical plexus – at the neck.
2. Brachial plexus – at the root of upper limb.
3. Lumbar and sacral plexuses – in the lower abdomen and pelvis.

CERVICAL PLEXUS

Formed by ventral rami of C_1 to C_4 nerves in the neck. Its branches supply skin and muscles of neck and lower part of head.

BRACHIAL PLEXUS

Formed at the root of neck and axilla by the ventral rami of C_5 to T_1 nerves (Fig. 11.9).

C_5 and C_6 roots join to form upper trunk

C_7 continues as middle trunk

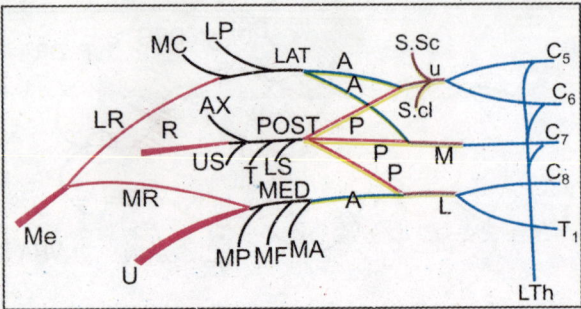

Fig. 11.9: Brachial Plexus

US	- Upper Subscapular Nerve
LS	- Lower Subscapular Nerve
T	- Thoraco Dorsal Nerve
MF	- Medial Cutaneous Nerve of Forearm
MA	- Medial Cutaneous Nerve of Arm
MP	- Medial Pectoral Nerve
S.Sc	- Suprascapular Nerve
S.Cl	- Nerve to Subculavius
L.Th	- Long Thoracic Nerve

C_8 and T_1 roots join to form lower trunk

Each trunk divides into anterior and posterior divisions.

All posterior divisions join to form posterior cord.

Anterior divisions of upper and middle trunks join to form lateral cord.

Anterior division of lower trunk continues as medial cord.

Branches are as shown in the figure.

C5 to T1	- Ventral Rami of C_5 toC_8 and T1 Spinal Nerves
U	- Upper Trunk
M	- Middle Trunk
L	- Lower Trunk
A,A,A	- Anterior Divisions
P, P, P	- Posterior Divisions
LAT	- Lateral Cord
POST	- Posterior Cord
MED	- Medial Cord
LR	- Lateral Root of Median Nerve
MR	- Medial Root of Median Nerve
Me	- Median Nerve
U	- Ulnar Nerve
R	- Radial Nerve
LP	- Lateral Pectoral Nerve
MC	- Musculocutaeous Nerve
AX	- Axillary Nerve

MAJOR TERMINAL BRANCHES

1. Median nerve

Root value - $C_{5,6,7,8}$ and T_1

Arises by two roots - medial and lateral, from the medial and lateral cords of brachial plexus. From the axilla it descends through upper arm in relation to the brachial artery. Below the elbow, it leaves the cubital fossa by passing between the two heads of pronator teres. Descends among the flexor muscles of forearm. Enters the hand by passing deep to flexor retinaculum. Divides into terminal branches in the hand. Course, branches and distribution as shown in. (Fig. 11.10)

Applied anatomy

Median nerve can be injured due to a supra- condylar fracture of humerus or a wound above the wrist or due to compression in the carpal tunnel, deep to flexor retinaculum.

Lesion of median nerve causes paralysis of muscles supplied by it. So Flexion at wrist is weak and also flexion at interphalangeal joints of first three fingers is affected. There is wasting of thenar muscles and the thumb remains adducted – similates "ape thumb".

Carpal tunnel syndrome

Due to compression of the nerve in the carpal tunnel. Results from tenosynovitis or arthritis. There will be wasting of thenar muscles and altered sensation of lateral 3 ½ fingers.

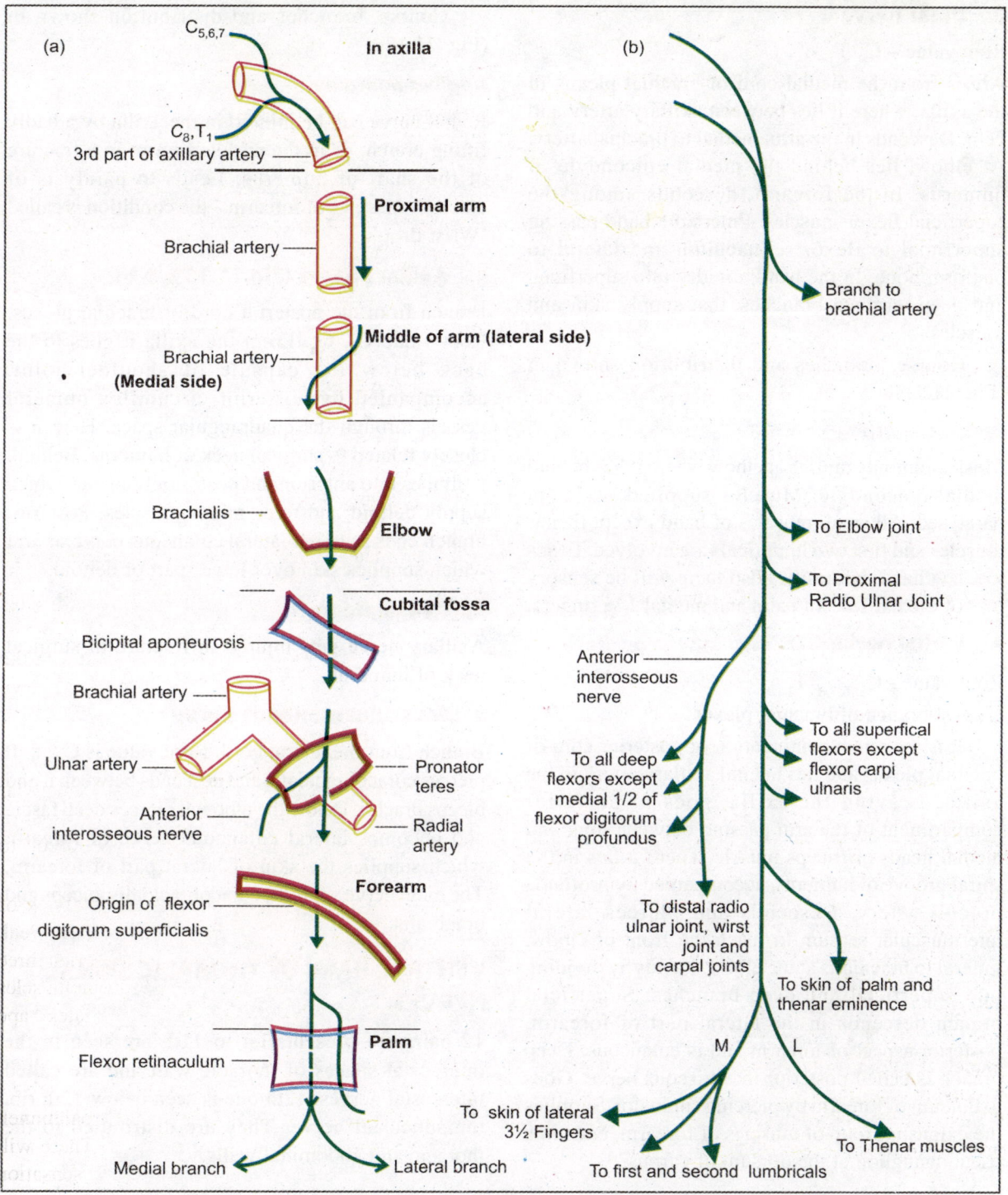

Fig. 11.10: Median Nerve (a) Course and Realations (b) Branches and Distribution

2. Ulnar nerve

Root value – C_8, T_1

Arises from the medial cord of brachial plexus in the axilla, where it lies between axillary artery and vein. Descends in the arm, medial to brachial artery. At elbow, lies behind the medial epicondyle of humerus. In the forearm, descends among the superficial flexor muscles. Enters the hand passing superficial to flexor retinaculum and lateral to pisiform bone. In the hand, divides into superficial and deep terminal branches, that supply skin and muscles.

Course, branches and distribution shown in (Fig. 11.11)

Applied anatomy

Most commonly injured at elbow where it lies behind medial epicondyle. Muscles supplied by it get paralysed. All small muscles of hand except thenar muscles and first two lumbricals are involved. Leads to Claw hand deformity. Also there will be sensory loss of medial $1/3^{rd}$ of palm and medial 1 ½ fingers.

3. Radial nerve

Root value - $C_{5,\,6,7,8}$, T_1

Largest branch of brachial plexus

It is the direct continuation of posterior cord of brachial plexus and lies behind axillary artery in the axilla. Leaving the axilla, goes to posterior compartment of the arm passing between long and medial heads of triceps muscle. There it lies in the spiral groove of humerus, accompanied by profunda brachii artery. Descends and pierces lateral intermuscular septum to reach the front of elbow. Lateral to brachialis at the elbow, it ends by dividing into superficial and deep branches. Superficial branch descends in the lateral part of forearm, posterior aspect of forearm and is cutaneous. Deep branch is called posterior interosseous nerve. Goes to dorsum of forearm by piercing supinator. Supplies the extensor group of muscles of forearm, ends in a pseudoganglion at the dorsum of carpus.

Course, branches and distribution shown in (Fig. 11.12.)

Applied anatomy

Radial nerve can be injured in the axilla by a badly fitting crutch, or in the middle of arm in a fracture of the shaft of humerus. Leads to paralysis of extensor muscles of forearm – the condition is called 'Wrist drop'.

4. Axillary nerve (Fig.11.13 a & b)

Branch from the posterior cord of brachial plexus. Root value C_5, C_6. From the axilla it goes to the back below the capsule of shoulder joint, accompanied by posterior circumflex humeral vessels through the quadrangular space. Here it is closely related to surgical neck of humerus. Behind, it divides into anterior and posterior branches which supply deltoid and teres minor muscles. Posterior branch ends as upper lateral cutaneous nerve of arm which supplies skin over lower part of deltoid.

Applied anatomy

Axillary nerve gets injured in fracture of surgical neck of humerus.

5. Musculocutaneous nerve

Branch from the lateral cord. Root value is $C_{5,6,7}$. It pierces coracobrachialis and descends between it and biceps brachii. Below the elbow it pierces deep fascia and becomes lateral cutaneous nerve of forearm which supplies the skin of lateral part of forearm. The main nerve supplies coracobrachialis, biceps and brachialis.

VENTRAL RAMI OF THORACIC SPINAL NERVES

12 pairs are present. 1st to 11th are seen in the intercostal spaces of thoracic wall and are called intercostal nerves. 12th one is seen below 12th rib, the subcostal nerve. They are distributed to the thoracic and abdominal walls.

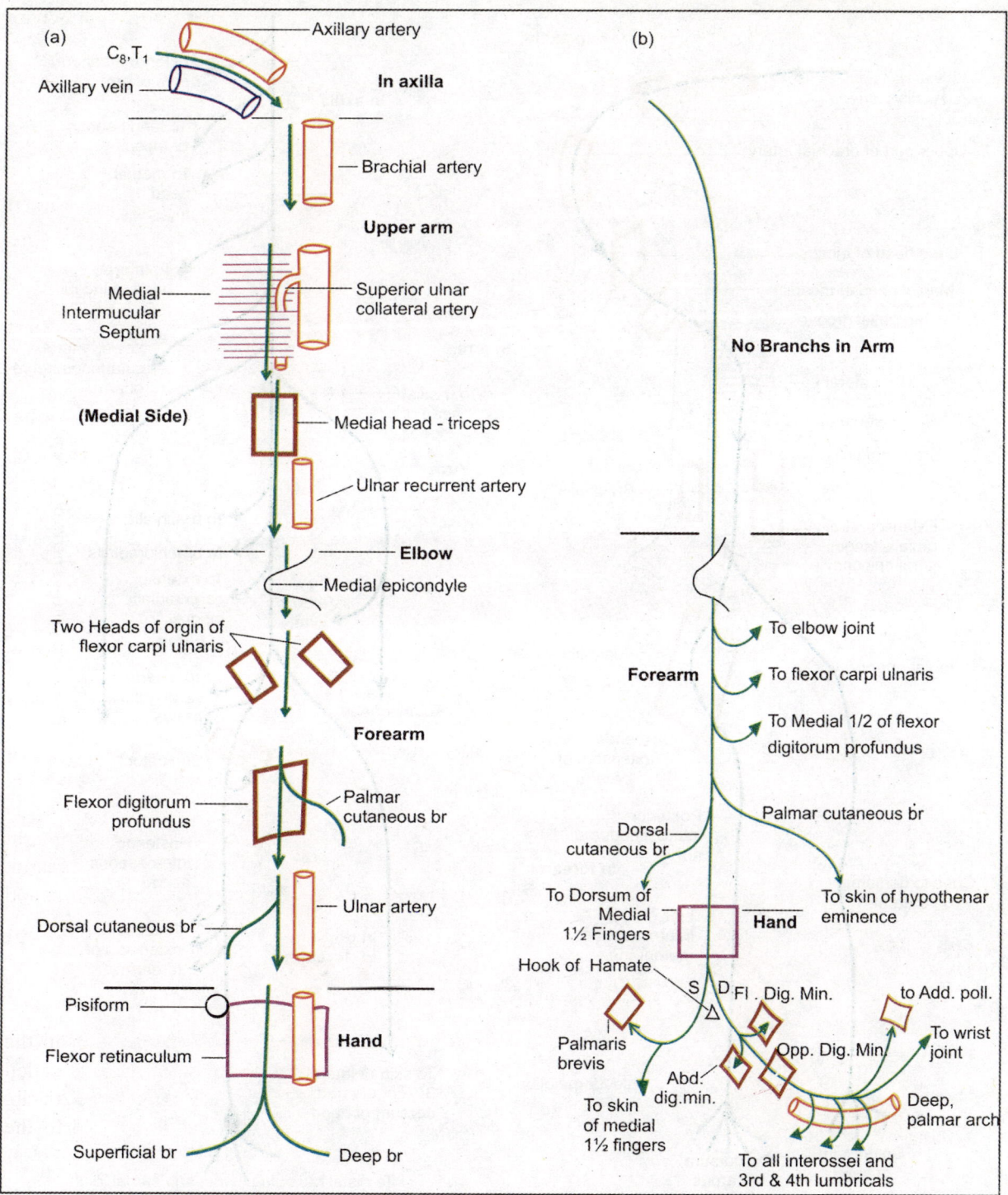

Fig. 11.11: Ulnar Nerve (a) Course and realations (b) Branches and distribution

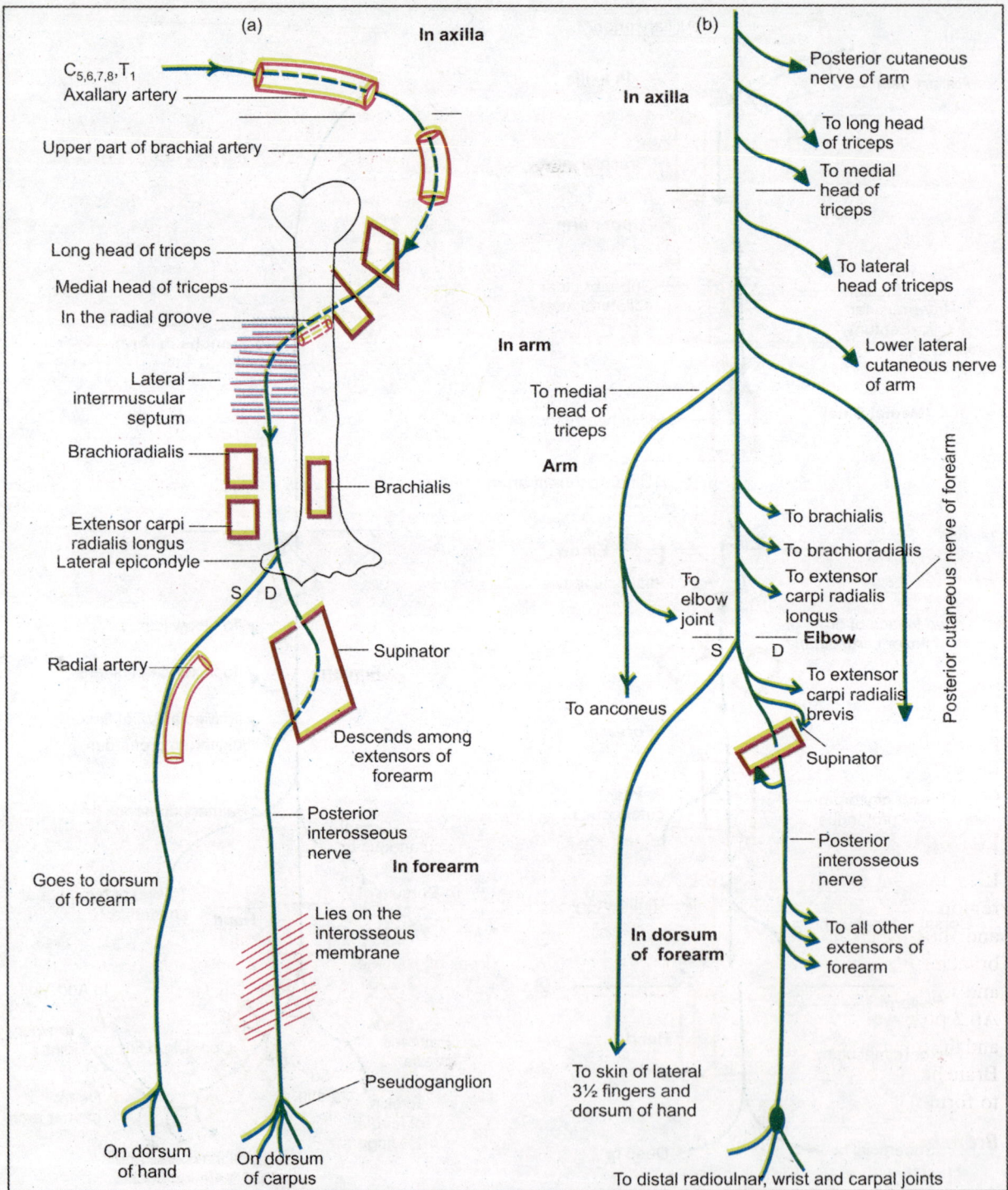

Fig. 11.12: Radial Nerve (a) Course and relations (b) Branches and distribution

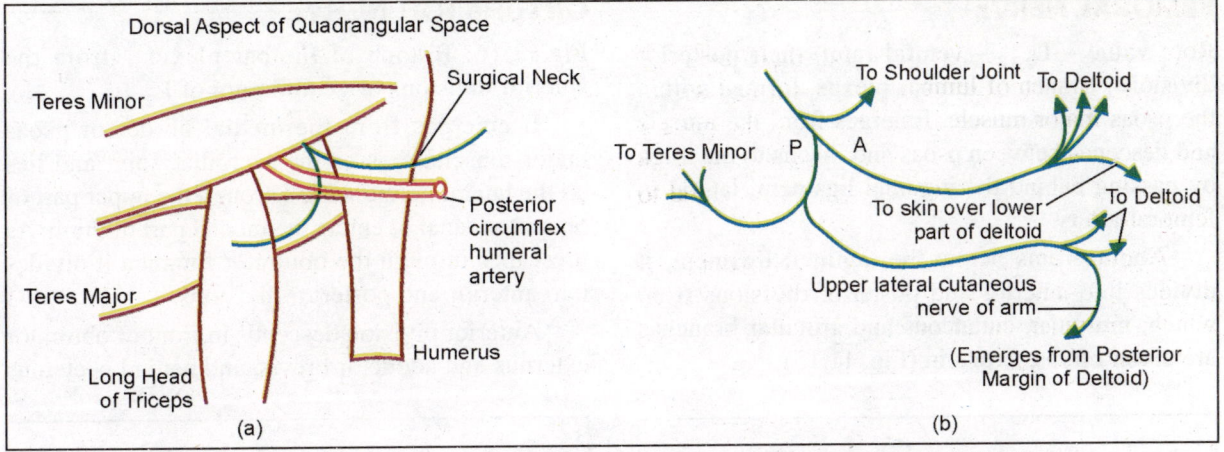

Fig. 11.13: Axillary Nerve(C-$_{5,6}$) (a) Course and relations (b) Branches and distribution

All these ventral rami are connected to the sympathetic ganglia through short connecting branches – grey and white rami communicantes.

VENTRAL RAMI OF LUMBAR SPINAL NERVES

Ventral rami of L_1 to L_4 form lumbar plexus within the psoas major muscle. L_5 joins with part of L_4 to form a nerve trunk – lumbosacral trunk, which takes part in the formation of sacral plexus. Branches from the lumbar and sacral plexus supply the lower part of anterior abdominal wall and lower limb.

LUMBAR PLEXUS (Fig. 11.14)

Lies in the posterior abdominal wall, in lumbar region. Major part of L_1 divides into iliohypogastric and ilioinguinal nerves. A branch from L_1 joins a branch from L_2 to form genitofemoral nerve. L_2, L_3, and L_4 divide into anterior and posterior divisions. All 3 posterior divisions join to form Femoral nerve and the three anterior divisions form Obturator nerve. Branches form posterior divisions of L_2 and L_3 join to form lateral cutaneous nerve of thigh.

Branches

1. Iliohypogastric – L_1 – to lower part of anterior part of abdominal wall.

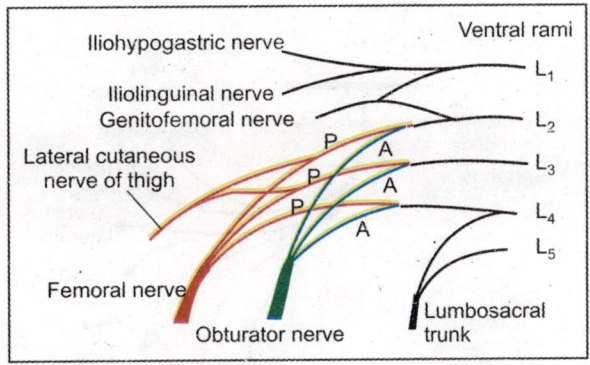

Fig.11.14

2. Ilioinguinal – L_1 – passes through inguinal canal to skin of groin and scrotum.

3. Genitofemoral - L_1, L_2 - Genital branch supplies cremaster muscle. Femoral branch supplies a small area in front of thigh.

4. Lateral cutanious nerve of thigh – L_2, L_3 - to lateral surface of thigh.

5. Femoral nerve – $L_{2,3,4}$ – goes behind inguinal ligament to the thigh.

6. Obturator nerve – $L_{2,3,4}$ – passes through obturator foramen to medial side of thigh.

7. Lumbosacral trunk - $L_{4,5}$ – takes part in sacral plexus.

8. Muscular branches

FEMORAL NERVE

Root value – $L_{2,3,4}$ – ventral rami, their posterior divisions. Branch of lumbar plexus, formed within the psoas major muscle. Emerges from the muscle and descends between psoas and iliacus to the thigh by passing behind the inguinal ligament, lateral to femoral artery.

About 4 cms below the inguinal ligament, it divides into anterior and posterior divisions from which, muscular, cutaneous and articular branches are given off, as shown in (Fig. 11.15)

OBTURATOR NERVE

Fig.11.16. Branch of lumbar plexus - from the anterior divisions of ventral rami of $L_{2, 3 \& 4}$.

It emerges from the medial border of psoas major muscle, crosses the sacroiliac joint and lies on the lateral pelvic wall. Through the upper part of obturator canal, it enters the medial part of thigh. As it escapes through the obturator foramen it divides into anterior and posterior divisions.

Anterior division descends in front of obturator externus and adductor brevis, and behind pectenius

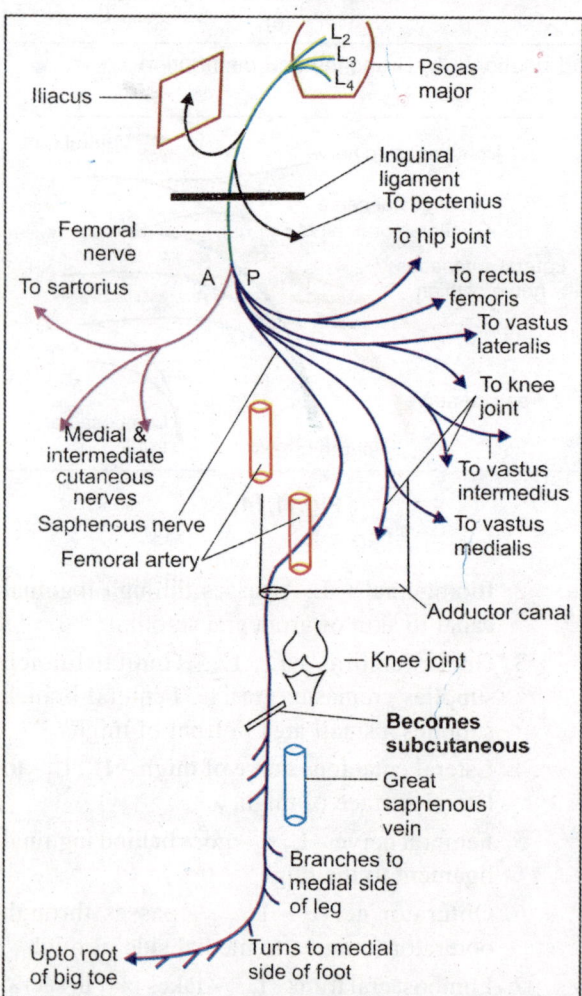

Fig. 11.15: Branches of Femoral Nerve

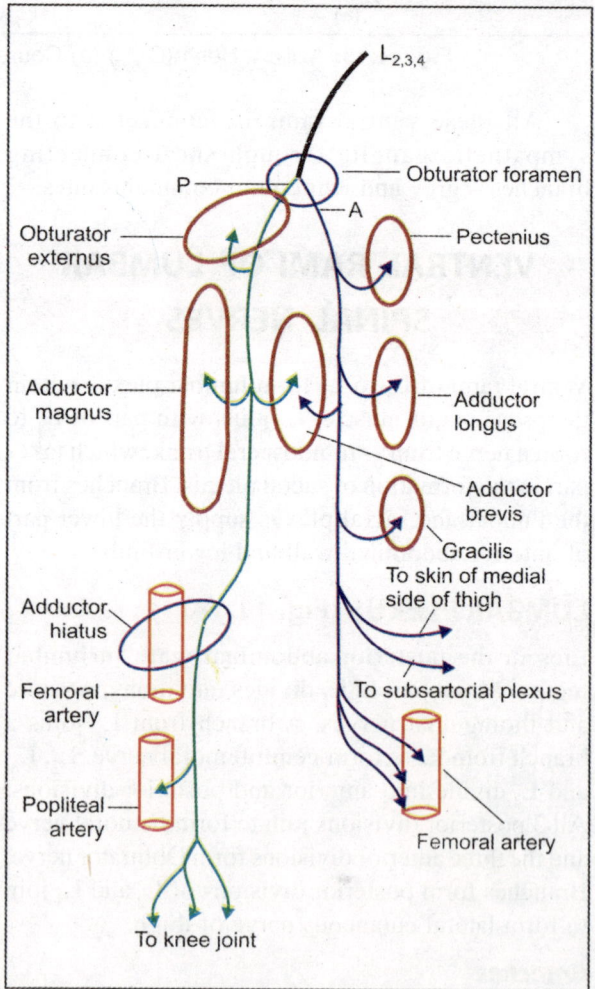

Fig. 11.16: Obturator Nerve

and adductor longus. Ends as a small branch to supply femoral artery.

Posterior division pierces obturator externus and descends behind adductor brevis and in front of adductor magnus. Terminates by passing through adductor hiatus to supply knee joint.

VENTRAL RAMI OF SACRAL NERVES

They emerge through the anterior sacral foramina and take part in the formation of sacral and coccygeal plexuses.

Sacral plexus (Fig. 11.17)

Lies in the posterior pelvic wall. Formed by lumbosacral trunk (L_4 and L_5) and upper 4 sacral nerves. Each nerve divides into anterior and posterior divisions. Posterior divisions of L_4, L_5, S_1 and S_2 join to form the common peroneal part of sciatic nerve. Anterior divisions of $L_{4,5}$, S_1, S_2 and S_3 nerves join to form tibial part of sciatic nerve. Branches from S_{-2}, S_3 and S_4 join to form pudental nerve.

Other branches are:

1. Superior gluteal nerve (L_4, L_5 and S_1)

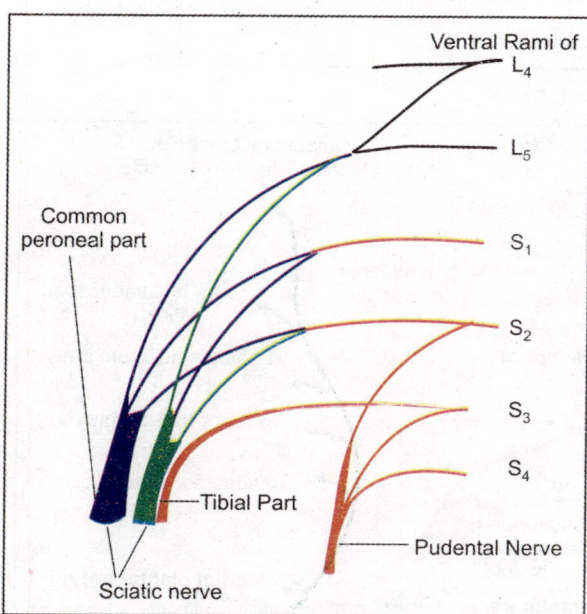

Fig. 11.17: Sacral Plexus

2. Inferior gluteal nerve (L_5 S_1 and S_2)
3. Posterior cutaneous nerve of thigh (S_1, S_2 and S_3)
4. Muscular branches.

SCIATIC NERVE

Fig.11.18. Root value L_4 to S_3.

Thickest nerve in the body. From the pelvis reaches gluteal region through greater sciatic foramen and lies deep to gluteus maximus. Descends in the back of thigh. At the junction between middle and lower 1/3rd of thigh, it ends by dividing into tibial and common peroneal nerves.

Branches from sciatic nerve:

1. From the tibial part to hamstring muscles.
2. From common paroneal part to short head of biceps.
3. To hip joint.
4. Terminal branches – tibial and common paroneal nerves.

1. Tibial nerve - ($L_{4,5}$ $S_{1,2,3}$) (Fig. 11.18)

One of the terminal branches of sciatic nerve, descends through popliteal fossa. Then to the leg, descends deep to gastrocnemius and soleus. Lies over tibialis posterior with posterior tibial artery. Behind medial malleolus, deep to flexor retinaculum, divides into its terminal branches – medial and lateral plantar nerves. Branches and distribution are shown in figure 11.18

Applied anatomy

Injury is rare. If occurs flexors of leg and intrinsic muscles of the sole arc paralysed.

Medial Plantar Nerve

Fig.11.19. Begins as one of the two terminal branches of tibial nerve, under the flexor retinaculum. Runs anteriorly in the medial part of sole accompanied by medial plantar artery. Ends by dividing into plantar digital branches, sensory to, medial 3 ½ toes. Branches, shown in the figure.

Lateral Plantar Nerve

Fig. 11.19. Begins deep to flexor retinaculum as one of the two terminal branches of tibial nerve. Crosses the sole accompanied by lateral plantar artery to lateral side and at the base of 5th metatarsal bone divides into superficial and deep branches. Branches, and distribution, shown in figure.

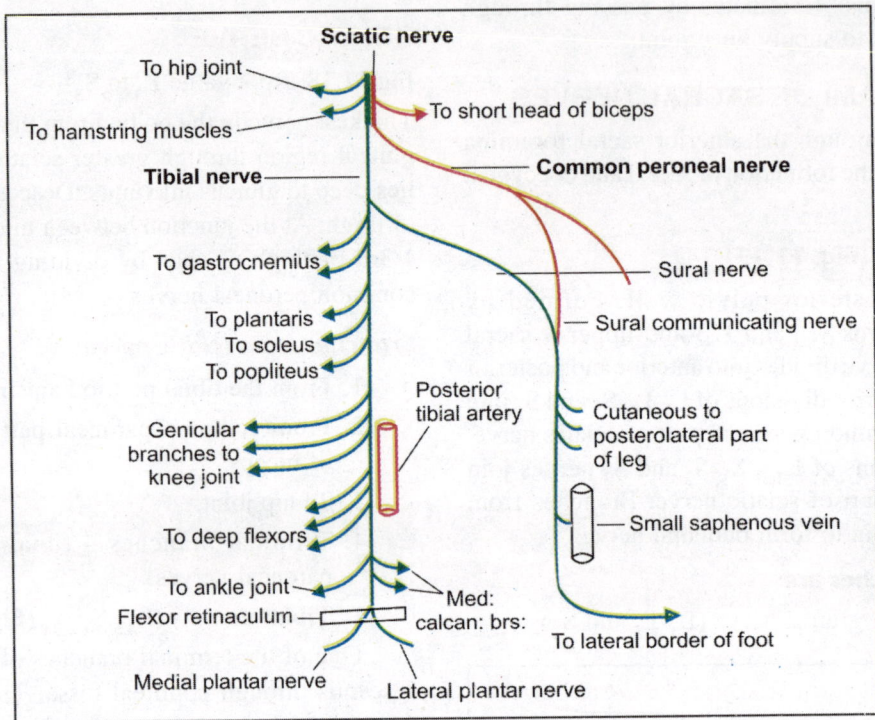

Fig. 11.18. Tibial nerve

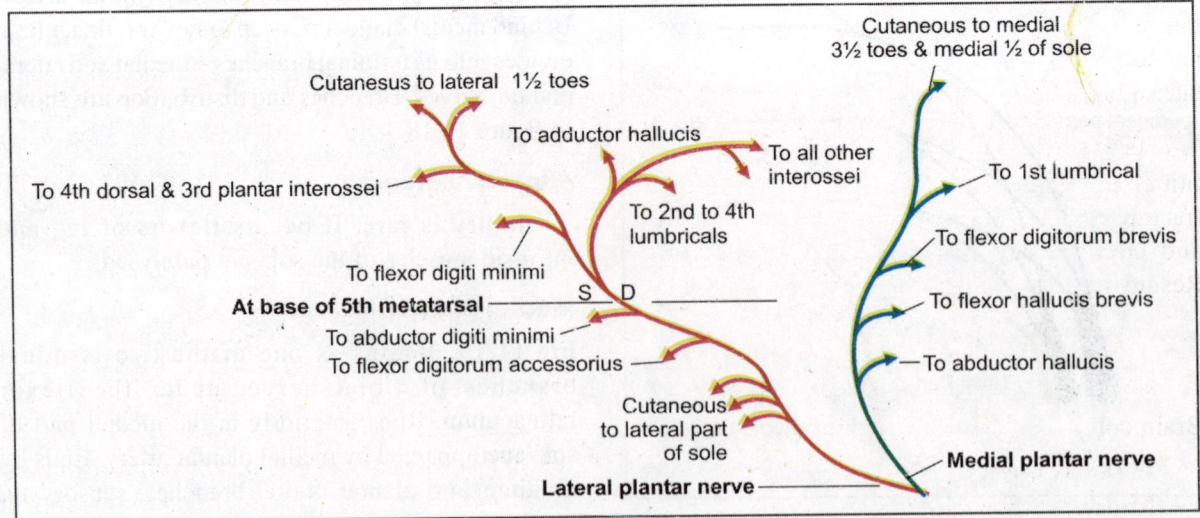

Fig. 11.19

Common peroneal nerve (Fig. 11.20)

Root value $L_{4,5} S_{1,2}$. From its origin from the sciatic nerve near the upper angle of popliteal fossa, descends along medial border of biceps femoris, to reach head of fibula. Then deep to peroneus longus, winds round neck of fibula and divides into superficial and deep peroneal nerves.

Branches from the trunk of common peroneal nerve are:

1. Sural communicating nerve.
2. Lateral cutaneous nerve of calf.
3. To knee joint.

Deep peroneal nerve

Begins as a branch of common peroneal nerve deep to proximal part of peroneus longus at the neck of fibula. It is the nerve of anterior compartment of leg. Descends deep in the anterior compartment accompanied by anterior tibial artery, on the interosseous membrane. In front of ankle joint, ends by dividing into lateral and medial branches. Branches and distribution, shown in (Fig.11.20)

Superficial peroneal nerve

One of the two terminal branches of common peroneal nerve and is the nerve of lateral compartment of leg. Descends between peroneus longus and brevis. Becomes cutaneous in the lower part of leg and ends by dividing into medial and lateral branches. Distribution, shown in (Fig.11.20)

Applied anatomy

Injury to common peroneal nerve is common in fracture of upper end of fibula. Muscles of anterior and lateral compartments of leg get paralysed. Results in 'foot drop'.

BRAIN

Brain consists of (Fig.11.21)

Fore brain,

Mid brain and

Hind brain

Forebrain is formed by 2 cerebral hemispheres (right and left), interconnected by corpus callosum.

Hind brain is formed of medulla oblongata (which is continuous with spinal cord below), pons and cerebellum.

Midbrain comes between forebrain and hind brain.

Medulla, pons and midbrain together form the brain stem.

Cerebellum is situated behind the brainstem and connected by superior, middle and inferior cerebellar peduncles to midbrain, pons and medulla.

The brain contains cavities – the ventricles, in which cerebro spinal fluid (CSF) is produced by choroid plexus. They are – two lateral ventricles, one in each cerebral hemisphere, one III ventricle, in the midline between the two hemispheres and a IV ventricle, in the hind brain. (Fig. 11.22)

The two lateral ventricles communicate with the III ventricle through the interventricular foramina. III ventricle is continuous below with the narrow cavity of midbrain – the cerebral aqueduct which opens below into the IV ventricle. IV ventricle is continuous below with the narrow central canal of the lower medulla and spinal cord.

C.S.F escapes into the subarachnoid space through 3 foramina present in the roof of IV ventricle.

MEDULLA OBLONGATA

It is about 3 cms long, below continuous with the spinal cord at the level of foramen magnum. It is conical in shape, broader above where it joins the pons. The central canal of spinal cord continues into the medulla, but it widens at the upper part of medulla to form the IV ventricle.

Surface features (Fig. 11.23 & 11.24)

Anteriorly and posteriorly along the midline, the medulla shows an anterior median fissure and a posterior median sulcus, both being continuous with similar features on spinal cord.

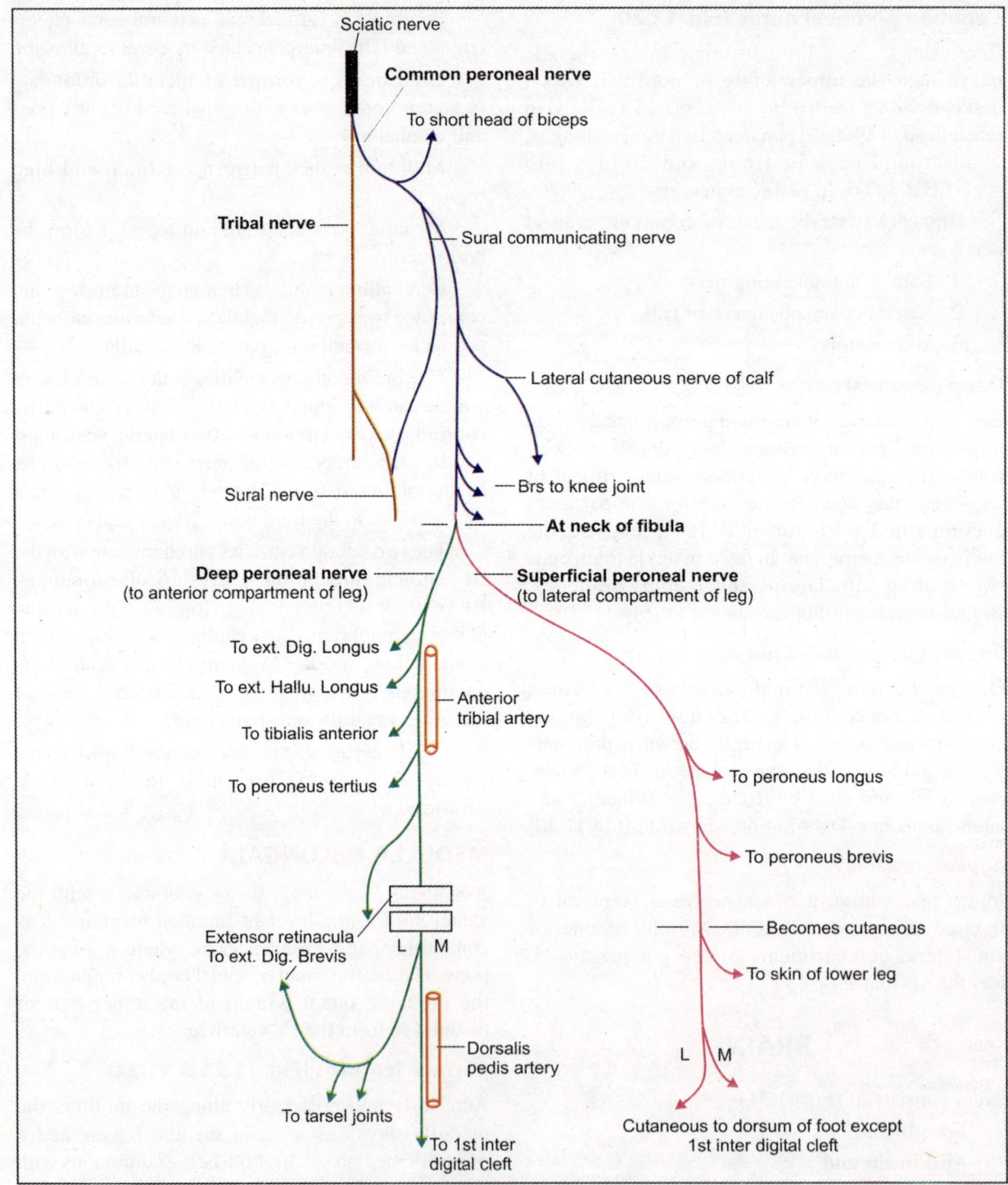

Sciatic nerve

Common peroneal nerve

To short head of biceps

Tribal nerve

Sural communicating nerve

Lateral cutaneous nerve of calf

Brs to knee joint

Sural nerve

At neck of fibula

Deep peroneal nerve
(to anterior compartment of leg)

Superficial peroneal nerve
(to lateral compartment of leg)

To ext. Dig. Longus

To ext. Hallu. Longus

Anterior
tribial artery

To tibialis anterior

To peroneus tertius

To peroneus longus

To peroneus brevis

Extensor retinacula
To ext. Dig. Brevis

L   M

Becomes cutaneous

To skin of lower leg

Dorsalis
pedis artery

L   M

To tarsel joints

To 1st inter
digital cleft

Cutaneous to dorsum of foot except
1st inter digital cleft

Fig. 11.20: Common peroneal nerve

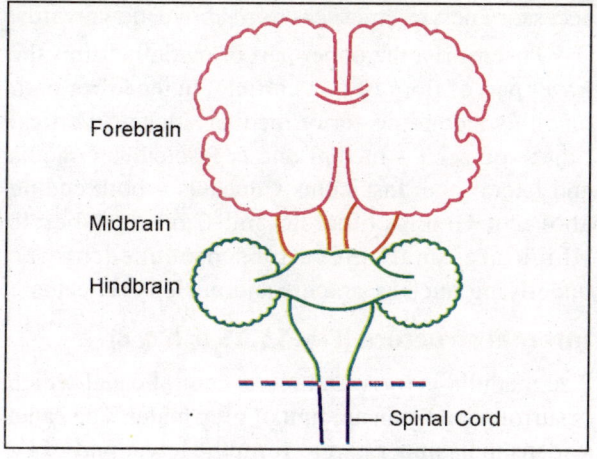

Fig. 11.21: Parts of brain

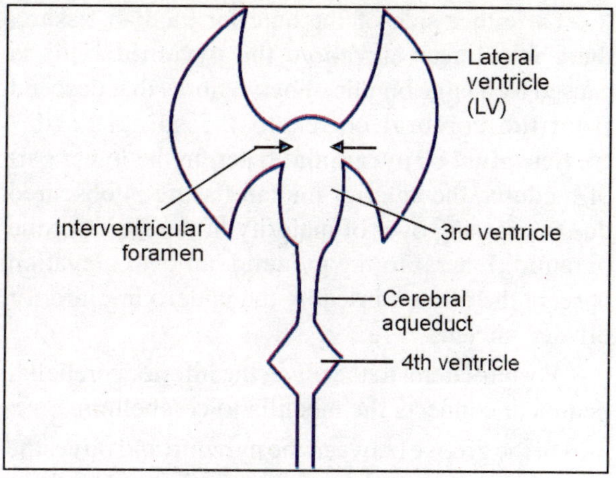

Fig. 11.22: Ventricles of brain

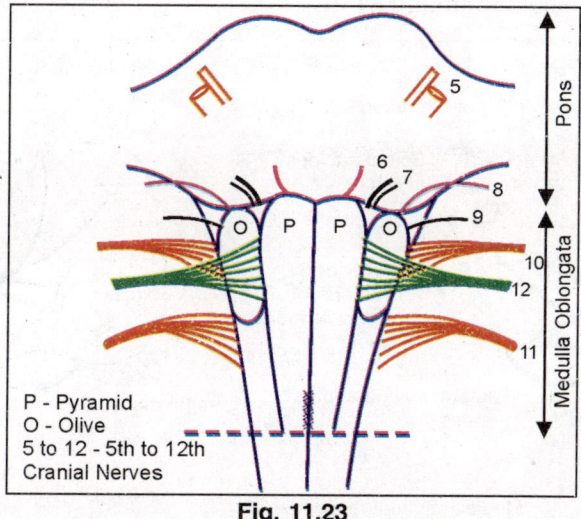

P - Pyramid
O - Olive
5 to 12 - 5th to 12th
Cranial Nerves

Fig. 11.23

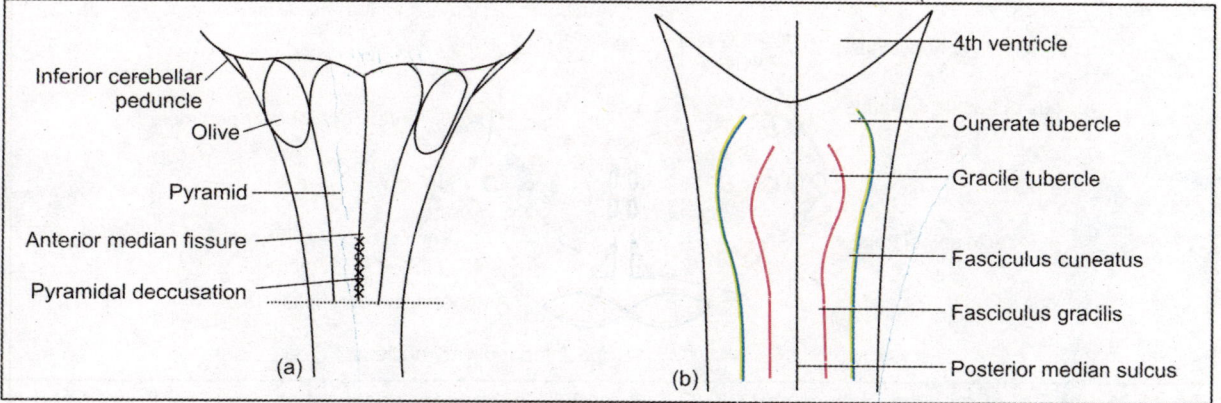

Fig. 11.24: (a) Medulla - Anterior aspect, (b) Medulla - Posterior aspect

On either side of the anterior median fissure, there is a linear elevation, the **pyramid.** This is caused by a large bundle of nerve fibres that descend from the cerebral cortex to the spinal cord – **corticospinal or pyramidal tract**. In the lower part of medulla, the anterior midian fissure is obscured due to crossing over of majority of the fibres of the pyramid. Lateral to the pyramid, an oval elevation is seen, the **olive**, caused by the underlying inferior olivary nucleus.

Posterolateral to the olive, the inferior cerebellar peduncle connects the medulla to cerebellum.

In the groove between the pyramid and olive, the rootlets of XII cranial nerve emerge. Lateral to olive, the glossopharyngeal, vagus and cranial part of accessory nerves emerge – from above, downwards.

Posteriorly, the upper part of medulla forms the lower part of floor of IV ventricle. In the lower part, on either side of posterior median sulcus, 2 vertical ridges are seen – medial one is fasciculus Gracilis and lateral one, fasciculus Cuneatus – both ending above in Gracile tubercle and Cuneate tubercle which are small elevations produced by the underlying nucleus gracilis and nucleus cuneatus.

Internal structure (Fig. 11.25 a, b & c)

The medulla is traversed by its central canal which is surrounded by an amount of grey mater. The canal widens in its upper part to form the lower part of IV ventricle.

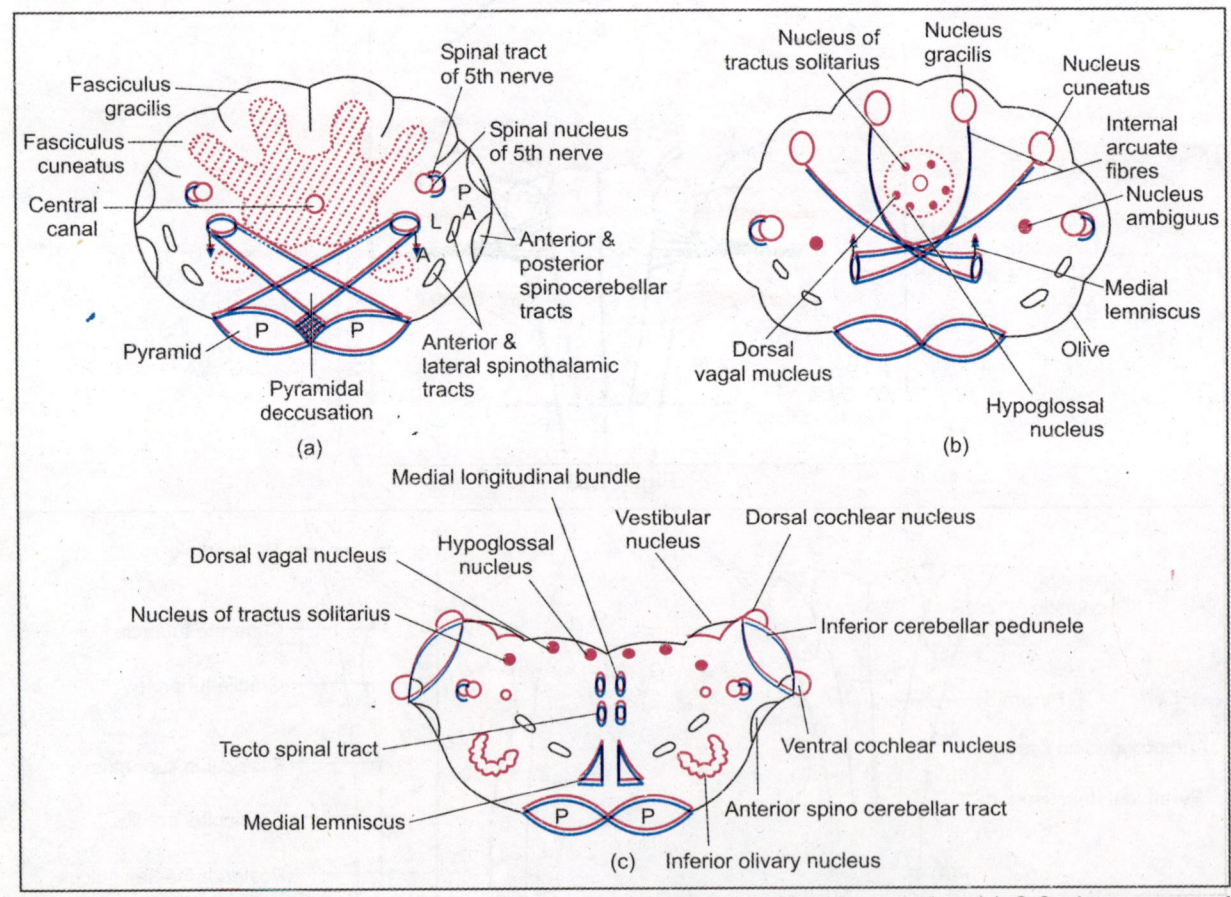

Fig. 11.25: (a) C.S of medulla - Lower part, (b) C.S of medulla at sensory deccusation, (c) C.S of upper part of medulla

Majority of the corticospinal fibres in the pyramid decussate in the lower part and descend through spinal cord as lateral corticospinal tract. Uncrossed fibres form anterior corticospinal tract.

Inferior olivary nucleus underlying the olive is seen as a crenated mass of grey mater.

From the gracile and cuneate nuclei fibres arise and cross over within the medulla as internal arcuate fibres and ascend towards thalamus as a band of white fibres - medial lemniscus. Also the anterior and lateral spinothalamic tracts ascend through the medulla.

Following cranial nerve nuclei are seen in the medulla.

Hypoglossal nucleus

Dorsal vagal nucleus

Nucleus of spinal tract of V nerve.

Nucleus of Tractus solitarius – common for VII, IX & X nerves.

Nucleus ambiguus – common for IX, X & XI nerves. Vestibular & cochlear nuclei near its junction with pons.

PONS

It is the region above the medulla and below the midbrain. About 2.5 cms in length. Behind it, cerebellum is situated, separated from it by the IV verticle. (Fig. 11.26 a)

Pons has a ventral bulging part, the basilar part and a dorsal part, the tegmentum. Posterior surface of the dorsal part forms floor of IV ventricle.

Internal structure (Fig. 11.26 b)

Basilar part is constituted by vertical fibres, horizontal fibres and collections of neurons – pontine nuclei. Vertical fibres descend from the cerebral cortex. Of these, the corticopontine fibres relay in the pontine nuclei and their fibres proceed as horizontal fibres towards cerebellum. Laterally, near the cerebellum, they form a compact bundle, middle

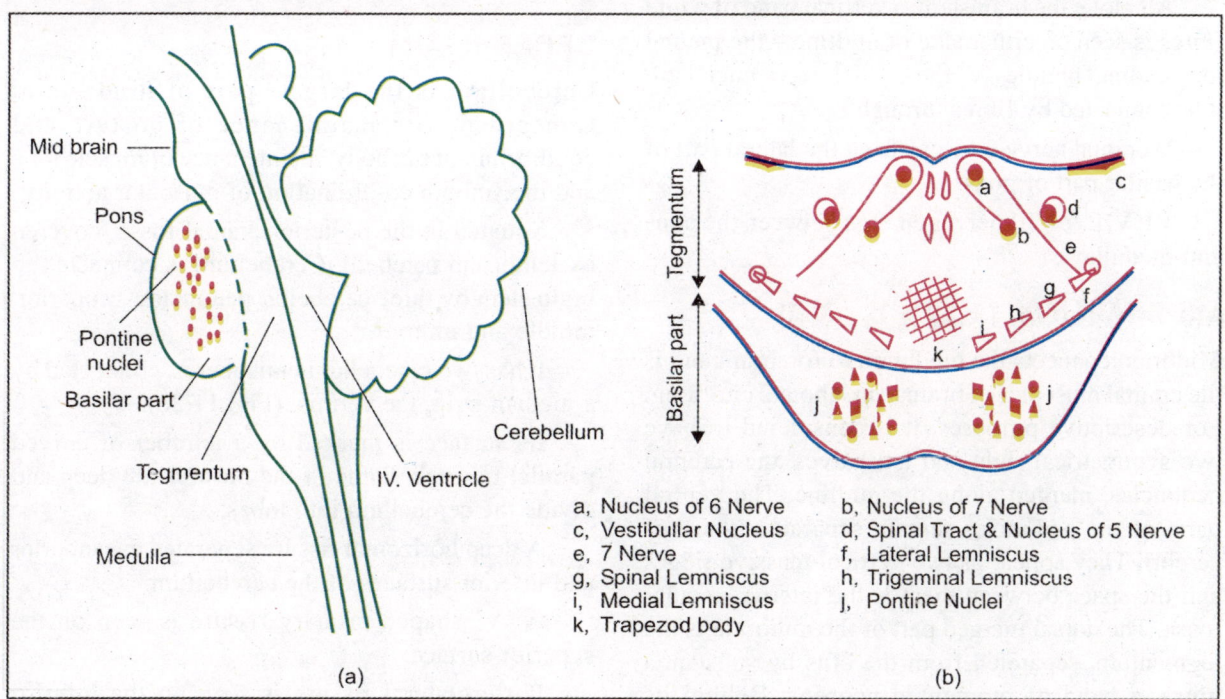

a, Nucleus of 6 Nerve	b, Nucleus of 7 Nerve
c, Vestibullar Nucleus	d, Spinal Tract & Nucleus of 5 Nerve
e, 7 Nerve	f, Lateral Lemniscus
g, Spinal Lemniscus	h, Trigeminal Lemniscus
i, Medial Lemniscus	j, Pontine Nuclei
k, Trapezod body	

(a)

(b)

Fig. 11.26: (a) Sagital section of brain stem with cerebellum (b) C.S of pons

cerebellar peduncle. The corticospinal and corticonuclear fibres descend to the medulla.

Anterior aspect of the dorsal part shows a conspicuous mass of transverse fibres crossing the midline – the trapezoid body. They are fibres in the auditory pathway, coming from the cochlear nuclei. Fibres from the trapezoid body ascend to midbrain as lateral lemniscus.

Lateral to the trapezoid body, there are the other ascending sensory fibre tracts - medial lemniscus, trigeminal leminiscus and spinal lemniscus.

In the lower aspect of the dorsal part, the nuclei of abducent and facial nerves are seen. Facial nerve fibres hook around the adbucent nucleus (facial colliculus) before the nerve emerges out. Laterally, the nucleus of spinal tract of trigeminal nerve and still laterally, vestibular nuclei extend into the posterior part of the lower part of pons.

Above in the dorsal part, the main sensory and motor nuclei of V nerve are seen.

All along the brainstem, a vertical band of white fibres is seen on either side of midline – the medial longitudinal bundle. All the cranial nerve nuclei are interconnected by fibres through it.

V cranial nerve emerges from the lateral part of the basilar part of pons.

VI, VII, & VIII nerves emerge between the pons and medulla.

MIDBRAIN (Fig. 11.27 a, b, c & d)

Midbrain connects the hindbrain to forebrain and is the cranial most part of brainstem, about 2 cms long. For descriptive purposes, it is considered to have two symmetrical right and left halves, the cerebral peduncles, merged along the midline. The ventral parts of the peduncles remain separate - the crus cerebri. They appear as two vertical massive ridges and the space between them is the interpeduncular fossa. The dorsal merged part of the midbrain is the tegmentum, separated from the crus by substantia nigra, a band of pigmented neurons. Behind its centre, the tegmentum is traversed by the cerebral

aqueduct connecting III ventricle above and IV ventricle below. The aqueduct is surrounded by an amount of grey mater- central grey mater. The part dorsal to the aqueduct is tectum.

Crus cerebri is formed of the descending fibres from cerebral cortex to lower levels.

Tectum consists of two pairs of colliculi - one pair of superior colliculus and one pair of inferior colliculus. They contain the corresponding nuclei. Superior colliculus is a visual reflex centre and inferior colliculus is a centre in the auditory pathway.

Through the tegmentum, pass the various ascending sensory tracts – lemnisci. At the level of superior colliculus, tegmentum has an oval mass of grey mater, the red nucleus. Red nucleus and substantia nigra are parts of extrapyramidal system.

Midbrain contains the nuclei of III and IV cranial nerves in the central grey mater. III nerve emerges through the ventral part and IV nerve through the dorsal part. The mesencephalic nucleus of V nerve also is seen in the central grey mater.

CEREBELLUM

Cerebellum is the largest part of hind brain. Concerned with maintenance of posture and equilibrium of the body, maintenance of muscle tone and the smooth co-ordination of muscular activity.

Situated in the posterior cranial fossa, covered by tentorium cerebelli. Cerebellum is connected to brain stem by three cerebellar peduncles – superior, middle and inferior.

It has two cerebellar hemispheres, connected by a median strip, the vermis. (Fig. 11.28)

Its surface is marked by a number of curved parallel fissures. Some of the fissures are deep and divide the cerebellum into lobes.

A deep horizontal fissure separates the superior and inferior surfaces of the cerebellum.

A 'V' shaped primary fissure is seen on the superior surface.

Posterolateral fissure is seen on the inferior surface.

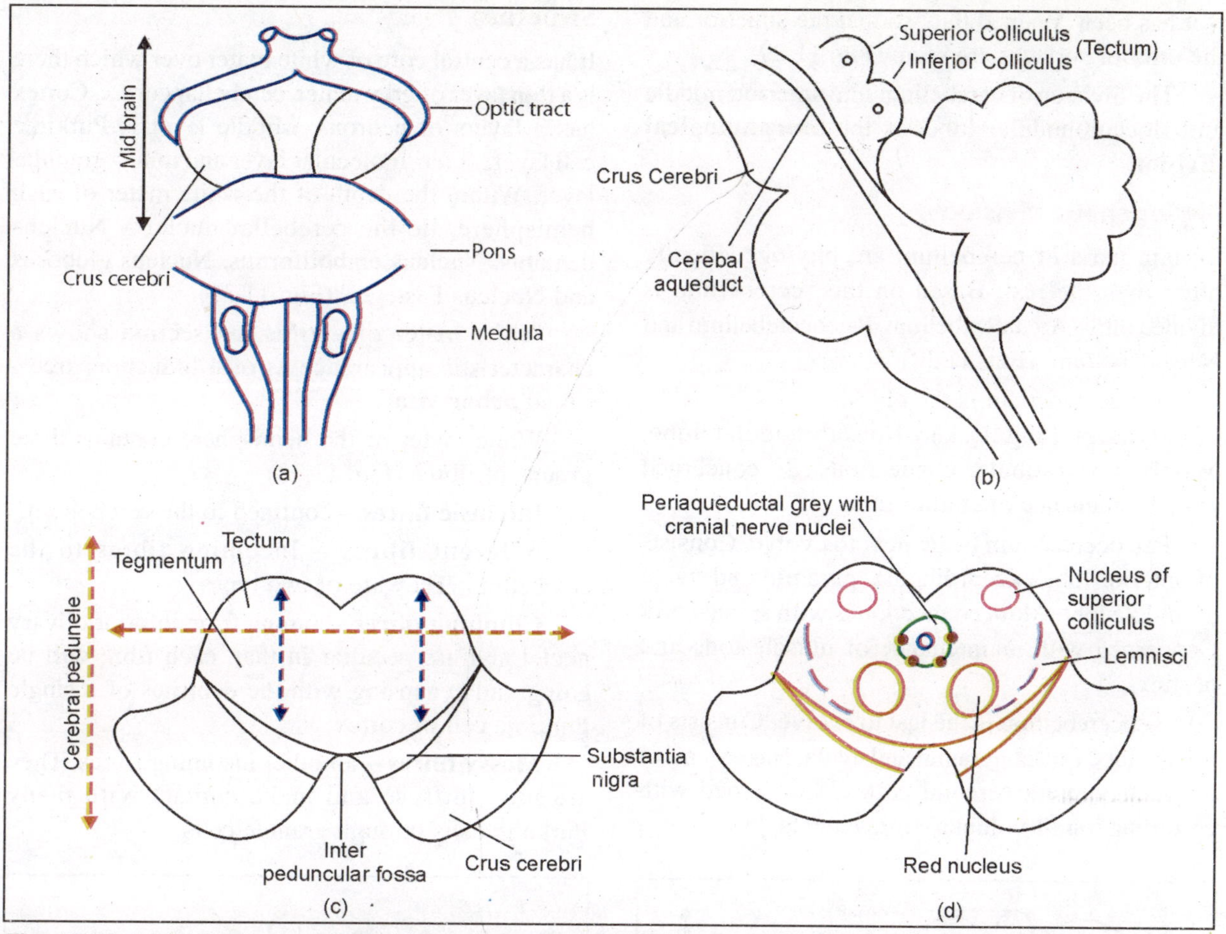

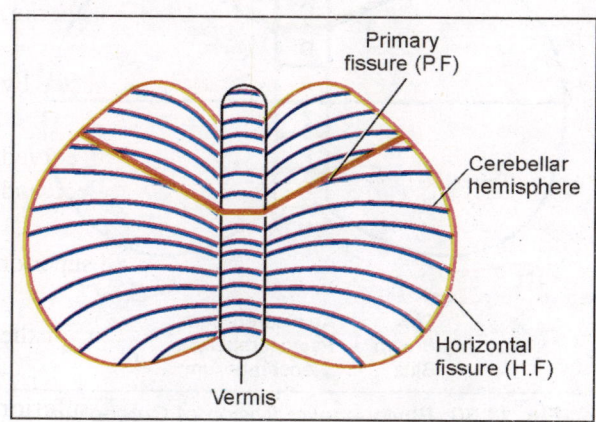

Fig. 11.27: (a) Midbrain ventral view (b) Midbrain sagital section (c) C.S of midbrain - parts (d) C.S. of midbrain - Superior colliculus level

Fig. 11.28: Cerebellum - Upper surface

The primary fissure and posterolateral fissure divide the cerebellum into three lobes.

Part anterior to primary fissure is anterior lobe.

Part between primary and posterolateral fissure is middle (or posterior) lobe.

Remaining part – flocculonodular lobe.

Fissures divide the vermis also into parts named as - Lingula, Central lobule, Culmen, Declive, Folium – on the superior surface and Tuber, Pyramid, Uvula and Nodule on the inferior surface.

To show the various subdivisions of cerebellum in a single diagram, here we represent the organ as if it has been "opened out" so that the superior and the inferior surfaces are seen. (Fig. 11.29)

The division of cerebellum into anterior, middle and flocculonodular lobes is the **morphological division.**

Phylogenetic division

Certain parts of cerebellum are phylogenetically older than the rest. Based on this, cerebellum is divided into – Archicerebellum, Paleocerebellum and Neocerebellum. (Fig. 11.30)

Archicerebellum is the oldest.

Consists of Lingula and flocculonodular lobe. Mainly has vestibular connections. So concerned with maintenance of equilibrium.

Paleocerebellum is the next to evolve. Consists of anterior lobe except lingula, pyramid and uvula of middle lobe. Main connection is with spinal cord. Concerned with maintenance of muscle tone and posture.

Neocerebellum is the last to evolve. Consists of middle lobe except pyramid and uvula. Has extensive connections with cerebral cortex. Concerned with co-ordination of voluntary movements.

Structure

It has a central core of white mater over which there is a thin layer of grey mater, cerebellar cortex. Cortex has 3 layers of neurons. Middle layer is Purkinje cell layer, outer- molecular layer and inner- granular layer. Within the depth of the white mater of each hemisphere, lie the cerebellar nuclei – Nucleus dentatus, Nucleus emboliformis, Nucleus globosus and Nucleus Fastegei. (Fig. 11.31)

White mater of vermis, on section shows a characteristic appearance as of a branching tree - called **arbor vitae.**

White mater of the hemisphere contains three groups of fibres (Fig. 11.32)

Intrinsic fibres – confined to the cerebellum.

Afferent fibres – Incoming fibres to the cerebellum. They are of two types:-

Climbing fibres - coming from inferior olivary nuclei and are peculiar in that, each fibre will be going and synapsing with the dentrites of a single Purkinje cell of cortex.

Mossy fibres – all other incoming fibres. They are more diffuse and make contact with many Purkinje cells through granule cells.

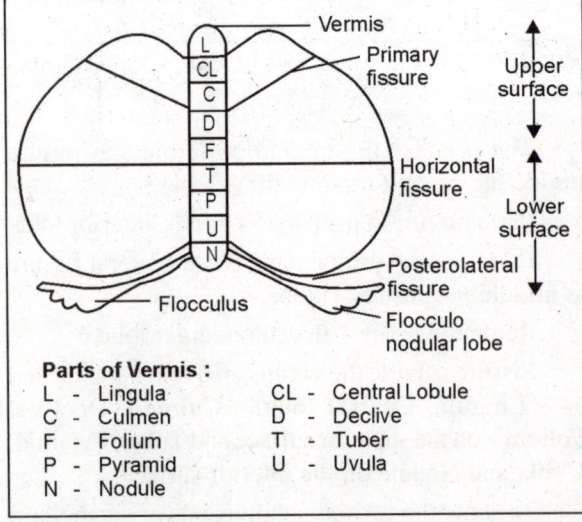

Parts of Vermis :

L	- Lingula	CL	- Central Lobule
C	- Culmen	D	- Declive
F	- Folium	T	- Tuber
P	- Pyramid	U	- Uvula
N	- Nodule		

Fig. 11.29: Schematic Diagram to Show the Features of Upper & Lower Surfaces of Cerebellum

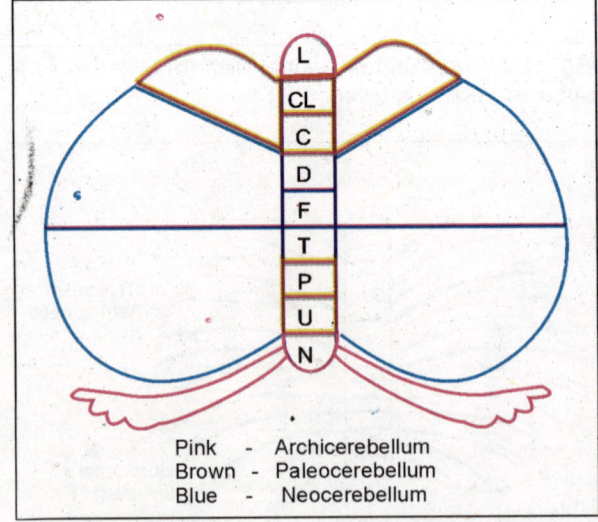

Pink - Archicerebellum
Brown - Paleocerebellum
Blue - Neocerebellum

Fig. 11.30: Phylogenetic division of Cerebellum

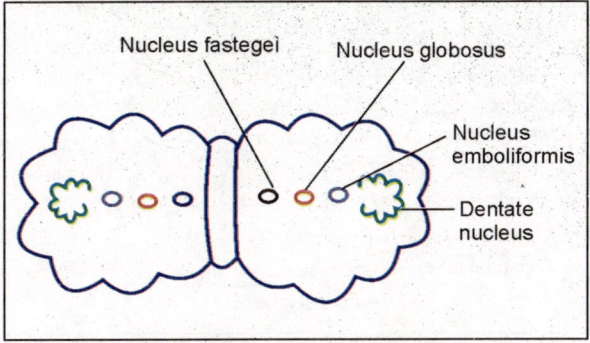

Fig. 11.31: Cerebellar Nucei

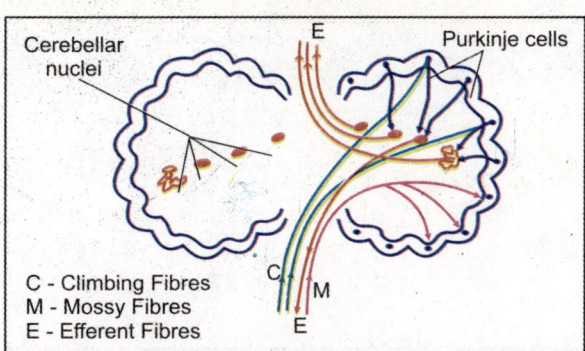

Fig. 11.32: Afferent & Efferent Fibres of Cerebellum

Efferent fibres - the cerebellar output begins as axons of Purkinje cells. They go and synapse with the cerebellar nuclei. Their axons go out as efferent fibres.

Afferent and efferent fibres pass through the three cerebellar peduncles. Through these fibres, Cerebellum is connected to Cerebrum, Thalamus, Red nucleus, Vestibular nuclei, Sensory tracts of spinal cord and Reticular formation. Inferior peduncle contains mostly afferent fibres from lower centres, middle peduncle contains pontocerebellar fibres and superior peduncle contains mostly efferent fibres to higher centres.

Functions and dysfunctions

Functions

- Co-ordination of muscular activity.
- Maintenance of equilibrium and posture.
- Maintenance of muscle tone.

Effects of dysfunction

- Disturbance in equilibrium and posture. Patient stands on a wide base, has tendency to fall to the side of lesion, sways on standing and has a staggering gait.
- Disturbance in muscle tone – Muscles become soft, tendon reflexes are reduced but sustained, muscles tire easily.
- Muscular in co-ordination – Asynergia - muscle groups fail to work harmoniously.

Dysmetria – control of range of movements is lost.

Dysdiadakokinesis – inability to do alternate rapid movements.

Intension tremor.

Nystagmus

Scanning speech - slurring speech.

CEREBRUM

Cerebrum (forebrain) is the largest and most rostral part of brain, occupies major part of cranial cavity.

It has right and left hemispheres separated by a median deep longitudinal fissure and partially connected by the Corpus callosum. Fig. 11.33

Each cerebral hemisphere has in its central core – Thalamus, Hypothalamus and related structures which together is known as Diencephalon. The remaining outer major part of the hemisphere is known as Telencephalon. The cavity of the diencephalon is the median III ventricle and of the telencephalon, the right and left lateral ventricles.

The cerebral hemisphere has got three poles: (Fig. 11.34.)

1. Frontal pole – anteriorly,
2. Occipital pole – posteriorly,
3. Temporal pole – anteroinferiorly.

It has got three surfaces –

1. Superolateral,
2. Medial and

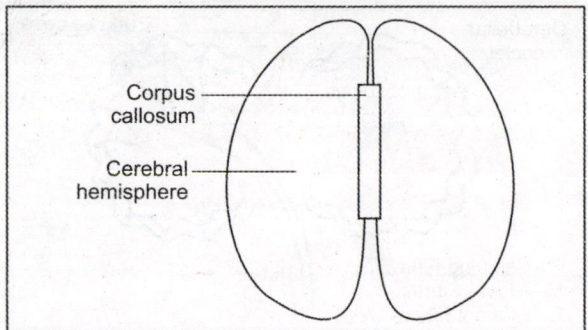

Fig. 11.33

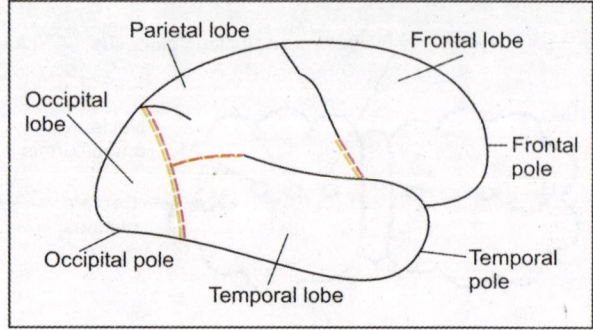

Fig. 11.34

3. Inferior.

Surfaces are not even, but present a number of grooves called sulci which separate the intervening ridge like regions called gyri.

Certain of the sulci are so prominent that they divide the cerebral hemisphere into lobes. They are the central and lateral sulci on the superolateral surface and the parieto-occipital and calcarine sulci on the medial surface. They divide the cerebrum into:

Frontal lobe,

Occipital lobe,

Temporal lobe and

Parietal lobe as shown in the Figure. 11.34.

Major sulci and gyri and functional areasm (Fig. 11.35 a,b,c)

Sulci

(a) On the superolateral surface

1. Central sulcus,

2. Precentral sulcus,

3. Post central sulcus,

4. Lateral sulcus, (has a stem, anterior horizontal ramus, anterior ascending ramus and posterior ramus).

5. Superior temporal sulcus,

6. Inferior temporal sulcus,

7. Intra parietal sulcus,

8. Superior frontal sulcus,

9. Inferior frontal sulcus and

10. Lunate sulcus.

(b) On the medial surface and posterior part of inferior surface-

1. Parieto-occipital sulcus,

2. Calcarine sulcus,

3. Cingulate sulcus,

4. Collateral sulcus,

5. Rhinal sulcus,

6. Occipito-temporal sulcus.

(c) On the anterior (orbital) part of inferior surface

1. Olfactory sulcus,

2. Orbital sulcus (H – shaped).

Gyri

(a) On supero-lateral surface:

1. Pre central gyrus (a),

2. Post central gyrus (b),

3. Superior, middle and inferior temporal gyri (f, g, h),

4. Superior, middle and inferior frontal gyri (c, d & e).

(b) On medial surface and posterior part of inferior surface :

1. Cingulate gyrus,

2. Cuneus,

3. Lingual gyrus,

4. Para-hippocampal gyrus.

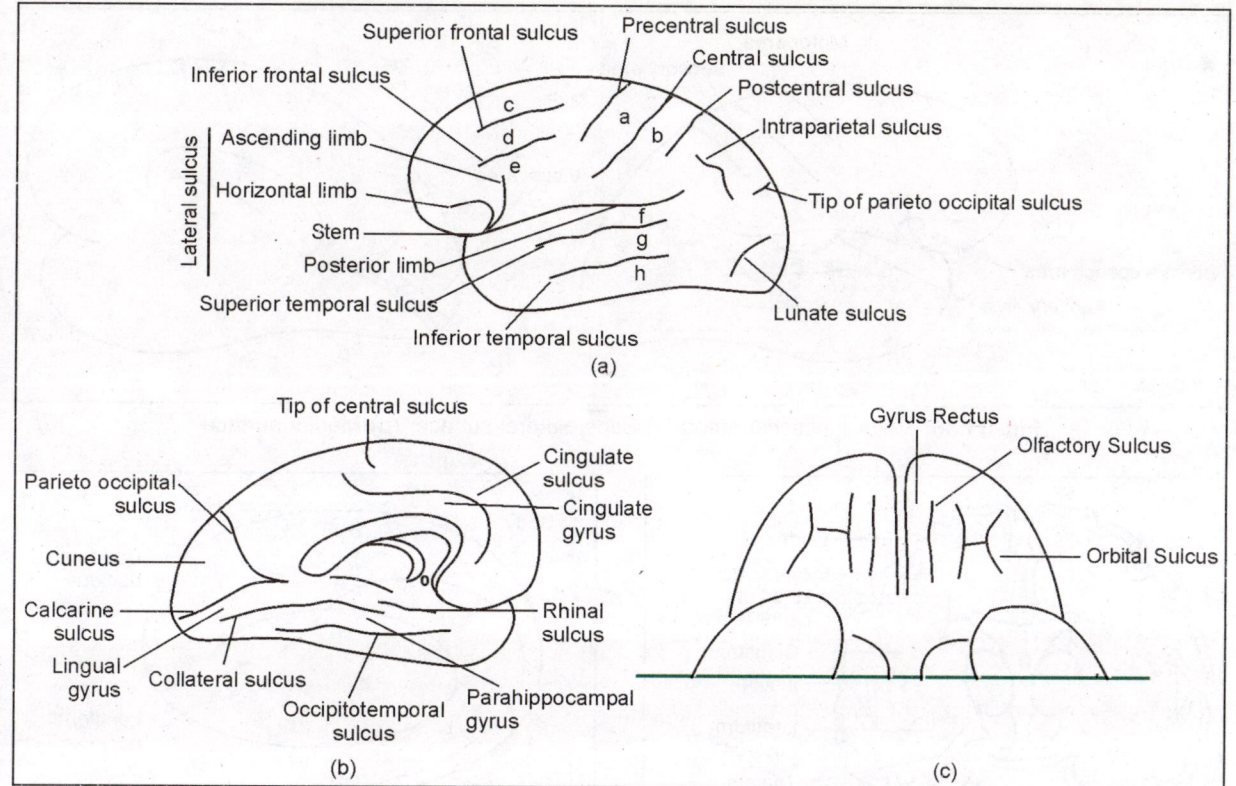

Fig. 11.35: Major sulci & gyri (a)Superolateral surface, (b) Medial surface (c) Anterior part of inferior surface

(c) On anterior part of inferior surface :

1. Gyrus rectus,
2. Anterior, posterior, medial and lateral orbital gyri

Major functional areas (Fig. 11.36 a&b)

1. Motor area – in precentral gyrus,
2. Sensory area – in postcentral gyrus,
3. Auditory area – in the inferior wall of postcrior ramus of lateral sulcus,
4. Speech area – between the anterior ascending ramus and posterior ramus of lateral sulcus,
5. Visual area – in the walls of calcarine sulcus.

Insula

Deep to the stem of lateral sulcus, there is a part of cerebral cortex, called Insula. During development of cerebrum, the surrounding regions overgrew this part, which thus got hidden from the surface. The surrounding parts of cerebrum are called opercula.

Structure of cerebral hemisphere

Cerebral hemisphere has an outer thin layer of grey matter, the cerebral cortex. Thickness varies between 1.5 to 4.5 cms in different regions and has different types of neurons arranged in layers. The various functional areas are located in different regions of the cortex.

Deep to the cortex, the cerebrum has white matter formed of nerve fibres. Masses of grey matter, the basal nuclei, lie in the depth of the white matter. (Fig. 11.37)

Medial to these, in the deep part of the cerebrum lie the parts of diencephalon – Thalamus, Hypothalamus and Subthalamus. (Fig. 11.37)

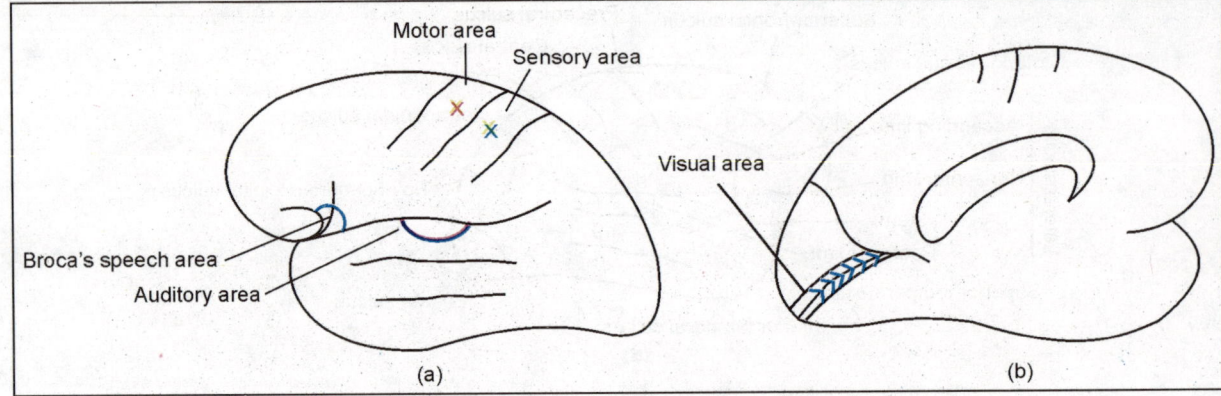

Fig. 11.36: Major functional areas (a) Superolateral surface, (b) Medial surface

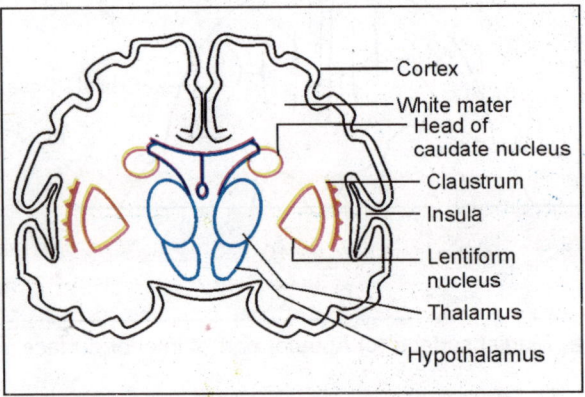

Fig. 11.37: Coronal Section of brain

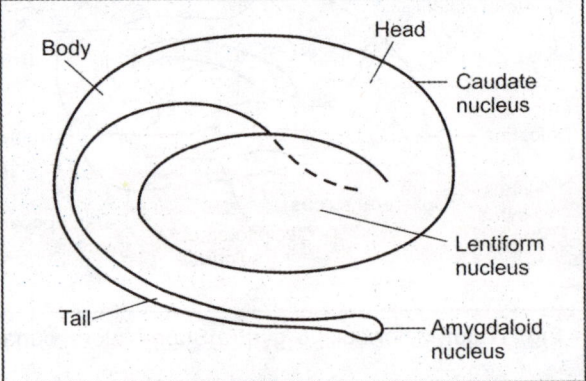

Fig. 11.38: Parts of Basal Ganglia

Basal Ganglia (Fig. 11.38 & 11.39)

They are masses of grey mater that lie in the deep inferior part of cerebrum, lateral to the thalamus.

They are:

1. Caudate nucleus,
2. Lentiform nucleus – Putamen & Globus pallidus
3. Amygdaloid nucleus,
4. Claustrum.

Caudate nucleus and lentiform nucleus together form the Corpus striatum.

Caudate Nucleus

It is a large 'C' shaped mass of grey mater closely related to the lateral ventricle and lies lateral to the thalamus. It has a head, body and tail.

Head is continuous with the putamen of lentiform nucleus. Amygdaloid nucleus is seen at the tip of the tail (Fig. 11.38).

Lentiform Nucleus

It is a wedge shaped mass of grey mater, lying lateral to thalamus and caudate nucleus, separated from them by the internal capsule. Its lateral part is putamen and medial part, globus pallidus (Fig. 11.39).

Claustrum

It is a thin lamina of grey mater which lies lateral to lentiform nucleus.

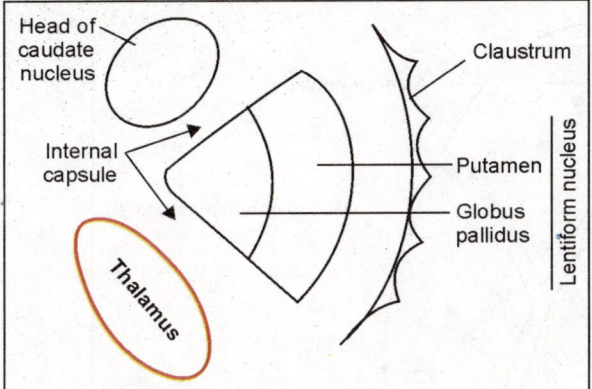

Fig. 11.39: Relations of basal ganglia (horizontal section)

Functions

Basal nuclei are connected to cerebral cortex, thalamus, substantia nigra and brain stem. Through these connections they influence the motor cortex and motor centres in the brain stem, and thus control and regulate the voluntary muscular movements.

Dysfunction of basal nuclei and substantia nigra leads to Parkinson's disease.

DIENCEPHALON

Within the cerebrum, there is a deep central part, the diencephalon. Parts of diencephalon of right and left hemispheres enclose a narrow midline cavity, the III ventricle.

Diencephalon consists of thalamus, hypothalamus, subthalamus and epithalamus.

Thalamus

Thalamus forms the major part of diencephalon. It is the great sensory relay station. Ascending sensory pathways carrying various sensations from the whole of the body (except olfactory sensation) reach the nuclei in the thalamus and relay there. Thence they are projected to the sensory cortex of cerebrum.

Thalamus is an ovoid mass of grey mater with a narrow anterior end and an expanded posterior end called pulvinar. Lies on either side of the III ventricle

and laterally it is separated from the lentiform nucleus by internal capsule.

On the posterior surface of pulvinar, there are two small swellings, the medial and lateral geniculate bodies. Medial one is a part of auditory pathway and lateral one, a part of visual pathway.

The grey mater of thalamus is divided by a 'Y' shaped sheet of white mater, the internal medullary lamina, into anterior, medial and lateral parts. Each part contains a number of important nuclear groups. (Fig. 11.40)

The nuclear groups are :-

(a) **in the ventral aspect of lateral part :**
1. Nucleus Ventralis Posterolateralis (V P L)
   Receives general sensations from the body except face.
2. Nucleus Ventralis Posteromedialis (V P M)
   Receives general sensations from face and also taste sensation.
3. Ventral Anterior Nucleus (V A)
4. Ventral Intermediate nucleus (V I)

(b) **in the dorsal aspect of lateral part :**
1. Lateral Dorsal Nucleus (L D)
2. Lateral Posterior Nucleus (L P)
3. Pulvinar (P)

(c) **in the anterior part:** Anterior nuclei (A).

(d) **in the medial part:** Medial Dorsal nucleus (M D)

(e) **on the medial surface:** Midline nuclei (M)

(f) **on the lateral surface:** Reticular nuclei (R)

(g) **in the internal medullary lamina:** Intra Laminar nuclei (I L)

(h) **on the posterior surface:**
1. Nucleus of Medial Geniculate Body
2. Nucleus of Lateral Geniculate Body

Lesion of thalamus results in loss of sensations on the opposite half of the body - usually due to vascular accidents – haemorrhage or thrombosis in thalamus.

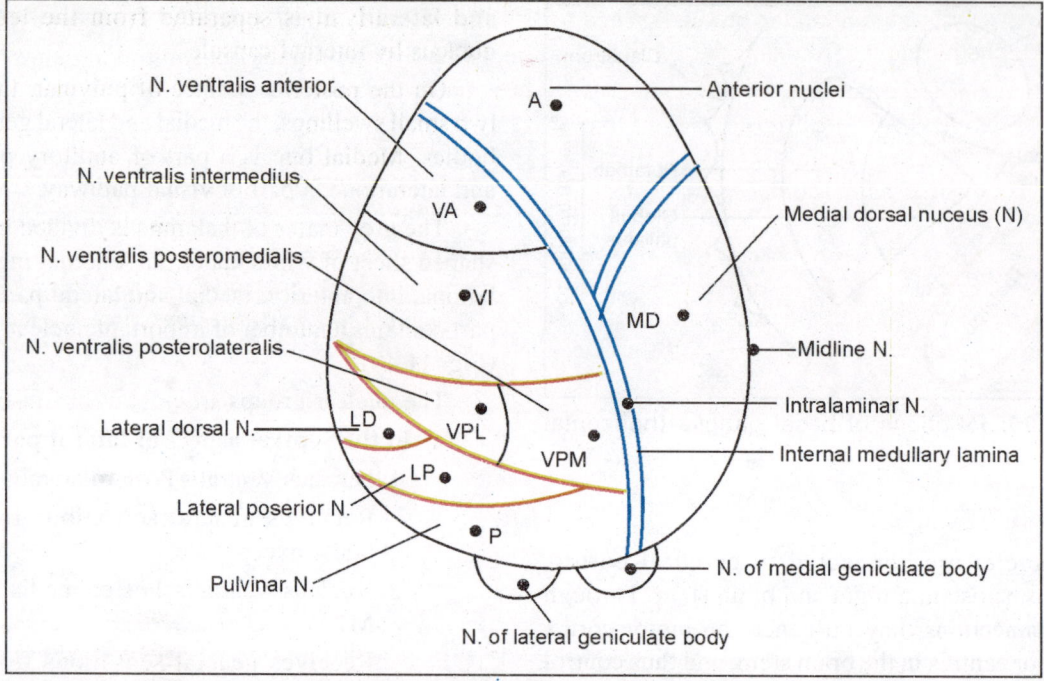

N. ventralis anterior

N. ventralis intermedius

N. ventralis posteromedialis

N. ventralis posterolateralis

Lateral dorsal N.

Lateral poserior N.

Pulvinar N.

A — Anterior nuclei

VA

VI

MD — Medial dorsal nuceus (N)

LD — Midline N.

VPL — Intralaminar N.

LP — Internal medullary lamina

VPM — N. of medial geniculate body

P

N. of lateral geniculate body

Fig. 11.40: Thalamic nuclei

Hypothalamus

It is a part of diencephalon, located below the thalamus, separated from it by the hypothalamic sulcus. Although a small part, it has got great functional importance. It controls the emotional states of the individual, the autonomic nervous system and the endocrine system. It regulates the body temperature, influences sleep, food and water intake and genital functions.

It is divided into different regions :-

1. Preoptic region – adjacent to lamina terminalis.
2. Supraoptic region – above optic chiasma.
3. Tuberal region -- includes infundibulum, tuber cinerium and region above it.
4. Mamillary region – includes mamillary bodies.

These regions contain important nuclear groups. They are:

1. Preoptic
2. Paraventricular
3. Dorsomedial
4. Ventromedial
5. Infundibular
6. Posterior
7. Supraoptic
8. Lateral
9. Tuberomamillary
10. Lateral tuberal
11. Supra chiasmatic.

The supra optic nucleus produces ADH (vasopressin) and paraventricular nucleus produces oxytocin. These secretions (neuro secretions) are carried along the axons of the neurons and are released into the sinusoids in neurohypophysis.

Hypothalamus directly influences the functions of pituitary gland. The infundibular nucleus produces release factors or release inhibiting factors which reach the adenohypophysis through capillaries.

These hormones induce or inhibit the production and release of various hormones from anterior pituitary.

The functional importance of hypothalamus is also due to its connections with different regions like limbic system, reticular formation, autonomic centres of the brainstem, spinal cord, cerebral cortex, thalamus and pituitary gland.

Subthalamus

This lies between the thalamus and tegmentum of midbrain, behind the hypothalamus. Apart from the subthalamic nucleus, it also includes cranial ends of red nucleus and substantia nigra of mid brain. It has connections with corpus striatum and hence involved in the control of muscular activity.

Epithalamus

Consists of habenular nuclei and pineal gland. Habenular nucleus is a small nucleus behind the thalamus. It is a centre of integration of olfactory, visceral and somatic pathways.

Pineal gland is a small gland connected to diencephalon posteriorly by a small stalk. It has no neurons, but specialized cells called pinealocytes, secretions of which exert inhibitory influences on the activities of other endocrine glands. Melatonin is a component of its secretion.

Limbic system

It includes certain regions of grey mater of brain arranged roughly in a ring like manner. They are:

1. Hippocampus
2. Dentate gyrus
3. Parahippocampal gyrus
4. Subcallosal gyrus
5. Cingulate gyrus
6. Amygdala
7. Habenular nuclei
8. Hypothalamic nuclei
9. Anterior thalamic nuclei
10. Septal nuclei
11. Uncus

The alveus, fimbria, fornix, mamillothalamic tract and stria terminalis constitute the connecting fibre pathways of this system.

Functions

1. Hippocampus is concerned with recent memory. Its lesion results in inability to store memory (anterograde amnesia).
2. Limbic system is concerned with emotional behaviour related to fear, anger and sexual activity.
3. It has a major role in the control of visceral functions.
4. It controls the activities of procuring food and eating behaviour.

RETICULAR FORMATION

It consists of a diffuse network of nerve cells and fibres, deeply placed in the CNS - from spinal cord to the cerebrum. Along it, neurons are grouped to form nuclei. The reticular formation is placed among the ascending and descending fibre tracts and the nuclei. It is reciprocally connected to all parts of the brain. It influences the motor cranial nerves, nuclei of brainstem and anterior horn cells of spinal cord. It is closely related and connected by collaterals with the ascending sensory tracts. Sensory information received in reticular formation through these is projected to different parts of cerebral cortex. This forms Ascending Reticular Activating System (ARAS) which is responsible for the level of alertness, wakefulness and consciousness of the individual. By means of its vast connections, other functions are :-

1. It influences and controls the muscle tone.
2. Controls the autonomic nervous system and the endocrine system.
3. Certain parts of reticular formation in medulla has influence on cardiovascular and respiratory functions – (through the connections of reticular formation with dorsal nucleus of vagus).

Blood supply of brain

Brain is richly supplied with blood. Neurons undergo irreversible damage within 7 minutes of cessation of blood supply. Vascular lesions are responsible for neurological disorders more than any other cause.

Brain gets its blood supply from two pairs of arteries – vertebral and internal carotid. (Fig. 11.41)

Inside the cranium the two vertebral arteries join to form basilar artery that lies on the surface of pons. At the upper border of pons it divides into two posterior cerebral arteries.

On the under surface of brain, at the interpeduncular fossa, the two internal carotid arteries divide into anterior cerebral and middle cerebral arteries. At the site of bifurcation, each internal carotid artery gives off a posterior communicating artery which goes posteriorly to join the posterior cerebral artery. The two anterior cerebral arteries are connected by a short anterior communicating artery. Thus a ring of arteries – Circulus arteriosus or Circle of Willis is formed at the base of brain. Branches from the circle supply the cerebrum, and branches from vertebral and basilar arteries supply the brainstem and cerebellum.

Branches:

1. Cortical branches

Cortical branches from the anterior, middle and posterior cerebral arteries ramify on the surface of the cerebrum and supply the cortex. They anastomose freely and the distribution is as follows. (Fig. 11.42 a, b & c)

On the superolateral surface - a narrow strip about 2.5cms broad along the superior border upto parieto-occipital sulcus is supplied by anterior cerebral artery. A similar strip along the inferior

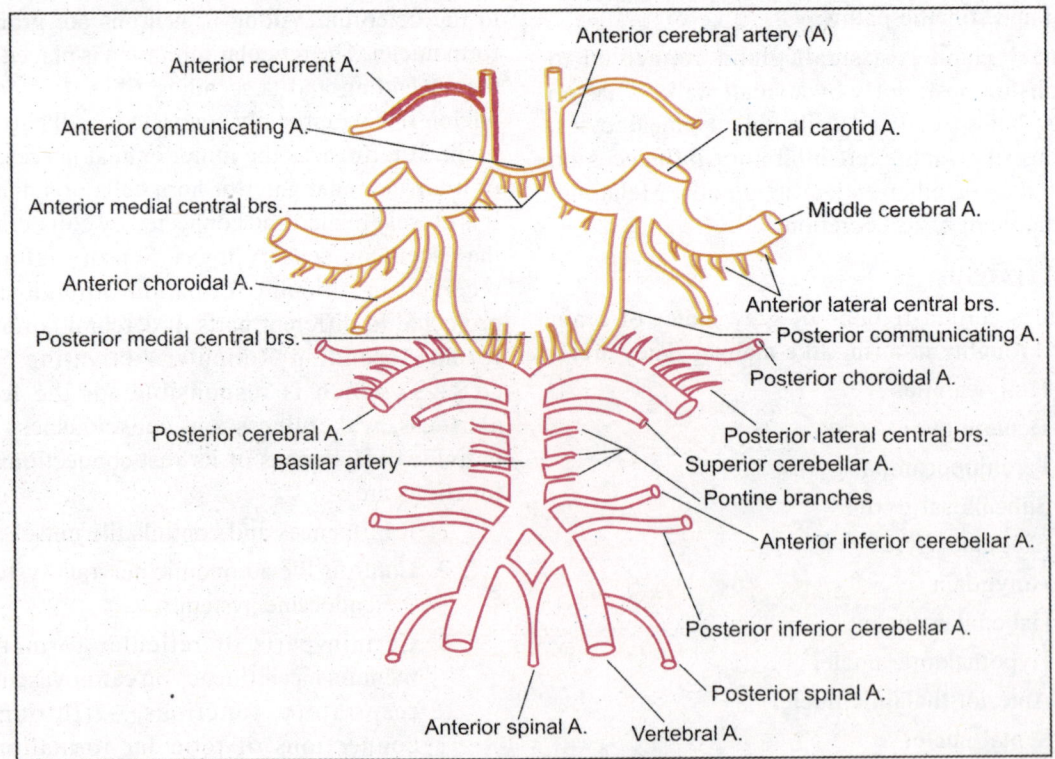

Fig. 11.41: Circle of willis

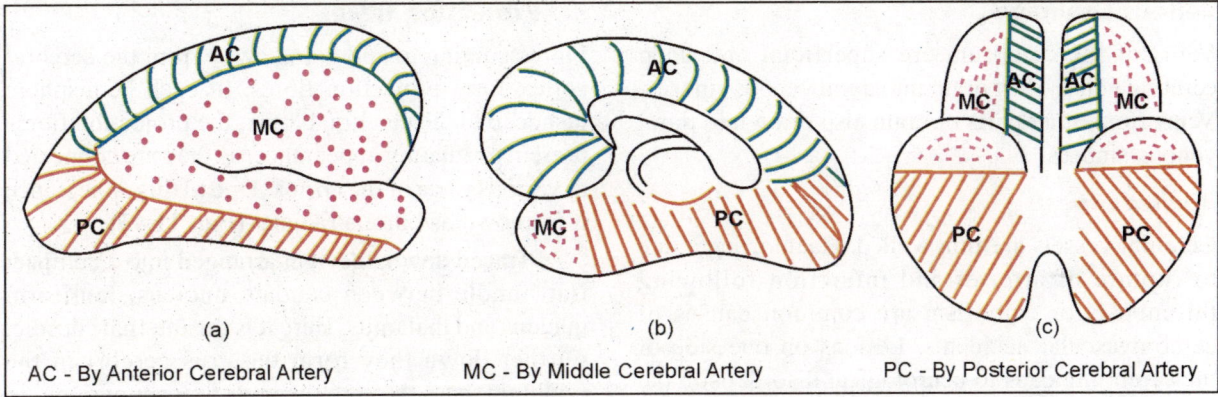

AC - By Anterior Cerebral Artery   MC - By Middle Cerebral Artery   PC - By Posterior Cerebral Artery

Fig. 11.42: (a) On Superolateral Surface, (b) On Medial Surface, (c) On Inferior Surface

border in the inferior temporal gyrus, upto and including occipital lobe, is supplied by the posterior cerebral artery. Remaining major part is supplied by middle cerebral artery.

On the medial surface – major part is supplied by anterior cerebral artery except the occipital lobe which is supplied by posterior cerebral artery and the temporal lobe which is supplied by middle cerebral artery.

On the inferior aspect – the tentorial surface is supplied by the posterior cerebral artery except at the temporal pole which is supplied by the middle cerebral artery. The orbital surface, in its lateral part by middle cerebral artery and in its medial part by anterior cerebral artery.

2. Central branches

They penetrate deep into the brain and supply the deeper parts. They do not show much anastamosis and are practically end arteries. There are four sets :-

(i) Anteromedial – from anterior cerebral and anterior communicating arteries.

(ii) Anterolateral – from middle cerebral artery. They are called striate arteries, and there are medial and lateral striate arteries. One among the lateral striate arteries, has a longer course and is more susceptable to haemorrhage, is

known as Charcot's artery of cerebral haemorrhage.

(iii) Posteromedial–from posterior cerebral and posterior communicating arteries.

(iv) Posterolateral – from posterior cerebral arteries.

3. Anterior choroidal artery

– a branch from internal carotid artery at its termination.

4. Posterior choroidal artery

– from posterior cerebral artery.

5. Anterior recurrent (Hubner's) artery

– from anterior cerebral artery.

Apart from these, branches from the vertebral and basilar arteries are:

(i) Anterior and posterior spinal arteries.

(ii) Posterior inferior cerebellar artery
   - both from vertebral artery.

(iii) Anterior inferior cerebellar artery.

(iv) Pontine arteries.

(v) Superior cerebellar artery.

(iii), (iv) & (v) from basilar artery.

These branches supply the neighbouring parts of brain.

Venous Drainage

Veins of the cerebrum are superficial and deep cerebral veins. They drain into dural venous sinuses. Veins from other parts of brain also drain into dural venous sinuses.

Applied aspects

Cerebral vessels are thin walled. Haemorrhage due to rupture of arteries and infarction following thrombosis or embolism are common causes of cerebrovascular accidents. Lesions on one side of the cerebrum leads to neurological disorders on the opposite half of the body. This depends upon the region of brain affected and the type of vascular lesion.

WHITE MATER OF BRAIN

Deep to the thin layer of grey mater - the cerebral cortex, the cerebral hemispheres have the white mater. It is composed of myelinated axons - nerve fibres, supported by neuroglia.

White mater is classified into three groups -

1. Association fibres

They run between different regions of the same hemisphere.

    (a) Short association fibres – connect adjacent gyri.

    (b) Long association fibres – connect distant parts of the hemisphere. (*e.g.*, uncinate fasciculus - runs between temporal and frontal poles, superior longitudinal bundle, inferior longitudinal bundle.)

2. Commissural fibres

They connect corresponding regions of the two hemispheres.

    (a) Corpus callosum

    (b) Anterior commissure

    (c) Posterior commissure

    (d) Habenular commissure

3. Projection fibres

Fibres coming to and going away from the cerebral cortex form projection fibres. In each hemisphere just deep to the cerebral cortex, the projection fibres present a radiating appearance, as they are connected to various parts of the cortex. Due to this appearance it is known as corona radiata. (Fig. 11.43)

Traced down, they get arranged into a compact flat bundle between caudate nucleus, lentiform nucleus and thalamus. Here it is the internal capsule. Further down they form the crus cerebri in the midbrain, pass through the pons to form pyramid in the medulla and finally reach the spinal cord as cortico spinal tract. Along its extent, fibres of this lengthy bundle of projection fibres are connected to most of the subcortical centres – thalamus, hypothalamus, basal ganglia, cranial nerve nuclei and the nuclei of the brain stem.

Internal capsule

A part of projection fibres. (Fig. 11.44)

It is a compact flat bundle of white mater, between the thalamus and caudate nucleus medially and lentiform nucleus laterally. Above – continuous with corona radiata and below with crus cerebri.

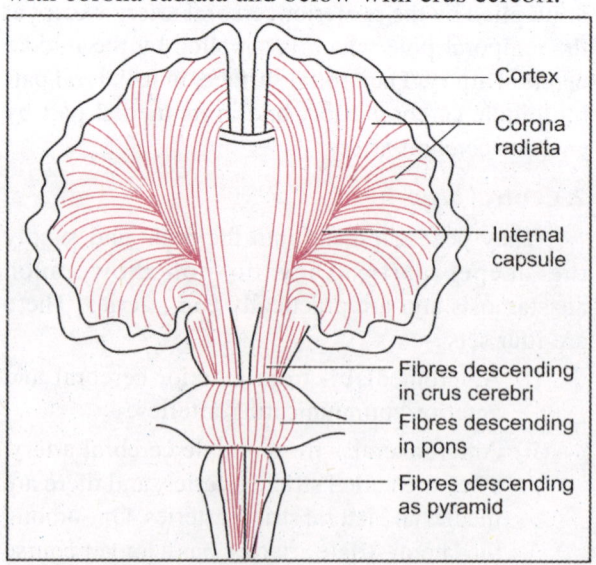

Fig. 11.43: Projection Fibres

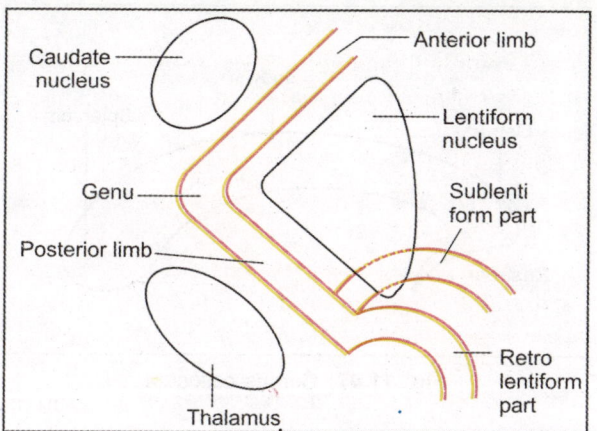

Fig. 11.44: Parts & Relations of Internal Capsule

In its position between thalamus, caudate nucleus and lentiform nucleus it is bent into a '<' shaped band. So it has an anterior limb, genu and posterior limb. Some fibres of the internal capsule lie behind the lentiform nucleus – it is the retrolentiform part. Some fibres lie beneath the lentiform nucleus – the sublentiform part. (Fig. 11.43 & Fig. 11.44)

Different groups of fibres occupy specific regions in the internal capsule, as shown in the figure (Fig 11.45). Auditory radiation (inferior thalamic radiation) occupy the sublentiform part and visual radiation (posterior thalamic radiation) occupy the retrolentiform part (Fig. 11.45).

Blood supply

Central / striate branches from the circle of Willis reach the internal capsule. Arteries supplying different parts of internal capsule are as shown. (Fig. 11.46)

Clinical importance

Internal capsule can be involved in vascular accidents like haemorrhage or embolism. Because of high concentration of fibres along internal capsule, even a small vascular lesion in it can cause widespread neurological symptoms on the opposite side of the body.

Corpus callosum (Fig. 11.47 to 11.49)

This thick bundle of white mater is the largest commissure of brain. When the two hemispheres are separated by a sagital section, the corpus callosum presents as a curved structure on the medial surface of the hemisphere.

Its curved anterior end is the genu. A narrow band extends from the genu – the rostrum. Major central part is the body. Body ends posteriorly in a thick curved part, the splenium.

Corpus callosum is closely related to the lateral

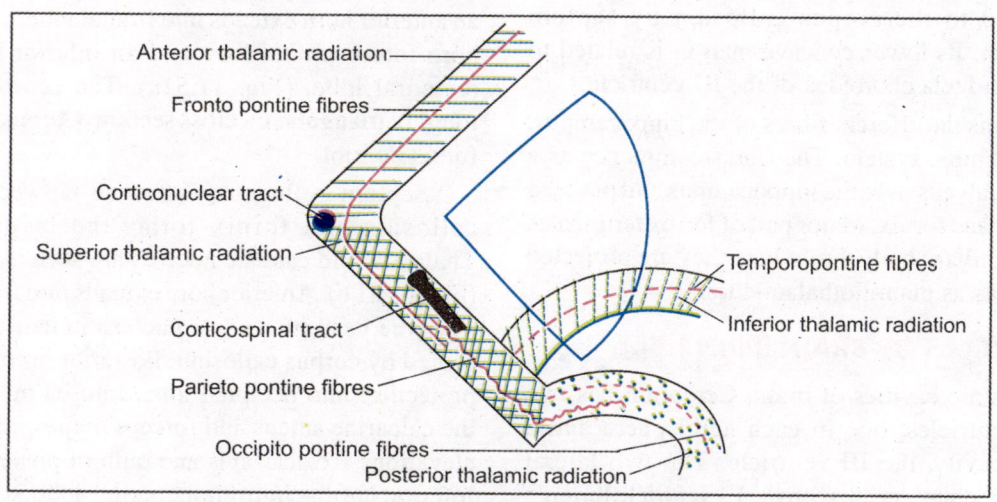

Fig. 11.45: Arrangement of Fibre Tracts in Internal Capsule

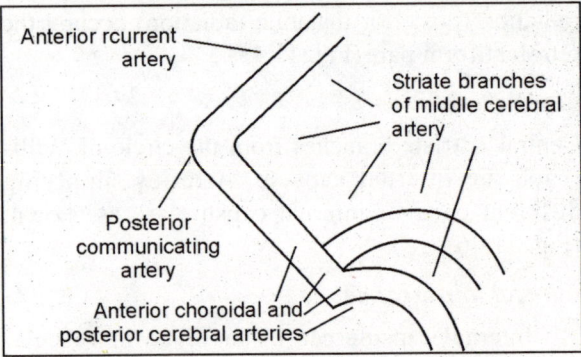

Fig. 11.46: Blood Supply of Internal Capsule

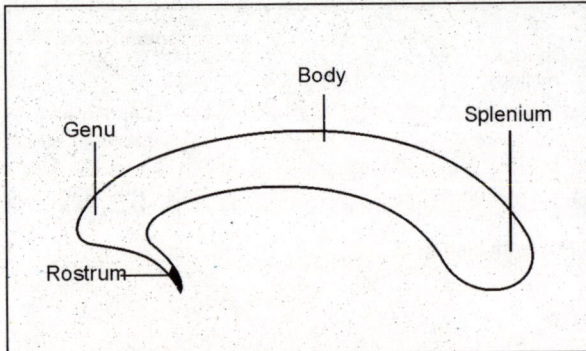

Fig. 11.47: Corpus callosum

ventricles and partly forms their roof. Septum pellucidum is attached to its under surface. Almost all parts of the two hemispheres are interconnected by the fibres of corpus callosum. Fibres that pass through the genu connect similar regions of the two frontal lobes; these constitute a 'U' shaped band called forceps minor. Fibres that pass through splenium connect the two occipital lobes and form a larger 'U' shaped band – forceps major. Fibres that pass through the body pass laterally and curve inferiorly forming a flat band – tapetum. (Fig. 11.48)

Fornix (Fig. 11.49)

It is seen as a curved bundle of fibres on the medial surface of the hemisphere. Its upper surface is connected to the corpus callosum by septum pellucidum. Its lower concave margin is related to the roof and tela choroidea of the III ventricle.

It forms the efferent fibres of the hippocampus, a part of limbic system. The fibres commence as a thin layer, alveus over the hippocampus and proceed as fimbria and fornix. Major part of fornix terminates in the mamillary body. From here they are projected to thalamus as mamillothalamic tract.

VENTRICLES OF BRAIN (Fig.11.50)

Ventricles are cavities of brain. Cerebrum has two lateral ventricles, one in each hemisphere and a midline cavity, the III ventricle. The two lateral ventricles communicate with the III ventricle through

the interventricular foramina of Luschka. The III ventricle is continuous posteriorly with the cerebral aqueduct, the cavity of the mid brain. The aqueduct opens into the IV ventricle, the cavity of hind brain. Below the IV ventricle is continuous with the narrow central canal of medulla and spinal cord, which ends below in a small dilatation called the terminal ventricle.

The ventricles are lined by ependyma and cerebrospinal fluid (CSF) is secreted in them by the choroid plexus which project into them.

Lateral ventricle

It is a 'C' shaped cavity. Its main central part is the body which occupies the parietal lobe. From the body an anterior horn extends into frontal lobe, a posterior horn into occipital lobe and an inferior horn into temporal lobe. (Fig. 11.51a). The central part is roughly triangular on cross section. Corpus callosum forms its roof.

Septum pellucidum attached between corpus callosum and fornix forms the medial wall. Thalamus and caudate nucleus are seen in the floor. (Fig. 11.51 b). Anterior horn extends into frontal lobe - has the head of caudate nucleus in its floor and is roofed by corpus callosum. Posterior horn is a short projection into occipital lobe. Into its medial wall, the calcarine sulcus and forceps major produce two elevations – calcar avis and bulb of posterior horn. Inferior horn – into the temporal lobe is a narrow

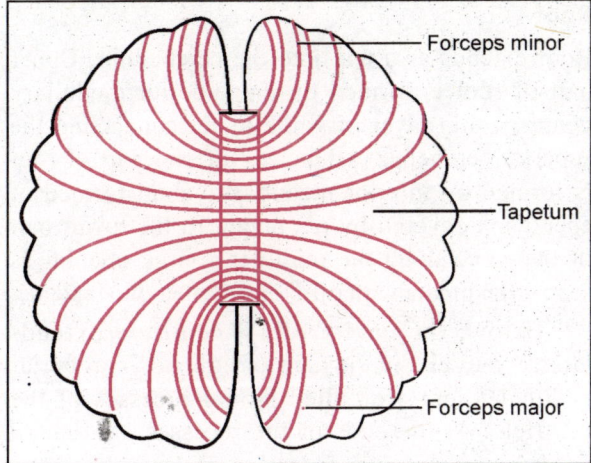

Fig. 11.48

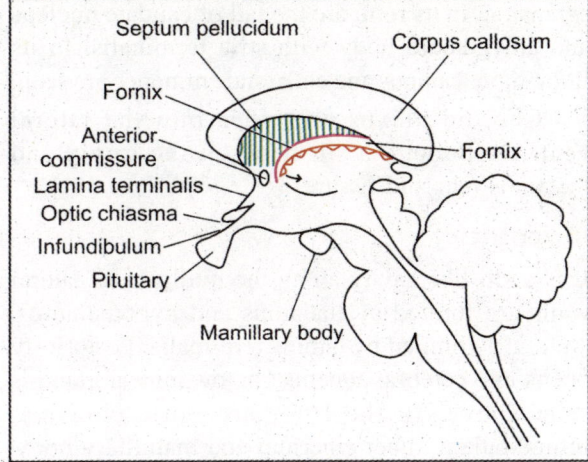

Fig. 11.49: Medial Surface of Deeper Part of Cerebrum

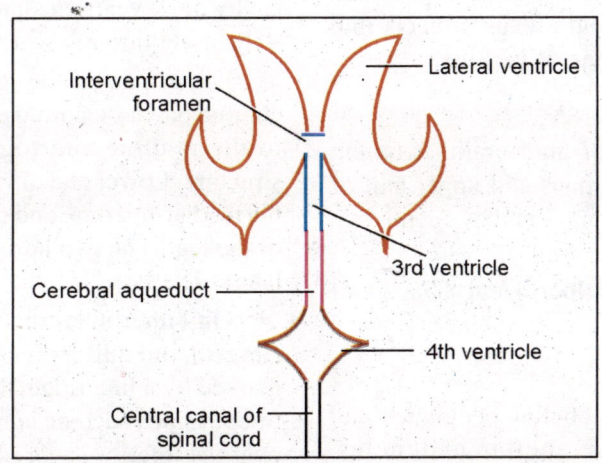

Fig. 11.50: Schematic Diagram of Ventricles of Brain

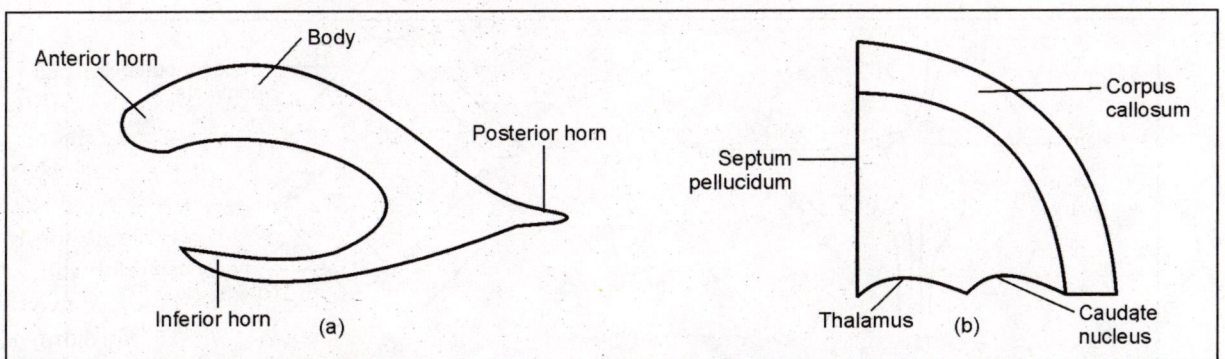

Fig. 11.51: Lateral Ventricle (a) Parts, (b) C.S Through Body of Lateral Ventricle

extension. In its roof, are the tail of caudate nucleus and amygdaloid body with stria terminalis. In its floor, hippocampus and collateral eminence are seen.

Choroid plexus protrudes into the lateral ventricle through a slit between the fornix and thalamus (choroid fissure).

III ventricle

It is a slit like cavity along the midline. Its lateral walls are formed by thalamus and hypothalamus. Anteriorly limited by lamina terminalis. Posteriorly opens into cerebral aqueduct below, pineal gland is seen above. In the floor are optic chiasma, infundibulum, tuber cinerium and mamillary body. Roof is thin, formed of ependyma covered by a double layered vascular piamater (tela choroidea). Through the roof, the choroid plexus projects into the III ventricle, on either side of midline.

IV ventricle

IV ventricle is the cavity of hind brain. It is tent shaped, situated behind the pons and upper half of medulla, in front of cerebellum; lined by ependyma. (Fig. 11.52 a)

It has a diamond shaped floor, a tent shaped roof and lateral boundaries.

Lateral boundaries

Upper part by superior cerebellar peduncles and lower part by inferior cerebellar peduncles. (Fig. 11.52 b)

Roof

Roof extends as a tent into the cerebellum. Upper part of roof is formed by the superior medullary velum, a thin layer of white mater connecting the superior cerebellar peduncles. Inferior part of roof is formed by inferior medullary velum formed of ependyma covered by pia mater. In the lower part of the roof, along the midline, a large opening is seen – the median aperture or foramen of Magende.

Below, the cavity of IV ventricle extends laterally over the surface of inferior cerebellar peduncles and are called lateral recesses of the ventricle. At the ends of the recesses, the lateral apertures are seen – foramina of Luschka. Thus through one median and two lateral apertures, the cavity of IV ventricle opens into subarachnoid space – the route through which CSF reaches the space.

Lower part of the roof of IV ventricle has the choroid plexus. Choroid plexus of both sides lie close to the midline and together form a 'T' shaped structure. Lower end of vertical limb of 'T' reaching the median aperture and upper end reaching the apex of the tent. The two horizontal limbs extent into the lateral recesses.

On either side, the line along which the roof (inferior medullary velum) touches the floor is marked by a line/ridge, the taenia. Below, the taenia of both sides become continuous at a curved margin over the inferior angle of the floor and is called the obex.

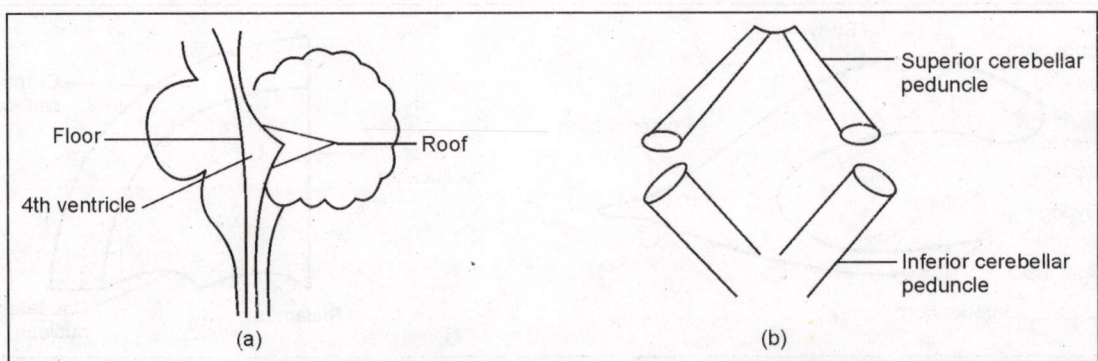

Fig. 11.52: (a) IV ventricle, (b) Lateral Boundaries

Floor of IV ventricle (Fig. 11.53)

Formed by the posterior surfaces of pons and upper half of medulla. It is known as rhomboid fossa, due to its shape.

Along the midline, there is a vertical groove, the median sulcus. On either side of it, a vertical ridge is seen, medial eminence, limited laterally by a groove, sulcus limitans.

Area lateral to sulcus limitans is the vestibular area, overlying the vestibular nuclei.

At the upper end of sulcus limitans, a pigmented area is seen, the locus ceruleus, produced by underlying pigmented neurons – substantia ferruginea.

Above the middle part of the medial eminence, a rounded prominence is seen on either side, facial colliculus, caused by the underlying abducent nucleus, curved over by facial nerve.

Above the facial colliculus, the sulcus limitans expands to form a triangular superior fovea. Below the facial colliculus, the floor is traversed horizontally by strands of nerve fibres – stria medullaris. They come from the arcuate nuclei on the surface of the pyramid, emerge through the median sulcus and go through the inferior cerebellar peduncle to the cerebellum.

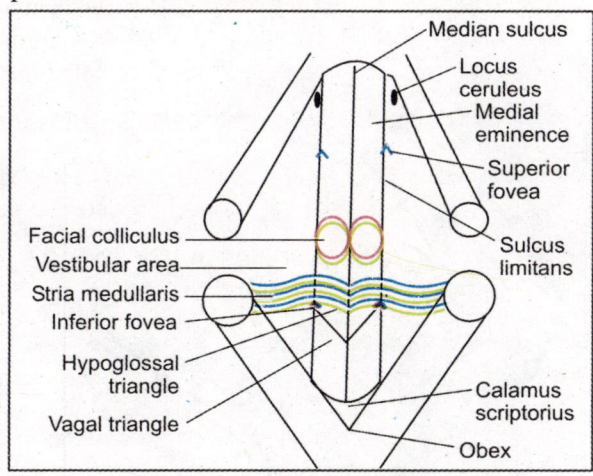

Fig. 11.53: Floor of 4th Vertricle

Below the stria, the sulcus limitans expands into a triangular area, inferior fovea. Area medial to the inferior fovea is the hypoglossal triangle, overlying its nucleus. Area below the fovea is the vagal triangle, overlying dorsal vagal nucleus. Vagal triangle is crossed by an oblique translucent ridge – funiculus separens, a small area lateral to which is called area postrema. The lower end of the floor of the ventricle, overlapped by obex, resembles in shape of a pen's nib – hence called Calamus scriptorius. (Fig. 11.53)

Choroid plexus

Choroid plexuses are structures which project into the ventricles and secrete CSF. It is formed by vascular fringes of piamater (tela choroidea) invaginating into the ependyma (covered by ependyma).

Cerebro Spinal Fluid (CSF)

CSF is a clear colourless fluid that circulates in the sub-arachnoid space around brain and spinal cord. It is secreted by the choroid plexus of ventricles of brain. CSF of IV ventricle reaches the III ventricle through interventricular foramina. From the III ventricle, it reaches the IV ventricle through cerebral aqueduct. Through the three apertures in the IV ventricle, CSF reaches the sub-arachnoid space and circulates around brain and spinal cord. Circulation of CSF is enhanced by the pulsations of arteries present in the space. Arachnoid villi are small diverticula of sub-arachnoid space and a number of them are grouped to form **arachnoid granulations** which project into the dural venous sinuses. Through them CSF is absorbed into the venous blood.

Samples of CSF can be withdrawn for diagnostic, investigative or therapeutic purposes by doing lumbar puncture.

Normal volume of CSF is about 140 ml.

Abnormal increase of CSF produces hydrocephalus, due to either more secretion or due to obstruction to the flow.

OLFACTORY TRACT (Fig. 11.54)

Sensory receptors for smell – olfactory cells are situated in the roof of the nasal cavity and forms olfactory epithelium. The central processes of these cells constitute the olfactory nerve fibres which enter the cranial cavity, through the cribriform plate of ethmoid bone. They end in a small ovoid body, the olfactory bulb, situated on the orbital surface of the frontal lobe of cerebral hemisphere. It is the collection of several types of cells (the largest being mitral cells). Olfactory nerve fibres synapse with the cells of olfactory bulb. Their central processes proceed back as a flat band, the olfactory tract. It reaches the anterior perforated substance and divides into medial and lateral striae.

The axons pass through the lateral olfactory stria and end in the primary olfactory cortex of cerebrum, formed of periamygdaloid and prepiriform areas. Some fibres of the olfactory tract pass through the medial olfactory stria to the opposite olfactory bulb.

Fibres arising from the primary olfactory cortex are projected to the secondary olfactory cortex, the entorhinal area (area 28), formed of uncus and part of parahippocampal gyrus. The primary and secondary olfactory cortex are responsible for olfactory sensation, which is not reaching thalamus directly.

OPTIC (VISUAL) PATHWAY) (Fig. 11.55)

The II cranial nerve - optic nerve is formed by the axons of ganglion cells of retina of the eye, and they carry visual sensation. Optic nerve leaves the orbit through optic canal. The two optic nerves unite to form the optic chiasma, at the base of brain. At the optic chiasma, fibres coming from the nasal half of the retina of both eyes cross over and fibres from the temporal halves remain uncrossed. The crossed and uncrossed fibres leave the optic chiasma as optic tract, around the cerebral peduncles of midbrain.

Fibres in the optic tract reach the lateral geniculate body of thalamus. Most of the fibres synapse with the neurons there and a few pass to the

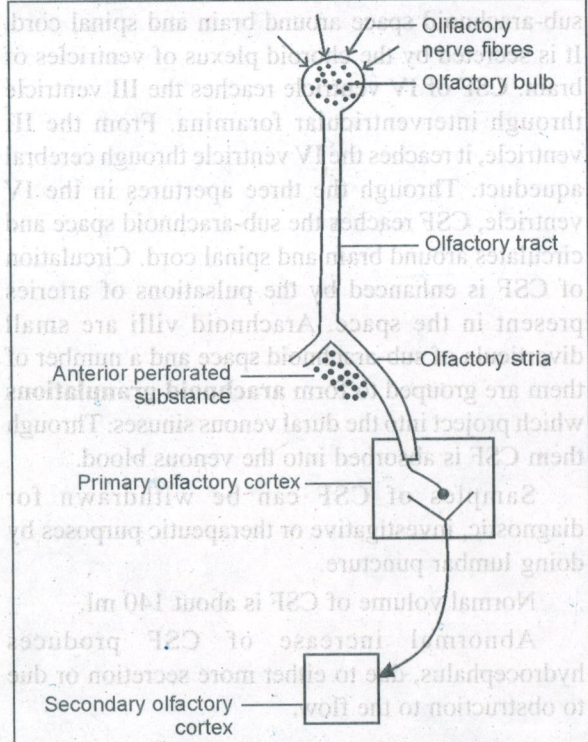

Fig. 11.54: Olfactory Tract

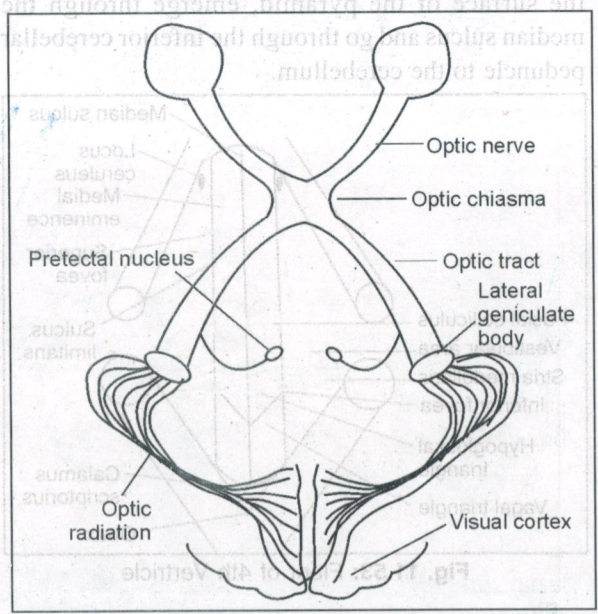

Fig. 11.55: Visual Pathway

superior colliculus and pretectal nucleus of midbrain. These connections are concerned with light reflexes.

From the lateral geniculate body, visual pathway emerges as the optic radiation. The fibres are axons of neurons of lateral geniculate body. Optic radiation passes through the retrolentiform part of internal capsule and reaches the visual cortex of cerebrum which is located in relation to calcarine sulcus.

CRANIAL NERVES

There are twelve pairs of cranial nerves. They emerge from the brain and leave the cranial cavity through foramina. Except the 10th nerve all others are distributed to the head and neck. The 10th nerve, apart from head and neck, supplies the thoracic and abdominal organs.

The nerves are : (Fig. 11.56)

1. Olfactory
2. Optic
3. Oculomotor
4. Trochlear
5. Trigeminal
6. Abducent
7. Facial
8. Vestibulocochlear
9. Glossopharyngeal
10. Vagus
11. Accessary
12. Hypoglossal

The cranial nerves have their nuclei deep in the brain – sensory, motor or parasympathetic. The fibres emerge from the brain attached to the brainstem.

1. Olfactory nerve

It is the nerve of the sense of smell. The fibers arise from the olfactory receptor cells of nasal cavity. They reach the olfactory bulb and tract on the undersurface of the frontal lobe of cerebrum. The tract ends in the olfactory cortex in the brain.

2. Optic nerve

Nerve of vision. Fibers arise as axons of ganglion cells of retina. They form the optic nerve and optic tract and finally reach the visual cortex of cerebrum as optic radiation.

3. Oculomotor nerve

It is a motor nerve. Nuclei - It has a main motor nucleus and a parasympathetic nucleus, both located in the upper part of midbrain. Nerve emerges from between the two cerebral peduncles of midbrain. Runs anteriorly in relation to cavernous sinus.

Distribution – The nerve enters orbit through superior orbital fissure and divides into branches. Motor fibres supply the levator muscle of the upper eyelid (levator palpebrae superioris) and the voluntary muscles of the eyeball except superior oblique and lateral rectus.

Parasympathetic fibres relay in the ciliary ganglion and postganglionic fibres supply two of the smooth muscles of eyeball, Sphincter pupillae and ciliaris.

4. Trochlear nerve

It is a motor nerve. Nucleus – located in the midbrain at the level of inferior colliculus. This slender nerve emerges from the dorsal surface of midbrain.

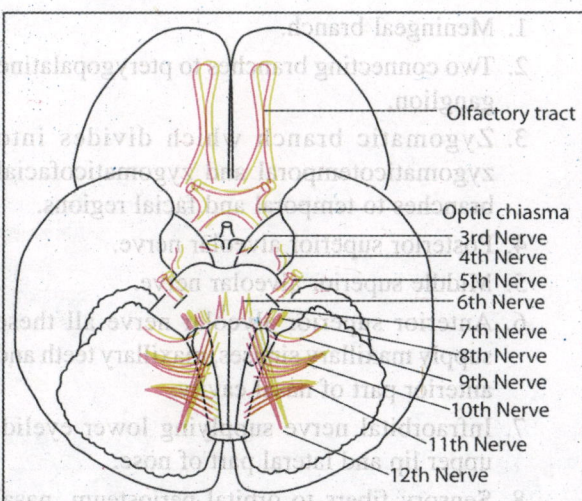

Olfactory tract
Optic chiasma
3rd Nerve
4th Nerve
5th Nerve
6th Nerve
7th Nerve
8th Nerve
9th Nerve
10th Nerve
11th Nerve
12th Nerve

Fig. 11.56: Base of Brain-Attachment of Cranial Nerves

Course and distribution

Runs in relation to cavernous sinus and enters orbit through superior orbital fissure. Supplies the superior oblique muscle of eyeball.

5. Trigeminal nerve

It is the largest cranial nerve and has got three divisions - ophthalmic nerve, maxillary nerve and mandibular nerve. Ophthalmic and maxillary are purely sensory and mandibular is a mixed nerve with both sensory and motor fibers.

Nuclei

1. Main sensory nucleus – in the pons.
2. Main motor nucleus – in the pons.
3. Mesencephalic nucleus – extends upto the midbrain, from sensory nucleus.
4. Nucleus of spinal tract – extends down to the upper two segments of spinal cord, from sensory nucleus.

The nerve emerges from the ventral surface of pons and has a large sensory root and a small motor root. Sensory root reaches the trigeminal ganglion and the three divisions leave the ganglion (Fig. 11.57). Motor root joins the mandibular division.

Opthalmic nerve

Course and distribution

Ophthalmic nerve passes through cavernous sinus, comes out of cranial cavity through superior orbital fissure, enters the orbit after dividing into its three terminal branches (Fig. 11.58) – lacrimal, frontal and nasociliary nerves.

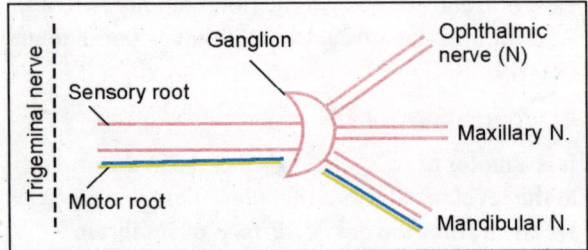

Fig. 11.57: Trigeminal Ganglion

Lacrimal branch receives postgangloinic secretomotor fibers to lacrimal gland from the zygomatico temporal nerve (branch of maxillary). These fibers are given to the lacrimal gland and the nerve ends by supplying lateral part of upper eyelid.

Frontal branch divides into supra trochlear and supra orbital branches which supply frontal air sinus, medial part of upper eyelid, forehead and scalp.

Nasociliary branch gives off:

1. A connecting branch to ciliary ganglion.
2. Long ciliary nerves to eyeball.
3. Posterior ethmoidal nerve – to ethmoidal and sphenoidal air sinuses.
4. Anterior ethmoidal nerve –to nasal cavity. and lower part of nose.
5. Infratrochlear nerve – to medial parts of eyelids, lacrimal sac and upper part of nose.

Maxillary nerve (Fig.11.59)

Passes through cavernous sinus, leaves the cranium through foramen rotundum, crosses the upper part of pterygopalatine fossa and enters the floor of orbit through inferior orbital fissure. Traverse infra orbital groove and canal and finally appears on the face through infraorbital foramen as infraorbital nerve.

Branches are

1. Meningeal branch.
2. Two connecting branches to pterygopalatine ganglion.
3. Zygomatic branch which divides into zygomaticotemporal and zygomaticofacial branches to temporal and facial regions.
4. Posterior superior alveolar nerve.
5. Middle superior alveolar nerve.
6. Anterior superior alveolar nerve all these supply maxillary sinuses, maxillary teeth and anterior part of nasal cavity.
7. Infraorbital nerve supplying lower eyelid, upper lip and lateral part of nose.
8. Sensory fibers to orbital periosteum, nasal cavity, pharynx and palate pass through pterygopalatine ganglion.

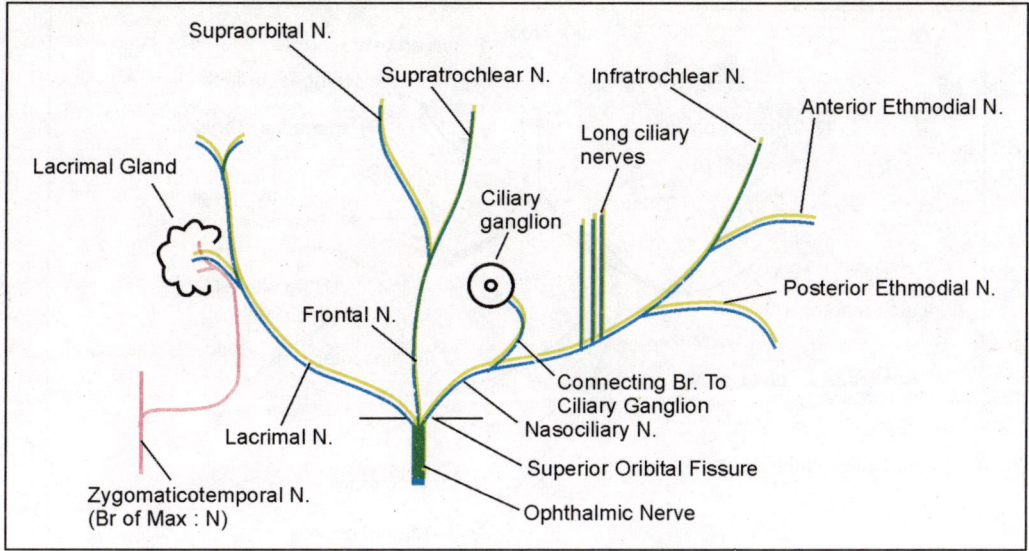

Fig. 11.58: Branches of Ophthalmic Nerve

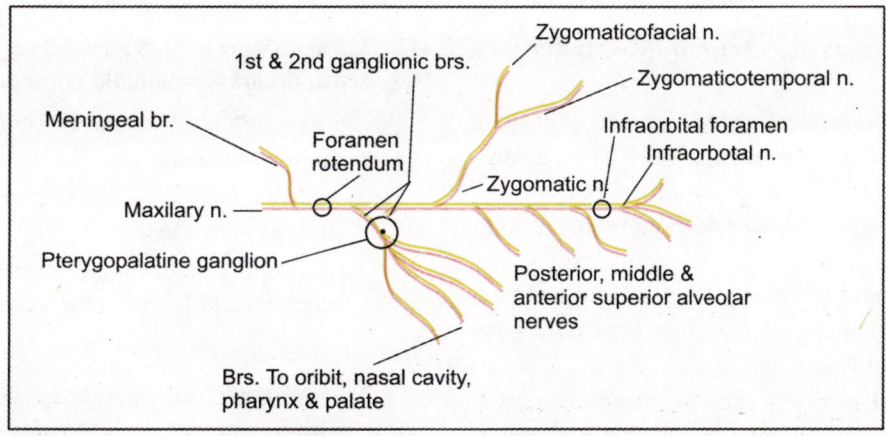

Fig. 11.59: Branches of Maxillary Nerve

Mandibular nerve (mixed nerve) (Fig. 11.60)

Leaves the cranium through foramen ovale. Just outside the foramen, the sensory root is joined by the motor root and trunk of the nerve is formed in the infratemporal fossa. Trunk divides into anterior and posterior divisions.

Branches are: From the trunk

1. Meningeal branch

2. Nerves to medial pterygoid, tensor palatini and tensor tympani

3. Connecting branch to otic ganglion.

From the anterior division (Mostly motor branches) –

1. Temporal branches to temporalis.

2. Nerves to lateral pterygoid and masseter.

3. Buccal branch (sensory).

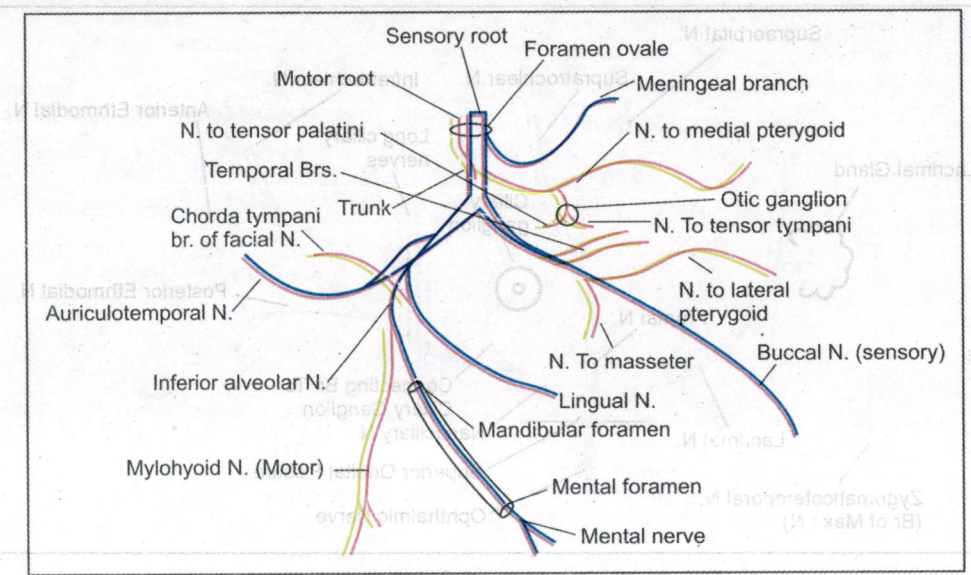

Fig. 11.60: Branches of Mandibular Nerve

From the posterior division (Mostly sensory branches):

1. Auriculotemporal nerve – to parts of auricle, external acoustic meatus, parotid gland, temporomandibular joint and temporal region

2. Inferior alveolar nerve – enters mandibular canal through mandibular foramen and gives branches to mandibular teeth. Its terminal part emerges through mental foramen as mental nerve to skin of chin and lower lip.

3. Lingual nerve – sensory to anterior two-thirds of tongue and floor of mouth. It also conveys taste sensation from anterior two-third of tongue to chorda tympani and preganglionic fibres from chorda tympani to submandibular ganglion.

4. Mylohyoid nerve – motor to mylohyoid and anterior belly of digastric. (Only motor branch from posterior division – arises from inferior alveolar nerve).

6. Abducent nerve – A small motor nerve. Nucleus is situated in the pons. Nerve emerges from between pons and medulla. Supplies the lateral rectus muscle of eyeball.

7. Facial nerve : It is a mixed nerve with motor, sensory and parasympathetic components.

Nuclei – located in the pons (Fig. 11.62)

1. motor nucleus

2. sensory nucleus – upper part of nucleus of tractus solitarius,

3. parasympathetic nuclei–superior salivatory nucleus and lacrimatory nucleus.

Course and distribution

The motor root and sensory root (nervus intermedius) emerge together from the ventral surface of brain stem, between pons and medulla.

It enters the petrous part of temporal bone through internal acoustic meatus together with vestibulocochlear nerve. Within the bone, the nerve runs in a bony canal - facial canal. First it is directed laterally, then turns posteriorly and finally turns downwards in relation to the internal and middle ears. As it turns posteriorly, there is a dilatation, the sensory Geniculate ganglion.

While it descends in the facial canal behind the middle ear, it gives of the branch to stapedius and chorda tympani. Finally it emerges through stylomastoid foramen. (Fig. 11.61) It enters the parotid gland and divides into terminal branches, that appear on the face.

Motor fibres supply the muscles of facial expression, muscles of scalp, stapedius, stylohyoid and posterior belly of digastric.

Sensory fibres bring taste sensation from anterior 2/3rd of tongue via chorda tympani.

Parasympathetic fibres from superior salivatory nucleus supply the submandibular and sublingual salivary glands. Fibres from lacrimatory nucleus supply the lacrimal gland.

Lesion of facial nerve below stylomastoid foramen leads to facial paralysis of same side(Bell's palsy). Supranuclear lesion leads to contralateral facial paralysis, below the level of eye.

8. Vestibulocochlear nerve: It is the nerve of hearing and equilibrium. Vestibular part is concerned with equilibrium. Cochlear part is concerned with hearing.

Nuclei

Vestibular nuclei situated in the lower part of pons and upper part of medulla, in the floor of IV ventricle.

Cochlear nuclei situated at the upper end of medulla.

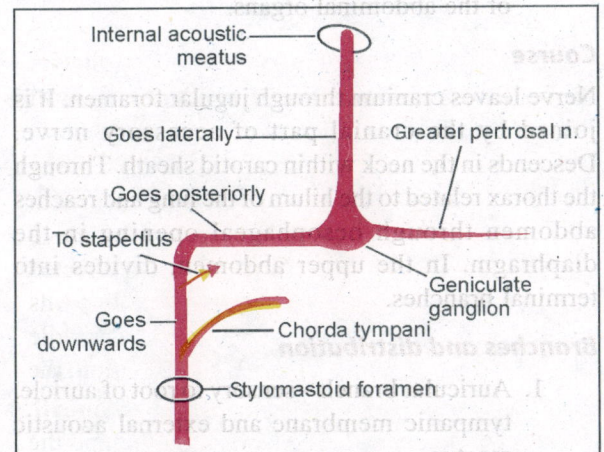

Fig. 11.61: Intrapetrous Course of Facial Nerve

The nerve emerges from the ventral aspect of brain stem between pons and medulla.

Vestibular nerve brings nerve impulses from the utricle and saccule and semicircular canals of internal ear. These impulses provide information regarding positions and movements of head. Vestibular nerve fibres are central processes of the neurons of the vestibular ganglion in the internal acoustic meatus. Vestibular nuclei are connected to the cerebellum, spinal cord and cerebral cortex. These help in maintenance of equilibrium and balance.

Cochlear nerve brings impulses concerned with sound from the organ of corti of cochlea. They are central processes of the spiral ganglion of the cochlea. From the cochlear nuclei, the fibres ascend through the lateral leminiscus and medial geniculate body and reach the auditory cortex as auditory radiation.

9. Glossopharyngeal nerve: A Mixed nerve. Emerges from the anterolateral surface of medulla, lateral to olive. Has the following components –

1. Motor – supplies stylopharyngeus muscle.
2. Sensory – to pharynx and posterior 1/3rd of tongue, soft palate and tonsil.
3. Special sensory – taste from the posterior 1/3rd of tongue and circumvallate papillae.
4. Parasympathetic –secretomotor to parotid gland.

Nuclei

Located in the medulla. (Fig 11.62)

Motor – upper end of nucleus ambiguus.

Sensory – common with spinal nucleus of trigeminal nerve.

Special sensory – middle part of the nucleus of tractus solitarius.

Parasympathetic – inferior salivatory nucleus.

Course and distribution

The nerve emerges from the medulla lateral to the olive. Leaves the skull through jugular foramen. In the upper part of the neck, it has two sensory ganglia.

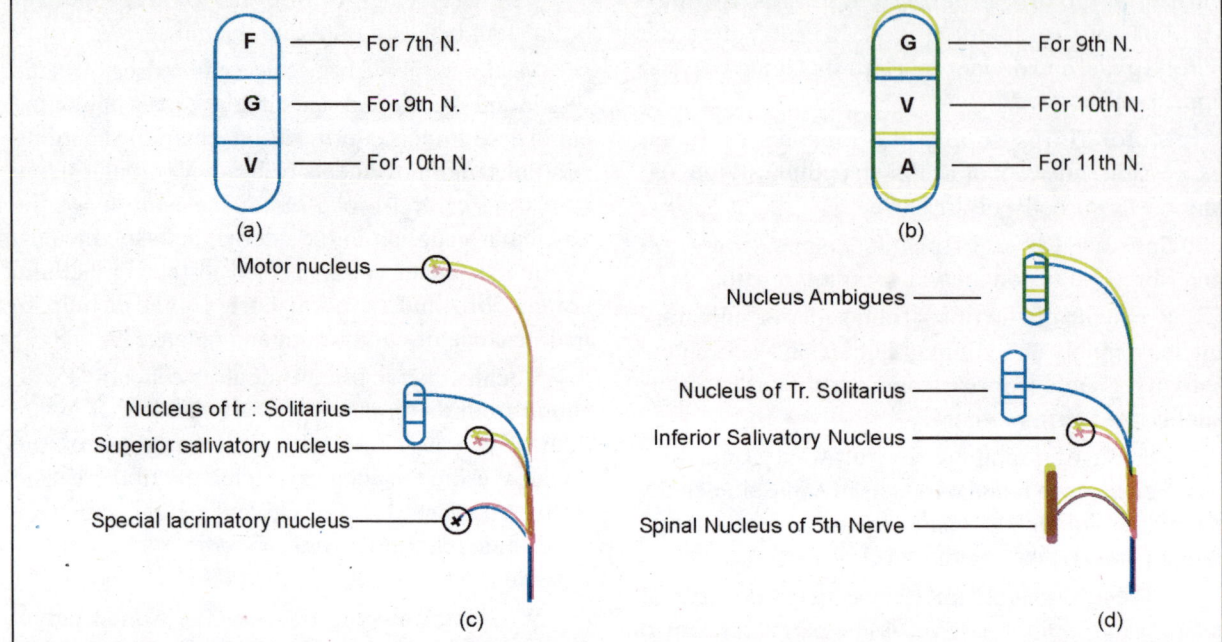

Fig. 11.62: (a) Nucleus of Tractus Solitarius (b) Nucleus Ambiguus (c) Facial Nerve (d) Glossopharyngeal N.

It gives off the tympanic branch which carries preganglionic secretomotor parasympathetic fibres to reach otic ganglion, for the supply to parotid gland. Branch to stylopharyngeus also is given in the upper part of the neck. Then it enters the pharynx between superior and middle constrictor muscles and gives off terminal branches to mucosa of pharynx and posterior 1/3rd of tongue.

10. Vagus nerve: Mixed nerve with motor and sensory fibres. Attached to the medulla lateral to the olive, below IX nerve. Vagal branches supply pharynx, soft palate, larynx, thoracic and abdominal organs.

Nuclei – located in the medulla.

1. Motor nucleus – middle part of nucleus ambiguus. Fibres from it supply the pharyngeal and laryngeal muscles.
2. Sensory nucleus – part of spinal nucleus of trigeminal nerve. Sensory fibres are distributed to root of auricle and external acoustic meatus.
3. Special sensory nucleus – lower part of nucleus of Tractus solitarius. The fibres bring taste sensation from posterior most part of tongue.
4. Parasympathetic nucleus – dorsal vagal nucleus. Fibres supply the thoracic and most of the abdominal organs.

Course

Nerve leaves cranium through jugular foramen. It is joined by the cranial part of accessory nerve. Descends in the neck within carotid sheath. Through the thorax related to the hilum of the lung and reaches abdomen through oesophageal opening in the diaphragm. In the upper abdomen, divides into terminal branches.

Branches and distribution

1. Auricular branch – sensory to root of auricle, tympanic membrane and external acoustic meatus.
2. Superior laryngeal nerve – Its internal

laryngeal branch is sensory to upper ½ of mucosa of larynx and carries taste sensation from posterior part of tongue. Its external laryngeal branch is motor to cricothyroid muscle of larynx.

3. Pharyngeal branches – main motor nerves to muscles of pharynx except stylopharyngeus. They contain fibres from cranial part of accessory nerve. They also supply palatine muscles except tensor palati. Pharyngeal branches form a pharyngeal plexus with sympathetic fibres, on the wall of pharynx. From the plexus the branches are distributed.

4. Reccurent laryngeal nerve – it is sensory to mucosa of lower ½ of larynx and motor to all laryngeal muscles except cricothyroid.

5. Parasympathetic branches – its cardiac, pulmonary, gastric and coeliac branches take part in the formation of cardiac, pulmonary, superior hypogastric and coeliac plexuses with branches of sympathetic nerves. Branches from the plexuses supply thoracic and abdominal organs.

11. Accessory nerve: A motor nerve. Has two roots – cranial root and spinal root.

Nuclei

Cranial root – lower part of nucleus ambiguus.

Spinal root – ventral grey horn of the spinal cord from C_1 to C_6 level.

Course and distribution

The cranial root is attached as rootlets to medulla, lateral to olive, inferior to vagus nerve. It runs towards jugular foramen. Spinal root ascends to cranium through foramen magnum and joins the cranial root for a while. The accessory nerve emerges out of cranium through jugular foramen. Immediately the cranial root separates from the nerve and joins the vagus. Its branches are distributed through the pharyngeal and laryngeal branches of vagus. Spinal root supplies sternocleidomastoid and trapezius muscles.

12. Hypoglossal nerve: A motor nerve, to the tongue muscles. Attached to medulla as rootlets between pyramid and olive.

Nucleus

In the lower part of medulla.

Course and distribution

Emerges from the brain on the ventral aspect of medulla, comes out of cranium through hypoglossal canal. In the neck it curves medially in front of great vessels of the neck, then lies over hyoglossus muscle, reaches the tongue and branches are distributed to muscles of tongue except palatoglossus.

Parasympathetic Ganglia Connected to Cranial Nerves. (Fig. 11.63 a,b,c,d).

(a) Otic Ganglion

Located in infratemoral fossa, connected structurally to mandibullar Nerve, but functionally connected to 9th nerve. Preganglionic fibres arise from inferior salivatory nucleus in brain stem. Pass through 9th nerve, its tympanic branch, tympanic plexus and through lesser petrosal nerve, reach the ganglion, relay there. Post Ganglionic fibres pass through auriculotemporal br. of mandibular nerve and reach the parotid gland. These fibres are secretomotor to the gland

(b) Sub mandibular ganglion.

Situated in Submandibular region structurally connected to lingual nerve, but functionally connected to facial nerve. Preganglionic fibres arise from superior salivatory nucleus in brain stem, pass through facial nerve, leave it through its chorda tympani branch and reach the lingual br. of mandibular nerve. The nerve carries the fibres to the ganglion which relay in it. Postganglionic fibres are distributed to sumandibullar and sulingual glands, and are secretomotor to them.

(c) Ciliary Ganglion

Located in the orbit structurally connected to nasociliary nerve, branch of ophthalmic nerve, but functionally connected to oculomotor nerve. Preganglionic fibres arise from Edinger - Westphal

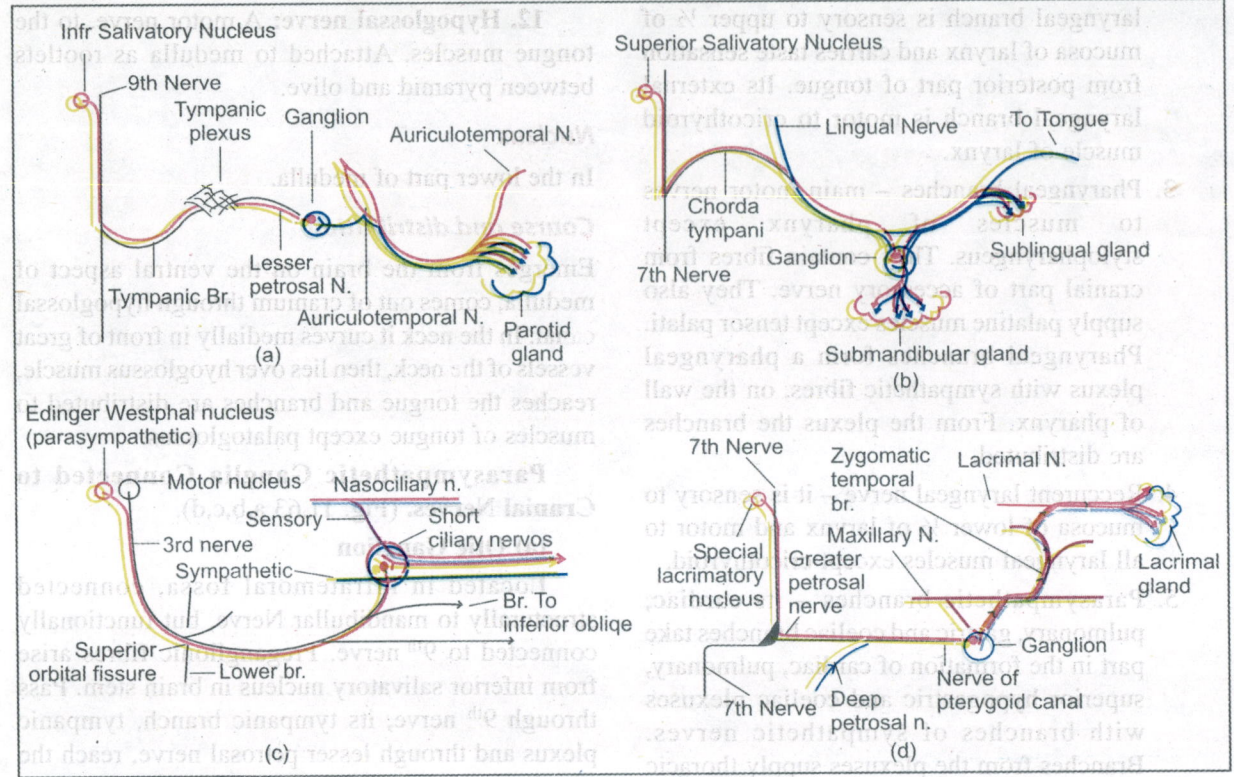

Fig. 11.63: (a) Otic Ganglion (b) Submandibular Ganglion (c) Ciliary Ganglion (d) Pterygopalatine Ganglion

nucleus, pass through 3rd Nerve, enters orbit, go through its lower branch and nerve to inferior oblique. From it reach the ganglion and relay there. Postganglionic fibres pass throuth short ciliary nerves to reach the eye ball. They supply sphinctor pupillae and ciliaris muscles. Sensory and sympathetic fibres also pass throuth the ganglion.

(d) Pterigopalatine Ganglion.

Situated in the pterygopalatine fossa, structurally connected to maxillary nerve, but functionallu connected to facial nerve. Preganglionic fibres arise from special lacrimatory nucleus, pass through facial nerve, leave it throuth its greater petrosal br. This nerve is joined by deep petrosal nerve and nerve of pterygoid canal is formed. This carries the fibres to ganglion which realy there. Postglonic fibres pass through the 2nd ganglionic branch of maxillary nerve,

throuth its zygomatic br. and zygomatico temporal br. The fibres reach the lacrimal branch of ophthalmic nerve through a connecting branch. They are distributed to the lacrimal gland and are secretomotor.

AUTONOMIC NERVOUS SYSTEM

Nerves of this system supply the thoracic, abdominal and pelvic organs, blood vessels, smooth muscles and exocrine glands of the body.

It has two parts – **Sympathetic and Parasympathetic**.

Generally sympathetic and parasympathetic parts have opposite effects for a particular stimulus. For example, sympathetic nerve stimulation causes dilatation of the pupil and parasympathetic stimulation causes constriction of the pupil. Action of sympathetic part is as if preparing the body for an emergency, *e.g.*, heart rate increases, blood pressure rises, pupil dilates, peristalsis decreases, sphincters close etc. Parasympathetic activity leads to slowing of heart rate, peristalsis increases, sphincters open etc.

Central part of autonomic nervous system

1. In the cerebrum, hypothalamus and limbic system – these are regions controlling visceral functions.
2. Centres in the reticular formation of brain stem.
3. In the spinal cord, intermediate horns of grey mater from T_1 to L_2 segments and grey mater of S_2 to S_4 segments.

Peripheral part of autonomic nervous system

Consists of the autonomic – sympathetic and parasympathetic – nerves, plexuses and the associated ganglia.

Sympathetic part

It is larger than parasympathetic part. Has two long nerve trunks – the sympathetic trunks located on either side of the vertebral column, extending from the base of skull to the coccyx. Each appears as a knotted thread, due to the presence of ganglia along them. About 22 pairs of ganglia are seen:

3 in cervical region

11 in thoracic region

4 in lumbar region and

4 in sacral region

The two trunks meet at the ganglion impar in front of coccyx.

The sympathetic trunks are connected to the spinal nerves by a series of short connecting branches called white and grey rami communicantes. The preganglionic neurons which give off the efferent fibres of the sympathetic system are located in the intermediolateral grey horn of spinal cord, present in the thoracic and upper two lumbar segments. (Fig. 11.64)

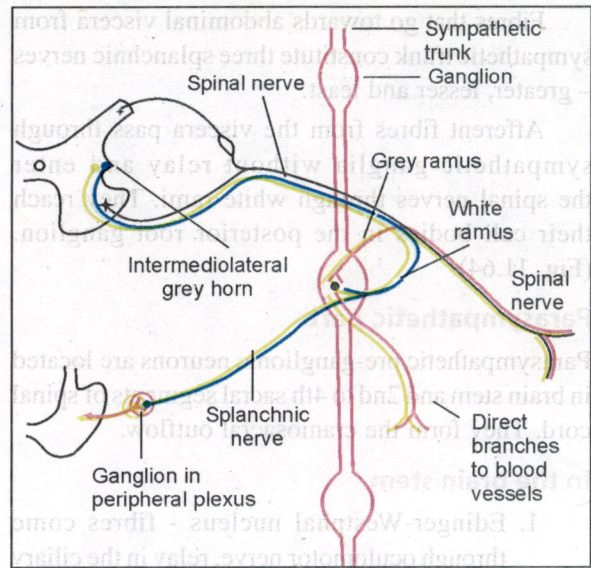

Fig. 11.64: Sympathetic Nerve and Trunk

The fibres originating in these neurons emerge through the spinal nerve and are carried along the white ramus to the sympathetic trunk. Further fate of the fibres is either of the following:

1. They synapse in the neurons of the corresponding ganglion. Post-ganglionic fibres pass back to the spinal nerve through grey ramus communicates, and are distributed to the smooth muscle of skin, blood vessels and to sweat glands. Some post-ganglionic fibres may go direct to the blood vessels.

2. After reaching the sympathetic trunk, they do not relay there, pass directly medially towards the organs or viscera. They synapse with neurons of smaller ganglia of peripheral plexuses located near the organs in the thorax, abdomen or pelvis and thence post-ganglionic fibres reach the organs. Such plexuses are cardiac plexus, pulmonary plexus, coeliac plexus, mesenteric plexus and hypogastric plexus. They all contain parasympathetic fibres from vagus also.

Fibres that go towards abdominal viscera from sympathetic trunk constitute three splanchnic nerves – greater, lesser and least.

Afferent fibres from the viscera pass through sympathetic ganglia without relay and enter the spinal nerves through white rami. They reach their cell bodies in the posterior root ganglion. (Fig. 11.64)

Parasympathetic part

Parasympathetic pre-ganglionic neurons are located in brain stem and 2nd to 4th sacral segments of spinal cord. They form the craniosacral outflow.

In the brain stem

1. Edinger-Westphal nucleus - fibres come through oculomotor nerve, relay in the ciliary ganglion. Post-ganglionic fibres supply the smooth muscles of eye ball – sphincter pupillae and ciliaris.

2. Superior salivatory nucleus – fibres pass through facial nerve, relay in the sub-mandibular ganglion. Post-ganglionic fibres supply submandibular and sublingual salivary glands.

3. Inferior salivatory nucleus – fibres pass through glossopharyngeal nerve, relay in the otic ganglion. Post-ganglionic fibres supply parotid gland.

4. Lacrimatory nucleus – fibres pass through facial nerve, relay in the pterygopalatine ganglion. Post-ganglionic fibres supply lacrimal gland.

5. Dorsal vagal nucleus – fibres pass through vagus nerve. The parasympathetic fibres of vagus descend to thorax and abdomen, relay in the neurons of the thoracic and abdominal autonomic plexuses (cardiac, pulmonary, coeliac, hypogastric). Post-ganglionic fibres supply thoracic and abdominal organs.

In the spinal cord

Pre-ganglionic neurons are in the grey mater of 2nd to 4th sacral segments of spinal cord. Their axons emerge through anterior roots of sacral spinal nerves and leave the spinal nerves to form pelvic splanchnic nerves. They relay in the neurons of the pelvic autonomic plexuses and supply pelvic organs.

Afferents

Like sympathetic, parasympathetic afferents have their cell bodies in the posterior root ganglia of sacral spinal nerves or the sensory ganglia of cranial nerves. Their peripheral processes receive impulses from the viscera and central processes enter the CNS.

Single Best Response – M.C.Qs

1. Length of spinal cord is about
   (a) 25 cms
   (b) 35 cms
   (c) 45 cms
   (d) 55 cm

2. Vertebral level of lower and spinal cord is
   (a) T_{12}
   (b) L_1
   (c) L_2
   (d) L_3

3. Number of pairs of spinal nerves attached to spinal cord is
   (a) 20
   (b) 21
   (c) 30
   (d) 31

4. Filum terminale is formed of
   (a) Pia mater
   (b) Arachnoid mater
   (c) Dura mater
   (d) Nervous tissue

5. Following are pial modifications except
   (a) Cauda equina
   (b) Ligamenta denticulata
   (c) Filum terminale
   (d) Linea splendens

6. Wrist drop' is due to injury of
   (a) Median nerve
   (b) Ulnar nerve
   (c) Axillary nerve
   (d) Radial nerve

7. Nerve that passes deep to flexor retinaculum is
   (a) Median nerve
   (b) Radial nerve
   (c) Ulnar nerve
   (d) Deep branch of ulnar nerve

8. Palmar & dorsal interossei are supplied by
   (a) Superficial branch of ulnar nerve
   (b) Deep branch of ulnar nerve
   (c) Radial nerve
   (d) Median nerve

9. Musculocutaneous nerve is a branch from
   (a) Radial nerve
   (b) Ulnar nerve
   (c) Median nerve
   (d) Branchial plexus

10. Cutaneous nerve to Ist interdigital cleft of foot is
    (a) Deep peroneal nerve
    (b) Superficial peroneal nerve
    (c) Sural nerve
    (d) Saphenous nerve

11. Root value of femoral nerve is
    (a) L_1, L_2, L_3
    (b) L_2, L_3, L_4
    (c) L_3, L_4, L_5
    (d) L_3, L_4

12. Sural nerve is a branch of
    (a) Sciatic nerve
    (b) Femoral nerve
    (c) Tibial nerve
    (d) Common peroneal nerve

13. Hind brain is formed of the following except
    (a) Medulla oblongata
    (b) Pons
    (c) Midbrain
    (d) Cerebellum

14. Pyramid of Medulla is formed by
    (a) Corticospinal tract
    (b) Inferior olivary nucleus
    (c) Anterior spinothalamic tract
    (d) Lateral spinothalamic tract.

15. Red nucleus is present in
    (a) Medulla oblongata
    (b) Pons
    (c) Lower part of Midbrain
    (d) Upper part of midbrain

16. Nucleus that does not belong to cerebellum is
    (a) Dentate
    (b) Olivary
    (c) Emboliform
    (d) Globose

17. Primary motor area of brain is in
    (a) Precentral gyrus
    (b) Post central gyrus
    (c) Superior temporal gyrus
    (d) Superior frontal gyrus

18. Visual area in brain is in relation to
    (a) Parieto-occipital sulcus
    (b) Calcarine sulcus
    (c) Collateral sulcus
    (d) Orbital sulcus.

19. The nucleus that does not belong to Basal Ganglia is
    (a) Caudate nucleus
    (b) Lentiform nucleus
    (c) Red nucleus
    (d) Amygdaloid nucleus

20. In internal capsule, corticospinal tract occupies
    (a) Anterior limb
    (b) Posterior limb
    (c) Retrolentiform part
    (d) Sublentiform part

21. Abducent nerve supplies
    (a) Lateral rectus
    (b) Medial rectus
    (c) Superior oblique
    (d) Inferior oblique.

22. Otic ganglion is seen connected to
    (a) Maxillary nerve
    (b) Ophthalmic nerve
    (c) Mandibular nerve
    (d) Lingual nerve

23. Only muscle supplied by glossopharyngeal nerve is
    (a) Styloglossus
    (b) Stylopharyngeus

(c) Palatopharyngeus
(d) Palatoglossus.
24. Hypoglossal nerve supplies muscles of
(a) Tongue
(b) Pharynx
(c) Soft palate

(d) Larynx
25. Largest commissure of brain is
(a) Anterior commissure
(b) Posterior commissure
(c) Hebanular commissure
(d) Corpus callosum

M.C.Qs - Answers

1. (c), 2. (b), 3. (d), 4. (a), 5. (a), 6. (d), 7. (a), 8. (b), 9. (d), 10. (a), 11. (b), 12. (c), 13. (c), 14. (a), 15. (d), 16. (b), 17. (a), 18. (b), 19. (c), 20. (b), 21. (a), 22. (c), 23. (b), 24. (a), 25. (d)

Essays

I. Describe the spinal cord and its blood supply.
II. Draw labelled diagrams to show the major sulci, gyri and functional areas of cerebral cortex.
III. Name the different types of white mater of brain and describe internal capsule.
IV. Describe the cranial nerves in brief.
V. Describe the lateral ventricle.
VI. Draw labelled diagram of floor of IV ventricle.
VII. With the help of labeled diagram give the formation of circle of Willis.
VIII. Draw labeled diagrams to show blood supply to the 3 surfaces of brain.
IX. Describe the formation of Brachial plexus.
X. Describe the Radial nerve.
XI. Describe the common peroneal nerve.
XII. Describe the femoral nerve.

Short Notes

1. Medulla oblongata
3. Midbrain
5. Thalamus
7. Facial nerve
9. Ulnar nerve
12. Median nerve
14. Obturator nerve

2. Cerebellum
4. Corpus callosum
6. Basal ganglia
8. Circle of Willis
10. Spinal nerve
13. Axillary nerve
15. C.S.F.

12 Embryology and Elementary Genetics

GENERAL EMBRYOLOGY

General embryology is the study of early stages of development of human.

GAMETOGENESIS

Formation of ovum or sperm in the gonads (ovary is female and testis is male)

In the female, oogenesis.

In the male, spermatogenesis.

Human somatic cell has 46 chromosomes. The gametes should have 23 chromosomes only, so that at fertilisation, when ovum and sperm fuse to form zygote, the normal number 46 is obtained. To achieve this, during gametogenesis the germ cells undergo reduction division, meiosis.

OOGENESIS

Formation of ovum in the ovary is known as oogenesis. Before a female child is born, when it is growing in the uterus of its mother, its developing ovary contains early germ cells, primordial germ cells which multiply and differentiate into oogonia. Oogonia undergo changes for the formation of ova.

They multiply by mitosis and differentiate into primary oocytes, during the intrauterin period.

Formation of graafian follicle (Fig. 12.1)

When the child is born, its ovary contains numerous primary oocytes which have completed the prophase of first meiotic division. Instead of going into metaphase they enter into a resting phase- Dictyotene stage.

Oocytes are surrounded by a layer of follicular cells- together they are called primary follicles.

Between oocyte and follicular cells, a layer of amorphous material appears- Zona pellucida.

The follicular cells multiply and become multilayered – membrana granulosa.

Among the granulosa cells, fluid filled cavity appears. The fluid- liqor folliculi- increases in volume. The follicle enlarges and oocyte with some surrounding cells (cumulus oophorus) gets pushed to one end. Thus a mature graafian follicle is formed.

The ovarian stromal cells surrounding the graafian follicles differentiate into glandular tissue- theca externa and theca interna. Theca interna is vascular and secretes oestrogen.

As the graafian follicle is mature the primary oocyte completes the first meiotic division and two cells are formed. One is large- the secondary oocyte and the smaller one is first polar body seen between cell wall of secondary oocyte and zona pellucida. Immediately the secondary oocyte prepares for second meiosis which will be completed only at fertilization.

The process of growth and maturation of graafian follicle is under the influence of F.S.H from anterior pituitary.

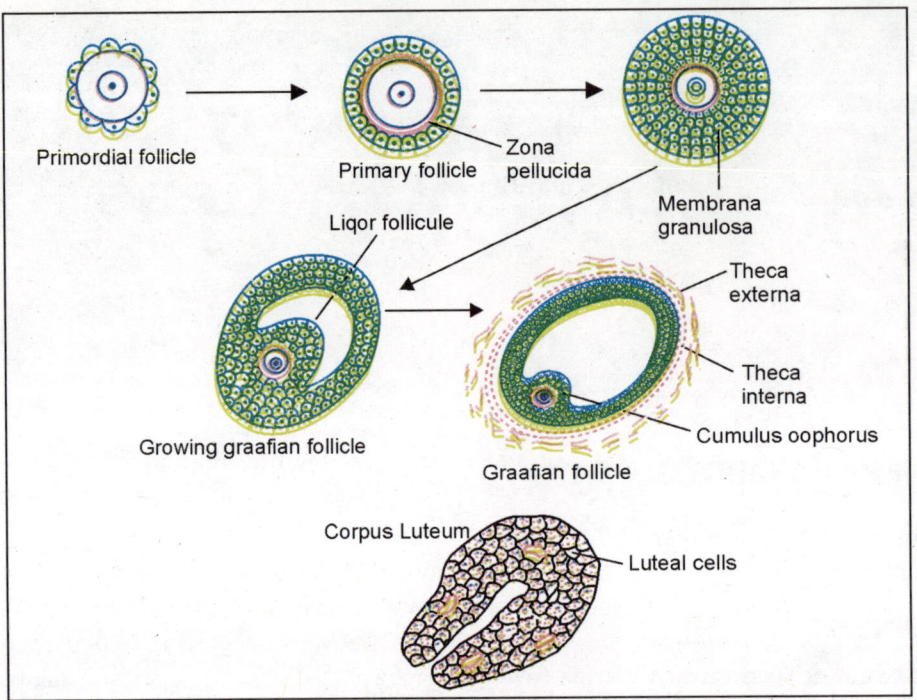

Fig. 12.1: Oogenesis

Ovulation

The mature graafian follicle is seen close to the surface of ovary. It ruptures and the secondary oocyte-ovum with the surrounding cells is liberated out into the peritoneal cavity. It is sucked into the fallopian tube by fimbriae.

The process of liberation of a mature ovum from an ovary is ovulation. Each ovary liberates an ovum during alternate months.

Corpus Luteum

After ovulation wall of graafian folicile collapses, granulosa cells enlarge and get changed into luteal cells with lutein pigments inside them. It gets vascularised and a corpus luteum is formed. It secretes progesterone. These changes are influnced by L.H from anterior pituitary.

If fertilization occurs, corpus luteum grows into corpus luteum of pregnancy; otherwise it undergoes degeneration and forms corpus albicans.

These changes constitute an **ovarian cycle**.

Uterine cycle (Menstrual cycle)

Wall of uterus has three layers. (Fig. 12.2) Outer to inner, they are perimetrium, myometrium and endometrium. The endometrium undergoes cyclical structural changes once in 28 days – this constitutes uterine cycle. Uterine cycle starts with the menstrual bleeding – Menstrual phase- which lasts for 4–7 days. During this phase, major part of the thickness of endometrium is shed off with menstrual blood and only a thin layer of endometrium persists.

Next is the proliferative phase which lasts upto about 14th day. During this phase, the full thickness of endometrium is rebuilt from the persisting part under the influence of oestrogen from ovary. Then ovulation occurs and ovary secretes progesterone also. Next 14 days of uterine cycle is secretory phase. Now under the influence of oestrogen and progesterone, the uterine endometrium becomes

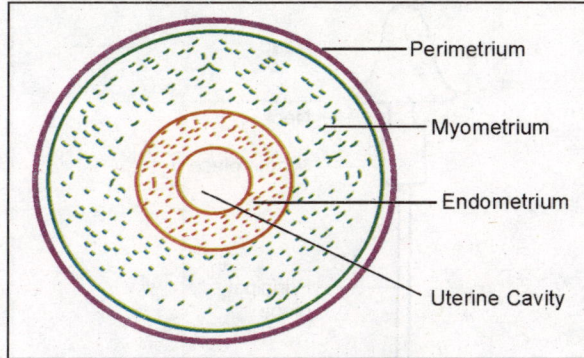

Fig. 12.2: C.S. of uterus

highly vascular, soft and velvetty and the endometrial glands start secreting. The endometrium is ready to receive a fertilized egg. If fertilization has not occurred, at the end of secretory phase i.e., 14 days after ovulation, endometrium breaks down causing menstrual bleeding.

SPERMATOGENESIS

Spermatogenesis means formation of spermatozoa (sperms) in the testes in the male. Testes have a coiled system of ducts- seminiferous tubules. Spermatozoa develop inside these tubules.

Between seminiferous tubules, there are a few scattered cells- interstitial cells of Leydig which secrete the male hormone- testosterone.

The early germ cells in the testes start developing into sperms only by the time of puberty. Changes undergone by primordial germ cells during spermatogenesis are described in two phases (Fig. 12.3).

I Phase of **cell growth and multiplication**

II Phase of **cell metamorphosis. (spermiogenesis)**

Phase I

Changes: Inside the seminiferous tubules,

1. Primordial germ cells multiply and differentiate into spermatogonia.
2. Spermatogonia differentiate into larger cells, primary spermatocytes.

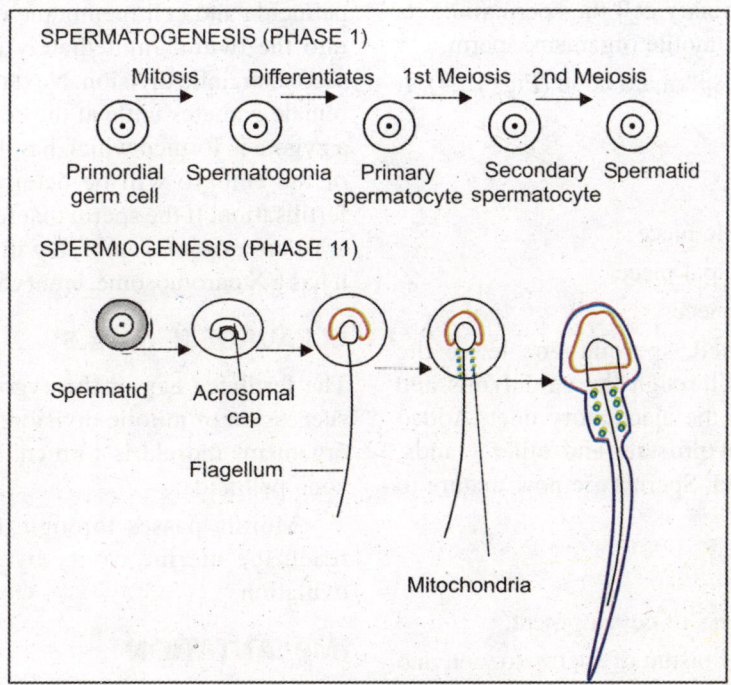

Fig. 12.3: Spermatogenesis

3. Primary spermatocytes undergo first meiotic division to form secondary spermatocytes.

4. Secondary spermatocytes quickly undergo second meiosis to form spermatids. They remain in contact with the supporting cells of Sertoli inside the tubules.

Phase II (spermiogenesis)

Spermatids undergo metamorphic changes to become spermatozoa.

Changes:

1. Golgi apparatus changes into an acrosomal cap over the nucleus.
2. A flagellum grows out of the cell.
3. Mitochondria get arranged around the proximal part of flagellum.
4. Cytoplasm condenses around flagellum and mitochondria to form middle piece.
5. Nucleus condenses into sperm head.
6. Rest of cell organelles and cytoplasm get discarded.

Thus a simple ordinary cell the spermatid gets metamorphosed into a motile organism, sperm.

The structure of a spermato zoon (Fig. 12.4). It has a **head and a tail**.

Head

	Neck
Tail	Middle piece
	Principal piece
	End piece

When fully formed, spermatozoa leave the supporting cells, pass through the epididymis and vas deferens to reach the ejaculatory duct. Added with the secretions of prostate and other glands, seminal fluid is formed. Sperms are now mature to fertilise the egg.

FERTILISATION

First stage in the process of development.

It is the process of fusion of spermatozoon and ovum to form zygote. Normally it takes place in the ampulla of fallopian tube.

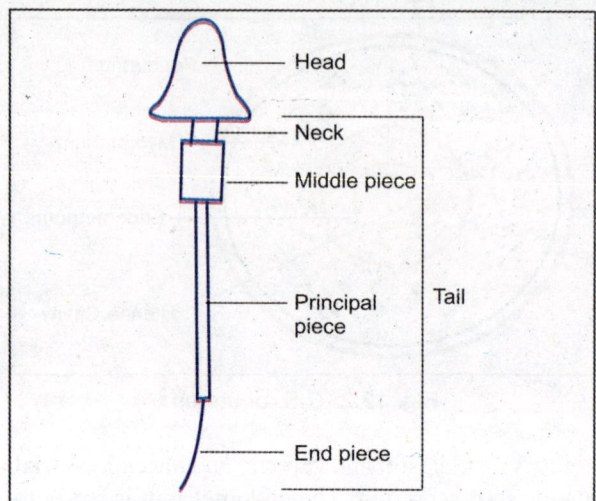

Fig. 12.4: Spermatozoon (Sperm)

Ovum liberated from the ovary is taken into fallopian tube through its fimbriated end. Of the numerous spermatozoa deposited in the vagina at a single ejaculation, only a few reach the fallopian tube by their motility. One of them peierces the zona pellucida and cell membrane of the oozyte to enter into the ovum. Immediately ovum completes the second meiotic division. Next the nuclei of male and female gametes unite at the centre of the ovum and a zygote is formed which has 46 chromosomes. Sex of the embryo will be determined at the time of fertilisation. If the sperm that fertilizes the ovum has a Y chromosome, embryo will be male (XY) and if it has a X chromosome, embryo will be female (XX).

CLEAVAGE (Fig. 12.5)

The fertilized egg or the zygote undergoes a rapid succession of mitotic division. Thus a multicellular organism- morula is formed. It is still covered by zona pellucida.

Morula passes through the fallopian tube to reach the uterine cavity by about 4th day after ovulation.

IMPLANTATION

In the uterine cavity, the zona pellucida starts disintegrating. Fluid from uterine cavity enters

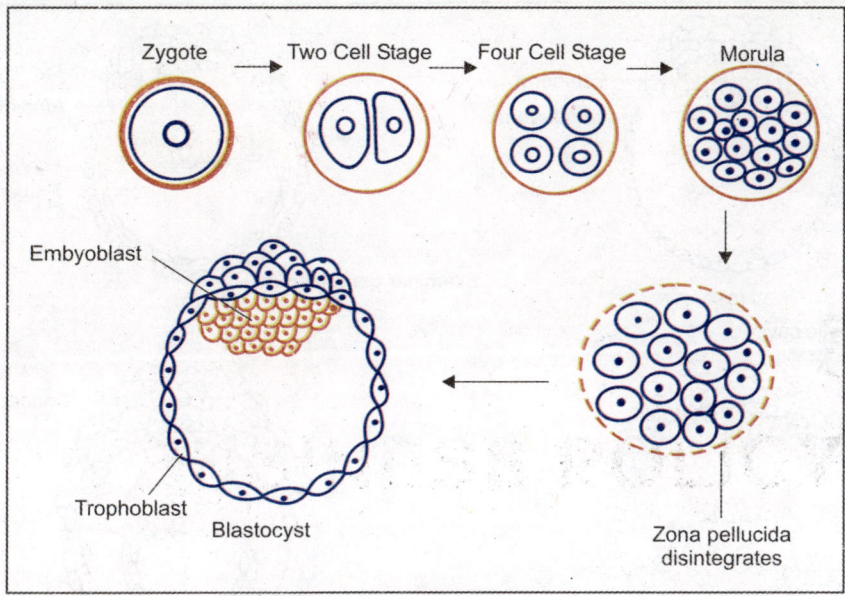

Zygote → Two Cell Stage → Four Cell Stage → Morula

Embyoblast

Trophoblast

Blastocyst

Zona pellucida
disintegrates

Fig. 12.5

between the cells of morula.. Thus morula changes into a blastocyst which has an outer layer of cells- **trophoblast** and inner cell mass, **embryoblast.** Embryoblast will develop into embryo proper. Trophoblast will give rise to placenta and related structures.

Blastocyst penetrates into the uterine endometrium, by about 6th or 7th day after fertilization. This is implantation. Normal site of implantation is, into the endometrium, along the posterior wall, near the fundus of uterus.

Abnormal sites of implantation

1. Inside uterus- near internal os
2. Outside uterus
   (a) In the tube- tubal pregnancy
   (b) In the ovary
   (c) In the peritoneum
   (d) In the pouch of Douglas.

Decidua

The modified endometrium of pregnancy is called decidua. Decidua at the site of implantation is called decidua basalis, which thickens to form decidual

plate and together with chorionic villi will form placenta. Decidua that covers the implanted chorionic sac is called decidua capsularis. Decidua lining the remaining part of uterine cavity is decidua parietalis. Decidua is shed off with the membranes at child birth.

FORMATION OF BILAMINAR GERM DISC (Fig. 12.6)

Changes of blastocyst after implantation: The embryoblastic cells differentiate into two layers.

1. A layer of flat cells- endoderm
2. A layer of columnar cells- ectoderm

These two layers of cells form a circular disc- Bilaminar germ disc.

FORMATION OF AMNIOTIC CAVITY AND YOLK SAC

Bilaminar germ disc gets separated from the trophoblastic cells by a cavity- amniotic cavity. Into this, amniotic fuild is secreted by amniogenic cells which roof the cavity. Below the germ disc, the inner surface of trophoblast gets lined by a layer of cells-

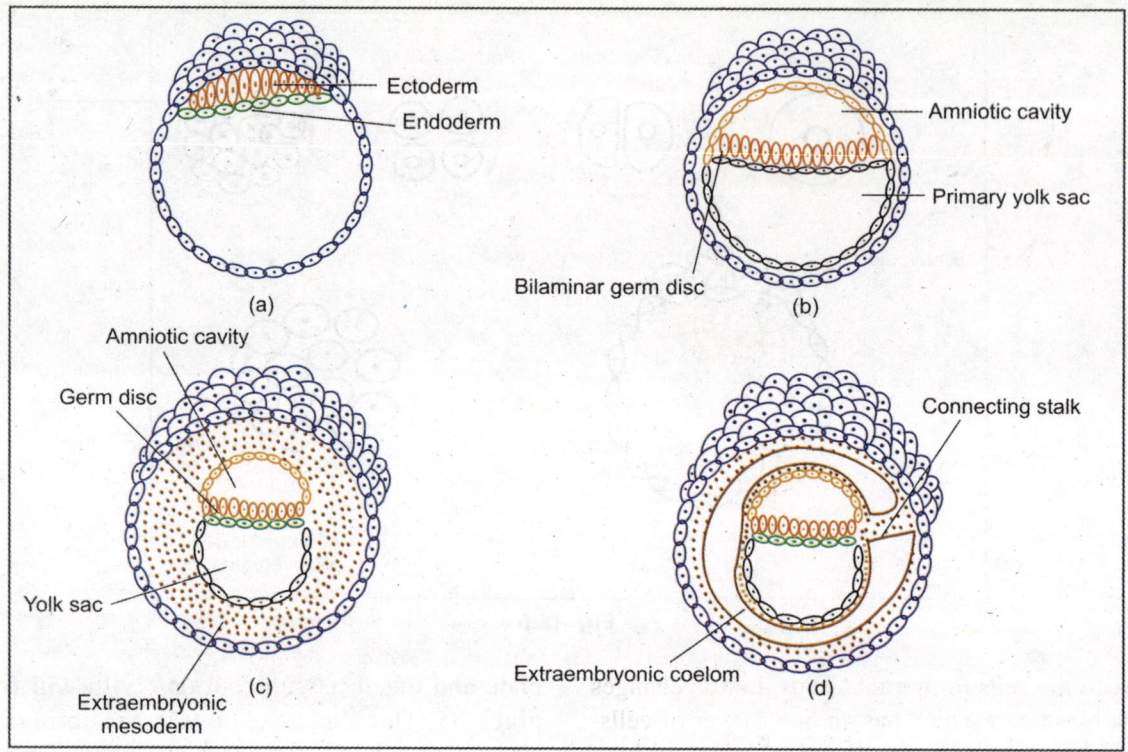

Fig. 12.6

Heusser's membrane. Now the cavity is called primary yolk sac.

EXTRA EMBRYONIC MESODERM (Fig. 12.6)

The amniotic cavity, the primary yolk sac and the intervening germ disc get separated from the trophoblast by an amount of loose connective tissue, extra embryonic mesoderm. A space or cavity develops in the extra embryonic mesoderm, extra embryonic coelom. Thus extra embryonic mesoderm is divided into extra embryonic somatopleuric mesoderm and extra embryonic splanchnopleuric mesoderm. A strip of etra embryonic mesoderm persists connecting the germ disc and the two cavities to the trophoblast-connecting stalk. The trophoblast, lined on its inner surface by etra embryonic somatopleuric mesoderm is called **chorion**.

PROCHORDAL PLATE

Towards the future anterior end of the circular germ disc, endoderm shows a localized thickening – prochordal plate.

Secondary yolk sac

Primary yolk sac becomes lined on its inner surface by a layer of cells derived from endoderm.(Heusser's membrane) Now it is the definitive or secondary yolk sac.

Changes in the trophoblast

During this time after implantation, from the trophoblast, a multinucleated cytoplasmic mass (syncytium) differentiates and grows into the uterine endometrium at the **site** of implantation. This is called Syncytiotrophoblast. Remaining part of trophoblast is called Cytotrophoblast.

In the Syncytium, small spaces called lacunae appear which later grow into larger spaces. As the syncytium grows deeper into uterine endometrium, it erodes the uterine endometrial vessels and maternal blood from uterine vessels flow into lacunae of syncytium. (First sign of uteroplacental circulation) cytotrophoblast develops columns of cells which project into syncytium- trophoblastic villi. (chorionic villi)

These villi float in maternal blood in enlarged lacunae – intervillous spaces.

Later during third and fourth weeks of development, cytotrophoblastic- chorionic villi grow deeper and reach the endometrium (decidual plate) which is thickened here. The chorionic villi, decidual plate and syncytium with its lacunae will develop into the placenta. Connecting stalk will form the umbilical cord.

PRIMITIVE STREAK AND INTRA-EMBRYONIC MESODERM (Fig. 12.7)

In the caudal part of germ disc, the ectodermal cells along the midline multiply in a localized area and form a small elevation – primitive streak. As cell multiplication continues, the rounded primitive streak becomes linear, directed towards prochordal plate.

Now the circular embryonic disc becomes oval and pear shaped. Multiplying cells of primitive streak migrate into the plane between ectoderm and endoderm and there they form another layer that is Mesoderm.

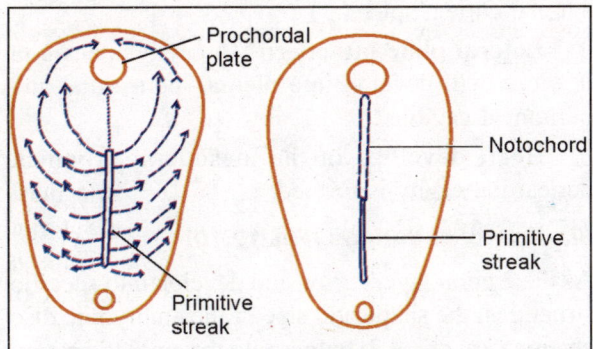

Fig. 12.7

Thus the germ disc becomes trilaminar except at prochordal plate. From the ectoderm, endoderm and mesoderm, the whole embryo will be developed.

NOTOCHORD (Fig. 12.7 b)

From the anterior end of primitive streak, the invaginating cells form a cord like process which extends towards and upto prochordal plate, between ectoderm and endoderm. This forms notochord, which is the central axis for the embryonic disc, around which the vertebral column will develop.

DERIVATIVES OF GERM LAYERS

4th to 8th week (embryonic period)

Now all the three germ layers- ectoderm, endoderm and mesoderm are formed. Each will give rise to specific tissues and organs of the body.

All the main organ systems are established during this period.

Shape of the embryo changes much and major external features are recognizable at the end of this period.

I.   Derivatives of ectoderm (Fig. 12.8)

1. Ectoderm overlying the notochord thickens and develops into a neural plate which later sinks and forms neural tube. Neural tube comes to lie deep to ectoderm along midline. (A group of cells which lie on either side of neural tube forms neural crest.)

   Anterior end of neural tube develops into brain. Remaining part will develop into spinal cord.

   Neural crest derivatives: Ganglion cells

   Adrenal medulla

   Neurolemma cells (Schwann cells)

   Pia and arachnoid cells

   Odontoblasts

   Branchial cartilage cells

   Melanoblasts

2. Lens of eye

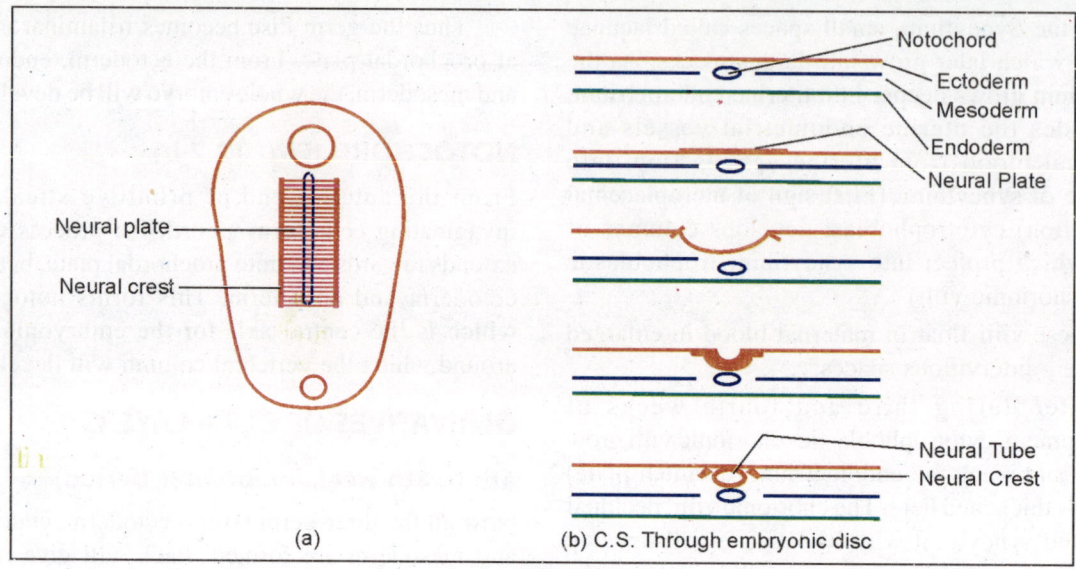

(a)

(b) C.S. Through embryonic disc

Fig. 12.8

3. Structures in internal ear.
4. Remaining part of ectoderm develops into the general body covering:-
   (a) Epidermis of skin and its derivatives as hair, nail, sweat and sebaceous glands, mammary gland.
   (b) Epithelium of oral and nasal cavities.
   (c) Epithelium of lower end of anal canal and terminal parts of genitourinary tracts.
   (d) Sensory epithelium of eye, ear and nose.
   (e) Enamel of teeth.

II. Derivatives of mesoderm (Fig. 12.9)

Intraembryonic mesoderm gets differentiated into 3 parts from medial to lateral – Paraxial, intermediate and lateral plate mesoderm.

Paraxial mesoderm: Gets segmented into cubical masses called Somites – about 42 to 44 pairs.

Somites give rise to :

Vertebral column

Dermis and subcutaneous tissue

Skeletal muscles

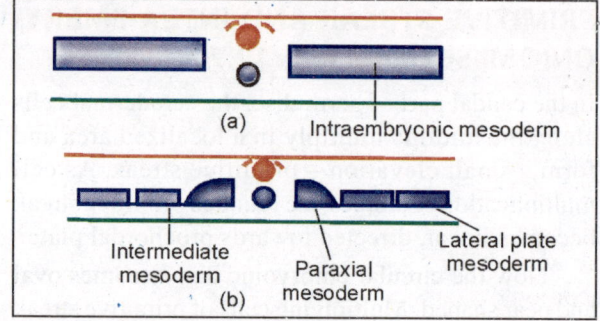

Fig. 12.9

Intermediate mesoderm:

Gives rise to urogenital organs – kidney, gonads, adrenal cortex, spleen.

Lateral plate mesoderm: A cavity appears in it which will develop into pleural, pericardial and peritoneal cavities.

Heart develops in the mesoderm in which pericardial cavity is formed.

III. Fate of endoderm (Fig. 12.10)

As the 3 germ layers grow and develop into specific structures, the shape and size of the embryonic disc change very much. It bulges into the amniotic cavity

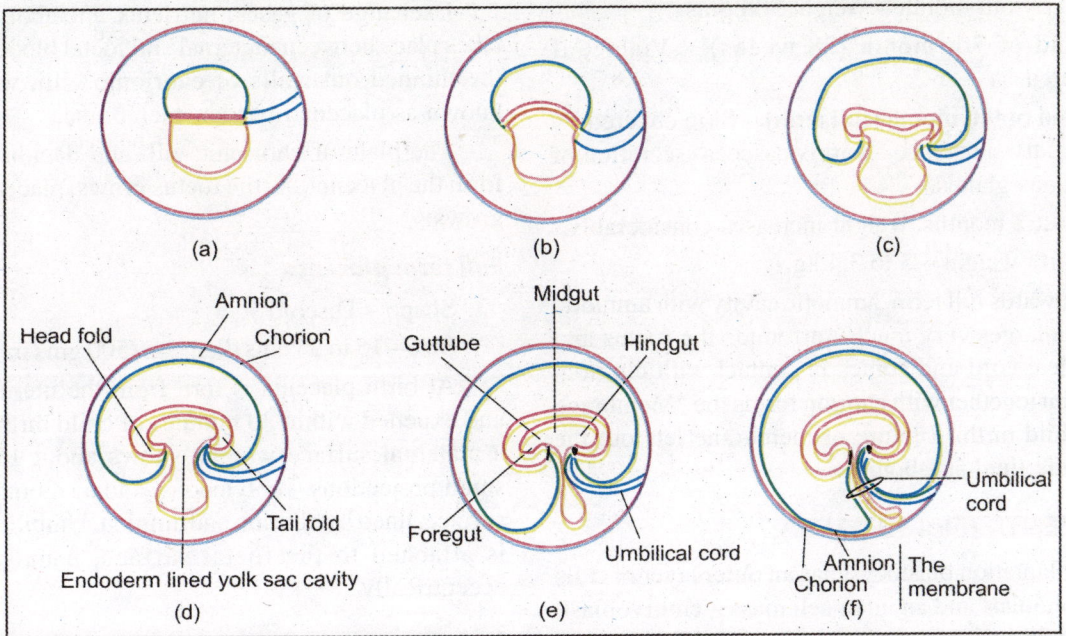

Fig. 12.10

and further undergoes foldings. A head fold, tail fold and 2 lateral folds are formed. The folds gradually constrict off the embryo from yolk sac and the characteristic shape of the embryo is formed.

Due to the foldings, the part of endodermal yolk sac which lies near the germ disc becomes incorporated into the embryo. This forms a tube like gut – Primitive gut which has the cranial end – foregut, middle part – mid gut and caudal part – hindgut. All parts of alimentary tract and associated glands develop form gut tube. Caudal end of gut tube is cloaca from which urinary bladder, urethra, rectum and upper anal canal develop. Thus the endoderm develops into:

- Epithelial lining of gut tube.
- Respiratory organs, auditory tube, middle ear.
- Thyroid, parathyroid, tonsil, Thymus.
- Liver, Pancreas.
- Urinary bladder and urethra.

GROWTH OF FOETUS AND TERM OF PREGNANCY

4th to 8th weeks – Embryonic period. The 3 germ layers give rise to tissues and organs.

9th week to full term – Foetal period. Maturation of organs and tissues and rapid growth of the body.

Period of gestation – 280 days or 40 weeks after the onset of last menstrual bleeding or 38 weeks after fertilization.

Growth changes

Early 5th week – Limb buds appear

3rd month – Face becomes human looking. External genitalia develop so that ultrasound shows sex of embryo.

End of 3rd month – Muscular activity begins.

End of 4th month – movements recognized by mother.

5th month – Fine hair over the body – Lanugo hair.

Early 6th month – Weight 500 gms

End of 7th month (28 weeks) – Viable, if delivered.

End of 9th month (full term) – Skin covered by white fatty substance – vernix cascosa- secretion of sebaceous glands.

Last 2 months, weight increases considerably.

Birth weight – 3 to 3.4 kg.

Towards full term, amniotic cavity with amniotic fluid enlarges very much, surrounds the foetus and umbilical cord and comes in contact with chorion. Amnion together with chorion forms the "Membrane " at child birth. Rupture of membrane lets out the amniotic fluid at labour.

PLACENTA (Fig. 12.11)

At implantation blastocyst has an outer layer of cells – Trophoblast and an inner cell mass – embryoblast. Embryoblast dfevelops into embryo and Trophoblast is involved in the formation of placenta.

At the site of implantation, trophoblast changes into cytotrophoblast and syncytiotrophoblast. The cytotrophoblastic cells multiply to form villous projections, chorionic villi.They grow into uterine endometrium – decidua. Chorionic villi develop a core of mesoderm containing foetal blood vessels. Villi become surrounded by maternal blood from endometrial blood vessels, in intervillous spaces. Cytotrophoblstic layer of villi gradually disappears.

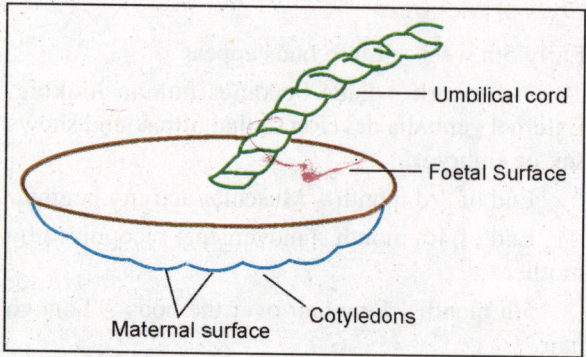

Fig. 12.11: Placenta

Exchange of gases, nutrients, metabolites etc, takes place between meternal and foetal blood across the thinned out walls of chorionic villi, which is known as placental barrier/ membrane.

The plate of chorionic villi and decidual plate form the placenta. As the foetus grows, placenta also grows.

Full term placenta

Shape – Discoid

Size – 15 to 25 cms diameter, 500 gms in weight.

At birth placenta is torn from the uterine wall and expelled within 30 minutes of child birth. It has a maternal surface whicvh shows about 15 to 20 small projections – cotyledons, and a smooth foetal surface, lined by chorion and amnion. Umbilical cord is attached to the foetal surface, usually a bit eccentrically.

UMBILICAL CORD

In early days of development the embryonic disc, at its caudal end is attached to the chorion by connecting stalk, formed of extra embryonic mesoderm. Later this connecting stalk gets transferred into umbilical cord.

As the embryonic disc grows into the embryo and foetus, the site of attachment of connecting stalk comes to lie on the ventral aspect of the foetus, at the umbilicus. Other end of it is attached to the foetal surface of placenta. It becomes covered by amnion as pregnancy advances. Extra embryonic mesoderm of connecting stalk gets changed into Wharton's jelly, a loose mesenchymal connective tissue. Umbilical cord contains two umbilical arteries and one umbilical vein in the Wharton's jelly.

At full term, umbilical cord is about 54 cm long – long enough to allow the foetus to float freely in the amniotic fluid. It shows a marked spiral torsion, due to unequal lengths of the blood vessels in it or due to foetal movements. Short umbilical cord can cause difficulty at child birth. A too long cord also is dangerous as it may form ties or can encircle the child's neck.

AMNIOTIC CAVITY (amnion)

Amniotic cavity is formed as early as the formation of bilaminar embryonic disc. It gets filled with amniotic fluid and the quantity of fluid increases as pregnancy advances. By 38 weeks it becomes 1 litre. The amniotic cavity surrounds the growing foetus and umbilical cord. By full term the amnion with its covering somatopleuric mesoderm comes in contact with inner surface of chorion and the chorionic cavity is obliterated; amnion + chorion form the 'membrane'. If the quantity of Amniotic fluid is less, the condition is called oligamnios. If the quantity is excess it is called hydramnios. For diagnosis of any suspected anomaly of the foetus amniotic fluid is withdrawn (amniocentesis) and investigated.

TWINNING

Human twins are of two types:

1. Monozygotic twins – Identical twins
2. Dizygotic twins – Unlike twins

Triplets, quadreplets and higher multiple pregnancies are not very common.

Monozygotic twins

Develop from a single fertilized ovum. They result due to splitting of zygote at early days of development. They look identical, of same sex, same blood group, same finger prints etc. – similar in all respects.

Conjoined twins result due to incomplete splitting and separation of the axial region of germ disc. (Fig. 12.12).

Example

1. Thoracopagus
2. Pygopagus
3. Craniopagus
4. Siamese twins – Only a skin bridge will be connecting the two foetuses.

Dizygotic twins

Most common type of twinning. Results from

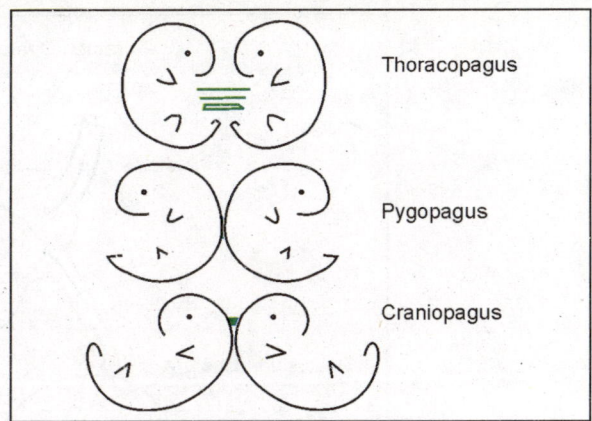

Fig. 12.12: Twinning

simultaneous shedding of two ova which get fertilized by two sperms. They resemble each other only as brother or sister of different ages. Sex may be same or different.

Foetal circulation (Fig. 12. 13)

Pure blood from placenta comes through umbilical vein. In the liver it gets bypassed to inferior vena cava through ductus venosus. Reaches the right atrium of heart through inferior vena cava. Passes through foramen ovale to left atrium. Through left atrioventricular orifice, goes to left ventricle. Through aortic orifice goes to arch of aorta and through its branches supplies the upper half of the body. Then it goes to descending aorta. Impure blood reaching right atrium through superior vena cava comes to right ventricle. Passes through pulmonary artery and then through ductus arteriosus to aorta. Impure blood from aorta passes through umbilical arteries, through umbilical cord to reach placenta for purification.

Changes after birth

After birth, placental blood flow ceases. Ductus arteriosus closes. Blood from pulmonary artery flows to 2 lungs and returns to left atrium. Thus pressure in left atrium increases and foramen ovale closes. Umbilical arteries and umbilical vein obliterate.

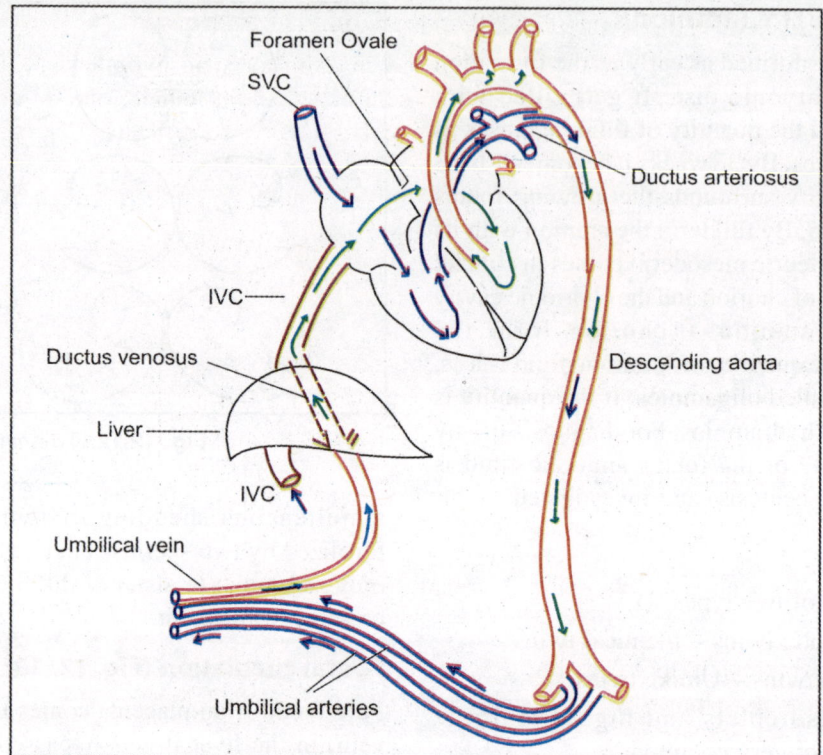

Fig. 12.13: Foetal circulation

GENETICS

No two persons are alike. Brothers and sisters from the same parentage differ in physical features and mental faculties. This can be explained by principles of genetics.

Genetics is the science of heredity. Transmission of inherited characters from generation to generation is known as heredity.

When a character or trait appears at least in 3 successive generations, it is called a hereditary character. When it appears only in one generation it is called a familial character. Characters are transmitted like this by genes in chromosomes of the cells.

To study the principle of genetics, it is essential to have a clear picture of human chromosomes and genes.

CHROMOSOMES

During inter-phase, chromosomes in nuclei appear as highly extended filaments forming a diffuse network, collectively called chromatin. The chromatin may be either dispersed and poorly staining- euchromatin or clumbed and densely staining- heterochromatin.

During cell division, chromosomes shorten much and appear as separate ones. In human, for somatic cell chromosomal number is 46 – diploid number. For gametes, chromosomal number is 23 – haploid number.

The 46 chromosomes appear in 23 pairs. Paring is between chromosomes that are identical in every respect. That is the two members are homologous. One member in each pair is paternal and the other, maternal in origin.

Of the 23 pairs in somatic cells, 22 pairs are between homologous chromosomes in male and females. These are autosomes. 23rd pair is of sex chromosomes. In female two similar (or homologous chromosomes) X chromosomes constitute the 23rd pair. But in male, the 23rd sex chromosome pair is formed of 2 dissimilar chromosomes- X and a small y. It is the Y chromosome of the male gamete that determines sex of the embryo.

All female gametes (ova) contain only X chromosomes. Male gametes (spermatozoa) contains either X or Y chromosomes. So at fertilization, sex of embryo is as shown in (Fig. 12.14)

SEX CHROMATIN OR BARR BODY (Fig. 12.15)

It is observed that the nuclei of female cells differ from those of male cells in that, there is a heterochromatic body in contact with the nuclear membrane. This is present in interphase and disappears at cell division. Barr and Bertram in 1949 stated that this was the sex chromatin (Barr body) and appears as a planoconvex dark structure beneath the nuclear membrane, or as a small drumstick attached to the nucleus.

The frequency at which this is seen in females varies from tissues to tissues. In amniotic or chorionic cells, it is 95%, in neurons 85% and in oral smears 25-30%.

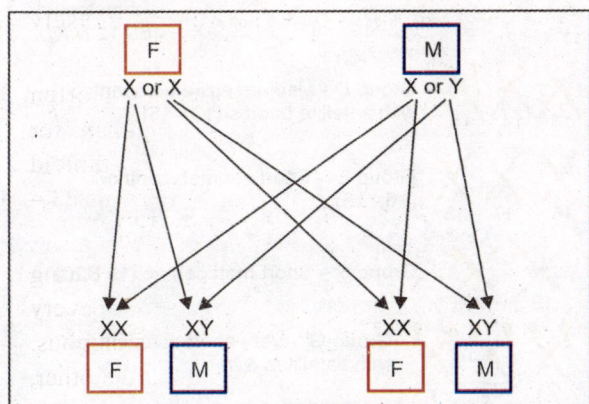

Fig. 12.14

LYON HYPOTHESIS

According to Lyon hypothesis, out of the two X chromosomes in female, one is highly coiled and inactive, so heterochromatic. This appears as the Barr body. Its other uncoiled euchromatic partner carries out all necessary synthetic functions.

STRUCTURE OF CHROMOSOMES (Fig. 12.16)

In early cell division, chromosomes are short and thick. Each consists of two parallel filaments-chromatids joined at the centromere.

Types (Fig. 12.17)

1. Metacentric chromosome – Centromere at the middle.
2. Submetacentric chromosome – Centromere not at the middle, but nearer to one end.
3. Acrocentric chromosome – Centromere near one end.
4. Telocentric chromosome – Centromere at one end.

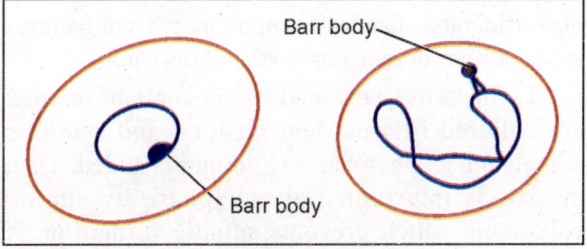

Fig. 12.15

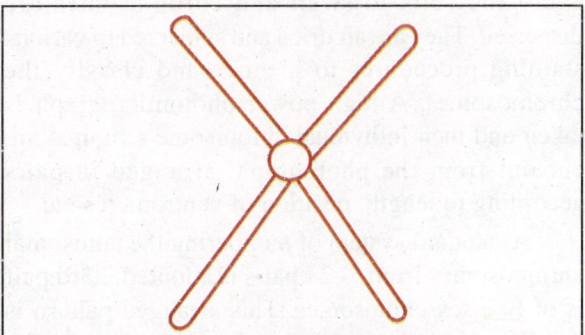

Fig. 12.16. Chromosome

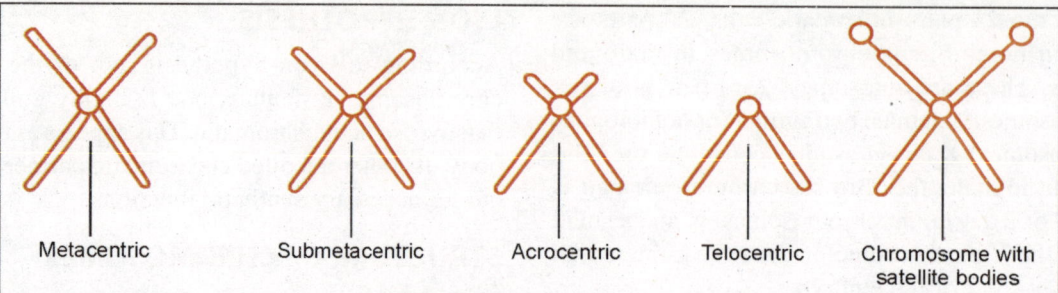

Fig. 12.17: Chromosomes

5. Chromosomes with satellite bodies – There is a constriction near one end of each chromatid.

Y chromosome is a small acrocentric one (smallest one). X chromosome is medium sized submeta-centric one.

CLASSIFICATION OF HUMAN CHROMOSOMES

Since a number of genetic abnormalities are directly related to the chromosomal patterns the characterisation or Karyotyping of chromosomes is of considerable diagnostic importance. Their features are best seen in metaphase of cell division.

Living cells from blood samples or bone marrow are cultured in a nutrient medium and a miotic stimulant *e.g.*, phytohaemagglutinin is added. Then mitosis is interrupted at metaphase by adding colchicine which prevents spindle formation. A hypotonic solution of sodium citrate is added to cause the cells to swell and chromosomes are dispersed. They are air dried and subjected to various staining procedures to identify and classify the chromosomes. A high power photomicrograph is taken and then individual chromsome's figures are cut out from the photograph, arranged in pairs according to length, position of centromeres etc.

A standard system of numbering the autosomal chromosomes from 1–22 pairs is adopted. 23rd pair is of two sex chomsomes. This arranged pattern is the Karyotype i.e., it is the chromosome set of a somatic cell. Process is called Karyotyping and reveals the number and gross structure of chromosomes.

Based on Karyotyping, chromosomal pairs are classified into 7 groups from A to G in the order of decreasing lengths. Thus 7 major groups (A–G) of human chromosomal pairs are present. This was presented in a genetic conference held in Denvur in 1960 hence called Denvur system of classification. (Fig.12.18)

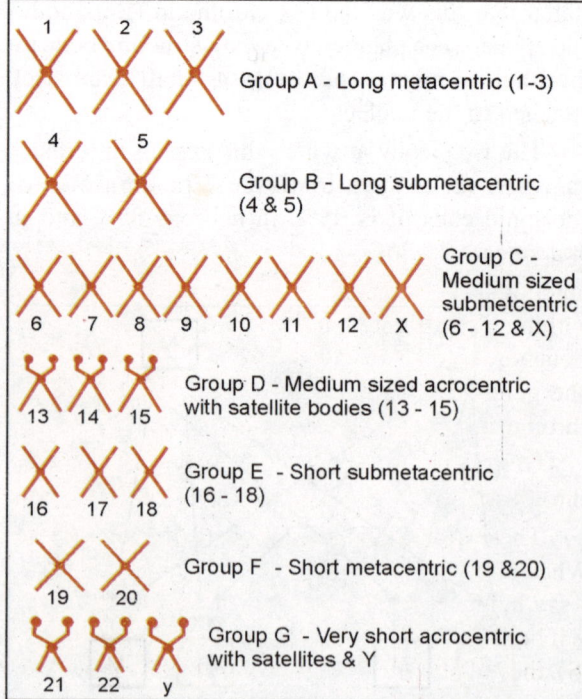

Fig. 12.18: Karyotyping of chromosomes

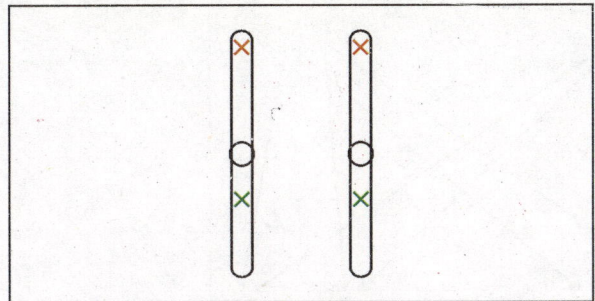

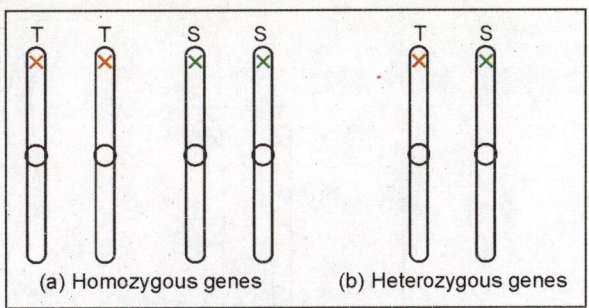

Fig. 12.19: Alleles

(a) Homozygous genes   (b) Heterozygous genes

Fig. 12.20

1. Group A – Long metacentric chromosomes. ·1–3
2. Group B – Long submetacentric chromosomes, 4 and 5
3. Group C – Medium sized submetacentric chromosomes, 6–12 and X
4. Group D – Medium sized acrocentric with satellite bodies, 13–15
5. Group E – Short submetacentric, 16–18
6. Group F – Short metacentric, 19 and 20
7. Group G – Very short acrocentric with satellites and Y chromosomes, 21, 22 and Y.

GENES

Chromosomes are formed of DNA and proteins. Variable lengths of DNA in a chromosome constitute genes. They are ultramicroscopic structural and functional units of hereditary characters, contained within chromosomes, in linear series as fine beads. Genes are the carriers of biological information from one generation to next. Position of a gene in the chromosome is called Locus.

Genes occupying identical loci in a pair of chromosomes are called allelomorphs or alleles.

These allelic genes regulate specific characters. When allelic genes regulating a particular character – say height, work in the same direction (similarly) ie if both are for tallness (T) or both are for Shortness (S), they are called Homozygous genes (Fig. 12.20). When they work in different direction, they are called heterozygous genes.

Dominant gene (Fig. 12. 21a) is the one which expresses its character always, ie; when the alleles are either homozygous or heterozygous. T is dominant here and S is recessive.

Recessive gene (Fig. 12.21b) is the gene which can express its character only when the alleles are homozygous.

Carrier gene- (Fig. 12.21a) A heterozygous recessive gene can act as a carrier. A heterozygous tall person (T and S) is a carrier of shortness gene, which may be expressed in a subsequent generation. When both parents are heterozygous tall, possibilities of height of offspring: (Fig. 12.22)

SEX LINKED GENE

Sex chromosome X or Y, besides containing genes for sex characters for determining sex, they also contain genes for body characters. These somatic genes, conveyed by sex chromosomes are called sex linked genes.

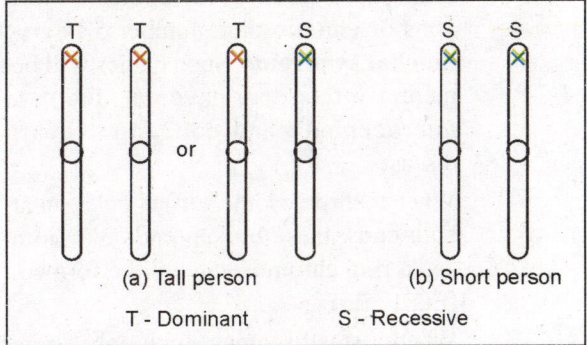

(a) Tall person   (b) Short person

T - Dominant   S - Recessive

Fig. 12.21

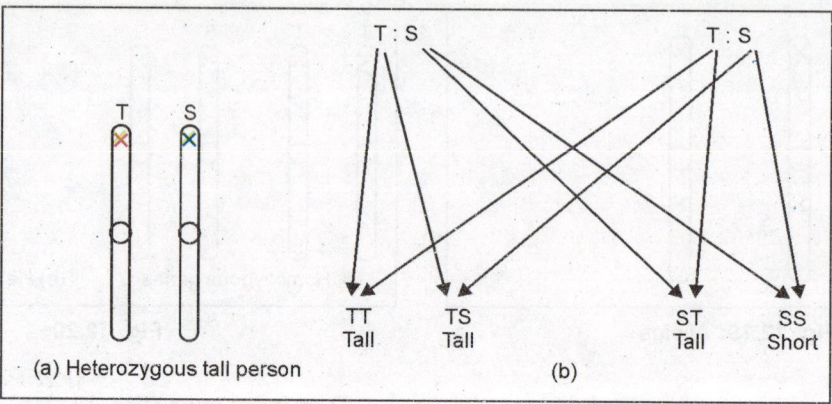

Fig. 12.22

Inheritance of genes present on sex chromosomes is known as sex linked inheritance. In sex linked inheritance, the genes involved are carried in X chromosomes. Hence called X linked inheritance. *e.g.*, Haemophilia, colour blindness. The only example of Y linked trait is hairy pinna.

CHROMOSOMAL ABNORMALITIES

They can be numerical or structural and both cause spontaneous abortion or abnormal baby.

1. **Structural abnormalities:** Normally occur due to breakage of segments of chromosomes. Cause may be viral infection, drug intake or exposure to radiation of the mother. The abnormalities are:

   (a) Deletion – Breaking away of a portion of a chromosome. (Fig.12.23a). The syndrome caused by deletion of short arms of chromosome number 5 is **cri-du-chat syndrome**. Such babies will be mentally retarded, have cat like cry, microcephaly and congenital heart disease.

   When a chromosome suffers deletion at both ends, these broken ends may join and a ring chromosome will be formed. (Fig.12.23)

   When a small segment with only a few contigous genes is deleted, the result is

Angelman syndrome – if the deletion is of maternal chromosome. The child has mental retardation, poor motor activity, excessive laughter and cannot speak. If inherited from parental chromosome the condition is **Prader-willi syndrome**

   (b) Inversion – The broken segments of chromosomes reattaches in a reverse order.

   (c) Translocation – Breakage occurs in 2 chromosomes and broken segments get exchanged and join the other chromosomes.

2. **Numerical anomalies:** The normal diploid human somatic chromosomal member is 46, i.e. 2n and of gametes is haploid is 23 i.e. n. If chromosomal number in a cell is not 46, but 45 or 47, the condition is called Aneuploidy. This is due to nondisjunction of chromosomes during cell division. ie Chomosomes fail to separate at anaphase and both members of a pair go to one of the daughter cells. The cell with 45 chromosome numbers - Monosony and that with 47 numbers - Trisony. Abnormalities are:

   (a) **Trisomy 21: Down syndrome.** Patient will have 47 chromosome and the extra one is 21 chromosome.

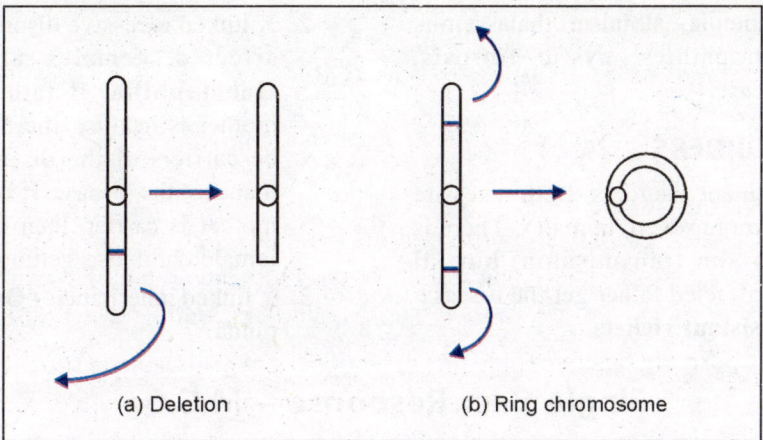

(a) Deletion   (b) Ring chromosome

Fig. 12.23

Features: Mental retardation, flat occiput and face, medial epicanthic folds, slanding eyes, short and flat bridge of nose, small ears, hypotonia, cardiac anomalies, premature aging. A transverse palmar crease may be seen.

(b) Klinefelter syndrome: Found in males. He will have an additional X chromosome- XXY (total 47). Barr body may be present. Person will be taller than normal. Gynaecomastia and hypogonadism are present. Usually has normal intelligence; sometimes mild mental retardation is seen. Facial hair growth is less and has a coarse voice.

(c) Turner syndrome: Here condition is monosomy ie only 45 chromosomes. 44 + X is the genotype. Female with absence of ovaries. She will be short statured, has webbed neck. Secondary sex characteristics are underdeveloped. Skeletal deformation may be present. Although has normal intelligence, behaves like a child.

(d) Triplex syndrome: Trisomy, female. She has an extra X chromosome and shows 2 Barr bodies. Has infantile character.

Of the autosomally transmitted abnormalities, Down syndrome and cri-du-chat syndrome are most common. The common sex chromosome anomalies are Turner syndrome and Klinefelter syndrome.

GENE ABNORMALITIES

Changes that influence gene functions are mutations. Mutations can occur in somatic cells or gametes. Abnormalities caused by transmition of a single mutant gene show either autosomal or sex linked inheritance.

Autosomal disorders

1. Autosomal dominant disorder – These diseases appear in each generation and male and female are affected. It is manifested late in life. Usually affected one has an affected parent. Sometimes neither parent is affected and spontaneous mutation may be a cause. e.g., Huntington's chorea, Achondroplasia, Marfan syndrome, Brachydectily, Neuro-fibromatosis, Myotinic dystrophy.

2. Autosomal recessive disorders – They appear early in life, both sexes are equally affected. May not be manifested in some generations. Incidence is more in children born in consanguineous marriages. *e.g.,*

sickle cell anemia, albinism thalassemia, haemoglobinopathies, cystic fibrosis, Wilson's disease.

SEX LINKED DISORDERS

1. X linked dominant disorders- Both sexes are affected, but more severe in males. There is no father to son transmission, but all daughters of affected father get the disease. *e.g.*, vit **D-resistant rickets**

2. X linked recessive disorder- Only males are affected, females are carriers. *e.g.*, **Haemophilia**. If father is affected and mother is healthy, the female children will be carriers of the disease and males will manifest the disease. If father is affected and mother is carrier, then there is a chance of female child also getting the disease.

3. Y linked inheritance – Only example is hairy pinna.

Single Best Response – M.C.Qs

1. Growing oocyte in a follicle is immediately surrounded by
   (a) Cumulus oophorus
   (b) Zona pellucida
   (c) Membrana granulosa
   (d) Liqor folliculi

2. Secondary occyte completes 2nd meiotic division.
   (a) As soon as it is formed
   (b) Just before ovulation
   (c) After ovulation
   (d) At fertilization

3. Progesterone is secreted by
   (a) Graafian follicle
   (b) Corpus luteum
   (c) Ovarian stromal cells
   (d) Uterine endometrium

4. Spermiogenesis is undergone by
   (a) Spermatogonia
   (b) Primary spermatocytes
   (c) Secondary spermatocytes
   (d) Spermatids

5. Somites are formed from
   (a) Ectoderm
   (b) Endoderm
   (c) Paraxial mesoderm
   (d) Intermediate mesoderm

6. Wharton's jelly is found in
   (a) Umbilical cord
   (b) Placenta
   (c) Amniotic fluid
   (d) Yolk sac

7. Average diameter of a normal placenta is
   (a) 5-10 cms
   (b) 10-15 cms
   (c) 15-25 cms
   (d) 25-3 cms

8. Following are correct about Barr body except.
   (a) It is found in nuclei of female cells
   (b) It is seen during interphase
   (c) It is one of the 2 X chromosomes
   (d) It is euchromatic, uncoiled and active

9. In numerical chromosomal abnormalities, condition with monosomy is
   (a) Down syndrome
   (b) Klinefelter's syndrome
   (c) Turner syndrome
   (d) Triplex syndrome

10. Haemophilia is a
    (a) Autosomal dominant disorder
    (b) Autosomal recessive disorder
    (c) X-linked dominant disorder
    (d) X-linked recessive disorder.

M.C.QS - ANSWERS

1. (b), 2. (d), 3. (b), 4. (d), 5. (c), 6. (a), 7. (c), 8. (d), 9. (c), 10. (d)

ESSAYS

I. Describe the stages of Oogenesis

II. Describe the stages of spermatogenesis

SHORT NOTES

1. Graafian follicle

2. Corpus luteum

3. Implantation

4. Blastocyst

5. Notochord

6. Placenta

7. Umbilical cord

8. Down Syndrome

9. Klinefelter's syndrome

10. Karyotyping

Index